The Cancer Registry CASEbook

Coding • Abstracting • Staging • Exercises

Second Edition

Volume II

Challenging Sites

Head and Neck Cancer
Cervix Cancer
Corpus Cancer
Ovarian Cancer
Central Nervous System Tumors
Malignant Lymphomas

April Fritz, BA, RHIT, CTR

Contributing Authors
Denise Harrison, BS, CTR
Louanne Currence, RHIT, CTR
Meryl Leventhal, MA, RHIT, CTR
Katheryne Vance, BA, CTR
Annette Hurlbut, RHIT, CTR

September 2011

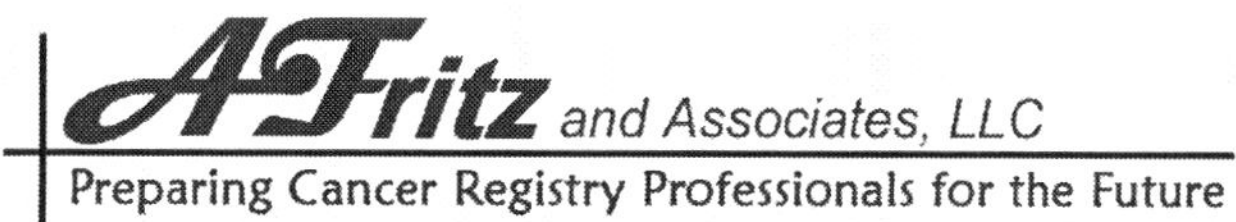

A.Fritz and Associates, LLC
21361 Crestview Road
Reno, NV 89521
www.afritz.org

Volume II
First edition published 2008
Second edition published 2011

While the information in this book is believed to be accurate at the time of publication, the editors accept no legal responsibility for any errors or omissions that may be made. A.Fritz and Associates, LLC, makes no warranty, express or implied, with respect to the material contained in this book.

Cancer treatment, and consequently cancer abstracting and coding, is constantly in flux. Over time, parts of this book may become out of date. Therefore, updates and errata will be posted as needed at **www.afritz.org/casebook**. Please check there periodically for notification of changes to the CASEbook. Questions and comments may be sent to **casebook@afritz.org**.

Additional copies of this book may be ordered from www.afritz.org.

The image of Leonardo DaVinci's Vitruvian Man on the cover is a reminder of every registrar's capabilities. Just as Leonardo illustrated the writings of the ancient Roman architect Vitruvius, who described the proportions of the human body, registrars record the measure of man by coding, abstracting, and staging the presence of malignancy in the human body.

CONTENTS BY SECTION

Contents by Section, continued

Contents by Section, continued

Contents by Section, continued

9. Malignant Lymphoma

FOREWORD TO VOLUME II

The Cancer Registry CASEbook series originally came about because my desk was too small. As I wrote in the Foreword to Volume I,

After layering my Collaborative Staging Manual
on my Multiple Primary and Histology Coding Rules
on my site-specific coding guidelines
on my SEER Summary Staging book
on my ICD-O-3 book
on my TNM Staging Manual
on my FORDS Manual
and then needing my CS Manual again,
I began to wish that someone would compile all the important abstracting information into one reference.

The CASEbook series has two purposes: first, to serve as a text for several courses Cancer Information Management (CIM) Programs at various community colleges, as well as other training and education programs for beginning registrars, and second, to provide a reference manual for working cancer registrars. Volume I of the CASEbook included introductory chapters on ICD-O-3, Summary Stage, TNM, Collaborative Staging and the Multiple Primary and Histology Coding rules, plus the five cancer sites that comprise about 60% of the caseload in most registries: colorectum, breast, lung, prostate and bladder. Volume II of the CASEbook consists of several overview or reference chapters and site-specific chapters on six of the more challenging primary cancers.

The overview/reference chapters are:
- Abstracting Information in Text Fields
- Acronyms, Initialisms and Abbreviations
- Diagnostic Tests and Tumor Markers
- The Lymphatic System

The site-specific chapters are:
- Head and Neck cancers
- Cervix cancer
- Corpus cancer
- Ovary cancer
- Central Nervous System tumors
- Malignant Lymphomas

Each site-specific chapter includes information about anatomy of the site and its regional nodes and adjacent structure, ICD-O-3 topography and morphology codes, the disease process for the site, diagnostic tests, surgery codes and other types of treatment, and discussion of the rules and codes for all of the staging and coding manuals in effect as of January 1, 2011. These are:

International Classification of Diseases for Oncology, third edition
SEER Summary Staging Manual 2000
AJCC Cancer Staging Manual, seventh edition
Collaborative Staging Manual, version 02.03.02
2007 Multiple Primary and Histology Coding Rules
Multiple Primary and Histology Coding Rules (2007)
Hematopoietic and Lymphoid Neoplasm Case Reportability and Coding Rules (2010)

As you may know by now, CASEbook stands for **C**oding, **A**bstracting, **S**taging, and **E**xercises, and there are lots of exercises in the book. Each of the site-specific chapters includes twelve one-page cases to code and stage, as well as the answers with rationales. The exception is the head and neck chapter where there are eighteen cases to code and stage. All of the cases and answers have been alpha- and beta-tested during several semesters of SBCC's coding and staging course, as well as in recent Principles of Oncology training programs. Of course, there will always be room for interpretation, so if you don't agree with an answer, please feel free to contact me at casebook@afritz.org. Updates and any errata will be posted at www.afritz.org/casebook.

The *Cancer Registry CASEbook* contains a great deal of information originally developed by others. I tried not to repeat the content of standard references like ICD-O, CS, and TNM; rather, my intent is to point out special issues or explain things in a different way. The CASEbook should be used as a companion to standard registry reference manuals. Much of the content has come from previous versions of registry training materials, such as the *Registrar's Key to Abstracting* that I used for several years in my Principles of Oncology Training Program. I am grateful for Meryl Leventhal's site-specific materials for her Santa Barbara City College abstracting classes and materials developed by Chris Casagrande-Wilborn and Katheryne Vance, who were the first instructors of SBCC's cancer coding and staging course. Dianne Hultstrom was my co-author on the *Workbook for Staging of Cancer, second edition*, and some of her work has been adapted for the CASEbook. My concern in writing this is that I have forgotten to acknowledge other colleagues whose training materials contributed to the body of resources used to create the CASEbook.

The Internet is a wonderful research tool as well. Many of the illustrations and general cancer facts, including the 'usual' treatments by stage, were found on websites around the world. Credit has been given—and permissions obtained—wherever possible for illustrations in the manual. Public domain graphics and medical clip-art collections provided many of the anatomy illustrations that I adapted to registrar needs.

Most importantly, I want to thank my registrar colleagues and contributing authors for their repeated reviews and valuable input and comments on these chapters. Louanne Currence, RHIT, CTR, is my co-teacher for Principles of Oncology; Meryl Leventhal, MA, RHIT, CTR, and Katheryne Vance, BA, CTR, were faculty colleagues at SBCC. Denise Harrison, BS, CTR, who has taken over as director of the SBCC CIM Program and instructor for coding and staging course, is one of the editors of the second edition and reviewed the chapters with fresh eyes. A major contributor to the Diagnostic Tests and Tumor Markers chapter and my proofreader with the incredibly sharp eyes is my friend and helper on many projects, Annette Hurlbut, RHIT, CTR. Thank you all for your contributions to this book.

Volume I was a tremendous success as far as self-published registry references go. Volume II tackles some of the more problematic sites—head and neck, lymphoma, CNS tumors and female genital sites. These sites are ones where the rules aren't as straightforward or where there's something a little different about the primary site. Due to all the changes that took effect in registry coding and rules starting in 2010, more than 75 pages of new content has been added to the second edition of Volume II. Volume III—less common sites like biliary tract, upper gastrointestinal tract, testis, melanoma, and more—is under development.

CASEbook users, please share your comments with me. I welcome your suggestions and additional hints, abstracting guidelines and other keys to make all registrars' lives easier.

April Fritz, RHIT, CTR
Virginia City Highlands, Nevada
September 2011
casebook@afritz.org

ACKNOWLEDGMENTS

In many publications, the references and acknowledgments are included at the back of the book. In this case, however, I believe that the many sources of cancer facts and abstracting guidelines should be listed up front. I certainly appreciate all of the work that went into developing these references, for without them, registrars would not have come as far as they have. My sources for *The Cancer Registry CASEbook* include, but are not completely limited to:

AJCC Cancer Staging Atlas, American Joint Committee on Cancer, Springer, New York, 2006.

AJCC Cancer Staging Manual, seventh edition, American Joint Committee on Cancer, Springer, New York, 2009, and previous editions, including the *Manual for Staging of Cancer*, AJCC.

Cancer Topics website, National Cancer Institute. www.cancer.org/cancertopics.

Collaborative Stage Data Collection System Coding Instructions, parts I and II, version 02.03.02, Collaborative Stage Version 2 Work Group. Published by American Joint Committee on Cancer (Chicago, IL). Updates are posted on www.cancerstaging.org/cstage.

Facility Oncology Registry Data Standards (FORDS) Manual. Commission on Cancer of the American College of Surgeons, Chicago, 2011 with updates, and previous editions.

Hematopoietic and Lymphoid Neoplasm Case Reportability and Coding Manual and Hematopoietic Data Base. National Cancer Institute, Surveillance, Epidemiology and End Results (SEER) Program, Bethesda, MD, 2010. www.seer.cancer.gov/tools/heme.

International Classification of Diseases for Oncology, third edition. April Fritz, Constance Percy, et al., editors. World Health Organization, 2000, and previous editions.

Multiple Primary and Histology Coding Rules, National Cancer Institute, Surveillance, Epidemiology and End Results (SEER) Program, Bethesda, MD, 2007 with updates. www.seer.cancer.gov/registrars

Professional Review for Tumor Registrars: A Study Guide, fourth edition. Gayle Clutter, CTR, Patricia Bentley, CTR, Jean Byers, CTR, and April Fritz, ART, CTR. Florida Tumor Registrars Association, 2004. www.fcra.org.

SEER Summary Staging Manual 2000. SEER Program, National Cancer Institute. NIH Publication No. 01-4969, 2001.

TNM Classification of Malignant Tumours, seventh edition. International Union Against Cancer (UICC). Edited by L. Sobin and Ch. Wittekind. Wiley-Liss, New York, 2009.

TNM Supplement: A Commentary on Uniform Use, third edition. International Union Against Cancer (UICC). Edited by Ch. Wittekind, F.L. Greene, et al. Wiley-Liss, New York, 2003.

Other references not commercially available

Training materials prepared for state and national registrars workshops by April Fritz and others

The Registrar's Key to Abstracting (reference for early years of the Principles of Oncology for Cancer Registrars training program), April Fritz.

Materials for various Cancer Information Management courses offered by Santa Barbara City College, California.

Page left blank.

ABSTRACTING INFORMATION IN TEXT FIELDS

Meryl Leventhal, MA, RHIT, CTR

The cancer abstract is the foundation for all other registry functions, whether in a hospital registry or a central registry. The information recorded on the abstract must be complete, timely and accurate in order to be useful. Cancer registry abstracting chronicles ***pertinent*** information about the patient and the site-specific disease process from the time a diagnosis of cancer is established until the end of the patient's life. Information collected and reported on the abstract is performed in accordance with guidelines established by the reporting facility and all regulatory agencies to which the facility reports its data. This chapter describes the text fields on the registry abstract—what to document and the most concise way to document the information.

Cancer registry abstracting is the process of creating a succinct summary or synopsis of the medical record of a cancer patient. The *abstract* is the document created, usually in computerized, analyzable form. Most of the information on a cancer registry abstract is stored in coded form for ease of data retrieval and analysis. However, there are drawbacks to working with only coded cancer information, such as

- accidentally transposing numbers, thereby storing incorrect information, such as 8072 versus 8720
- researchers may not recognize cases abstracted on the basis of ambiguous terminology
- if nonspecific codes are used, valuable information may be lost
- unusual occurrences may generate computer edit messages that could easily be explained, such as a 36 year old patient with prostate cancer
- visual editors and researchers may not be able to recognize true anomalies in the data because of the codes selected

To facilitate the quality review of cancer abstracts at the central registry level and to provide a greater level of detail for researchers and others using cancer abstracts, all coded information stored in the abstract should be justified in text. In fact, text validation of codes is required by most central registries. The North American Association of Central Cancer Registries (NAACCR) standard 3.2.2 states that "Text information **should** be included in the registry's dataset in computerized form along with the data codes to facilitate quality control."

There are a number of benefits to documenting codes with text, including

- reduction of query-backs on data edits
- explanation of unusual codes or circumstances
- clarification of code choices
- verification of edit checks

Proper documentation of codes is both a skill and an art. While there are style elements for recording text that are unique to each abstractor, the text information on the abstract is only valuable if it is digitized (recorded in a coded field) for electronic retrieval. Although it is possible to scan text fields to retrieve information, it is a difficult process and not all types of registry software have this capability. However, if there are questions regarding the coded data, text can explain or justify the choice of codes.

This chapter describes the text documentation standards of the California Cancer Registry, which has the highest quality control and data accuracy standards in the world. Although code validation requirements for other central registries may not be as stringent, these guidelines should serve as a model for registrars who desire to make their abstracts useful to researchers and other reviewers who use cancer registry data on a regular basis.

The following general guidelines apply to recording text information.

1. **All coded data fields must have text support recorded on the abstract. In other words, record text to validate coded data fields.**
    - Fields that must have text verification include patient race and other demographics, primary site, histology, extent of disease, and treatment.
    - The few data fields that do not need text support include date of birth, social security number, and medical record number.
    - Text fields should be completed by the abstractor. Text that is generated by the computer is not acceptable.
2. **Record *pertinent* site-specific cancer information.**
    - Record positive and negative findings that validate the primary site, histology, extent of disease and treatment.
    - There is no requirement to record information in the diagnostic workup, lab work or treatment fields if it has no bearing on the cancer.
3. **Complete text fields before assigning codes.**
    - Insure that all coded fields are substantiated in the text fields.
    - Recorded text information is then converted by the abstractor into numerical values, or codes, to permit electronic data retrieval of the text information.
4. **Record text information in a consistent, organized manner.**
    - Even though it is difficult to search text, if information is listed in specified order, it is easier to find.
    - Record the information documented on the abstract in an *organized* manner in text fields using a software program designed for collection, analysis and interpretation of this data. The text fields available in registry software vary among vendors. The common text fields—and what to record in them—are discussed below.
    - Use the same format for dates throughout the abstract and for every abstract. Refer to the section on acceptable date formats.
    - If information is missing from the medical record, identify what is missing, for example, "race not stated."
5. **Record text in a concise manner.**
    - Space is usually at a premium on most computerized abstract forms. Some registry software programs allow unlimited storage of text information, but usually only a limited amount of text is transmitted to the central registry. Recording the most pertinent information first will assure that it will be transmitted to the central registry.
    - Complete sentences are not required—or necessary—on the abstract.
    - Key phrases are separated by punctuation, either periods (.) or semicolons (;), as allowed by the registry software program.
    - Use *standard* medical abbreviations for text to save space. Refer to the abbreviations lists in the next chapter of this book, avoiding abbreviations that may have different meanings in different contexts.
    - If the registry software allows, avoid using all capital letters as this text is difficult to read. Use either all lower case or a combination of upper and lower case.

6. **Additional guidelines and comments**
   - Do not repeat the same information in multiple text fields.
   - Additional comments can be continued in empty text fields, including Remarks. For text documentation that is continued from one text field to another, use asterisks or other symbols to indicate the connection with preceding text.
   - Avoid including irrelevant information.
   - Do not include information that the registry is not authorized to collect.

SUGGESTIONS FOR CONCISE TEXT AND SUCCESSFUL ABBREVIATIONS

- Leave out articles, such as 'a,' 'an,' and 'the.'
- Leave out verbs (complete sentences not needed).
- Use numeric symbols with distinct meanings, such as +, &, –, #, @, as the software allows.
- Use standard abbreviations whenever possible.
- To create an abbreviation

To create an abbreviation	*Example*	*Meaning*
∘ Use the first syllable of the word	col	colon
∘ Add letters as needed to clarify	colect	colectomy
∘ Leave out vowels	brst	breast
∘ Use the first letters of words in a phrase	LN	lymph node
∘ Add 's' to make the abbreviation plural	LNs	lymph nodes
∘ Use just enough letters to recognize the term	endosc	endoscopy
∘ Use apostrophes to shorten term	cont'd	continued

- When in doubt, *write it out.*

DATE FORMATS

Every procedure, diagnostic test, and significant event should have a date associated with it. Every date also has a date flag associated with it. The central registry or the registry software vendor will determine how the date (and any missing information) should be recorded and stored. For example, the registry coding manual may say that unknown dates are filled with 9s, such as 02/99/2011 to indicate that the exact day is not known. Follow the instructions for your software, and use the same format for all abstracts.

Acceptable formats

mmddyyyy	02092011
mmddyy	020911
mm/dd/yyyy	02/09/2011
mm/dd/yy	02/09/11
m/d/yyyy	2/9/2011
m/d/yy	2/9/11
m/dd/yy	2/14/11

Unacceptable formats

mdyyyy	292011
mmdyyyy	0292011
mmdyy	02911

Data storage formats

yyyymmdd	20110209	complete year-month-day
yyyymm	201102	missing day information
yyyy	2011	unknown month and day

Date Flags

Date flags were added to the registry data base effective with 2010 cases. Date flags record codes that explain why information is missing from the date field. For example, if a patient has surgery in February of 2011 but the exact day is unknown, the date is stored in the database as 201102__ __ (the last two digits are blank). The vendor's software may allow the abstractor to record the date in 'natural' format (month, day, and year with some symbol indicating missing information) and in the background transpose the date for storage into the year-month-day format. The date flag to explain missing information may be coded directly by the abstractor or may coded automatically by the software. Examples of codes used in most date flags are displayed in Table 1.

Table 1. Examples of Codes Used In Date Flag Fields

10 = No information
Example: unknown if tx done

11 = No proper value
Example: tx not done

12 = Proper value applicable but not known
Example: test done, date unknown

15 = Information not available, maybe later
Example: tx planned, not started as of last date of contact

Blank = Valid date provided

TEXT FIELDS

The NAACCR Data Dictionary (*Volume II Data Standards and Data Dictionary,* version 12.2) defines 20 text fields used on cancer registry abstracts. This chapter will focus on seven that document the patient workup and diagnostic procedures, in the following order:

- History and Physical Exam
- X-rays and Scans
- Endoscopy (Scopes)
- Lab Tests and Tumor Markers
- Operative Report
- Pathology Report
- Remarks

HISTORY AND PHYSICAL EXAM TEXT FIELD

(NAACCR Field #2520 Text—DX Proc—PE; 1000 characters)

This text field documents the history of the current tumor and the clinical description of the tumor.

The History and Physical Exam (H&P) Report, commonly referred to as the H&P in the medical record, includes pertinent medical events leading up to the reason for admission for this cancer. In addition to the H&P, physical exam findings may be found in physician or clinic progress notes and consultation reports.

HISTORY OF PRESENT ILLNESS

The patient's history of the present illness (HPI) sets the stage for the rest of the abstract. The presenting symptoms or chief complaint provide clues to the type and extent of the diagnostic work-up and/or treatment you should expect to find. For example, if a patient presents with signs and symptoms of advanced disease, you would expect to find a complete metastatic work-up that you might not find if the patient presents with localized disease. Documentation of symptoms is not a requirement for central registries, but is useful information to record if the facility registry is used extensively by researchers, physicians, or medical students. If the registry software program has a separate History field, record the patient's symptoms there.

History and Physical Exam Text Field, *continued*

PHYSICAL EXAM FINDINGS

The physical exam documents what the physician sees, feels, hears, and even smells in relation to the specific cancer. In addition to the H&P report, physical exam findings may be found in physician or clinic progress notes and consultation reports.

Record only information that describes the ***location, size or extension of the primary cancer site*** as well as the "diagnostic impression" if stated.

You will not necessarily find documentation for all of the information listed below. These are guidelines as to the type of information ***typically*** found in the patient's record.

Date of exam

- Documents whether the exam was done prior to admission and establishes the point of reference for documentation of symptoms
- If this field documents an exam before admission, record the date if known, or "PTA" (prior to admission).

Primary site

- Palpability (any mass that can be felt)
- Size in centimeters; if a descriptive term is given, such as "cancer the size of a walnut", document this and convert the description to centimeters when recording tumor size per the conversion chart in the Collaborative Stage Data Collection System Coding Instructions, Appendix 1
- Location including subsite(s), lobe(s), quadrant(s)
- Laterality

Lymph nodes

- Anatomic location or name
- Palpability, fixation, matting, mobility of accessible lymph nodes
- Size of largest involved lymph node
- Laterality
- Number of involved lymph nodes in relation to primary tumor

Extent of disease

- Extent of tumor spread/invasion to other tissues or adjacent organs and lymph nodes by direct extension of tumor or distant site involvement. Examples: ascites; pleural effusion.
- Neurological findings (indicates brain or spinal metastases), abdominal or pelvic masses

Admitting impression/admitting diagnosis if stated by examining physician

- Provides working diagnosis and an indication of the kinds of tests that might be done to confirm the diagnosis

What NOT to Record in the History and Physical Exam Text Field

- ***Every detailed presenting symptom***
  Space is limited on the abstract form. Recording non-essential/non-contributory text is time consuming and is of little value unless the information can be captured in a coded data field.
- ***Other medical conditions***
  The patient's overall medical condition certainly impacts decisions relating to the diagnostic work-up and eventual treatment. The only exception is when other medical conditions (COPD; MI; Diabetes; Hypertension, etc) impact the patient's ability to undergo diagnostic procedures and/or treatment.

History and Physical Exam Text Field, *continued*

Example: a patient with severe COPD may not be able to withstand a surgical procedure due to compromised respiratory status. In the surgery treatment field (not the H+P), record that surgery is contraindicated due to severe COPD.

- ***Previous surgery(ies)***
  For example, a TAH/BSO is non-contributory for colon cancer and should not be recorded on the abstract.
- ***Family history, smoking history, alcohol history***
  This information has value only if your computerized software can capture and retrieve the information in a coded field or if your state collects this information.
- ***Planned work-up***
  Do not record in the H&P "planned work-up" (lumpectomy planned). If performed, this information will be recorded in the appropriate text field (s) on the abstract.

What to select and record on the abstract (record in this order)

- Date of History and Physical Exam
- Age, sex and race/ethnicity of patient
  History of Present Illness (HPI) or Chief Complaint (CC) stated concisely
  - Is the patient being admitted to diagnose cancer?
  - Is the patient being admitted to diagnose and treat cancer?
  - Is the patient being admitted to treat cancer that has been diagnosed and/or treated prior to this admission?
- Patient history of previous malignancies and/or benign/uncertain behavior CNS tumors
- Pertinent site-specific signs and symptoms are optional; if recorded, these should be stated concisely
- Pertinent *positive* site-specific findings that describe the primary site and any other involved organs. Record positive findings before negative findings.
  - Location
  - Size of tumor
  - Extent of disease (regional extension, involved nodes, and distant metastases)
- Pertinent *negative* site-specific findings, particularly those that pertain to staging. For example, negative axillary lymph nodes on physical exam are important to document for clinical N status for breast cancer, but it is not necessary to document a lymph node exam of the entire body by subsite (supraclavicular, cervical, inguinal, etc.) for a breast case.

The following data fields can be documented in the History and Physical Exam text field:

- Date of First Contact
- Admission Date and Flag
- Facility Referred From
- Date of Initial Diagnosis (if diagnosed prior to admission) and Flag
- Primary Site
- Laterality
- Histology (if diagnosed prior to admission)
- Class of Case
- Sequence Number
- Summary Stage
- CS Tumor Size
- CS Extension
- CS Lymph Nodes
- CS Mets at Dx
- Patient demographics:
  - Age at Diagnosis
  - Race 1-5
  - Spanish/Hispanic Origin
  - Sex

Sample Report #1
History and Physical Exam Report (Breast Cancer)

Admit date: 05/06/2011

History of Present Illness
Biopsy proven Rt breast CA. Self-discovered mass in right breast last month. Mammogram performed on April 15 revealed malignant appearing LIQ lesion of the right breast. Needle biopsy performed at Ocean View Surgery Center on April 30 revealed adenocarcinoma. Today, a hard mass in the inner lower quadrant of the right breast is palpated.

Past History Mumps 1960; Thyroid cancer diagnosed and treated 1968

Medications Synthroid

Habits Denies alcohol and tobacco

Occupation Office worker, Global Oil Corp.

Marital Married 25 years; three children

Birthplace Michigan

Family History Maternal grandmother had breast and colon cancer

General
Healthy female; Height: 5' 2"; Weight: 153 pounds; Blood Pressure: 130/70

Review of Systems

Head/Neck: Within normal limits; Wears corrective lenses for reading
Cardiorespiratory: Occasional SOB when climbing hills or steps; no history of asthma; denies chronic cough, hemoptysis, chest pain, ankle swelling
GI: Occasional post-prandial gas; good appetite; regular bowel movements; denies any history of blood loss
GU: Occasional cough/ sneeze incontinence; denies pain, burning, frequency
GYN: G3 P3; LMP April 15

Physical Exam
Eyes, Nose, Mouth, Throat, Neck: Neg
Heart: Regular sinus rhythm; no murmurs
Chest: Clear to percussion and auscultation
Abdomen: Soft, nontender; no masses, surgical scars
Pelvic: Recent exam within normal limits
Breasts: 3cm mass lower inner quadrant right breast; prominent skin retraction; left breast WNL
Axillae: Negative

Impression: Carcinoma Rt breast **Plan:** Lumpectomy

PRACTICE 1
Sample History and Physical Exam Report *(See Sample Report #1)*

From the sample H&P Exam Report, identify the pertinent medical events leading up to the reason for admission and the pertinent physical exam findings for the site-specific cancer and write them in concise form for the abstract.

Pertinent information from the sample H&P Exam Report:

- Admission to treat cancer that has been diagnosed prior to this admission
    - Rt breast needle biopsy performed at Ocean View Surgery Center on April 30 revealed adenocarcinoma

Practice 1, *continued*

- History of previous malignancies.
    - Thyroid cancer diagnosed and treated 1968
- Description of primary site
    - Location/laterality: Rt breast
    - Subsite: lower inner quadrant
    - Tumor size/description 3cm; prominent skin retraction
- Description of accessible Regional Lymph Nodes
    - Axillae: neg
- Extent of disease
    - Left breast wnl
- Admitting impression
    - Carcinoma Rt breast

The history and physical exam findings would be recorded on the abstract as:

- 05/06/11 58YO WF with bx proven Rt breast CA at Ocean View Surgery Center on 4/30/11; Thyroid ca dx/tx 1968. Rt Breast: 3cm mass LIQ; prominent skin retraction; Lt breast: wnl; Axillae: neg; Imp: CA Rt breast [206 characters including spaces]

RADIOLOGY PROCEDURES (X-RAYS AND SCANS) TEXT FIELD

(NAACCR field #2530 TEXT—DX PROC—X-RAY/SCAN; 1000 characters)

Radiologic tests (x-rays, scans, other imaging procedures) are performed to establish the diagnosis of cancer (identify the primary site) and to evaluate the extent of cancer involvement. If the physician indicates on the test request that the exam is to rule out cancer, the radiologist may make a statement regarding whether the patient has cancer or no cancer.

More often than not, the ordering physician does not indicate the reason for the test so the radiology findings can include everything and anything. **Do not record** non-cancer specific findings on the abstract. If the radiologist indicates that the exam is "normal" you can record "wnl" (within normal limits) on the abstract. An exam may be negative for cancer but if other non-cancer related findings are described (such as arthritis or pulmonary disease) you can't really say that the exam is normal or negative. You can record "negative for mets" or "negative for cancer."

Common Radiology Procedures (see also the Diagnostic Tests chapter)

- *X-rays*—record a "picture" of a body part using ionizing radiation
    - Chest x-ray (record initial chest x-ray on all patients as this may document CS Mets at Dx)
    - Bone series
    - Metastatic series
- *Computed Tomography (CT)/Computerized Axial Tomography (CAT)*—non-invasive examination of soft tissues of the body; records "slices" of the body with an x-ray scanner that are integrated by computer to give a cross-sectional image
- *Magnetic Resonance Imaging (MRI)*—imaging of the interior of the body without using x-rays or other types of ionizing radiation; capable of showing fine detail of different tissues
- *Positron emission tomography (PET) scan*—provides an image of metabolic function; more sensitive than CT scan; differentiates between malignant and non-malignant tumors; accurately assess location and extent of malignant disease; detects occult disease; provides a whole body view and earlier detection of recurrent cancer

Radiology Procedures Text Field, *continued*

- Other radiography (examples)
  - *Cystography/cystogram*—radiographic examination of the bladder
  - *Mammography/mammogram*—radiographic examination of the breasts
- *Ultrasonography*
- Nuclear medicine scans—imaging of organs involving administration of a radioactive tracer
  - *Brain Scan*
  - *Bone Scan*
  - *Liver/spleen Scan*

What to select and record (record in this order)

- For procedures relevant to primary site: date, type of procedure, site(s) being studied
  - If there are multiple procedures, record in chronological order.
  - If there are multiple procedures performed on the same date, record the date once. Separate the procedures with a period (.) or semi-colon (;).
    Example: 12/19/2010 CXR: wnl; IVU: neg
- Pertinent site-specific findings, both positive and negative, noted by the radiologist that describe the primary site in terms of location, size and extent of disease.

You will not necessarily find documentation for all of the information listed below; these are guidelines as to the type of information *typically* documented in the report.

Primary site
- Tumor Size
- Location including subsite(s)
- Lobe(s)
- Quadrant(s)
- Laterality

Lymph nodes
- Size of largest involved lymph node
- Location
- Laterality
- Number of involved lymph nodes in relation to primary tumor

Extent of disease
- Extent of tumor spread/invasion to other tissues or adjacent organs and lymph nodes by direct extension or distant site involvement

Diagnostic impression per radiologist

The following data fields can be documented with the Radiology Procedures Text Field:
- Date of Initial Diagnosis and Flag
- Diagnostic and Staging Procedures (RxSumm-Dx/Stg Proc)
- Primary Site
- Laterality
- Histology
- Collaborative Stage variables
- Summary Stage

Sample Report #2
Diagnostic Radiology Reports

A. Chest X-Ray (Breast Cancer)

Date: 5/4/2011

Exam: Chest X-ray

Clinical History: Pre-op CXR

Findings: Single AP view shows lung fields to be clear of active infiltrates.

Impression: Negative exam

B. CT Scan (Colon Cancer)

Date: 12/28/2011

Exam: CT Chest, Abdomen, Pelvis

Clinical Information: Colorectal CA

Pre contrast imaging of the liver was first performed. The chest, abdomen, and pelvis was then scanned following contrast injection.

There is an osseous lesion of a rib with associated pleural thickening in the right mid to upper posterolateral chest consistent with metastatic lesion and correlating with increased metabolic activity in this area on PET scan of 12/14/07.

The mediastinum is free of adenopathy. No pulmonary nodules are demonstrated.

There is nodularity along the lesser curvature of the stomach, in the porta hepatis, and in the mesentery consistent with mesenteric adenopathy. Adenopathy involves the retroperitoneum as well. The findings correlate with increased metabolic activity on recent PET scan.

C. Bone Scan (Prostate Cancer)

Date: 11/11/2011

Exam: Bone Scan

Clinical Hx: 57 year old man with CAP [carcinoma of prostate]; rule out bone mets

Procedure: Following the IV administration of 20.4mCi of Tc-00n MDP, images of the skeleton were obtained in anterior and posterior projections two hours later using the large field of view gamma camera and whole body scanning table.

Findings: The bone scan demonstrates degenerative changes in the shoulder and hip joints, but no areas of increased activity to suggest metastasis to the skeleton. The remainder of the axial and appendicular skeleton was unremarkable. Both kidneys and urinary bladder were visualized normally.

Impression: Negative bone scan for metastatic disease.

PRACTICE 2

Sample Radiology Reports ***(See Sample Report #2)***

From each of the three sample radiology reports, identify the pertinent exam findings for the site-specific cancer and write them in concise form for the abstract.

Pertinent Imaging Findings

A. Chest X-ray Report

- Diagnostic impression per radiologist opinion: Negative exam

The **Chest X-Ray text** would be recorded on the abstract as

- 05/04/11 CXR: neg

B. CT Scan Report

- Sites examined: Chest, abdomen, pelvis
- Lymph nodes and extent of disease
  - Sites of metastatic disease: rib lesion and pleural thickening
  - Status of lung and chest lymph nodes: no lymphadenopathy in mediastinum, no nodules in lung
  - Status of retroperitoneal lymph nodes: extensive lymphadenopathy in lesser curvature, porta hepatis, mesentery and retroperitoneum

The **CT Scan text** would be recorded on the abstract as

- 12/28/11 CT Chest, Abd, Pelvis: osseous lsn of a rib c/w mets; mediastinum: no LAD; no pulm nodules; nodularity along lesser curvature stomach in porta hepatis and mesentery c/w LAD; retroperitoneum: LAD

C. Bone Scan Report

- Type of procedure/purpose: rule out bone mets
- Diagnostic impression: negative bone scan for metastatic disease

The **Bone Scan text** would be recorded on the abstract as:

- 11/11/2011 BSc: neg for mets

ENDOSCOPY PROCEDURES TEXT FIELD

(NAACCR Field #2540 TEXT—DX PROC—SCOPES; 1000 characters)

An endoscopy procedure involves the use of an instrument to examine the interior of a canal, hollow organ, or body cavity. Examples include:

- Bronchoscopy—examination of the bronchi in the lungs
- Colonoscopy—examination of the colon
- Cystoscopy—examination of the bladder
- Mediastinoscopy—examination of the space between the lungs, the mediastinum

What to select and record (record in this order)

- Date and type of procedure
  - If there are multiple procedures, record in chronological order.
  - If there are multiple procedures performed on the same date, record the date once. Separate the procedures with a period (.) or semi-colon (;).

Endoscopy Procedures Text Field, *continued*

- Pertinent site-specific findings both positive and negative noted by the endoscopist that describe the primary site in terms of location, size and extent of disease.

You will not necessarily find documentation for all of the information listed below; these are guidelines as to the type of information *typically* documented in the report.

Primary site

- Size
- Location including subsite(s)
- Lobe(s)
- Quadrant(s)
- Laterality

Lymph nodes

- Size of largest involved lymph node
- Location
- Laterality
- Number of involved lymph nodes in relation to primary tumor

Extent of disease

- Extent of tumor spread/invasion to other tissues or adjacent organs and lymph nodes by direct extension or distant site involvement
  Note: An endoscopic examination of a tube such as the bronchus cannot assess involvement of areas and tissues outside the tube. The report may describe narrowing from a mass outside the tube but the endoscopist cannot see the mass itself if it is outside the tube (extrinsic).

Diagnostic impression according to the endoscopist

The following data fields can be documented in the Endoscopy Procedures text field:

- Date of Initial Diagnosis and Flag
- Date of 1st Positive Bx and Flag
- Diagnostic and Staging Procedures (RxSumm-Dx/Stg Proc)
- Diagnostic Confirmation
- Primary Site
- Laterality
- Histology
- Collaborative Stage variables
- Summary Stage

PRACTICE 3
Sample Endoscopy Report ***(See Sample Report #3)***

From the sample endoscopy reports, identify pertinent findings for the site-specific cancer and write them in concise form for the abstract.

Sample Report #3
Endoscopy Report

A. COLONOSCOPY (Colon cancer)

Exam date:	July 4, 2011
Clinical Information:	55 yr old male; Iron deficiency anemia
Medications:	Demerol 50 mg IV before procedure Midazolam HCL 1.5mg IV before procedure
Procedure:	Rectal exam: normal. The endoscope was passed without difficulty to the cecum confirmed by ileocecal valve. Retroflexion was performed. The quality of the preparation was excellent.
Findings:	There was a 3 cm sessile mass present in the cecum. Multiple biopsies were obtained. There were numerous medium diverticula present in the sigmoid colon.
Complications:	None
Impression:	Sessile mass in cecum Numerous medium divertiula in sigmoid colon
Recommendation:	Surgery consult; Await pathology from biopsies.

B. CYSTOSCOPY (Bladder Cancer)

Date:	August 8, 2011
Pre-op Dx:	Huge bladder tumor with hematuria
Post-op Dx:	Golf-ball size bladder tumor with hematuria right side of the urinary bladder close to the trigone area, unable to identify the ureteral orifice.
Operation:	Cystoscopy with transurethral resection of the bladder
Procedure:	Inside of the bladder was inspected with the cystoscopy which showed a cauliflower type of huge bladder tumor about a golf ball-type in size. It bled quite easily. The tumor was resected with the rectoscope down to the muscle layer. The tumor was completely removed. The bladder was irrigated with normal saline with 24- French three way 30 cc balloon inserted.

Pertinent Endoscopy Findings

A. Colonoscopy (Colon cancer)

- Primary site; tumor size: 3 cm sessile mass present in the cecum.

The colonoscopy text would be recorded on the abstract as:

- 07/04/11 C'scope/bx: 3cm sessile mass in cecum

B. Cystoscopy (Bladder)

- Primary site: Rt side urinary bladder close to trigone; unable to identify ureteral orifice
- Tumor size: Golf-ball size

The cystoscopy text would be recorded on the abstract as:

- 08/08/11 Cysto: Golf-ball size bladder tumor Rt side of bladder close to trigone area, unable to identify ureteral orifice

LABORATORY TESTS/TUMOR MARKERS TEXT FIELD

(NAACCR Field #2550 TEXT—DX PROC—LAB TESTS; 1000 characters)

Laboratory test(s) and tumor markers are performed to establish the diagnosis of cancer or the presence of metastatic disease, to document characteristics of the cancer, or to predict some aspect of the natural history of the cancer.

A lab test is the microscopic examination of the cells of the blood, blood-forming tissues, or other body fluids looking for changes in the structure of and/or numbers of various types of cells or natural body chemicals. Examples of common lab tests include

- CBC (complete blood count)
- LFT (liver function test)
- PFT (pulmonary function test) (lungs)
- Urinalysis (urine)
- LDH (lactate dehydrogenase—assesses multiple body systems)

Tumor markers are substances released by tumor cells into blood, urine, tissue, body fluids or in chromosomes that can be site-specific or histology-specific, performed to

- Screen for or detect malignancies
- Monitor response to treatment or relapse
- Determine extent of disease
- Provide prognostic information

Examples of tumor markers and their uses include

- Breast—estrogen receptor assay (ERA), progesterone receptor assay (PRA), HER2 overexpression, all of which help predict the patient's response to various systemic therapies
- Prostate—prostate-specific antigen (PSA), an indicator of potential tumor spread outside the prostatic capsule
- Melanoma—mitotic rate, an estimate of the growth rate
- Colon and rectum—KRAS, a predictor of response to certain chemotherapy drugs

These and many other tumor markers are also coded in site-specific factors of the Collaborative Stage Data Collection System (CS). They are described in more detail in the site-specific chapters of the CASEbooks.

Tumor markers are NOT used to establish or confirm the diagnosis of cancer unless there is a physician statement that the patient has cancer based on the tumor marker result.

- Record only lab tests and tumor markers pertinent to the cancer being abstracted.
  Examples: A man with kidney cancer may have a PSA. Do not record the PSA because it is not pertinent to his kidney cancer.
  A colon cancer patient may have a hemoglobin and hematocrit that show anemia resulting from the cancer, but it is not necessary to record the blood work values.

Where to look for lab tests/tumor markers

- Laboratory reports
- Attachments or addenda to pathology reports
- History and physical exam report
- Progress notes
- Consultation reports

Lab Tests/Tumor Markers Text Field, *continued*

The test may not be a separate document in the medical record. If the test was performed outside the hospital, the result may be reported by the clinician in the H&P or consultation report.

What to select and record (record in this order)

- Date of test(s) was performed
- Name of test(s)
- Test result(s)
- Normal test value/range recorded in parenthesis
- If multiple tests are performed, record in chronological order.

The following data fields may be documented in the Lab Tests and Tumor Markers field:

- Primary Site
- Grade
- Diagnostic Confirmation
- Presence of metastases
- Collaborative Stage variables (site-specific factors)
- Date of Initial Diagnosis and Flag

PRACTICE 4

Sample Lab Report ***(See Sample Report #4)***

From each of the two sample **Lab Reports**, identify pertinent findings for the site-specific cancer and write them in concise form for the abstract.

Sample Report #4
Laboratory Report

A. Prostate Specific AG (Prostate Cancer)

Date collected: 11 August 2011

	Abnormal	Normal	Ref-Range Units
PSA :	High 10.10		< or = 2.5 ng/mL

Age-related PSA Normal Values

Age (yrs)	Normal Value (ng/mL)
49 or less	Less than or equal to 2.5
50-59	Less than or equal to 3.5
60-69	Less than or equal to 4.5
70 or greater	Less than or equal to 6.5

B. CEA (Colon Cancer)

Date collected: 02 November 2011
CEA: 1.0 (normal)

Pertinent Lab Test and Tumor Marker Findings

A. PSA Report

- Test result: 10.10 (high, abnormal)
- Reference range (≤ 2.5 ng/ml)

The PSA text would be recorded on the abstract as:

- 08/11/11 PSA: 10.10 (High; nl <2.5)

Practice 4, *continued*

B. CEA Report

Pertinent findings from the sample **CEA Report**:

- Test result: 1.0 (normal)

The CEA text would be recorded on the abstract as

- 11/02/11 CEA:1.0 (normal)

OPERATIVE FINDINGS TEXT FIELD

(NAACCR Field #2560 TEXT—DX PROC—OP; 1000 characters)

If cancer of an internal organ is suspected, direct access to it may require a surgical procedure. Exploratory surgery may be performed to determine whether or not a cancerous condition exists and the degree to which the cancer may have affected other organs and structures within the observed area. Biopsies may be performed. Exploratory surgery may be followed immediately by definitive surgery or the exploration may indicate a cancer so extensive that definitive surgery is ruled out.

Surgical procedures (the technique) are described in an operative report. The report *usually* lists the pre- and post-operative diagnoses, the name of the procedure and the operative findings.

Operative findings are the observations of the surgeon—what the surgeon actually sees when the patient is opened and explored. Operative findings may also be listed in the "Op note" or in the progress notes. If the operative findings are not enumerated, they may be "scattered" through the body of the report, so be sure to skim through the report to identify the findings.

Operative findings may include

- Description of the exact location of the primary tumor
- Tumor size
- Extent to which the tumor has or has not spread beyond the primary site
- Residual tumor tissue, tumor tissue that was not/could not be removed

Operative findings/observations must be recorded on the abstract as they may be the most complete assessment of the malignancy, especially when the tumor is not completely excised or when no definitive surgery is performed. For example, an operative report might reveal liver and lymph node metastasis that were not seen on imaging but were observed by surgeon at time of abdominal surgery.

If operative findings are not documented, record **"**technique only**"** in the operative findings text field on the abstract. This indicates that the only documentation in the medical record is how the surgery was performed.

Operative findings are *not*

- Step by step procedures performed (what the surgeon did), in other words the "technique"
- Endoscopy findings (record in Endoscopy field)
- Pathologic findings (record in Pathology field)

What to select and record (record in this order)

Observations of the surgeon that describe

Primary site

- Size
- Location including subsite(s), lobe(s), quadrant(s)
- Laterality

Operative Findings Text Field, *continued*

Lymph nodes

- Size of largest involved lymph node
- Location
- Laterality
- Number of involved lymph nodes in relation to primary tumor

Extent of disease

- Organs or tissues that are removed
- Invasion into other tissues or adjacent organs or lymph nodes
- Biopsies or resections of regional or metastatic sites
- Evidence of multiple tumors and multiple sites of origin
- Discontinuous spread to distant organ or lymph node
- Stage at diagnosis if stated by physician
- Record presence and site of any gross tumor not resected by surgeon

The following data fields may be documented in the Operative Findings text field:

- Date of 1st Positive Bx and Flag
- Date of Initial Diagnosis and Flag
- Diagnostic and Staging Procedures (RxSumm-Dx/Stg Proc)
- Diagnostic Confirmation
- Primary Site
- RX Hosp—Dx/Stg Proc
- RX Summ—Surg Prim Site
- Collaborative Stage variables
- SEER Summary Stage

PRACTICE 5
Sample Operative Report *(See Sample Report #5)*

From the sample **Operative Report**, identify pertinent findings for the site-specific cancer and write them in concise form for the abstract.

Sample Report # 5
Operative Report (Colon Cancer)

DATE OF OPERATION: 11/20/11

SURGEON: M.R. Carson, MD

PRE OP DX: Right colon cancer

POST OP DX: Right colon cancer; Metastatic colon cancer to left lobe of liver

OPERATION PERFORMED: Laparoscopic segmental ileocecal resection

ANESTHESIA: General

EBL: Less than 100 ml

INDICATIONS FOR SURGERY: Colonoscopy revealed mass in the cecum which was biopsy proven to be a cecal cancer.

Sample Report # 5—Operative Report, continued

DETAILS OF OPERATION: The patient received preoperative antibiotics and was placed supine. General anesthesia was given per endotracheal tube. Bilateral sequential compression devices were placed on her legs and a Foley catheter was placed. The patient's abdomen was prepped and draped in the usual fashion.

A small incision was made above the umbilicus. The Veress needle was inserted into the peritoneal cavity, and its position was confirmed using the aspiration and saline test. Pneumoperitoneum was established using carbon dioxide. The Veress needle was removed followed by insertion of the 5 mm trocar and then followed by the camera, which was a 5 mm 45 degree laparoscope.

Laparoscopically, the abdomen was inspected. In the left lobe of the liver, there were noted to be four suspicious lesions. A picture was taken of this. There was one lesion near the edge of the left lobe of the liver. A true cut biopsy was performed of this and the frozen section was positive for metastatic colon cancer to the liver. There was no lesion seen on the right lobe.

Because of the metastatic nature of this disease to the liver, it was felt that performing a full right hemicolectomy was not indicated because of the spread to the liver. Therefore it was decided to perform a segmental resection of the ileal cecum because the patient has a history of anemia.

A size #5 mm trocar was placed in the right upper quadrant and also a size #5 mm trocar was placed in the left lower quadrant. Using a grasper and a sonosurge, the white line of Toldt was open lateral to the right colon. The terminal ileum was also mobilized. The cecum and ascending colon were able to mobilize medially. The patient was placed in the left side position and in Trendelenburg's. The patient was placed in the head up position with the left side down. The right hepatic flexure was mobilized by dividing the hepatocolic ligament with the sonosurge. This then mobilized the hepatic flexure. The right transverse colon was mobilized as well. The duodenum was visualized. The right colon was mobilized to the midline as much as possible.

The terminal ileum and ascending colon were well mobilized and easily able to be brought up to the abdominal wall. The rest of the surgery was performed extracorporally. The camera was removed.

An incision was made transversely in the right mid-abdomen 1cm above the umbilicus. The muscles were divided in the usual fashion. A large wound protector was placed. The ascending colon and the cecum were then able to be pulled out of the abdomen. There was noted to be a lymph node near the cecum which was included with the specimen. The descending colon, hepatic flexure and the terminal ileum were than able to be brought out extracorporally.

The ascending was divided in the mid-ascending colon. The terminal ileum was divided 3cm proximal to the ileoceal valve. The mesentery to this portion of the bowel was divided between clamps and suture ligated with 2-0 silk suture. The specimen was removed off of the field. The two ends of the bowel were brought together, and there was good blood supply to the bowel. Both bowel ends were pink and with no tension. Then a side-to-side functional end-to end anastomosis was created with a GIA-80 stapler followed by a TA-60 stapler. The anastomosis was checked before closing off the anastamosis. There was no bleeding. After the anastomosis was completed it was tested and it was patent.

The mesenteric defect was closed using interrupted 3 0 silk sutures. The bowel was placed back in the abdomen. The omentum was draped over the bowels. The abdomen was lifted upward with the retractor and the retroperitoneum was inspected. A dry pack was placed in the retroperitoneum and was left in place. There were no signs of active bleeding. The abdomen was irrigated copiously with saline and all of the irrigation was clear. All of the packs were removed as was the wound protector. The surgeon's gloves were changed and the wounds were closed in two layers using #1 Maxon suture. The wounds were irrigated and the skin was closed using staples.

The patient was extubated and transferred to the recovery room. The Foley catheter was left in place.

Practice 5, *continued*

Pertinent findings from the sample **Operative Report**:

- Extent to which the tumor has or has not spread beyond the primary site:
  - In the left lobe of the liver, there were noted to be four suspicious lesions. There was one lesion near the edge of the left lobe of the liver. There was no lesion seen in the right lobe.

The Operative findings text would be recorded on the abstract as:

- 11/20/11 4 suspicious lesions in Lt lobe of liver; one lesion near edge of Lt lobe of liver; no lesion seen on Rt lobe.

PATHOLOGY FINDINGS TEXT FIELD

(NAACCR Field #2570 TEXT—DX PROC—PATH; 1000 characters)

The most accurate methods for diagnosing cancer are microscopic examination of tissues (histology) removed from the site of a suspected cancer and/or microscopic examination of cells (cytology) contained in the fluid that bathes a suspected site. Histologic findings are recorded on the pathology report. Cytologic findings are recorded on the cytology report.

Microscopic Examination of Tissue (Histology)
A histologic examination may be made from a blood sample, a biopsy specimen, a surgical specimen, bone marrow specimen or at autopsy. The pathologist examines the gross tissue specimen. The findings are documented on the pathology report.

Blocks of tissue are cut from the specimen for further microscopic evaluation. The sample should include resection margins and lymph nodes if contained within the specimen. The tissues are fixed, hydrated and embedded in wax. Thin sections are cut, stained and mounted on glass slides. Different chemical stains are applied to help define cell type and structure (morphology/histology), behavior (in-situ or invasive), and grade or differentiation.

A biopsy specimen can be processed quickly by a frozen section technique or by routine fixation (permanent section) by H and E (Hematoxylin and Eosin) stain, which usually takes 48 hours to prepare.

Immunohistochemistry studies may be performed on tissue specimens. This involves staining tissue using specific antibodies that can be targeted to recognize specific components of the cell. This technique enables the pathologist to identify a type of tumor by substances it contains. These same substances can be used as tumor markers to identify cancer cells that may have spread to bone marrow or lymph nodes.

Molecular diagnostics are the biotech diagnostics including gene expression profiling, DNA/RNA analysis of minute amounts of genetic material in fetal and adult tissues and monoclonal antibodies.

Cytogenetics is the ability to detect classes of tumors and predict who will get cancer type and aggressiveness of cancer.

Procedures that yield tissue/pathology reports

- Biopsy report—sample of tissue excised to establish a diagnosis
- Aspiration biopsy—removal of tissue near surface of skin or deep-seated organs by means of suction through a hollow needle
- Incisional biopsy—removal of a piece or portion of tissue

Pathology Findings Text Field, ***continued***

- Core needle biopsy—removal of a core of tissue from a lesion or organ located deep in body
- Punch biopsy—punch technique used to obtain tissue
- Curettage—removal of tissue by scraping with a curette
- Bone marrow aspiration and biopsy (hematology)
- Excisional biopsy—removal of entire tumor with margin of normal tissue
- Partial/total removal of organ ("-ectomy")
- Autopsy report—all major organs of the body examined to correlate clinical and pathological findings and to identify missed diagnoses; the final diagnosis section of the report describes primary tumor, histology, extent of primary tumor, metastases based on histopathologic exam of tissues after death

Pathology Report Format
While pathology report formats vary among facilities, the content of the report is fairly standard. There may be more than one pathology report in the medical record. Record information from all pertinent pathology reports on the abstract in chronologic order.

The key sections of a pathology report are

1. Clinical/pre-operative diagnosis (as per attending physician)
2. Gross (macroscopic) description (what is seen without a microscope)
   - Size (the greatest dimension) of tumor, NOT size of specimen
   - Location of tumor within the organ
   - Single or multiple tumors
   - Other tissues removed or biopsied by surgeon
   - Number/names of removed lymph nodes-regional and distant
3. Microscopic description (what is seen through microscope)
   - Primary site
   - Histology: cell type, behavior, grade/differentiation
   - Single lesion, same behavior
   - Multiple lesions, single primary
   - Extent of disease/involvement of surrounding tissues: invasion of tumor into tissues within the primary site, invasion of tumor into adjacent anatomic structures
   - Status of lymph nodes: name of involved/uninvolved nodes, regional and distant, number positive, number examined, size of metastasis in involved lymph node(s)
   - Status of surgical margins
   - Discontinuous metastasis
4. Final pathologic diagnosis (a summary of the pathologist's observations)
   - Histologic type
   - Grade/differentiation
   - Summary of extent of disease

The College of American Pathologists (CAP) has published a series of documents called checklists, protocols, or synoptic reports. These documents provide formats for the inclusion of specific pieces of information for various types of procedures, such as breast core needle biopsy, partial mastectomy (lumpectomy) and mastectomy (total, modified radical or radical). The CAP protocols are very useful to clinicians and registrars because they provide clear descriptions of the extent of the cancer in a consistent format. The Commission on Cancer (COC) recommends that some sort of checklist format be used for cancer pathology reports in COC-approved cancer programs. In some facilities, the cancer protocol or synoptic report has replaced all or part of the text for the gross and microscopic examination in the pathology report.

Pathology Findings Text Field, *continued*

What information to select and record

Record pertinent findings both positive and negative, in a concise and uniform manner. Record positive findings before negative findings. Following a specified format insures that important details from the pathology report will not be omitted.

Suggested format (record in this order)

- Specimen date (date specimen was removed from the patient)
- Pathology report number
- Primary cancer site/tissue specimen source
- Histology/behavior/grade (include all modifying adjectives, such as predominantly, with features of, with foci of, elements of)
- Extent of disease within and beyond the primary site
- Tumor size (record only the greatest dimension of the tumor)
- Status of margins
- Lymph node involvement: number positive, number examined, name of lymph node chain if stated. Record as: #LNs positive/# of LNs examined (2+/4 Axillary LNs)
- Other tissue (s)/organ (s)
- Include any comments or reports from outside consultants

Microscopic Examination of Cells (Cytology)

Cells are continually shed from tissues that line the cavities and hollow organs of the body. These cells may float in the fluid which bathes or pass through the cavities. Fluid in a body cavity that can be aspirated indicates a pathological process, commonly malignant and/or metastatic.

Cells lining tissues can be sampled by scraping and examined as cytological preparations. Cells or fluids can be obtained by tapping or puncturing a body cavity, such as the pleura and peritoneum, and suctioning off the liquid through a needle or catheter. The microscopic examination of these cells is termed *exfoliative cytology*.

Where to look for documentation

Cells for study may be obtained from examination of cells, smears, fluids. Cytologic information is usually found on a cytology report but it may be submitted on a pathology report form (record as cytology) and labeled cytology findings. Some cytology specimens contain tissue (record as pathology). Some pathology/tissue specimens contain only cells or fluid aspirations (record as cytology).

Procedures that yield cells/cytology reports

- Fine needle aspiration (FNA)—removal of cells or fluid by suctioning through a hollow needle
- Thoracentesis—removal of fluid from the chest
- Abdominal paracentesis—removal of fluid from abdominal cavity
- Exfoliated (shedding) cells
- Washings—removal of fluid from an organ or structure to collect cells
- Brushings—brushing the lining of an organ to obtain cells
- Scrapings of cells from surface epithelium
- Pap smears—removal of cells from cervix (tip of uterus) using a tiny brush and small spatula
- Secretions
- Sputum cytology
- Urine
- Flow cytometry—analyzes the amount of DNA in tumor cells

Pathology Findings Text Field, *continued*

What to record (record in this order)

- Specimen date (date specimen was removed from the patient, not date report was finished)
- Specimen source
- Positive and/or negative findings
- If there is more than one cytology report, record them in chronologic order.

The following data fields can be documented in the Pathology Findings text field:

- Date of Initial Diagnosis and Flag
- Primary Site
- Laterality
- Histologic Type
- Grade
- Collaborative Stage variables
- Diagnostic confirmation

PRACTICE 6
Sample Pathology Report *(See Sample Report #6)*

From the sample **Pathology Report**, identify pertinent findings for the site-specific cancer and write them in concise form for the abstract.

Sample Report # 6
Surgical Pathology Report (Colon Cancer)

Date of Procedure	11/03/11
Date of Receipt	11/04/11
Date of Report	11/05/11
Pathology Report Number	S11-0507

SPECIMEN:
A. Ileocecum
B. Liver core bx

GROSS DESCRIPTION:
A. Received fresh is a right segmental resection specimen, 12cm in length x 5cm in diameter with terminal ileum, 3.5cm in length x 2.0cm in diameter, and grossly unremarkable vermiform appendix, 6.5cm in length x 0.5cm in diameter. Within the cecum is an irregular polypoid to somewhat ulcerated tan to tan-brown mass measuring approximately 5.7 x 4.0 x 1.6cm. The mass can be seen extending over the ileocecal valve; however, not into the ileum. The mass is 4cm from the proximal margin and 7.5cm from the distal margin. Sectioning reveals gross extension through the wall and to within 0.1cm of the serosal surface and soft tissue margin. Necrosis is not grossly identified. 5.5 cm from the distal margin is a small sessile polypoid lesion, 0.7 x 0.5 x0.1cm. No other mucosal lesions are identified. Sectioning of the fat reveals diffuse gross tumor Involvement and several probably grossly involved lymph nodes ranging in size from 0.2cm up to 1.0cm in greatest diameter. Representative sections are submitted as follow: A1, proximal and distal margins; A2, tumor showing deepest invasion; A3-A5, tumor; A6, small sessile polyp; A7 normal large bowel mucosa; A8, appendix; A9-16 probable lymph nodes.
B. Received in formalin is a core of gray-white tan soft tissue measuring 1.4 x 0.2cm.

MICRO AND FINAL DIAGNOSIS
A. Ileocecum, segmental resection:
Tumor type and grade: Moderately Differentiated Adenocarcinoma

Sample Report # 6—Surgical Pathology Report, continued

Anatomic Site:	Cecum
Tumor Size:	5.7cm
Resection Margins:	Proximal and distal resection margins free of tumor
Depth of Invasion:	Infiltrating muscularis propria into adjacent fibroadipose tissue
Pericolic LNs:	Multiple matted nodes, approximately 21; all nodes positive for metastatic tumor
Associated findings:	Portion of unremarkable appendix with adjacent serosal adipose tissue containing tumor nodule

B. Liver, left lobe, core biopsy:
Metastatic Moderately Differentiated Colonic Adenocarcinoma

Pertinent findings from the sample **Pathology Report**:

- The Micro and Final Diagnosis section of this pathology report is an example of the synoptic report or CAP protocol mentioned above.
- Ileocecum, segmental resection

Tumor type and grade:	Moderately Differentiated Adenocarcinoma
Anatomic Site:	Cecum
Tumor Size:	5.7 cm
Resection Margins:	Proximal and distal resection margins free of tumor
Depth of Invasion:	Infiltrating muscularis propria into adjacent fibroadipose tissue
Pericolic LNs:	Multiple matted nodes, approximately 21; all nodes positive for metastatic tumor
Associated findings:	Portion of unremarkable appendix with adjacent serosal adipose tissue containing tumor nodule

- Liver, left lobe, core biopsy
  Metastatic Moderately Differentiated Colonic Adenocarcinoma

The **Pathology Report** findings text would be recorded on the abstract as:

- 11/3/11 (S11-0507) Ileocecum: MD Adenoca Cecum infiltrating muscularis propria into adj fibroadipose tissue; TS: 5.7cm; Prox/Dist margs:neg; 21+/21 pericolic LNs; Liver bx: (+) mets

Sample Report # 7
Cytology Report (Lung Cancer)

Date:	October 19, 2011
Specimen Number:	C-14682
Type+Source of Specimen	Bronchial washings
Clinical Findings:	DOE [dyspnea on exertion]; Coughing up blood

Screening for Malignancy
( ) Negative
( ) Atypical
( ) Unsatisfactory
( ) Suspicious
(+) Positive

Comments:
Cells positive for small cell carcinoma

PRACTICE 7
Sample Cytology Report ***(See Sample Report #7)***

From the sample **Cytology Report**, identify pertinent findings for the site-specific cancer and write them in concise form for the abstract.

Pertinent findings from the sample **Cytology Report**
- Cells positive for small cell carcinoma

The **Cytology Report** findings text would be recorded on the abstract as:
- 10/19/11 C-14682 Bronch wash: (+) for small cell CA

TREATMENT TEXT FIELDS

The different treatment modalities have their own text fields in the cancer registry abstract, but each supports multiple coded data fields. The following are general guidelines for including information in the treatment text fields:
- Most treatment fields are 1000 characters in length. Although some registry software programs allow unlimited storage of text information, usually only a limited amount of text is transmitted to the central registry. Recording the most pertinent information first will assure that it will be sent to the central registry.
- If additional space is needed, continue the text in a remarks field by connecting the two fields with asterisks or other symbols.
- Use standard abbreviations.
- Do not rely on computer-generated text to fill the field based on the input code.
- Do not duplicate information in other fields, such as the Operative Findings and Pathology text fields.
- Avoid recording non-pertinent information, such as an incidental hernia repair or incidental appendectomy.
- If information is missing, note what is missing, such as "operative report not in record."
- Document all of the related data fields to the greatest extent possible.

SURGERY TEXT FIELD
(NAACCR Field #2610 RX TEXT-SURGERY; 1000 characters)

Surgery is the oldest type of cancer treatment. Surgical removal of the primary site has been the mainstay of cancer treatment for most cancers, completely excising the cancer offers the patient the greatest chance for cure if the cancer has a low tendency to metastasize.

Surgery may be performed to:
- Diagnose or stage disease
- Remove the primary cancer, surrounding lymph nodes, margin of normal tissue
- Remove residual, metastatic or recurrent lesions
- Relieve symptoms such as obstruction or nerve compression caused by the cancer (so-called bypass procedures)
- Restore or improve function (reconstruction)
- Improve appearance (cosmetic)
- Support radiation treatment
- Implant catheters that will be loaded with radioactive material

Surgery Text Field, *continued*

- Expose a tumor so that a large dose of radiation can be given directly to the tumor or the tumor bed (intra-operative radiation)
- Support chemotherapy
- Surgically implant a port, catheter or pump to deliver chemotherapy

Types of surgical procedures

- Total or partial removal of tumor tissue of primary or secondary site, with or without resection of regional nodes (excludes incisional biopsy, which cuts through tumor)
- Re-excision of a previously resected specimen performed to insure no residual tumor; surgery where the specimen does not contain tumor tissue
- Radical excision with/without lymph node dissection
- Excisional biopsy—removal of entire tumor and margin of normal tissue
- Electrocautery—malignant tissue burned by passage of electric current
- En bloc resection—tumor is removed along with a large area of surrounding tissues containing affected lymph nodes in one piece
- Exenteration—wide resection involving removal of tumor, its organ of origin and all surrounding tissue in the body space, such as the pelvis
- Debulking—cyto-reductive surgery (to decrease tumor mass)
- Cryosurgery—malignant tissue destroyed by freezing tissue
- Fulguration—bladder, rectum, skin tumors
- Laser surgery—specify whether tumor was vaporized with no pathology specimen or tumor was excised with the aid of a laser beam to cut into tissue and specimen was submitted for analysis
- Transurethral resection (endoscopic) of bladder or prostate tumor
- Reconstructive/rehabilitation surgery—procedures performed as first course of treatment that improve shape, appearance and/or function of body structures that are missing, defective, damaged or misshapen by cancer

What to select and record for the surgery field

- Date each surgical procedure performed
    - Record each procedure—excisional biopsy, wide excision, total organ removal, and so forth. Do not record aspiration biopsies or incisional biopsies in this field.
- Facility where each procedure performed
- Name of each surgical procedure
    - Read the entire operative report—don't just copy the name of the procedure. *Example:* The procedure may be titled "radical prostatectomy and laparoscopic lymph node dissection," but if the surgeon finds involved regional nodes, the prostatectomy may be cancelled. In such a case, the name of the procedure would be "laparoscopic lymph node dissection."

The following data fields can be documented in the Surgery text field:

- RX Date of Surgery and Flag
- RX Summ-Surg Prim Site
- RX Hosp-Surg Prim Site
- RX Summ Scope Reg LN Sur
- RX Hosp-Scope Reg LN Sur
- RX Summ-Surg Oth Reg/Dis
- Date of Initial RX-SEER and Flag

Surgery Text Field, *continued*

- Date of 1st Crs RX-CoC and Flag
- Site of Distant Met 1-3
- Reason for No Surgery
- RX Summ-Surgical Margins
- RX Hosp-Palliative Proc
- RX Summ-Palliative Proc
- Text-Place of Diagnosis

PRACTICE 8A

Using the information from the Operative Report (Sample Report #5), summarize the surgical treatment(s) in concise form for the surgery text field on the abstract.

The Surgery text field would be recorded on the abstract as

- 11/20/11 Laparosc segm ileocecal resect

RADIATION TEXT FIELDS
(NAACCR Field #2620 RX TEXT-RADIATION (BEAM); 1000 characters)
(NAACCR Field #2630 RX TEXT-RADIATION OTHER; 1000 characters)

Treatment of cancer using high energy radiation to kill cancer cells in the treatment area (so called target tissue) causes DNA double strand breaks which stops cell growth and cell division. Radiation dose, the amount of radiation absorbed by tissue (s), is referred to as gray (Gy) or centigray (cGy).

- one Gy=100 RADS (**R**adiation **A**bsorbed **D**ose was measurement used before 1985)
- one cGy=1 rad

Radiation is delivered in small doses called **fractions**. Giving treatment in small, repeated doses rather than a few large doses (fractionization) maximizes tumor destruction while minimizing damage to healthy tissues.

Radiation is delivered with two general techniques, **external beam** and **internal radiation** or **brachytherapy**. In certain cases, combination of external and internal radiation may be recommended.

External radiation treatment (also called Teletherapy)
External beam radiation is the most widely used type of radiation treatment. High-energy electromagnetic beams are delivered to the cancer site from the external source of the radiation via orthovoltage or supervoltage machines such as cobalt machines and linear accelerators (LINAC). There is no direct physical contact with the patient.

Treatment is delivered fractions over a prescribed period of time rather than a few large doses. The radiation oncologist will select the type and energy of radiation that is most suitable for each patient's cancer.

Methods of delivery/treatment modality (type of machine) include:

- Orthovoltage
- Photons
- Electrons
- Neutrons
- 3D conformal dose radiation

Radiation Text Fields, *continued*

- Intensity Modulated Radiation Therapy (IMRT)
- Protons
- Stereotactic radiosurgery (**Note:** this technique is radiation, not surgery)
- Intra-operative radiation therapy (IORT)

Internal radiation treatment (Brachytherapy)
Brachytherapy (brachy is Greek for short distance/close)—a technique in which radioactive material is inserted directly into or near the tumor. The radiation is emitted outward, unlike external beam radiotherapy, where radiation must pass through normal tissue in order to reach the tumor. High doses of radiation can be delivered in a shorter time to a small area without damaging normal tissues.

The radioactive sources (such as cesium, iridium, palladium, or iodine) are usually in the form of catheters, needles, wires, seeds, or rods. Placement of the radiation source is crucial as a high dose of energy is delivered to the immediate vicinity of the target and then decreases quickly with distance. Internal radiation may be delivered using low dose rate (LDR) or high dose rate (HDR) sources. Sometimes the material is left in the body (permanent brachytherapy). In this case, small beads or seeds containing the radioactive material are inserted into the tumor. The beads release radiation at the site of the tumor over a few days or weeks, after which they are no longer radioactive. This type of treatment is most commonly used for cancers of the head and neck, breast, uterus, thyroid, cervix, and prostate.

Methods of delivery include:

- Interstitial/internal radiation—implants, molds, seeds, rods, ribbons, or wires are placed directly inside/near the affected tissue on a temporary or permanent basis.
- Intracavitary radiation—a container of radioactive material is placed inside a body cavity, such as the uterus, vagina, or windpipe; this is always temporary.

Other internal radiation: Radioisotopes
Systemic radiation involves injecting radio-active isotopes either into a vein or into an organ. The individual types of radiation seek out and concentrate in tumor tissue anywhere in the body.

- Radioactive iodine (I-131)—given for some types of thyroid cancer
- Strontium-89 (metastron)—used to treat cancer that has spread to the bone

What to select and record

- Treatment start and stop dates
- Where treatment was given (facility)
- Other treatment information, for example, patient discontinued after 3 treatments
- Treatment summary, including
  - **Treatment Volume**—the area included in the radiation treatment, such as chest wall, mantle field, or pelvis
  - **Regional Treatment Modality**—the dominant modality of radiation therapy (see above) used to deliver the most clinically significant regional dose to the primary target site/primary tumor; include number of fractions and note if hyperfractionization used
  - **Boost Treatment Modality**—a supplemental dose of radiation targeted directly to the area of the tumor (treatment is directed/coned down to a specific area); it can be delivered either through external or internal radiation; include number of treatment fractions and note if hyperfractionization used
  - **Regional and boost dosages**—the amount of radiation received in centiGrays
  - If brachytherapy is given, include the type of non-beam radiation (seeds, intracavitary, radioisotope) and the radiation source (cesium, iodine, other)

Radiation Text Fields, ***continued***

- **Reason no radiation treatment** if no radiation treatment is performed
- **Radiation sequence with surgery**—the order in which radiation and surgical procedures were performed as part of the first course of treatment

The following data fields can also be documented in the Radiation text fields:

- Date of Initial RX-SEER and Flag
- Date of 1st Crs RX-CoC and Flag
- RX Summ-Radiation
- RX Hosp-Radiation
- RX Summ-Rad to CNS

Sample Report # 8
Radiation Therapy Treatment Summary Report

Date: 12/14/11

Clinical History: 18 year old male presented with a right anterior high cervical lymph. Biopsy on 7/10/11 revealed a diffuse B-cell malignant lymphoma, predominantly large cell type, with focal anaplastic features and apoptosis, intermediate to high-grade, CD20, 45, 79 A-positive, and BCL-1, 2 and S 100 negative. Status post CHOP x 3 cycles (10/2011). Stage IA.

CT of the chest on 7/28/11 revealed a 3.5 cm soft tissue mass in the anterior mediastinum probably representing thymic tissue. Gallium scan revealed a single focus of right upper neck activity near the angle of the mandible.

Blood work was essentially normal. A bone marrow was negative.

Received three cycles of CHOP chemotherapy. Referred for consolidative radiation therapy

Treatment Summary: Start date: 10/08/11 Completion date: 12/13/11
Area treated: Right neck, right supraclavicular fossa, right pre and postauricular and occipital lymph nodes

The right neck, supraclavicular fossa, pre and postauricular and occipital lymph nodes were treated to a dose of 3,600 centigray in 20 fractions over 29 calendar days. The right neck scar and tumor bed region were treated with an additional 900 centigray in five fractions. The right neck received a total dose of 4,500 centigray in 25 fractions of 36 calendar days.

The right neck supraclavicular fossa, pre and post auricular and occipital lymph nodes received 6 MV photons delivered via AP/PA portal fields, with the anterior field measuring 14.5 x 21 cm at 100 SAD, and the posterior field measuring 14.5 x 18.5 cm at 100 SAD. Custom blocks were utilized. The treatments were delivered to mid plan in 180 centigray per fraction.

The right neck scar and tumor bed region was treated with 9 MEV electrons delivered to D-max with a 6 . 10 cm cone en face at 100 SSD with custom cutout. The treatments were delivered in 180 centigray per fraction.

Treatment Course: The patient began treatments weighing in at 179 lbs, and completed treatments at 188 lbs. Hemograms were performed which revealed a WBC as low as 3.9. He did develop the usual and expected side-effects which included skin erythema without moist desquamation, slight dysphagia, fatigue, and right occipital scalp alopecia. He was given triple mixture for esophagitis as well as Aquaphor for the skin. He otherwise tolerated the radiation therapy treatments well. Patient is NED at this time.

Plan: Patient instructed to return in one month. He will notify us of any problems. He will continue with the skin care.

PRACTICE 8B

Sample Radiation Therapy Treatment Summary Report ***(See Sample Report # 8)***

From the sample **Radiation Therapy Treatment Summary Report**, identify pertinent findings for the site-specific cancer and write them in concise form for the abstract.

Pertinent findings from the sample **Radiation Therapy Treatment Summary Report**

- 10/08/11–12/13/11 Rt neck, supraclavicular fossa, pre and postauricular and occipital lymph nodes: treated to a dose of 3,600 centigray in 20 fractions over 29 calendar days. The right neck scar and tumor bed region were treated with an additional 900 centigray in five fractions. The right neck received a total dose of 4,500 centigray in 25 fractions of 36 calendar days.
- The right neck supraclavicular fossa, pre and post auricular and occipital lymph nodes received 6 MV photons delivered via AP/PA portal fields, with the anterior field measuring 14.5 x 21 cm at 100 SAD, and the posterior field measuring 14.5 x 18.5 cm at 100 SAD. Custom blocks were used. Treatments were delivered to mid plan in 180 cGy per fraction.
- The right neck scar and tumor bed region was treated with 9 MEV electrons delivered to D-max with a 6.10 cm cone en face at 100 SSD with custom cutout. The treatments were delivered in 180 centigray per fraction

The Radiation Therapy Treatment Summary findings text would be recorded on the abstract as:

- 10/8/11-12/13/11 Rt neck, SCLAV fossa, pre+post auricular, occipital LNs: 3600 cGy in 20 fractions, 6MV photons; 900 cGy in 5 fractions Rt neck scar+tumor bed region, 9MEV. Total: 4500 cGy.

CHEMOTHERAPY TEXT FIELD

(NAACCR Field #2640 RX TEXT-CHEMO; 1000 characters)

Traditional chemotherapy is systemic treatment in which chemical agents (other than hormones and biological response modifiers) are administered to attack and destroy cancer cells, interfere with cell growth and prevent cells from multiplying.

Combination chemotherapy—the use of two or more anti-tumor agents together—has proven more effective than single agent regimens for many cancers by attacking as many cancer cells as possible in various stages of replication while avoiding damage to normal tissues. The combination of drugs is called a **regimen**.

Drugs are given according to a written treatment plan called a **protocol** which details exactly how the drugs will be given. Often the drugs are given in a sequence over a week or more, then the patient takes no drugs for awhile while the bone marrow and other organs recover. Then the drugs are given again. This administration–rest timing is called a **cycle**. Most patients get more than one cycle of a regimen in the protocol.

Methods of administration include injection directly into a vein, catheter placed into an artery, orally in pill form, intracavitary (into an area of the body where fluid has accumulated), intrathecal (drugs given into cerebrospinal fluid), infusion.

What to information to select and record

- Treatment start date. Record in chronological order if multiple treatments
- Agent(s). Record the specific generic or trade name
- Record reason for no treatment if chemotherapy would be expected

Chemotherapy Text Field, *continued*

The best resource for identifying cancer-directed drug treatments (chemotherapy, hormone therapy, immunotherapy) is SEER*Rx, available free from www.seer.cancer.gov/tools/seerrx. Look up individual agents in SEER*Rx to verify that they are being administered as chemotherapy. Do not select chemical agents that achieve their effect through change of hormone balance (hormone therapy) or by affecting the patient's immune system (immunotherapy); record these in their designated fields (see below). The individual agents in a regimen can be looked up in the regimen section of SEER*Rx to sort out whether to record them as chemo, hormone or immunotherapy.

The following data fields can be documented in the Chemotherapy text field:

- Date of Initial RX-SEER and Flag
- Date of 1st Crs RX-CoC and Flag
- RX Summ-Chemo
- RX Hosp-Chemo
- RX Date-Systemic and Flag
- RX Date-Chemo and Flag

PRACTICE 9
Sample Medical Oncology Consult Report ***(See Sample Report # 9)***

From the sample **Medical Oncology Consult Report**, identify pertinent chemotherapy findings for the site-specific cancer and write them in concise form for the abstract.

Sample Report # 9
Medical Oncology Consult 8/7/11

History of Present Illness: This 18 year old college student is seen in consultation for evaluation of malignant lymphoma. The patient has felt well; there has been no fever or drenching sweat. His weight has been stable.

In mid June he became aware of a mass in the right neck while shaving. He felt no other masses or nodules. Evaluation by his primary physician revealed an upper anterior cervical lymph node on the right. On 7/10/08, the patient underwent incisional biopsy of right cervical mass which revealed a 4 x 4 cm necrotic lymph node.

The pathologic diagnosis: diffuse B cell malignant lymphoma, predominantly large cell type with focal anaplastic features and apoptosis; intermediate to high grade. Additional immunophenotyping showed again this to be a B cell malignant lymphoma, large cell type, CD20, CD45, and CD79 positive.

On 7/28/11, chemistry 7 panel and CBC were normal. Full chemistry 12 panel showed bilirubin 2.1 but was otherwise normal. Serum protein electrophoresis is pending at the time of this dictation. Platelet count was 135,000 on 6/14/11.

During and after the neck node biopsy procedure the patient had no excessive or prolonged bleeding.

Additional staging has been done: Gallium scan 8/1/11 showed single focus of right upper neck activity. CT of the abdomen and pelvis 7/28/11 were within normal limits.
CT of the chest 7/28/11 showed a 3.5 soft tissue mass in the anterior mediastinum, probably representing thymic tissue.

Medications: None

Family History: Maternal grandmother-throat cancer. Paternal grandfather-gastric cancer.

Sample Report # 9—Medical Oncology Consult, continued

Past History: No excessive bleeding after dental work. No TB, DVT, transfusions.

Habits: Never smoked or consumed alcohol.

Social History: Born in Minnesota. He attended high school there for two years then moved to California. He lives with his brothers and a sister. The patient currently is a student; he studies accounting.

Review of Systems: ENT- No change in vision or hearing. CHEST- No cough, dyspnea, chest pain. GI- No nausea or vomiting; no history of ulcer, liver, biliary disease. No hematemesis or melena. GU-No dysuria or frequency. MS- No bone pain. SKIN- No lesions. CNS- No headache, localizing paresthesia, weakness.

Physical Exam: WT 177 lbs; HT 68 inches; BP 132/66; P 61; RESP 16; T 98.6. Patient is alert, cooperative, anxious, pleasant, well-nourished, no acute distress. HEAD- Oropharynx negative. NECK- Supple. Thyroid not enlarged. LYMPHATICS- There is thickening in the right upper anterior cervical area at the site of the previous lymph node biopsy but I do not feel a discrete lymph node mass. There is no lymphadenopathy identifiable in other sites. THORAX- Normal configuration. BREASTS- No masses. LUNGS- Clear. HEART- Regular S1, S2, no murmur nor gallup. ABDOMEN- Flat, soft, no organomegaly nor focal mass nor tenderness. BACK- No spine nor CVA tenderness. GENITALIA- Normal uncircumsized penis and normal testes with no masses. RECTUM/ANUS- Not examined. EXTREMITIES- No edema nor joint deformity. NEUROLOGIC- Cranial nerves intact. Symmetric normal deep reflexes.

Assessment: The patient has diffuse B-cell malignant lymphoma, predominantly large cell type, with focal anaplastic features and apoptosis; intermediate to high grade. At present the disease appears to be limited to the right upper cervical lymph node area according to gallium scanning.

Recommendations: Additional staging including bilateral bone marrow biopsies as well as CT scanning of the neck for radiation treatment planning.

I would recommend treatment with chemotherapy consisting of CHOP for three cycles followed by radiation therapy. If there is evidence of disease in the bone marrow, then the patient would require CHOP chemotherapy followed by consideration for high dose therapy with stem cell support depending on the response to the CHOP chemotherapy.

We discussed in detail with the patient the current findings as well as the risks and benefits of treatment. The patient will return following completion of the staging studies.

Addendum: CHOP started 8/16/11; Completed 9/30/11

Pertinent findings from the sample **Medical Oncology Consult Report**:

- Chemotherapy consisting of CHOP for three cycles followed by radiation therapy. If there is evidence of disease in the bone marrow, then the patient would require CHOP chemotherapy followed by consideration for high dose therapy with stem cell support depending on the response to the CHOP chemotherapy
  Addendum: CHOP started 8/16/11; Completed 9/30/11

The Chemotherapy findings text would be recorded on the abstract as

- 08/16/11-9/30/11 CHOP

HORMONE TREATMENT TEXT FIELD

(NAACCR Field #2650 RX TEXT-HORMONE; 1000 characters)

Hormone treatment involves any kind of therapy which changes the patient's hormone balance by removing, blocking or adding hormones or anti-hormones. Steroids such as prednisone may be administered in combination with chemotherapy for lymphomas, leukemias and a few other cancers. In addition to including the steroid as part of the combination chemotherapy regimen, also record the steroid administration in the hormone field. **Do not record** steroids administered to inhibit the growth of the tumor, such as steroids given to improve appetite.

- The regimen "MOPP" is a combination of three chemotherapy agents plus prednisone (the last P is for prednisone).
- Record MOPP treatment regimen as combination chemotherapy in the chemotherapy field and also record prednisone in the hormone field.

If the hormonal effect is achieved by surgical removal of endocrine glands or by radiation to endocrine glands, record this treatment in the "Transplant/Endocrine Procedure" field (see below).

What information to select and record

- Treatment start date. Record in chronological order if multiple agents are administered.
- Agent (s). Record the specific generic or trade name and the type (anti-hormone, steroid)
- Record reason for no treatment if hormone therapy would be expected

Look up agents in SEER*Rx to verify that the agents are being used for hormone manipulation.

The following data fields can be documented in the Hormone text field:

- Date of Initial RX-SEER and Flag
- Date of 1st Crs RX-CoC and Flag
- RX Summ-Hormone
- RX Hosp-Hormone
- RX Date-Systemic and Flag
- RX Date-Hormone and Flag

PRACTICE 10

Sample Medical Oncology Consult Report ***(See Sample Report # 9)***

From the sample **Medical Oncology Consult Report**, identify pertinent hormone therapy findings for the site-specific cancer.

Pertinent findings from the sample **Medical Oncology Consult Report:**

- Chemotherapy consisting of CHOP for three cycles followed by radiation therapy. If there is evidence of disease in the bone marrow, then the patient would require CHOP chemotherapy followed by consideration for high dose therapy with stem cell support depending on the response to the CHOP chemotherapy
  Addendum: CHOP started 8/16/11; Completed 9/30/11

The Hormone findings text would be recorded on the abstract as

- 08/16/11-9/30/11 Prednisone (as part of CHOP)

IMMUNOTHERAPY/BIOLOGICAL RESPONSE MODIFIERS (BRM) TEXT FIELD
(NAACCR Field #2660 RX TEXT-BRM; 1000 characters)

Biological response modifiers (BRMs) are substances that do not directly destroy the cancer. Instead, they change the response of certain specific elements of the immune system to make it more effective against cancer. BRMs may be used to lessen the side effects caused by some cancer treatment.

The immune system makes proteins known as antibodies to attach to the antigens that are usually found on the surface of cells. The antigens can then be identified and destroyed by antibodies or other cells in the immune system. Antibodies appear to be a key element in the treatment of cancer.

Monoclonal antibodies (sometimes abbreviated as MoAbs, or MABs) are a type of natural or created antibody. MABs act in different ways on cancers.

- Some MABs cause the cancer to stop growing—these are cytostatic and coded as ***chemotherapy***.
- Some MABs are simply the delivery agent for a radioisotope or a cell toxin—these are coded as ***radiation therapy*** or ***chemotherapy***.
- At present, there are no cancer-directed monoclonal antibodies that stimulate the immune system to fight the cancer.
- Research each agent in SEER*Rx to determine where to record the agent on the abstract.

What information to select and record

- Treatment start date. Record in chronological order if multiple agents are administered.
- Agent (s). Record the specific generic or trade name

The following data fields can be documented in the BRM text field:

- Date of Initial RX-SEER and Flag
- Date of 1st Crs RX-CoC and Flag
- RX Hosp-BRM
- RX Date Systemic and Flag
- RX Summ-BRM
- RX Date-BRM and Flag

Immunotherapy/biological response modifier findings are recorded on the abstract in the same manner as the chemotherapy and hormone therapy information.

TRANSPLANT/ENDOCRINE PROCEDURES

What to select and record

Transplant procedures include:

- Bone marrow transplantation
- Peripheral stem cell transplantation—replaces blood-forming cells destroyed by cancer treatment

Hormone (Endocrine) Surgery/Hormone (Endocrine) Radiation is performed for hormonal effect for breast and prostate cancer only. Procedures include:

- Bilateral orchiectomy to reduce production of hormones in treatment of prostate cancer
- Endocrine radiation

Transplant and endocrine procedures do not have their own text field. Record any findings in the surgery text field.

OTHER THERAPY TEXT FIELD

(NAACCR Field #2670 RX TEXT-OTHER; 1000 characters)

"Other" therapy is any type of cancer-directed treatment that does not fit neatly into another treatment category. For example:

- Hyperbaric oxygen
- Blinded clinical trials
- Alternative therapy (only if no other cancer-directed treatment is given)
- Unproven treatments (sometimes known as cancer quackery)
- Treatments for reportable hematopoietic diseases (such as phlebotomy, transfusion, and aspirin) that do not meet the usual definition of cancer-directed treatment
- Any other cancer directed therapy that is not elsewhere classified.

What information to select and record

- Treatment start date. Record in chronological order if multiple "other" therapies are administered.
- Specific type of Other Therapy
    - Experimental therapy (describe)
    - Unproven therapy (describe)
    - Double blind clinical trial information (name of clinical trial)

The following data fields can be documented in the Other Therapy text field:

- Date of Initial RX-SEER and Flag
- Date of 1st Crs RX-CoC and Flag
- RX Summ-Other
- RX Date-Other and Flag
- RX Hosp-Other

Other Therapy findings would be recorded on the abstract in the same manner as the chemotherapy and hormone therapy information.

REMARKS

(NAACCR Field #2680 TEXT-REMARKS; 1000 characters)

The Remarks field allows the abstractor to record text for data fields and other information that is not captured elsewhere on the abstract. Examples include:

- Significant co-morbidities that limit or rule out cancer-directed treatment
- Alcohol and smoking history (if requested by facility clinicians or the state registry)
- Family history of cancer
- Personal history of cancer (especially if previous cancer was diagnosed in another state or prior to the registry's reference date)
- Place of birth
- Religion (if pertinent to case, such as Ashkenazy Jewish)
- Justification of over-ride flags not documented elsewhere

The Remarks field can also be used to continue other text fields. A simple way to show continuation is to use asterisks or other symbols at the end of the previous field and to start the remarks. For example,

PE field ... Lt breast: wnl; *** **Remarks field** ***Axillae: neg; Imp: CA Rt breast.

SUMMARY

As noted earlier, there are many other text fields associated with other items on the abstract. Among these are text fields for place of diagnosis, histology title, occupation, industry, and staging. The principles of consistency of formatting and the use of abbreviations should be applied to these fields as well.

The importance of documenting codes on the abstract in text fields cannot be over-emphasized. Text provides the patient's cancer information in a readable format. Whether it is called defensive abstracting or pro-active abstracting, including text on the abstract provides valuable information for quality control, recoding audits, researchers and other registry purposes. Text also documents unusual occurrences, and verifies edit check discrepancies. In short, text saves chart review time for the facility and the central registry whenever a question arises.

Page left blank.

Acronyms, Initialisms, and Abbreviations

This chapter of the Cancer Registry CASEbook is nothing but definitions for symbols, abbreviations (shortened words, such as ADM for admission), initialisms (abbreviations using the first letter of each word in a phrase, such as ADL for activities of daily living), and acronyms (abbreviations that form a word, such as AIDS for acquired immunodeficiency syndrome).

In the list, parentheses ( ) indicate a letter or term that is frequently associated with the letters and/or phrase. Square brackets [ ] provide additional information about the term. The terms are alphabetized by short version (first column) without regard to punctuation or capitalization that is part of the term. An asterisk (*) indicates a context sensitive abbreviation; use with caution. The list is extensive but not all-inclusive. Resources are cited at the end of the chapter.

In the table below, the final column indicates where the term may commonly be found in the medical record or cancer abstract, as follows:

Anatomy, including directional terms	Anat
Conditions, diseases, comorbidities	Cond
Grade, differentiation	Grad
Imaging and endoscopy	Imag
Laboratory tests, tumor markers, agents, and body chemicals	Labs
Miscellaneous	Misc
Pathology and cytology	Path
Procedure (diagnostic, therapeutic)	Proc
Report findings (discharge summary, H&P, consults, etc.)	Rpts

Individual facilities may have an official abbreviation list—usually maintained in the medical record/HIM department—that employees must abide by if they make any notes in the medical record. It may be helpful to the facility to add any common cancer terms used by the physicians. The facility's list and any official list provided by the central registry should be used if there is a discrepancy between those lists and this chapter.

NOTE: For drug abbreviations and chemotherapy regimen definitions, refer to SEER*Rx, the Cancer Registrar's Interactive Antineoplastic Drug Database, available from www.seer.cancer.gov/tools/seerrx. For organization and agency acronyms, see the list at the end of this chapter.

Symbols

–	Negative	Misc
#*	Number (if before a numeral)	Misc
#*	Pounds (if after a numeral)	Misc
/	Comparison	Misc
@	At	Misc
+	Positive	Misc
&	And	Misc
↓	Decreased	Misc
<	Less than; Decrease	Misc
≤	Less than or equal to	Misc
=	Equals	Misc
↑	Increased; Elevated	Misc
>	Greater/more than; Increase	Misc
≥	Greater/more than or equal to	Misc
3D	3 dimensional (conformal radiation therapy)	Proc
α; Α	alpha	Misc
β; Β	beta	Misc
γ; Γ	gamma	Misc
δ; Δ	delta	Misc
κ; Κ	kappa	Misc
λ; Λ	lambda	Misc
μ; Μ	mu	Misc
χ; Χ	chi	Misc

A

A&P	Auscultation & percussion	Rpts
A/P Resx	Anterior/posterior resection	Proc
ABC	Aspiration biopsy cytology	Path
ABCD	Asymmetry, borders, color, diameter [melanoma]	Rpts
ABD	Abdomen; abdominal	Anat
ABG	Arterial blood gases	Labs
ABMT	Autologous bone marrow transplant; Allogeneic bone marrow transplant; Allogenic bone marrow transplant	Proc
ABN	Abnormal	Rpts
ABS	Absent/Absence	Rpts
ABST	Abstract/Abstracted	Misc
AC	Adrenal cortex (also Adriamycin and Cytoxan regimen)	Anat
ACBE	Air contrast barium enema	Imag
ACH	Adrenal cortical hormone	Labs
ACID PHOS	Acid phosphatase	Labs
A-COLON	Ascending colon	Anat
ACTH	Adrenocorticotrophic hormone	Labs
ADENOCA	Adenocarcinoma	Path
ADH*	Antidiuretic hormone	Labs
ADH*	Atypical ductal hyperplasia	Path

ADJ	Adjacent	Rpts
ADL	Activities of daily living	Misc
ADM	Admit; Admission	Rpts
ADR	Adverse drug reaction	Rpts
ADT	Androgen deprivation therapy	Proc
AFF	Affirmative	Rpts
AFIB	Atrial fibrillation	Cond
AFLUTTER	Atrial flutter	Cond
AFP	Alpha fetoprotein	Labs
AFRT	Altered fractionation radiotherapy	Proc
AG	Antigen	Labs
AGC	Absolute granulocyte count	Labs
AGL	Acute granulocytic leukemia	Path
AHA	Acquired hemolytic anemia; autoimmune hemolytic anemia	Cond
AHF	Accelerated hyperfractionation	Proc
AI	Atrial stenosis/insufficiency/ incompetence	Cond
AIDS	Acquired Immunodeficiency Syndrome	Cond
AIHA	Autoimmune hemolytic anemia	Cond
AIL	Angiocentric immunoproliferative lesion; Angioimmunoblastic lymphadenopathy	Path
AILD	Angioimmunoblastic lymphaden-opathy with dysproteinemia	Path
AIN (III)	Anal intraepithelial neoplasia (grade III)	Path
AK(A)	Above knee (amputation)	Cond
AKA	Also known as	Rpts
ALB	Albumin	Labs
ALCL	Anaplastic large cell lymphoma	Path
ALK PHOS	Alkaline phosphatase	Labs
ALL	Acute lymphocytic leukemia; Acute lymphoblastic leukemia	Path
ALND	Axillary lymph node dissection	Proc
ALP	Alkaline phosphatase	Labs
ALS	Amyotrophic lateral sclerosis	Cond
AM	Before noon	Rpts
AMA	Against medical advice	Rpts
AMB	Ambulatory	Rpts
AMI	Acute myocardial infarction	Cond
AML	Acute myelogenous/monoblastic/ monocytic/myelocytic/myeloid leukemia	Path
AMM	Agnogenic myeloid metaplasia	Path
AMML	Acute myelomonoblastic leukemia	Path
AMP	Amputation	Cond
AMT	Amount	Rpts
ANAP	Anaplastic	Grad
ANC	Absolute neutrophil count	Labs
ANGIO	Angiography; angiogram	Imag
ANLL	Acute non-lymphocytic leukemia	Path
ANS	Autonomic nervous system	Anat
ANT	Anterior	Rpts
AODM	Adult-onset diabetes mellitus	Cond
AP*	Abdominal perineal	Anat
AP*	Anterior/posterior; anteroposterior	Rpts
AP(M)L	Acute promyelocytic leukemia	Path
AP*; APR	Abdominal perineal resection	Proc
APC	Atrial premature complexes	Cond
APP	Appendix	Anat
APPL'Y	Apparently	Rpts
APPROX	Approximately	Rpts
APUD	Amine precursor uptake and decarboxylation	Labs
ARC	AIDS-related condition/complex	Cond
ARD	AIDS-related disease	Cond
ARDS	Acute respiratory distress syndrome; Adult respiratory distress syndrome	Cond
ARF	Acute renal failure	Cond
ARRHY	Arrhythmia	Cond
ART	Artery; arterial	Anat
AS	Arteriosclerosis/Arteriosclerotic	Cond
ASA	Aspirin, Acetylsalicylic acid	Misc
ASAP	As soon as possible	Rpts
ASC	Ascending [colon]	Anat
ASCVD	Arteriosclerotic cardiovascular disease	Cond
ASHD	Arteriosclerotic heart disease	Cond
ASP	Aspiration	Cond
ASPVD	Arteriosclerotic peripheral vascular disease	Cond
AST	Androgen suppression therapy	Proc
A-STEN	Aortic stenosis	Cond
ASX	Asymptomatic	Rpts
ATCL	Angioimmunoblastic T-cell lymphoma	Path
ATLL	Adult T-cell leukemia/lymphoma	Path
ATN	Acute tubular necrosis	Cond
ATP	Adenosine triphosphate	Misc
ATR	Achilles tendon reflex	Rpts
AUT	Autopsy	Path
AV	Arteriovenous	Anat
AVF	Arteriovenous fistula	Anat
AVG	Average	Rpts
AVM	Arteriovenous malformation	Anat
AX	Axillary; axilla	Anat

B

BA	Barium	Imag
BAC	Bronchioalveolar carcinoma	Path
BAD	Bipolar affective disorder	Cond
BALT	Bronchial-associated lymphoid tissue (lymphoma)	Path
BCC	Basal cell carcinoma	Path
BCG	Bacillus Calmette-Guerin	Proc
BCR	Breakpoint cluster region [positive/negative]	Labs
BCS	Breast conserving/conservation surgery	Proc
BCT	Breast conserving therapy/ treatment	Proc
BD	Bile duct	Anat
BE	Barium enema	Imag
BF; B/F	Black female	Rpts
BHCG	Beta subunit human chorionic gonadotropin	Labs
BID	Twice a day	Rpts
BIL; BILAT	Bilateral	Rpts
BIRADS	Breast imaging reporting and data system	Imag
BK(A)	Below knee (Amputation)	Cond

BM*; B/M	Black male	Rpts
BM*	Bone marrow	Anat
BM*	Bowel movement	Rpts
BMA	Bone marrow aspiration	Path
BMB	Bone marrow biopsy	Path
BMI	Body mass index	Misc
BMT	Bone marrow transplant	Proc
BOD	Twice a day (daily)	Misc
BP	Blood pressure	Rpts
BPH*	Benign prostatic hyperplasia	Cond
BPH*	Benign prostatic hypertrophy	Cond
BPLND	Bilateral pelvic lymph node dissection	Proc
BRBPR	Bright red blood per rectum	Rpts
BRM	Biologic response modifier	Proc
BRO	Brother	Rpts
BRONCH	Bronchoscopy	Proc
BS*	Bone scan	Imag
BS*	Bowel sounds	Rpts
BS*; BRS	Breath sounds	Rpts
BSC	Bone scan	Imag
BSE	Breast self-examination	Rpts
BSO	Bilateral salpingo-oophorectomy	Proc
BT	Bladder tumor	Path
BUN	Blood urea nitrogen	Labs
BUS	Bartholin's, urethral, and Skene's glands	Anat
BV	Blood volume	Labs
BX	Biopsy	Proc

C

c̄	With	Rpts
C/O; CO	Complaining of; complains of	Rpts
C/W	Consistent with	Path
C1 - C7	Cervical vertebrae	Anat
CA*	Calcium	Labs
CA*	Cancer antigen; carbohydrate antigen	Labs
CA*	Carcinoma; cancer	Path
CA-125	Carbohydrate antigen 125	Labs
CABG	Coronary artery bypass graft	Cond
CAD	Coronary artery disease	Cond
CALLA	Common acute lymphoblastic leukemia antigen	Path
CAP(S)	Capsule(s)	Rpts
CAT; CAT scan	Computerized axial tomography (scan)	Imag
CBC	Complete blood count	Labs
CBD	Common bile duct	Anat
CC*	Chief complaint	Rpts
CC*	Cubic centimeter	Misc
CCRT	Concurrent chemoradiotherapy	Proc
CCU	Coronary care unit	Rpts
CD	Cluster of differentiation; Cluster designation	Path
CEA	Carcinoembyronic antigen	Labs
CF	Cystic fibrosis	Cond
CGL	Chronic granulocytic leukemia	Path
cGY	centiGray	Proc
CHD	Congenital heart disease	Cond
CHEMO	Chemotherapy	Proc
CHF	Congestive heart failure	Cond
CHG	Change	Rpts
CHR	Chronic	Rpts
CI	Confidence interval	Misc
CIG	Cigarettes	Rpts
CIN (III)	Cervical intraepithelial neoplasia (grade III)	Path
CIS	Carcinoma in situ	Path
CLL	Chronic lymphocytic leukemia	Path
CLR	Clear	Rpts
cm*	Centimenter	Misc
CM*	Costal margin	Anat
CMI	Cell-mediated immunity	Labs
CML	Chronic myeloid/myelogenous/ myelocytic leukemia	Path
CMML	Chronic myelomonocytic leukemia	Path
CMT	Combined modality therapy	Proc
CMV	Cytomegalovirus	Labs
CNS	Central nervous system	Anat
CO60	Cobalt 60	Proc
COLD	Chronic obstructive lung disease	Cond
CONT	Continue; continuous	Rpts
CONTRA	Contralateral	Rpts
COPD	Chronic obstructive pulmonary disease	Cond
CR	Complete remission/response	Rpts
CRC	Colorectal cancer	Path
CRF	Chronic renal failure	Cond
CRT	Conformal radiation therapy	Proc
CS*	Cesium	Proc
CS*	Collaborative stage	Misc
CSF*	Cerebrospinal fluid	Anat
C-SF*	Colony stimulating factor	Labs
C-Spine	Cervical spine	Anat
CT; CT scan; CTS	Computerized tomography scan	Imag
CTCL	Cutaneous T-cell lymphoma	Path
CUC	Chronic ulcerative colitis	Cond
CUP	Carcinoma of unknown primary	Path
CVA*	Cerebrovascular accident	Cond
CVA*	Costovertebral angle	Anat
CVD	Cardiovascular disease	Cond
CX	Cervix	Anat
CXR	Chest x-ray	Imag
CYC	Cycle [chemotherapy]	Proc
CYSTO	Cystoscopy	Proc
CYTO	Cytology	Path

D

D&C; D+C	Dilatation and curettage	Proc
DC	Discontinued	Rpts
DCBE	Dual/double contrast barium enema	Imag
DCIS	Ductal carcinoma in situ	Path
D-COLON	Descending colon	Anat
DD	Differential diagnosis	Rpts
DECR	Decreased; <	Rpts
DERM	Dermatology	Rpts
DES	Diethylstilbestrol	Proc
DESC	Descending [colon]	Anat
DFI	Disease free interval	Misc
DFS	Disease-free survival	Misc
DFSP	Dermatofibrosarcoma protuberans	Path

DIAM	Diameter	Misc
DIC	Disseminated intravascular coagulation/coagulopathy	Cond
DIFF	Differentiated	Grad
DIN	Ductal intraepithelial neoplasia	Path
DIS*; DISCH	Discharge	Rpts
DIS*	Disease	Rpts
D/C	Discharge	Rpts
DLBCL	Diffuse large B-cell lymphoma	Path
DLCL	Diffuse large cell lymphoma	Path
DM	Diabetes mellitus; diameter	Cond
DNA	Deoxyribonucleic acid	Labs
DNET	Dysembryoplastic neuroepithelial tumor	Path
DNI	Do not interrupt	Rpts
DNR	Do not resuscitate	Rpts
DOA	Dead on arrival	Rpts
DOB	Date of birth	Rpts
DOD	Date of death	Rpts
DoDx	Date of diagnosis	Rpts
DOE	Dyspnea on exertion	Cond
DR	[Medical] Doctor	Rpts
DRE	Digital rectal examination	Rpts
DS	Discharge summary; discharge	Rpts
DSRCT	Desmoplastic small round cell tumor	Path
DSS	Disease-specific survival	Misc
DTR	Deep tendon reflexes	Rpts
DVT	Deep vein thrombosis	Cond
DX	Diagnosis	Rpts
DZ	Disease	Rpts

E

E.G.	For example	Rpts
EBRT	External beam radiation therapy	Proc
ECC*	Endocervical curettage	Proc
ECC*	Enterochromaffin cell	Path
ECF	Extended care facility	Rpts
ECG; EKG	Electrocardiogram	Imag
EEG	Electroencephalogram	Imag
EENT	Eyes, ears, nose, throat	Rpts
EFGR	Epidermal growth factor receptor	Labs
EFS	Event-free survival	Misc
EG	Esophagogastric	Anat
EGBUS	External genitalia, Bartholin's gland, urethra and Skene's gland	Anat
EGD	Esophagogastroduodenoscopy	Imag
EGF	Endothelial growth factor	Labs
EGJ	Esophagogastric junction	Anat
EHR	Electronic health record	Misc
EIN	Endometrial intraepithelial hyperplasia	Path
EmBx	Endometrial biopsy	Proc
EMG	Electromyogram	Imag
EMP	Extramedullary plasmacytoma	Path
EMR*	Electronic medical record	Misc
EMR*	Endoscopic mucosal resection	Proc
ENL; ENLGD	Enlarged	Rpts
ENT	Ears, nose, and throat	Anat
EPE	Extraprostatic extension	Rpts
ER*	Emergency room	Rpts
ER*; ERA	Estrogen receptor assay	Labs
ERCP	Endoscopic retrograde cholangiopancreatography	Imag
ERT	Estrogen replacement therapy; External (beam) radiation therapy	Proc
ES	Extracapsular spread	Rpts
ESFT	Ewing sarcoma family of tumors	Path
ESRD	End stage renal disease	Cond
ESS	Endometrial stromal sarcoma	Path
ETOH	Alcohol	Rpts
EUA	Examination under anesthesia	Proc
EUS	Endorectal ultrasound; endoscopic ultrasound/ultrasonography	Imag
EVAL	Evaluation	Rpts
EXAM	Examination	Rpts
EXC Bx	Excisional biopsy	Proc
EXC(D)	Excision/excise(d)	Proc
EXP	Expired	Rpts
EXP LAP	Exploratory laparotomy	Proc
EXT*	Extension; extend	Path
EXT*	External	Rpts
EXT*	Extremity	Anat

F

F	Female	Rpts
F(M)H	Family (Medical) history	Rpts
FAB	French-American-British classification [myeloid diseases]	Path
FAP	Familial adenomatous polyposis [syndrome]	Cond
FB	Fingerbreadth	Rpts
FDC	Follicular dendritic cell	Path
FDG-PET	Fluorodeoxyglucose dual-head positron emission tomography	Imag
FISH	Fluorescence/fluorescent in situ hybridization	Labs
FL	Fluid	Rpts
FLIPI	Follicular lymphoma international prognostic index	Path
FLUORO	Fluoroscopy	Imag
FMMM	Familial atypical multiple mole melanoma [syndrome]	Rpts
FMOLES	Femtomoles [ER/PR measure]	Labs
FNA	Fine needle aspirate; fine needle aspiration	Proc
FNAB	Fine needle aspiration biopsy	Proc
FNAC	Fine needle aspiration cytology	Path
FOBT	Fecal occult blood test	Labs
FOM	Floor of mouth	Anat
FREQ	Frequent; Frequency	Rpts
FRX	Fractions [radiation therapy]	Proc
FS	Frozen section	Path
FSH	Follicle stimulating hormone	Labs
FTSG	Full thickness skin graft	Proc
FU	Follow-up	Rpts
FUO	Fever of undetermined/unknown origin	Cond
FVC	False vocal cord	Anat
FX	Fracture	Cond

G

GALT	Gut-associated lymphoid tissue (lymphoma)	Path
GB	Gallbladder	Anat
GBM	Glioblastoma multiforme	Path
GCT	Germ cell tumor	Path
GE*	Gastroenterostomy	Proc
GE*	Gastroesophageal	Anat
GEN	General; Generalized	Rpts
GERD	Gastroesophageal reflux disease	Cond
GHRF	Growth hormone releasing factor	Labs
GI	Gastrointestinal	Anat
GIST	Gastrointestinal stromal tumor	Path
GIT	Gastrointestinal tract	Anat
GM	Gram	Rpts
GR	Grade	Grad
GTD	Gestational trophoblastic disease	Path
GTT	Gestational trophoblastic tumor	Path
GU	Genitourinary	Anat
GVHD	Graft-versus-host disease	Cond
GY	Gray	Proc
GYN	Gynecology	Rpts

H

H&E	Hematoxylin and eosin	Path
H&P	History & Physical; History and physical	Rpts
H/A	Headache	Cond
H/O	History of	Rpts
H+N	Head and neck	Anat
HAART	Highly active antiretroviral therapy	Misc
HAI	Hepatic artery infusion	Proc
HAV	Hepatitis A (virus)	Cond
HBI	Hemibody irradiation	Proc
HBV	Hepatitis B (virus)	Cond
HCC	Hepatocellular carcinoma	Path
HCD	Heavy chain disease	Path
hCG	Human chorionic gonadotropin	Labs
HCT	Hematocrit	Labs
HCV	Hepatitis C (virus)	Cond
HCVD	Hypertensive cardiovascular disease	Cond
HD	Hodgkin's disease	Path
HDR	High dose rate	Proc
HDV	Hepatitis D (virus)	Cond
HEENT	Head, eyes, ears, nose, throat	Anat
HepA	Hepatitis A (virus)	Cond
HepB	Hepatitis B (virus)	Cond
HepC	Hepatitis C (virus)	Cond
HER2; HER-2; HER-2/neu	Human epidermal growth factor receptor 2	Labs
HEV	Herpes E virus	Cond
HGB	Hemoglobin	Labs
HGD	High grade dysplasia	Path
HGSIL; HSIL	High grade squamous intra-epithelial lesion	Path
HHV	Human herpes virus	Labs
HIAA; 5-HIAA; 6-HIAA	Hydroxyindoleacetic acid	Labs
HIFU	High intensity focused ultrasound	Proc
HIV	Human immunodeficiency virus	Cond
HNPCC	Hereditary nonpolyposis colon/colorectal cancer	Cond
HO; H/O	History of	Rpts
Ho:YAG	Holmium-yttrium-argon-garnet [laser]	Proc
Horm	Hormone therapy; hormone	Proc
HOSP	Hospital	Rpts
HPF	High-power field	Path
HPI	History of Present Illness	Rpts
HPV	Human Papillomavirus	Labs
HR; HRS	Hour; Hours	Rpts
HRPC	Hormone refractory prostate cancer	Cond
HRT	Hormone replacement therapy	Proc
HSM	Hepatosplenomegaly	Cond
HSV	Herpes simplex virus	Labs
HTLV(-III)	Human T-lymphotrophic virus (Type III); Human T-cell leukemia virus (Type III)	Labs
HTN	Hypertension	Cond
HVA	Homovanillic acid	Labs
HVD	Hypertensive vascular disease	Cond
HX	History (of)	Rpts
HYST	Hysterectomy	Proc

I

I	Iodine	Proc
I&D	Incision & drainage	Proc
IBC	Inflammatory breast carcinoma	Path
IBD	Inflammatory bowel disease	Cond
ICM	Intercostal margin	Anat
ICS	Intercostal space	Anat
ICU	Intensive care unit	Rpts
IDC*	Interdigitating dendritic cell	Path
IDC*	Invasive ductal carcinoma; Intraductal carcinoma	Path
IDDM	Insulin-dependent diabetes mellitus	Cond
I.E.	That is	Rpts
IG	Immunoglobulin	Labs
IGF; ILGF	Insulin-like growth factor	Labs
IHC	Immunohistochemical; Immunohistochemistry	Path
IHSS	Idiopathic hypertrophic subaortic stenosis	Cond
ILD	Interstitial lung disease	Cond
ILP	Isolated limb perfusion	Proc
IM*; IMC	Internal mammary chain (lymph nodes)	Anat
IM*	Intramuscular	Rpts
IMA	Internal mammary artery	Anat
IMP	Impression	Rpts
IMRT	Intensity modulated radiation therapy	Proc
INCL	Includes; Including	Rpts
INCR	Increase; >	Rpts
IND	Investigational new drug	Misc
INF	Inferior	Anat
INFILT	Infiltrating	Path
INT	Internal	Anat
INV	Invade(s); invading; invasion	Rpts

Acronyms

INVL	Involve(s); involvement; involving	Rpts
IORT	Intraoperative radiation therapy	Proc
IP	Inpatient	Rpts
IPI	International prognostic index	Path
IPPB	Intermittent positive pressure breathing	Proc
IPSI	Ipsilateral	Rpts
IPSID	Immunoproliferative small intestinal disease	Path
IRREG	Irregular	Rpts
IS	In situ	Path
ISADH	Inappropriate secretion of antidiurectic hormone	Cond
IT*	Information technology	Misc
IT*	Intrathecal	Anat
ITC	Isolated tumor cell	Path
ITP	Idiopathic thrombocytopenic purpura; Idiopathic thrombocytopenia	Cond
IV	Intravenous	Misc
IVC	Inferior vena cava	Anat
IVCA	Intravenous cholangiogram	Imag
IVIG	Intravenous immunoglobulin	Labs
IVP	Intravenous pyelogram	Imag
IVU	Intravenous urogram; Intravenous urethrogram	Imag

J

JRA	Juvenile rheumatic arthritis	Cond
JVD	Jugular venous distention	Cond

K

KG	Kilogram	Rpts
KLS	Kidney liver spleen	Anat
KPS	Karnofsky performance status	Rpts
KS	Kaposi sarcoma	Path
KUB	Kidneys, ureters, and bladder [x-ray]	Anat
KV	Kilovolt	Proc

L

L*	Liter	Rpts
L*; Lt; Ⓛ	Left	Rpts
L1 - L5	Lumbar vertebra	Anat
LAB	Laboratory	Labs
LAC	Laparoscopy-assisted colectomy	Proc
LAD*	Lymphadenectomy	Proc
LAD*; LAN	Lymphadenopathy	Cond
LAG	Lymphangiogram	Imag
LAK	Lymphokine activated killer (cell)	Labs
LAP	Laparotomy; Laparoscopy	Proc
LAR	Low anterior resection	Proc
LAT	Lateral	Rpts
LAV	Lymphadenopathy-associated virus	Labs
LB*	Large bowel	Anat
LB*	Pound	Rpts
LBBB	Left bundle branch block	Cond
LCH	Langerhans cell histiocytosis	Path
LCIS	Lobular intraepithelial neoplasia; Laryngeal intraepithelial neoplasia	Path
LCM	Left costal margin	Anat
LCNEC	Large cell neuroendocrine carcinoma	Path
LDH	Lactic dehydrogenase	Labs
LDR	Low dose rate	Proc
LE*	Lower extremity	Anat
LE*	Lupus erythrematosus	
LEEP	Loop electosurgical excision procedure	Proc
LFT	Liver function test	Labs
LG	Large	Rpts
LGD	Low grade dysplasia	Path
LGSIL; LSIL	Low-grade squamous intraepithelial lesion	Path
LHRH	Luteinizing hormone-releasing hormone	Labs
LINAC	Linear accelerator	Proc
LIQ	Lower inner quadrant	Anat
LKS(B)	Liver, kidney, spleen (bladder)	Anat
LLE	Left lower extremity	Anat
LLL	Left lower lobe	Anat
LLQ	Left lower quadrant	Anat
LMD	Local MD	Rpts
LMM	Lentigo maligna melanoma	Path
LMP*	Last menstrual period	Rpts
LMP*	Low malignant potential	Path
LN(S)	Lymph node(s)	Rpts
LND	Lymph node dissection	Proc
LOQ	Lower outer quadrant	Anat
LP	Lumbar puncture	Proc
LPN	Licensed practical nurse	Misc
LRG	Large	Rpts
LS	Lumbosacral	Anat
LS SCAN; L/S SCAN	Liver/spleen scan	Imag
LSN	Lesion	Rpts
LSO	Left salpingo-oophorectomy	Proc
L-SPINE	Lumbar spine	Anat
LT	Left	Rpts
LUE	Left upper extremity	Anat
LUL	Left upper lobe	Anat
LUOQ	Left upper outer quadrant	Anat
LUP ERYTH	Lupus erythematosus	Cond
LUQ	Left upper quadrant	Anat
LVI*	Lymphatic vessel invasion	Path
LVI*	Lymphovascular invasion	Path

M

M	Male	Rpts
MAB	Monoclonal antibody	Misc
MAL; MALIG	Malignant	Path
MALT	Mucosa-associated lymphoid tissue (lymphoma)	Path
MAND	Mandible; mandibular	Anat
MARG	Margin	Rpts
MAST	Mastectomy	Proc
MAT	Multifocal arterial tachycardia	Cond
MAX*	Maxilla; maxillary	Anat
MAX*	Maximum	Rpts
MC	Medical center	Rpts
MC(H)	Millicurie(hours)	Proc
MCC	Merkel cell carcinoma	Path

MCG	Microgram	Misc
MCI	Millicuries (on I-131 report)	Proc
MCID	Mixed combined immuno-deficiency	Cond
MCL*	Mantle cell lymphoma	Path
MCL*	Midclavicular line	Anat
M-CSF	Macrophage colony-stimulating factor	Labs
MCTD	Mixed connective tissue disease	Cond
MD*	Medical doctor	Rpts
MD*	Moderately differentiated	Grad
MDR	Multi-drug resistant; Multiple drug resistance	Cond
MDS	Myelodysplastic syndrome	Path
MED	Medicine; Medication	Rpts
MEN	Multiple endocrine neoplasia	Cond
MET; METS	Metastatic; Metastasis	Rpts
MEV	Million electron volts; Megavolt; Megaelectron volt	Proc
MF	Mycosis fungoides	Path
MFH	Malignant fibrous histiocytoma	Path
MG	Myasthenia gravis	Cond
MG(H)	Milligram (hours)	Proc
MGUS	Monoclonal gammopathy of undetermined significance	Path
MI	Myocardial infarction	Cond
MIBI	Methoxyisobutylisonitrile [scan]	Imag
MICRO	Microscopic	Path
MIN*	Minimum	Rpts
MIN*	Minute	Rpts
ML*	Middle lobe	Anat
ML*	Milliliter	Rpts
MLC	Multileaf collimator	Proc
mm*	Millimeter	Rpts
MM*	Multiple myeloma	Path
MMG	Mammogram	Imag
MMM	Myelofibrosis with myeloid metaplasia	Path
MMMT	Malignant mixed mesodermal tumor	Path
MMT	Mixed Mullerian tumor	Path
MOD	Moderate; Moderately	Grad
MOD DIFF	Moderately differentiated	Grad
MPD	Myeloproliferative disorder/disease	Path
M-PD	Moderate to poorly differentiated	Grad
MPNST	Malignant peripheral nerve sheath tumor	Path
MPVC	Multifocal premature ventricular contraction	Cond
MRCP	Magnetic resonance cholangiopancreatography	Imag
MRI	Magnetic resonance imaging	Imag
MRM	Modified radical mastectomy	Proc
MRND	Modified radical neck dissection	Proc
MRSA	Methicillin resistant staphylococcus aureus	Cond
MS	Multiple sclerosis	Cond
MSB	Mainstem bronchus	Anat
MSI	Microsatellite instability	Labs
MUGA	Multiple gated acquisition [scan]	Imag
MULT	Multiple	Rpts
MVP	Mitral valve prolapse	Cond
MWD	Moderately well differentiated	Grad
MX	Mammogram	Imag
MZL	Mantle zone lymphoma	Path

N

N&V	Nausea and vomiting	Cond
NA	Not applicable	Rpts
NAD	No active disease	Rpts
NBUVB	Narrow band ultraviolet B phototherapy (for mycosis fungoides)	Proc
Nd:YAG	Neodymium-yttrium-alluminum-garnet [laser]	Proc
NEC*	Neuroendocrine carcinoma	Path
NEC*	Not elsewhere classified	Rpts
NED	No evidence of disease	Rpts
NEG	Negative; (-)	Rpts
NEOPL	Neoplasm	Rpts
NET	Neuroendocrine tumor	Path
NEURO	Neurology	Rpts
NH	Nursing home	Rpts
NHL	Non-Hodgkin lymphoma	Path
NK	Natural killer (cell)	Path
NL	Normal	Rpts
NMR	Nuclear magnetic resonance [imaging]	Imag
NMSC	Non-melanoma skin cancer	Path
NOS	Not otherwise specified	Misc
NPC	Nasopharyngeal carcinoma	Path
NPL	Neoplasm	Path
NR	Not recorded	Rpts
NSCCA; NSCC	Non small cell carcinoma	Path
NSCLC	Non-small cell lung cancer	Path
NSE	Neuron-specific enolase	Labs
NSF	No significant findings	Rpts
NSGCT	Nonseminomatous germ cell tumor	Path
NST	No special type [breast histology]	Path
NV; N+V	Nausea and vomiting	Cond
NVD	Neck vein distention	Cond

O

OB	Obstetrics	Rpts
OBS	Organic brain syndrome	Cond
OBST	Obstructed; obstructing; Obstruction	Rpts
OP*	Operation	Proc
OP*	Outpatient	Rpts
OP REPORT; OP RPT	Operative report	Rpts
OR	Operating room	Rpts
ORTHO	Orthopedics	Rpts
OTO	Otology	Rpts
OZ	Ounce	Rpts

P

P&A	Percussion and auscultation	Rpts
P32	Phosphorus 32	Proc
PA*	Posteroanterior	Anat
PA*	Pulmonary artery	Anat
PAC	Premature atrial contraction	Cond

Acronyms

PAIN	Pancreatic intraepithelial neoplasia	Path
PALP	Palpated; palpable	Rpts
PAP*	Papanicolaou smear	Path
PAP*	Papillary	Path
PAP*	Prostatic acid phosphatase	Labs
PATH	Pathology	Path
PBSCT	Peripheral blood stem cell transplant	Proc
PCA	Patient-controlled analgesia	Proc
PCI; PCR	Prophylactic cranial irradiation/ radiation	Proc
PD	Poorly differentiated	Grad
PDT	Photodynamic therapy	Proc
PE	Physical exam	Rpts
PEDS	Pediatrics	Rpts
PERC	Percutaneous	Rpts
PERLA	Pupils equal and reactive to light and accommodation	Rpts
PERRLA	Pupils equal, round, reactive to light and accommodation	Rpts
PET	Positron emission tomography	Imag
PFNAB	Percutaneous fine needle aspiration biopsy	Proc
PI	Present illness	Rpts
PICC	Peripherally inserted central catheter	Proc
PID	Pelvic inflammatory disease	Cond
PIN (III)	Prostatic intraepithelial neoplasia (grade III)	Path
PLND	Pelvic lymph node dissection	Proc
PLT	Platelets	Labs
PM	After noon	Rpts
PMD	Personal/Primary medical doctor	Rpts
PMH	Past medical history	Rpts
PML	Promyelocytic leukemia	Path
PMP	Primary medical physician	Rpts
PNET	Primitive neuroectodermal tumor [CNS; see also PPNET]	Path
PO	Postoperative; Postoperatively	Rpts
POD	Postoperative day	Rpts
POEMS	Polyneuropathy, organomegaly, endocrine abnormalities, monoclonal gammopathy, skin changes [syndrome]	Cond
POOR DIFF	Poorly differentiated	Grad
PORT	Postoperative radiation therapy	Proc
POS	Positive; (+)	Rpts
POSS	Possible	Rpts
POST*	Posterior	Anat
POST*	Postmortem examination	Rpts
POST OP	Postoperative; Postoperatively	Rpts
PPD	Packs per day	Rpts
PPNET	Peripheral primitive neuroectodermal tumor	Path
PR*	Partial response	Rpts
PR*	Per rectum	Rpts
PR*; PRA	Progesterone receptor assay	Labs
PREOP	Preoperative; Preoperatively	Rpts
PREV	Previous	Rpts
PROB	Probable; probably	Rpts
PROC	Procedure	Proc
PROCTO	Proctoscopy	Proc
PRV	Polycythemia rubra vera	Path
PSA	Prostate specific antigen	Labs
PSAD	Prostate specific antigen density	Labs
PSADT	Prostate specific antigen doubling time	Labs
PSAV	Prostate specific antigen velocity	Labs
PSCT	Peripheral Stem Cell Transplant	
PSTT	Placental site trophoblastic tumor	Path
PT*	Patient	Rpts
PT*	Physiotherapy; Physical therapy	Proc
PTA	Prior to admission	Rpts
PTC	Percutaneous transhepatic cholecystogram/cholangiography	Imag
PTLD	Post-transplant lymphoproliferative disorder	Path
PUD	Peptic ulcer disease	Cond
PULM	Pulmonary	Anat
PUNLMP	Papillary urothelial neoplasm of low malignant potential	Path
PUVA	Psoralen and ultraviolet A	Proc
PV; P. vera; PCV	Polycythemia vera	Path
PVD	Peripheral vascular disease	Cond
PWA	Person with AIDS	Cond
PX*	Physical examination	Rpts
PX*	Prognosis	Rpts

Q

Q	Every	Rpts
QD	Every day	Rpts
QOL	Quality of life	Rpts
QUAD	Quadrant	Anat

R

r	Recombinant	Labs
R/O	Rule out	Rpts
R; Rt; Ⓡ	Right	Anat
RA	Radium	Proc
RAD*	Radiation absorbed dose; Radiation	Proc
RAD*	Radical	Proc
RAI*	Radioactive iodine	Imag
RAI*	Radioactive iodine [radiation therapy]	Proc
RALP	Robotic-assisted laparoscopic prostatectomy	Proc
RBBB	Right bundle branch block	Cond
RBC	Red blood cells	Labs
RCC	Renal cell carcinoma	Path
RCM	Right costal margin	Anat
RCT	Radiochemotherapy	Proc
RE	Regarding	Rpts
REAL	Revised European-American lymphoma [classification]	Path
REC'D	Received	Rpts
REG*	Regimen [chemotherapy]	Proc
REG*	Regular	Rpts
RESEC	Resection; resected	Proc
RESP	Respiration(s)	Rpts
RESPIR	Respiratory	Anat
RESX	Resection	Proc
RFA	Radiofrequency ablation	Proc

RHD	Rheumatic heart disease	Cond
RIA	Radioimmunoassay	Labs
RIQ	Right inner quadrant	Anat
RLE	Right lower extremity	Anat
RLL	Right lower lobe	Anat
RLQ	Right lower quadrant of abdomen	Anat
RMC	Regional medical center	Rpts
RML	Right middle lobe	Anat
RMS	Rhabdomyosarcoma	Path
RND	Radical neck dissection	Proc
RO; R/O	Rule out	Rpts
ROF	Review of outside films	Rpts
ROQ	Right outer quadrant	Anat
ROS*	Review of outside slides	Rpts
ROS*	Review of systems	Rpts
RP	Radical prostatectomy	Proc
RPLND	Retroperitoneal lymph node dissection	Proc
RRP	Radical retropubic prostatectomy	Proc
R-S	Reed-Sternberg (cell)	Path
RSO	Right salpingo-oophorectomy	Proc
RSR	Regular sinus rhythm	Cond
RT*	Radiation therapy	Proc
RT*;Ⓡ	Right	Anat
RT-PCR	Reverse transcriptase-polymerase chain reaction	Labs
RUDT	Respiratory and upper digestive tract	Anat
RUE	Right upper extremity	Anat
RUG	Retrograde urethrography	Imag
RUL	Right upper lobe (lung)	Anat
RUQ	Right upper quadrant (abdomen)	Anat
RX*	Medical prescription; Prescription drug	Rpts
RX*	Treatment; Therapy	Proc

S

s̄	Without	Rpts
S/P	Status post	Rpts
S1 - S5	Sacral vertebra	Anat
SAT	Saturation	Rpts
SATIS	Satisfactory	Rpts
SB	Small bowel	Anat
SBO	Small bowel obstruction	Cond
SBR	Scarff-Bloom-Richardson	Grad
SBRT	Stereotactic body radiation therapy	Proc
SCC*	Small cell carcinoma	Path
SCC*	Squamous cell carcinoma	Path
SCID	Severe combined immuno-deficiency syndrome	Cond
SCLC	Small cell lung cancer	Path
S-COLON	Sigmoid colon	Anat
SCT	Stem cell transplant	Proc
SES	Socioeconomic status	Misc
SGOT	Serum glutamic oxaloacetic transaminase	Labs
SGPT	Serum glutamic pyruvic trans-aminase	Labs
SH	Social history [personal habits, living situation, job]	Rpts
SHx	Surgical history	Rpts
SIADH	Syndrome of inappropriate secretion of antidiuretic hormone	Cond
SIG (COLON)	Sigmoid colon	Anat
SIL	Squamous intraepithelial lesion	Path
SLE	Systemic lupus erythematosus	Cond
SLN(D)	Sentinel lymph node (dissection)	Path
SM	Small	Rpts
SMA	Sequential multiple analysis [Biochemical profile]	Labs
SML BWL	Small bowel	Anat
SNF	Skilled nursing facility	Rpts
SO	Salpingo-oophorectomy	Proc
SOB	Shortness of breath	Cond
SOBOE	Short of breath on exertion	Cond
SOL	Space occupying lesion	Rpts
SPEC	Specimen	Path
SPECT	Single photon emission computed tomography	Imag
SQ*	Subcutaneous	Rpts
SQ*; SQUAM; SqCC	Squamous	Path
SRS	Stereotactic radiosurgery	Proc
SS	(SEER) Summary stage	Misc
S-SPINE	Sacral spine	Anat
SSS	Sick sinus syndrome	Cond
STG	Stage	Rpts
STS	Soft tissue sarcoma	Path
STSG	Split thickness skin graft	Proc
SUBCU; SUBQ; SUB-Q	Subcutaneous	Anat
SUBTOT	Subtotal	Rpts
SUMM	Summary	Rpts
SURG	Surgery, Surgical	Rpts
SUSP	Suspicious; suspected	Rpts
SUV	Standardized uptake value	Imag
SVAB	Stereotactic vacuum-assisted biopsy	Proc
SVC(S)	Superior vena cava (syndrome)	Cond
SX*	Surgery	Rpts
SX*	Symptoms	Rpts

T

T	Thoracic	Anat
T1 - T12	Thoracic vertebra	Anat
TAH	Total abdominal hysterectomy	Proc
TAH-BSO	Total abdominal hysterectomy with bilateral salpingo-oophor-ectomy	Proc
TB	Tuberculosis	Cond
TBI	Total body irradiation	Proc
TCC	Transitional cell carcinoma	Path
T-COLON	Transverse colon	Anat
TEF	Tracheoesophageal fistula	Cond
THE	Transhiatal esophagectomy	Proc
TIA	Transient ischemic attack	Cond
TIL	Tumor infiltrating lymphocyte	Labs
TID	Three times per day	Rpts
TME	Total mesorectal excision	Proc
TMJ	Temporomandibular joint	Anat
TNF	Tumor necrosis factor	Labs
TNM	Tumor-Node-Metastasis [staging system]	Misc
TOB	Tobacco	Rpts
TOT	Total	Rpts

TPE	Total pelvic exenteration	Proc
TPN	Total parenteral nutrition	Rpts
TRAM	Transverse rectus abdominal muscle (flap)	Proc
TRANS-COLON	Transverse colon	Anat
TRG	Tumor regression grade	Path
TRUS	Transrectal ultrasound	Imag
TS	Tumor size	Rpts
TSE	Testicular self exam	Rpts
TSH	Thyroid stimulating hormone	Labs
T-SPINE	Thoracic spine	Anat
TTE	Total thoracic esophagectomy	Proc
TTP	Thrombotic thrombocytopenia purpura	Cond
TULIP	Transurethral ultrasound-guided laser-induced prostatectomy	Proc
TUMT	Transurethral microwave thermo-therapy	Proc
TUNA	Transurethral needle ablation	Proc
TUR	Transurethral resection	Proc
TURBT	Transurethral resection of bladder tumor	Proc
TURP	Transurethral resection of prostate	Proc
TVC	True vocal cord	Anat
TVH	Total vaginal hysterectomy	Proc
TVS	Transvaginal ultrasound	Imag
TX*	Transplant	Proc
TX*	Treatment; Therapy	Rpts

— U —

UA	Urinalysis	Labs
UADT	Upper aerodigestive tract	Anat
UD	Undifferentiated	Grad
UE	Upper extremity	Anat
UGI	Upper gastrointestinal	Anat
UIQ	Upper inner quadrant	Anat
UNCB	Ultrasound-guided needle biopsy	Proc
UNDIFF	Undifferentiated	Grad
UNK	Unknown	Rpts
UOQ	Upper outer quadrant	Anat
UPJ	Ureteropelvic junction	Anat
URI	Upper respiratory infection	Cond
US; U/S	Ultrasound	Imag
USG	Ultrasonography	Imag
USO	Unilateral salpingo-oophorectomy	Proc
UTI	Urinary tract infection	Cond
UVJ	Ureterovesical junction	Anat

— V —

VAG	Vagina; Vaginal	Anat
VAG HYST	Vaginal hysterectomy	Proc
VAIN (III)	Vaginal intraepithelial neoplasia (grade III)	Path
VASC	Vascular	Rpts
VATS	Video-assisted thoracoscopic surgery	Proc
VE	Vaginal examination (manual examination)	Proc
VEGF	Vascular endothelial growth factor	Labs
VIN (III)	Vulvar intraepithelial neoplasia (grade III)	Path
VIPoma	Vasoactive intestinal polypeptide tumor	Path

— W —

W/	With	Rpts
W/O	Without	Rpts
W/U	Work-up	Rpts
WBC	White blood cells	Labs
WBR	Whole body radiation	Proc
WBRT	Whole brain radiotherapy	Proc
WD; WELL DIFF	Well differentiated	Grad
WF*; W/F	White female	Rpts
WF*; W/F	Working formulation [lymphoma]	Path
WHO	World Health Organization	Grad
WLE	Wide local excision	Proc
WM; W/M	White male	Rpts
W-MD	Well to moderately differentiated	Grad
WNL	Within normal limits	Rpts
WPW	Wolff-Parkinson-White syndrome	Cond

— X —

x	Times	Rpts
XR	Xray	Imag
XRT	Radiation therapy	Proc

— Y —

YLF	Yttrium-lithium-fluoride [laser]	Misc
YO; Y/O	Years old	Rpts
YR	Year	Rpts

— Z —

ZES	Zollinger-Ellison syndrome	Cond

Resources Used in Compiling This List

California Cancer Registry Volume I: Data Standards and Data Dictionary, Appendix M.2: Common Acceptable Abbreviations, May 2008. Downloaded from http://www.ccrcal.org/DSQC_Pubs/V1_2011_Online_Manual/Vol_01_11.htm

NAACCR Recommended Abbreviations List, in *Standards for Cancer Registries, Volume II: Data Standards and Data Dictionary, 16th Edition,* June 2011, Appendices C and G. Downloaded from http://www.naaccr.org/LinkClick.aspx?fileticket=r5CVvCn6dA4%3d&tabid=133&mid=473

Stedman's Oncology Words, Fifth Edition, Lippincott, Williams & Wilkins, 2006.

Lists of abbreviations compiled by CASEbook editors

Healthcare Organizations and Agencies and Other Registry Terms

AACCR American Association of Central Cancer Registries [in 1994, name was changed to "North American Association of Central Cancer Registries" (NAACCR) to include the Canadian Provinces' registries]
AACI American Association of Cancer Institutes
AACR American Association of Cancer Research
ABMTR Autologous Blood and Marrow Transplant Registry
ABTA American Brain Tumor Association
ACCC Association of Community Cancer Centers
ACE Association of Cancer Executives
ACoS American College of Surgeons
ACOSOG American College of Surgeons Oncology Group
ACR American College of Radiology
ACS American Cancer Society
ACTUR Automated Central Tumor Registry [Department of Defense registry software]
ADA American Dental Association
AFIP Armed Forces Institute of Pathology
AHA American Hospital Association
AHIC American Health Information Community
AHIMA American Health Information Management Association
AJCC American Joint Committee on Cancer
AMA American Medical Association
AMFAR American Foundation for AIDS Research
AOA American Osteopathic Association
APON Association of Pediatric Oncology Nurses
ART Accredited Records Technician (former title for Registered Health Information Technician {RHIT})
ASCO American Society of Clinical Oncology
ASH American Society of Hematology
ASPHO American Society of Pediatric Hematology/Oncology
ASPO American Society of Preventive Oncology
AST American Thoracic Society
ASTRO American Society for Therapeutic Radiology and Oncology
AUA American Urological Association

BCEDP Breast Cancer Early Detection Program
BRFSS Behavioral Risk Factor Surveillance System

caBIG Cancer Biomedical Informatics Grid
CALGB Cancer and Leukemia Group B
CAM Complememtary amd Alternative Medicine
CAP College of American Pathologists
CCCR Canadian Council of Cancer Registries
CCG Children's Cancer Group
CCR Central cancer registry; Canadian Cancer Registry
CCRA Certified Cancer Research Associate
CCS Canadian Cancer Society
CCSG Children's Cancer Study Group
CDC Centers for Disease Control and Prevention
CIM Cancer Information Management
CINA Cancer Incidence in North America
CI5 Cancer Incidence in 5 Continents
CIS Cancer Information Service
CLP Cancer Liaison Program
CMS Centers for Medicare and Medicaid Services (formerly HCFA)
COC Commission on Cancer
CP3R Cancer Programs Practice Profile Reports
CPAC Canadian Partnership Against Cancer
CPS Cancer Program Standards
CPT Current Procedural Terminology
CS Collaborative Stage Data Collection System
CSv2 Collaborative Stage Data Collection System, version 2
CSP Cancer Surveillance Program
CSS Cancer Surneillance System
CTR Certified Tumor Registrar

DAM Data Acquisition Manual (predecessor to ROADS manual)
DCO Death Certificate Only
DOH Department of Health
DRG Diagnostic Related Group

EBCTCG Early Breast Cancer Trialists' Collaborative Group
ECOG Eastern Clinical Oncology Group
EDITS Exchangeable-edits, Data-dictionary, and Information Translation Standard
EHR Electronic Health Record
EMR Electronic Medical Record
EOD Extent of Disease

FDA Food and Drug Administration
FIGO Federation Internationale de Gynecologie et Obstetrique
FIPS Facility Information Profile System (ACoS); Federal Information Processing Standards
FORDS Facility Oncology Registry Data Standards

GITSG Gastrointestinal Tumor Study Group
GOG Gynecologic Oncology Group

HCBR Hospital Comparison Benchmark Reports
HCFA Health Care Finance Administration (now CMS)
HCO Healthcare Organization
HEDIS Health Plan Employer Data and Information Set
HIM Health Information Management

HIPAA Health Information Portability and Accountability Act
HMO Health Maintenance Organization

IACR International Association of Cancer Registries
IARC International Agency for Research on Cancer
IBMTR International Bone Marrow Transplant Registry
ICD International Classification of Diseases
-9 -Ninth Revision
-10 -Tenth Revision
-CM -Clinical Modification
-O -for Oncology
-O-2 -for Oncology, Second Edition
-O-3 -for Oncology, Third Edition
IPA Independent Practice Association
IRB Institutional Review Board
IRSG Intergroup Rhabdomyosarcoma Study Group

JCAHO Joint Commission on Accreditation of Healthcare Organizations

MOTNAC Manual of Tumor Nomenclature and Coding
MP/H Multiple Primary and Histology Coding (rules that took effect 01/01/2007)
MSA Metropolitan Statistical Area

NAACCR North American Association of Central Cancer Registries
NAPBC National Accreditation Program for Breast Centers
NBCR National Board for Certification of Registrars (see NCRA)
NCCDPHP National Center for Chronic Disease Prevention and Health Promotion
NCCN National Comprehensive Cancer Network
NCDB National Cancer Data Base
NCHS National Center for Health Statistics
NCI National Cancer Institute
NCQA National Committee for Quality Assurance
NCRA National Cancer Registrars Association (formerly "National Tumor Registrars Association")
NDI National Death Index
NIH National Institutes of Health
NPCR National Program of Cancer Registries
NQF National Quality Forum
NSABP National Surgical Adjuvant Breast (and Bowel) Project
NWTSG National Wilms Tumor Study Group

OAA Outstanding Achievement Award
OCN Oncology Certified Nurse
ONS Oncology Nursing Society
ORTAT Operations Research and Technical Assistance Team

PDQ Physicians Data Query
POG Pediatric Oncology Group
PPO Preferred Provider Organization
PTCR Provincial and Territorial Cancer Registries (Canada)

QA Quality Assurance
QC Quality Control
QI Quality Improvement
QM Quality Management

RHIA Registered Health Information Administrator
RHIT Registered Health Information Technician
ROADS Registry Operations and Data Standards manual (Commission on Cancer)
RQRS Rapid Quality Reporting System
RRA Registered Records Administrator (former title for Registered Health Information Administrator {RHIA})
RSNA Radiologic Society of North America
RTOG Radiation Therapy Oncology Group

SEER Surveillance, Epidemiology, and End Results (Program)
SGO Society of Gynecologic Oncology
SIOP International Society of Pediatric Oncology
SMSA Standard Metropolitan Statistical Area
SNOMED Systematized Nomenclature of Medicine
SNOP Systematized Nomenclature of Pathology
SOCRA Society of Clinical Research Associates
SS Summary Stage
SSO Society of Surgical Oncology
SSSM2K SEER Summary Staging Manual 2000
SWOG Southwest Oncology Group

TJC The Joint Commission
TNM Tumor, Node, Metastasis (staging)

UDSC Uniform Data Standards Committee (of NAACCR)
UICC Union Internationale Contre le Cancer (International Union Against Cancer)
USDHHS United States Department of Health and Human Services
USDS US Cancer Statistics

WHI Women's Health Initiative
WHO World Health Organization

DIAGNOSTIC TESTS AND TUMOR MARKERS

This chapter consists of alphabetized lists of diagnostic tests and other measures of cancer information. The tests are grouped by source of information.

Dx Tests

SEQUENCE OF SECTIONS

Various studies include wording to note when determining whether a test confirms the presence of cancer and what is important to record on the abstract.

DEFINITIONS

Key words/possible involvement: terms which indicate possible involvement by tumor. Common terms are provided but the list is not all-inclusive.
Other words/no involvement: other terms seen in reports which indicate an abnormality but do not indicate a neoplastic process. Common terms are provided, but the list is not all-inclusive.
Key information: words or phrases to look for in the report of the study. Key information helps define the extent of disease.

The contributions of Annette Hurlbut, RHIT, CTR to this chapter are gratefully acknowledged.

PHYSICAL EXAM

PHYSICAL EXAM – Systematic review and record of findings of various body regions—head and neck, thorax, abdomen, lymph nodes, and extremities. Includes observation of all external surfaces and palpation of various portions of the body for the purpose of determining the consistency of the parts beneath the surface.
Key information: obvious lesions; palpable mass(es); ulceration; size (in centimeters or inches) and location (especially if tumor crosses midline) of primary tumor(s); swelling or enlargement of any masses or organs (organomegaly, hepatomegaly, splenomegaly, hepatosplenomegaly/HSM); skin changes; fixation of mass; invasion/erosion of bone; laterality, size and number of palpable lymph nodes, especially cervical, supraclavicular, axillary or inguinal; evaluation of cranial nerves; evidence of "frozen" pelvis. For lymphoma, involvement of lymph nodes (matted nodes, fixed vs. mobile, lymphadenopathy, enlarged, "shotty" nodes, palpable, enlarged, visible swelling). For central nervous system tumors, neurologic examination for signs and symptoms (which help identify the location of the tumor); vision changes; attention deficit; focal deficit (blindness, taste aberrations); tumor impingement on a specific nerve or structure; mass effect (light-headedness, loss of vision); evidence of increased intracranial pressure (edema, headache, nausea and vomiting); evidence of obstructive hydrocephalus.

DIGITAL RECTAL EXAM – Also called DRE, rectal exam, manual exam. Manual or digital examination of the lower portion of the rectum, perineum and surrounding tissues using a gloved finger inserted into the anus. During the exam-ination, the examining finger can feel the prostate gland.
Key words/possible involvement: nodularity, palpable tumor, induration, fixation of seminal vesicles, enlargement, firmness, lesion, fixation to surrounding tissues, neoplasm, malignancy, active bleeding
Other words/no involvement: no mention of prostatic abnormality during the exam; benign prostatic hypertrophy

EXAMINATION OF ABDOMEN
Key information: Masses and enlarged organs (organomegaly; hepatomegaly; splenomegaly); palpable lymph nodes; jaundice (yellowing of skin and eyes due to blockage of bile ducts)

NEUROLOGICAL EXAM – Also called neuro exam. A series of questions and tests to check brain, spinal cord, and nerve function. The exam checks a person's mental status, coordination, ability to walk, and how well the muscles, sensory systems, and deep tendon reflexes work.

PELVIC EXAM – Manual or speculum evaluation of cervix, vagina, rectum, external genitalia. Digital exam of the rectum and vagina is also called a rectovaginal exam

SCHILLER TEST – Examination of cells in the vagina and cervix. The exam can be peformed in a doctor's office. Iodine solution is swabbed on the walls of the cervix and vagina. Normal cells are stained brown. Abnormal cells do not absorb the solution and may appear to be pink or white.

VISUAL EXAMINATION – Also called indirect or mirror examination. Visualization of clinically accessible areas of the head and neck by viewing them in a mirror or through an endoscope (see also Diagnostic Studies—Endoscopy).

VISUAL FIELD EXAM –A test to determine any defects in the patient's vision, which in turn may reveal the location of a brain tumor. Visual field alterations caused by problems in different brain sites are unique.

X-RAYS

X-RAY – Also called radiograph, roentgenogram, plain films, routine x-rays, XR. General term for images produced on a special type of photographic film from high-energy electromagnetic waves of very short length that can penetrate the body. No contrast media or radioisotopes are used to enhance the image.

X-ray Series – X-ray examination that requires taking a number of pictures. A summary is usually provided in one report. See also Metastatic Work-up.

Key information: size and location of primary tumor; relationship of mass to other tissues, such as impingement or extension to another tissue (ribs, chest wall, pleura); elevation of diaphragm on one side (phrenic nerve paralysis); hilar or mediastinal involvement; enlargement or decrease in size of lung(s); opacity, such as atelectasis, pleural effusion or pneumonitis; masses in mediastinum and/or hilum of lung; involvement of distant sites

AIR CONTRAST X-RAYS – An x-ray that uses inflation with air to obtain a better outline of some parts of the body. The air can be inhaled, swallowed, injected, or ingested by drinking a carbonated beverage, after which the x-ray is taken. See also Barium Enema.

ANGIOGRAM – Also called angiography. X-ray study of the vascular system that is used to diagnose some cancers. An angiogram visualizes the blood vessels leading to an organ or areas of concern as well as the blood distribution within the organ. A contrast agent that will show up on an x-ray is injected into the blood vessels, usually through a catheter or tube.
Key words/possible involvement: hypervascularity, stricture, extrinsic mass, lesion, neoplasm, malignancy, opacification, nonvisualization
Other words/no involvement: no specific reference to visible abnormality in the vasculature of the liver; hepatic hemangioma, hamartoma, cyst or other references to benign conditions

ANGIOGRAPHY (CELIAC AND TRANSHEPATIC) – See Percutaneous Transhepatic Cholangiography.

ARTERIOGRAM – Also called arteriography. Radiographic visualization of arteries leading to an organ or areas of concern as well as the blood distribution within the organ. A contrast agent that will show up on an x-ray is injected, usually through a catheter or tube. See Angiogram for key words.

BARIUM ENEMA – Also called BE, double contrast barium enema, air contrast barium enema, air contrast study, pneumocolon, barium contrast study of the colon. Evaluation of the colon using contrast material (barium and/or air) inserted through the rectum.
Key words/possible involvement: lesion, irregular density, stricture, shouldered stricture, applecore lesion, filling defect, obstruction, stenosis, polyps, villous adenoma, fistula
Other words/no involvement: no visible abnormality in the colon, diverticulosis, megacolon, ulcerative colitis, Crohn's disease, abscess, or infectious process, or other benign conditions

BARIUM SWALLOW – See Upper GI Series.

BRONCHOGRAM – Also called bronchography. Views of the bronchial tree using contrast media.
Key words/possible involvement: lesion, irregular density, stricture, narrowing, blockage, shouldered stricture, applecore lesion, filling defect, protrusion, obstruction, fistula, extravasation, abnormal contour, bleeding
Other words/no involvement: no visible abnormality in the bronchi; inflammation, bronchitis, congenital abnormalities, spasm, edema, abscess, infectious process, or other benign conditions

X-rays, *continued*

CEREBRAL ANGIOGRAPHY – Also called brain angiogram. Invasive radiographic procedure that injects dye into cerebral vessels to determine the location of and blood flow to a brain tumor. The contrast material visualizes the blood vessels and helps determine the planes of resection.
Key words/possible involvement: stricture, mass, mass effect, extrinsic mass, metastases, filling defect, obstruction, space occupying lesion, neovascularization, vascular parisitization
Other words/no involvement: no specific reference to abnormality of the cerebral vasculature; references to cysts, hamartomas, angiomyolipomas, AVM (arteriovenous malformation)

CHEST X-RAY – Also called CXR, AP and PA chest films, chest radiographs, chest roentgenograms. Evaluation of the lungs and mediastinum.
Key words/possible involvement: lesion, irregular density, coin lesion, cannonball lesion, nodular lesion, cavitary lesion, homogenous parenchymal lesion with sharply defined margins, multiple opacities, multiple pulmonary nodules, unilateral hilar enlargement, pleural effusion, pleural masses, rib lesion with adjacent soft tissue mass, mediastinal mass, metastases, spiculated lesion
Other words/no involvement: calcifications, hamartomas, granulomas, bronchogenic cysts, vascular abnormalities, and other benign conditions

CHOLANGIOGRAM – Also called cholangiography, percutaneous cholangiogram, skinny needle cholangiogram, intravenous cholangiography, T-tube cholangiogram (a postoperative procedure). Sequential x-rays that evaluate the liver, gallbladder and bile ducts using contrast material injected intravenously.
Key words/possible involvement: hypervascularity, stricture, extrinsic mass, lesion, neoplasm, malignancy, opacification, nonvisualization
Other words/no involvement: no specific reference to visible abnormality in the organ; inflammatory process, foreign bodies, or other benign conditions

CHOLECYSTOGRAM – Also called cholecystography, oral gallbladder test. Radiologic study of the function of the gallbladder and bile ducts after an opaque medium has been introduced either orally or intravenously.

CINE-PHARYNGOESOPHAGRAM – Also called cineradiography. Serial (moving picture) x-rays of the aerodigestive tract. Allows dynamic (with motion) visualization of swallowing function, as well as strictures and other abnormalities.

CONTACT THERMOGRAM – See Thermography.

CYSTOGRAM – Also called cystography, double contrast cystogram. X-rays to visualize the bladder after the introduction of radiopaque contrast via urethral catheter. After the patient voids, air may be used as a second contrast agent.
Key words/possible involvement: stricture, mass, mass effect, metastases, lytic lesion, osteolytic lesion, blastic lesion, osteoblastic lesion, surface irregularities of bladder, filling defect in the bladder, non-functioning kidney, ureteral obstruction
Other words/no involvement: no specific reference to abnormality in the bladder

DIAPHANOGRAM – Also called diaphanography, transillumination, light scanning. A procedure that may be used in the diagnosis of breast cancer. A strong, cold beam of light is focused on the breast in a darkened room. An infrared camera is used, which will show, on a screen, differences that distinguish a solid tumor from a cyst that is filled with fluid.

DIGITAL MAMMOGRAPHY – Also called computerized mammogram, digital mammogram, digital breast radiography. Examination of the breast by using a computer along with the x-ray to get a finer resolution. Images are recorded on a computer rather than x-ray film.

X-rays, *continued*

DIGITAL RADIOGRAPHY – Radiology system that uses computers to convert the lighter and darker areas of the radiographic image into numbers and then translates these numbers into an image on a computer screen.

DUCTOGRAM – Also called galactogram. Injection of contrast material into a breast duct to evaluate whether there is an intraductal mass or to identify cause of nipple discharge.

DUODENOGRAM – Also called duodenography. Diagnostic contrast x-ray of the duodenum and the pancreas.

EEG (ELECTROENCEPHALOGRAM) – Measurement of electrical impulses from the brain by placing electrodes on the outside of the head to record brain activity. The usefulness of EEG has diminished in recent years because CT scanning yields more detail.
Key words/possible involvement: abnormal pattern, abnormal reading, abnormality
Other words/no involvement: no specific reference to abnormality in the brain, including references to abscesses, subdural hematomas, hematomas, cerebrovascular disease, cerebrovascular accident, infarction, trauma

ENTEROCLYSIS – Contrast examination of the small intestine. A small tube is passed through the upper gastrointestinal tract to the opening of the small intestine. Barium is released into the small intestine along with a substance that causes air. As the small intestine expands from the air, x-rays are taken to provide better images than small bowel follow through imaging (see below). See also Small Bowel Series.

ESOPHAGOGRAM – Also called esophagram, barium swallow, barium esophagogram, cineradiography; includes fluoroscopy of esophagus. Radiographic evaluation of the esophagus using contrast media. The x-rays are taken after the person drinks a solution that contains barium, which coats and outlines the esophagus on the x-ray.
Key words/possible involvement: lesion, irregular density, stricture, shouldered stricture, applecore lesion, filling defect, obstruction, fistula, extravasation, abnormal contour, bleeding
Other words/no involvement: no visible abnormality in the esophagus; normal peristalsis, diverticuli, inflammation, esophagitis, esophageal varices, congenital abnormalities, spasm, edema, abscess, infectious process, or other benign conditions

EXCRETORY UROGRAM – See IVP (Intravenous Pyelogram).

GASTROINTESTINAL SERIES – Also called GI series. Examination of the upper and lower digestive tract by x-ray after the administration of barium, a contrast medium. Barium outlines or highlights irregularities that are present.

HYSTEROGRAM – Also called hysterography, metrogram. Examination of the uterus by x-ray after the administration of a contrast medium. The dye is inserted via a catheter through the vagina and into the uterus.

INFUSION NEPHROTOMOGRAPHY – Radiologic visualization of the kidney by tomography after intravenous introduction of contrast medium. See also Nephrotomography.

IVP (INTRAVENOUS PYELOGRAM) – A series of x-rays that evaluate the structure and function of the kidney, ureters and bladder after radiopaque dye has been injected intravenously. Also called excretory urogram, pyelography. Excludes KUB (Kidney-Ureters-Bladder) radiography during which no dye is injected.
Key words/possible involvement: stricture, mass, mass effect, stricture, nonfunctioning kidney,

X-rays, *continued*

IVP (Intravenous Pyelogram), continued
metastases, lytic lesion, osteolytic lesion, blastic lesion, osteoblastic lesion, surface irregularities of bladder, filling defect in the bladder, ureteral obstruction
Other words/no involvement: no specific reference to metastases, lesion, or visible abnormality of the kidneys, ureters, or bladder

IVU (INTRAVENOUS URETHROGRAM) – Radiographs of the urethra after the injection of an opaque medium. See IVP for key words.

KUB (KIDNEYS-URETER-BLADDER) – X-rays to evaluate the status of the urinary system. No dye is injected during this procedure.
Key words/possible involvement: stricture, mass, mass effect, metastases, lytic lesion, osteolytic lesion, blastic lesion, osteoblastic lesion, surface irregularities of bladder, filling defect in the bladder, non-functioning kidney, nonvisualized kidney, ureteral obstruction
Other words/no involvement: no specific reference to visible abnormality in the urinary tract

LARYNGOGRAM – Also called laryngeal tomography, laryngography. Radiographic studies through various levels of the larynx.

LIENOGRAM – Also called lienography. X-ray that outlines the spleen after an injection of a contrast medium.

LIGHT SCANNING – See Diaphanogram.

LOWER GI SERIES – X-ray studies of the large bowel following rectal injection of barium. X-rays of the colon and rectum (lower gastrointestinal tract) that are taken after a person is given a barium enema. See also Barium Enema.

LYMPHANGIOGRAM – Also called pedal/bipedal lymphangiography, lymphography, LAG. Radiographic examination of the lymphatic system of the trunk by injecting dye into a lymphatic vessel in each foot to determine retroperitoneal involvement. The following areas should be visualized to adequately assess extent of disease: lymphatics of the legs, inguinal and iliac regions, and retroperitoneum including periarotic. Does not visualize the mesenteric, celiac or portal nodes. Since the advent of CT and MRI scanning, this invasive procedure is less frequently done.
Key words/possible involvement: area of increased density, area of enhanced contrast, space occupying lesion, diffuse nodularity, decreased uptake, decreased activity, lymphadenopathy, filling defect, lack of opacification, enlarged or foamy-looking nodes
Other words/no involvement: no specific reference to abnormality in the lymph nodes of the trunk

MAMMOGRAM – Includes unilateral (involved breast), bilateral (both breasts), contralateral (side not suspected of containing cancer), screening (routine of both breasts), diagnostic (very careful inspection of both breasts), magnification, spot compression tests. Radiographic examination of breasts to detect breast cysts or tumors, especially those that cannot be felt (palpable) by the fingers during a physical examination.
Key words/possible involvement: lesion, mass, nodular or irregular density, clustered calcification, spiculation, mammary duct distortion or asymmetry, skin or nipple thickening, enlarged lymph nodes
Other words/no involvement: no specific reference to visible abnormality in the evaluated breast

METASTATIC WORK-UP – Also called metastatic survey. Any imaging or other test to assess the presence of other primaries that may have caused a metastatic tumor; any imaging or other testing to look in organs distant from the primary site for evidence of metastases. Can include plain x-rays, scans, PET scans, MRI.

X-rays, *continued*

METROGRAM – See Hysterogram.

MIRALUMA TEST – See Scintimammogram in Nuclear Imaging section.

MYELOGRAM – Also called myelography. An x-ray of the spinal cord taken after an injection of dye into the space between meninges. A myelogram can identify a spinal cord tumor.

NEPHROTOMOGRAPHY – Radiographic evaluation of kidneys by taking films of serial, thin sections of renal tissue. Also called renal tomography, renal tomos. Excludes computerized tomography of the kidneys and plain x-rays of the kidneys. See also Infusion Nephrotomography.
Key words/possible involvement: lesion, irregular density, space occupying lesion, cavitary lesion, homogenous parenchymal lesion with sharply defined margins, multiple opacities, metastases
Other words/no involvement: no specific reference to visible abnormality in the lungs; references to calcifications, hamartomas, angiomyolipoma, granulomas, cysts, vascular abnormalities, and other benign conditions

PERCUTANEOUS TRANSHEPATIC CHOLANGIOGRAM – Also called PTC, celiac and transhepatic angiography. Evaluation of the liver and biliary tree using contrast material injected through the skin directly into the liver.
Key words/possible involvement: hypervascularity, stricture, extrinsic mass, lesion, neoplasm, malignancy, opacification, nonvisualization
Other words/no involvement: no specific reference to visible abnormality in the vasculature of the liver; hepatic hemangioma, hamartoma, cyst or other references to benign conditions

PLAIN FILMS – See X-ray.

PNEUMOCOLON – Air contrast enema. See Barium Enema.

PNEUMOENCEPHALOGRAM – Injection of air contrast into the cranial cavity to evaluate the midline brain (pituitary and cranial fossa) structures and the brain stem. This is a very dangerous procedure and is not used except in cases where a diagnosis cannot be reached any other way. The usefulness of pneumoencephalography has diminished in recent years because CT scanning or MRI yields more detail.

PORTOGRAM – Also called portography. Radiographic examination of the portal vein (the large vein that carries blood to the liver from the veins of the stomach, intestine, spleen, and pancreas). For greater visibility of the portal vein, a contrast substance is injected into the veins or spleen.

PYELOGRAM – Also called pyelography. See IVP (Intravenous Pyelography).

RADIOLOGIC EXAM – A general term for an examination that uses radiation or other imaging procedures to find signs of cancer or other abnormalities. Radiologic exams may use contrast or radioisotopes or other methods to visualize tumors or other areas of concern. Each type of radiologic exam has a specific name.

RENAL ANGIOGRAPHY – Also called digital intravenous angiography, digital fluorography, renal arteriography, renal venography, renal angiogram. Invasive radiographic procedure that injects dye into renal vessels to determine the location of and blood flow to a kidney tumor. The contrast material visualizes both the renal blood vessels and the collecting systems.
Key words/possible involvement: stricture, mass, mass effect, extrinsic mass, metastases, filling defect, obstruction, space occupying lesion, neovascularization, vascular parisitization
Other words/no involvement: no specific reference to abnormality of the renal vasculature; references to cysts, hamartomas, angiomyolipomas

X-rays*, continued*

RENAL FLOW STUDY – A fluoroscopic examination to check the flow of blood through the kidneys after contrast material has been injected into the veins.

RENOCYSTOGRAM – X-rays to visualize the bladder, ureters and kidneys after the introduction of intravenous radiopaque contrast material.
Key words/possible involvement: stricture, mass, mass effect, metastases, filling defect in the kidney or bladder, non-functioning kidney, ureteral obstruction
Other words/no involvement: no specific reference to abnormality in the urinary tract

RETROGRADE PYELOGRAM – Also called retrograde pyelography, retrograde urogram, retrograde urography. A series of x-rays to evaluate the upper urinary tract by using a cystoscope to insert catheters through ureters to the level of the renal pelvis and injecting radiopaque contrast dye tovisualize the renal pelvis, calyces and ureter of a kidney. Useful if IVP is inadequate due to nonvisualized kidney.
Key words/possible involvement: mass, stricture, lesion, filling defect, extrinsic mass, narrowing, metastases, non-functioning kidney
Other words/no involvement: no specific reference to visible abnormality in the urinary tract

ROENTGENOGRAPHY – An older term for radiography or x-rays. See X-ray.

SALPINGOGRAM – Also called salpingography. Radiologic study of the uterus and fallopian tubes.

SELECTIVE RENAL ARTERIOGRAM – Also called selective renal arteriography. Examination of the kidney's blood vessels by x-ray using a contrast substance injected into the bloodstream. See also Arteriogram.

SIALOGRAPHY – Also called Sialogram. Radiographic examination of the salivary ducts; not recommended as a diagnostic tool because of the possibility of introducing sepsis.

SKULL RADIOGRAPHS – X-rays of the bones of the skull to determine the presence of tumor and its effect on internal structures in the brain. Also called skull films.
Key words/possible involvement: midline shift, calcification, skull or sella turcica erosion, erosion of inner table, stricture, mass, mass effect, metastases, filling defect, obstruction (to cerebrospinal fluid flow), space occupying lesion
Other words/no involvement: no specific reference to abnormality of the cerebral vasculature; references to cysts, hamartomas

SMALL BOWEL FOLLOW THROUGH – Continuation of a barium swallow (see Upper GI Series) looking for problems in the small intestine by taking x-rays at regular intervals as the barium passes through the upper gastrointestinal tract.

SMALL BOWEL SERIES – Also called enteroclysis. Includes fluoroscopy of the small bowel. Excludes upper gastrointestinal series (UGI).
Key words/possible involvement: lesion, irregular density, stricture, shouldered stricture, applecore lesion, filling defect, obstruction, polyps, villous adenoma, bleeding, deformity of duodenum
Other words/no involvement: no visible abnormality in the small bowel; congenital atresia, regional enteritis, ulcerative colitis, Whipple's disease, sprue, lymphoid hyperplasia, malabsorption syndrome, intussusception, edema, abscess, or infectious process, or other benign conditions

STOMACH X-RAYS – Also called gastric radiography. Radiographic examination of the stomach. Also part of an upper GI series.
Key words/possible involvement: lesion, irregular density, stricture, shouldered stricture, filling defect, obstruction, fistula, extravasation, perforation, thickening of wall, abnormal contour, extrinsic

X-rays, *continued*

Stomach x-rays, continued
mass, bleeding, ulcer (unless described as benign or non-malignant), enlarged rugal folds, deformity of pylorus
Other words/no involvement: no visible abnormality; normal peristalsis, diverticuli, inflammation, varices, pyloric stenosis, gastritis, congenital abnormalities, foreign bodies, spasm, edema, abscess, infectious process, or other benign conditions

THERMOGRAPHY – Also called contact thermogram, graphic stress telethermometry. Examination of body tissue using an infrared camera to measure and display heat patterns. Abnormalities may show up as "hot" spots in the film, since the temperature of diseased or abnormal tissue is frequently higher than that of normal tissue. Used to diagnose breast cancer and other tumors.

TOMOGRAMS – Also called tomos or tomography, body section radiography, planigraphy, laminogram, laminography, stratigraphy. Evaluation of a plane or level of tissue (most commonly the larynx or paranasal sinuses) that can reveal tumor size, location, and extension into other structures. See also Whole Lung Tomograms, Nephrotomography and other site-specific tomography procedures.
Key words/possible involvement: mass, bony tumor involvement, obstruction, abnormal contour
Other words/no involvement: no visible abnormality; or reference to foreign body, inflammation, congenital abnormalities, edema, abscess, infectious process, or other benign conditions

TOMOSYNTHESIS (3D Mammography) – Similar to tomography of other sites (x-ray views in thin slices through tissue), tomosynthesis may allow detection of smaller lesions than standard mammograms. The patient lies face down on a special table with the breast projecting through a hole in the table while a mammography machine rotates around the breast taking images that are combined into a 3-dimensional picture.

TRANSILLUMINATION – See Diaphanogram.

UPPER GI SERIES – Also called UGI, double contrast Upper GI series, barium swallow. Radiographic examination of the esophagus, stomach and small bowel in one procedure.
Key words/possible involvement: lesion, irregular density, stricture, shouldered stricture, perforation, filling defect, obstruction, fistula, extravasation, thickening of wall, abnormal contour, extrinsic mass
Other words/no involvement: no visible abnormality; normal peristalsis, diverticuli, inflammation, congenital abnormalities, foreign bodies, spasm, edema, abscess, infectious process, or other benign conditions

URETHROGRAM – Also called urethrography. Examination of the urethra by x-ray for the presence of a tumor or suspicious area.

UROGRAM – Also called urography. Radiologic study of the urinary tract.

UTEROGRAPHY – See Hysterogram.

VENACAVOGRAM – X-ray of the renal (kidney) vein.

VENOGRAM – Also called venography. X-ray of any of the veins after administration by injection of a dye into a vein.

WHOLE LUNG TOMOGRAM – Radiographic evaluation of lungs by taking films of serial, thin sections of lung tissue. Also called whole lung tomography, chest tomos. Excludes computerized tomography of the lungs and plain x-rays of the lungs. See also Tomograms.

X-rays, ***continued***

Whole lung tomograms, continued
Key words/possible involvement: lesion, irregular density, coin lesion, cannonball lesion, nodular lesion, cavitary lesion, homogenous parenchymal lesion with sharply defined margins, multiple opacities, multiple pulmonary nodules, unilateral hilar enlargement, pleural effusion, pleural masses, rib lesion with adjacent soft tissue mass, mediastinal mass, metastases, spiculated
Other words/no involvement: no specific reference to visible abnormality in the lungs; references to calcifications, hamartomas, granulomas, bronchogenic cysts, vascular abnormalities, and other benign conditions

XEROGRAM – Also called xeroradiograph, xerography. An image of the body recorded on paper rather than on film; x-rays of soft tissues developed using the same image-producing process as the Xerox office copier machines.

XEROMAMMOGRAM – Also called xeromammography. Mammograms developed using the same image-producing process as the Xerox office copier machines.

OTHER IMAGING TECHNIQUES

Key information: size of primary tumor, extension to or involvement of other structures or organs, masses that press upon other organs, involvement of distant sites

1H-NUCLEAR MAGNETIC RESONANCE SPECTROSCOPIC IMAGING – Also called magnetic resonance spectroscopic imaging and proton magnetic resonance spectroscopic imaging. A noninvasive imaging method that provides information about cellular activity (metabolic information). It is used along with magnetic resonance imaging (MRI) which provides information about the shape and size of the tumor (spacial information).

COMPUTED TOMOGRAPHY – Also called CT scan, CAT scan, computerized tomography, computerized axial tomography scan, computerized scanning, computerized transaxial tomography, contrast enhanced CT, arterial portogram CT, helical computed tomography, spiral CT, incremental CT. A series of detailed radiographs of areas inside the body taken from different angles; the pictures are created by a computer linked to an x-ray machine. CT scanning is used for the examination of many parts of the body. The scan's images show cross-sectional 'slices' of the body that are each a millimeter thick. A composite image is created by the computer and photocopied. CT scanning provides an accurate picture of the extent of disease. CT scans are performed both with and without contrast media. CT scans can be taken of the head, chest, abdomen, pelvis, or the whole body.

COMPUTED TOMOGRAPHY COLOGRAPHY – Also called virtual colonoscopy, computed tomographic colonography, CTC. A method to examine the colon by taking a series of x-rays and using a computer to reconstruct 2D and 3D pictures of the interior surfaces of the colon from these x-rays. The pictures can be saved, manipulated to better viewing angles, and reviewed after the procedure, even years later.

ECAT SCAN (Emission Computerized Axial Tomography) – Diagnostic test similar to the CT scan. After radioactive material is administered to the patient, the ECAT scanner records the charged particles given off from deep within the body. The picture that is being taken is that of the inside of the organ that is being studied.

ELECTRICAL IMPEDANCE IMAGING (T-scan) – Examination of the breast for electrical conductivity, based on theory that breast cancer cells conduct electricity differently from normal cells. Helps in classifying tumors found on mammogram but not used as a screening tool.

Other Imaging Techniques, *continued*

FLUOROSCOPY – A technique for continuous or intermittent x-ray monitoring. An x-ray procedure that makes it possible to see internal organs in motion.

FUNCTIONAL MAGNETIC RESONANCE IMAGING – A noninvasive tool used to observe functioning in the brain or other organs by detecting changes in chemical composition, blood flow, or both.

HELICAL COMPUTED TOMOGRAPHY (SPIRAL CT SCAN) – Also called low-dose spiral CT or helical CT. A series of detailed images of areas inside the body created by a computer linked to an x-ray machine that scans the body in a spiral path. Low dose spiral CT is better at finding smaller abnormalities in the lungs than standard chest x-rays, but it also detects more abnormalities that need further investigation before ruling out malignancy. Low dose spiral CT is under clinical evaluation to see if it would be effective as a screening tool for lung cancer. See also Computed Tomography.

IMAGING (PRIMARY SITE) – General term for CT, tomography, magnetic resonance imaging (MRI) or nuclear magnetic resonance (NMR) scan, positron emission tomography (PET) of a suspected primary site of cancer.
Key words/possible involvement: area of increased density, area of enhanced contrast, area of high radioactivity, space occupying lesion, adenopathy, mass, enlargement, metastases
Other words/no involvement: no specific reference to visible abnormality, as well as references to calcifications, granulomas, vascular abnormalities, congenital anomalies, and other benign conditions

IMAGING, ABDOMEN – General term for abdominal x-rays, Kidney-Ureters-Bladder (KUB), abdominal flat plate, abdominal CT scan, MRI scan, nuclear scan of the abdominal cavity, PET scan. The following organs would be visualized during abdominal imaging: colon, small bowel, internal genital organs, retroperitoneum, urinary tract, skeletal structure of the lower trunk and possibly abdominal lymph nodes.
Key words/possible involvement: mass, lesion, distortion, displacement, area of increased density, area of enhanced contrast, area of high radioactivity, space occupying lesion, diffuse nodularity; decreased uptake, decreased activity, abnormal concentration (gallium scan)
Other words/no involvement: no specific reference to visible abnormality of the organs in the abdomen or retroperitoneum

IMAGING, ABDOMEN/PELVIS – General term for abdominal x-rays, Kidney-Ureters-Bladder (KUB), abdominal flat plate, abdominal CT scan, pelvic CT scan, MRI scan, nuclear scan of the abdominal cavity or pelvis, PET scan. The following organs would be visualized during an abdominal or pelvic scan: colon, small bowel, liver, internal genital organs, retroperitoneum, urinary tract, skeletal structure of the lower trunk, and possibly abdominal and pelvic lymph nodes.
Key words/possible involvement: mass, lesion, distortion, displacement, area of increased density, area of enhanced contrast, area of high radioactivity, space occupying lesion, diffuse nodularity; decreased uptake, decreased activity, abnormal concentration (gallium scan)
Other words/no involvement: no specific reference to visible abnormality of the organs in the abdomen, retroperitoneum, or pelvis

IMAGING, BONE – General term for skull films, bone scan, technetium (Tc99m) scan, CT scan of bone, metastatic skeletal survey, bone survey.
Key words/possible involvement: direct extension of tumor into any bone, lytic lesion, osteolytic lesion, blastic lesion, osteoblastic lesion, area(s) of increased uptake, bony destruction. *Exceptions*: use of these terms in conjunction with a (suspected) diagnosis of arthritis, fracture or osteomyelitis
Other words/no involvement: no specific reference to lesion or increased uptake

Other Imaging Techniques, ***continued***

IMAGING, BRAIN – General term for brain scan, CT scan of brain, technetium (Tc99m) brain scan, magnetic resonance imaging (MRI) of the brain, nuclear magnetic resonance (NMR) of the brain, head imaging. Isotope brain scans are useful for identifying meningiomas, glioblastomas, and large metastatic deposits.
Key words/possible involvement: translucent zone, low density zone, edema, mass effect, area of increased density, area of enhanced contrast, area of high radioactivity, space occupying lesion, diffuse nodularity; decreased uptake, decreased activity
Other words/no involvement: no specific reference to visible abnormality in the brain

IMAGING, CHEST – General term for lung scan, CT chest, perfusion scan of lung, ventilation scan of lung, lung tomography, magnetic resonance imaging (MRI) or nuclear magnetic resonance (NMR) scan of the lung, PET scan, bronchography. Chest imaging can also visualize the upper part of liver.
Key words/possible involvement: area of increased density, area of enhanced contrast, area of high radioactivity, space occupying lesion, hilar adenopathy, hilar or mediastinal mass, hilar enlargement, pleural effusion, multiple pulmonary nodules, pleural masses, rib lesion with adjacent soft tissue mass, mediastinal mass, metastases, masses or abnormalities in upper liver, spleen or adrenal glands.
Other words/no involvement: no specific reference to visible abnormality in the chest, lungs, mediastinum, liver, spleen and adrenal glands, as well as references to calcifications, hamartomas, granulomas, bronchogenic cysts, vascular abnormalities, and other benign conditions

IMAGING, LIVER/SPLEEN – General term for liver/spleen scan, technetium (Tc99m) scan of liver and spleen, gallium scan of liver. May include visualization of the adrenal glands and kidneys.
Key words/possible involvement area of increased density, area of enhanced contrast, area of high radioactivity, space occupying lesion, diffuse nodularity; decreased uptake, decreased activity, cold spot (liver scan); abnormal concentration (gallium scan)
Other words/no involvement: no specific reference to visible abnormality in the liver, spleen and adrenal glands

IMAGING, LUNG – General term for lung scan, CT chest, perfusion scan of lung, and ventilation scan of lung, whole lung tomography, magnetic resonance imaging (MRI) or nuclear magnetic resonance (NMR) scan of the lung, PET scan, bronchography. Excludes standard chest x-ray.
Key words/possible involvement: area of increased density, area of enhanced contrast, area of high radioactivity, space occupying lesion, hilar adenopathy, hilar mass, mediastinal mass, hilar enlargement, pleural effusion, multiple pulmonary nodules, pleural masses, rib lesion with adjacent soft tissue mass, metastases, masses or abnormalities in upper liver, spleen or adrenal glands.
Other words/no involvement: no specific reference to visible abnormality in the liver, spleen and adrenal glands, as well as references to calcifications, hamartomas, granulomas, bronchogenic cysts, vascular abnormalities, and other benign conditions

LOW DOSE SPIRAL CT – See Helical Computed Tomography.

MAGNETIC RESONANCE IMAGING (MRI) – Also called nuclear magnetic resonance imaging, NMR, functional magnetic resonance imaging. A procedure in which radio waves and a powerful magnet linked to a computer are used to create detailed pictures of areas inside the body. These pictures can show the difference between normal and diseased tissue. MRI makes better images of organs and soft tissue than other scanning techniques, such as CT or X-ray. MRI is especially useful for imaging the brain, spine, the soft tissue of joints, and the inside of bones.

Magnetic resonance angiography (MRA) – Evaluates structure of blood vessels in brain; useful in planning operation.

Other Imaging Techniques, ***continued***

Magnetic resonance imaging, continued

Magnetic resonance cholangiopancreatography (MRCP) – Uses MRI technology to evaluate bile ducts; less invasive than ERCP (see ERCP under Endoscopy) and does not require contrast agent.

MAGNETIC RESONANCE SPECTROSCOPIC IMAGING – Also called MRSI, magnetic resonance spectroscopy, and proton magnetic resonance spectroscopic imaging. A noninvasive imaging method that provides information about cellular activity (metabolic information). It is used along with magnetic resonance imaging (MRI), which provides information about the shape and size of the tumor (spacial information). See also 1H-nuclear magnetic resonance spectroscopic imaging.

NUCLEAR MAGNETIC RESONANCE (NMR) – See Magnetic Resonance Imaging.

PERFUSION MAGNETIC RESONANCE IMAGING – Also called magnetic resonance perfusion imaging. A special type of magnetic resonance imaging (MRI) that uses an injected dye in order to see blood flow through tissues.

POSITRON EMISSION TOMOGRAM (PET) – Also called PET scan, positron emission tomography. Specialized scan that permits investigation of glucose metabolism and thus measures chemical compounds of the body. A small amount of radioactive glucose (sugar) is injected into a vein, and a scanner is used to make detailed, computerized pictures of areas inside the body where the glucose is used. Because cancer cells often use more glucose than normal cells, the pictures can be used to find cancer cells in the body.

SCAN – A general term for a view or image of the interior of the body that can show abnormalities in structure and function of brain, pelvis, liver, spleen, adrenal glands, or other organs and structures for evidence of primary lesions and/or distant metastases. Includes computer-assisted techniques such as CT, magnetic resonance imaging (MRI), nuclear magnetic resonance (NMR) and positron emission tomography (PET), as well as nuclear scanning procedures requiring the ingestion of radioisotopes such as gallium, technetium (Tc99m), iodine (I-131). See also Nuclear Imaging, below. In CT scanning, an x-ray machine linked to a computer is used to produce detailed pictures of organs inside the body. MRI scans use a large magnet connected to a computer to create pictures of areas inside the body.
Key words/possible involvement: area of increased density, area of enhanced contrast, area of high radioactivity, space occupying lesion, diffuse nodularity, decreased uptake, decreased activity, mass effect
Other words/no involvement: no specific reference to visible abnormality of the organs assessed as part of the scan

SINGLE-PHOTON EMISSION COMPUTED TOMOGRAPHY (SPECT) – A special type of computed tomography (CT) scan in which a small amount of a radioactive drug is injected into a vein and a scanner is used to make detailed images of areas inside the body where the radioactive material is taken up by the cells. SPECT can give information about blood flow to tissues and chemical reactions (metabolism) in the body.

SPIRAL CT SCAN – See Helical Computed Tomography and Computed Tomography.

NUCLEAR IMAGING

BONE SCAN – Also called BS. Generation of bone images on a computer screen or on film showing metastatic lytic (destructive) lesions or blastic (overgrowth of bone) lesions of bone. A small amount of radioactive material is injected into a blood vessel and travels through the bloodstream; it collects in the bones and is detected by a scanner.

BRAIN SCAN – Scan using radioisotopes injected intravenously to show location or size of a tumor and associated vascular structures within and around the brain.

GALLIUM SCAN – Radiographic imaging of the body that measures the amount of the radioisotope gallium concentrated in a specific part of the body. It is most useful in detecting nodal disease above the diaphragm. A gallium scan also may be done to determine whether cancer has spread (metastasized) to other areas of the body, or to monitor the effectiveness of cancer treatment. Also called: Gallium-67 scintigraphy, Ga67 scan, high dose (8-11 mCi) gallium scan.
Key words/possible involvement: area of increased density, area of enhanced contrast, area of high radioactivity, space occupying lesion, diffuse nodularity, decreased uptake, decreased activity
Other words/no involvement: no specific reference to visible abnormality of the organs in the abdomen, retroperitoneum, or pelvis

IMMUNOSCINTIGRAPHY – A procedure in which antibodies labeled with radioactive substances are given to the person. An image is taken of sites in the body where the antibody localizes.

KIDNEY SCAN – Examination of the structure of the kidneys after administration of a small dose of a radioactive substance. A scanner starts taking pictures when the substance reaches the major arteries and continues taking pictures about every 5 minutes for about half an hour.

LIVER/SPLEEN SCAN – Also called liver cell function scan, technetium scan of liver and spleen, gallium scan of liver. Radioisotope scan used to indicate the location or size of a tumor and associated vascular structures in and around liver/spleen.

LUNG SCAN – Examination of the lungs after administration of a small amount of harmless radioactive substance administered intravenously.

LYMPHOSCINTIGRAPHY – A method used to identify the sentinel lymph node (the first draining lymph node near a tumor). A radioactive substance that can be taken up by lymph nodes is injected at the site of the tumor, and a doctor follows the movement of this substance on a computer screen. Once the lymph nodes that have taken up the substance are identified, they can be removed and examined to see if they contain tumor cells. See also Sentinel Lymph Node Biopsy and Lymph Node Mapping in Pathology section.

MAMMOSCINTIGRAPHY – See Scintimammography.

MIBG SCINTIGRAPHY – A radioisotope (Iodine-131) scan done exclusively to diagnose neuroectodermally derived tumors (neuroblastoma, ganglioneuroma, pheochromocytoma) in childhood. Higher doses of radioisotope may be used as therapy.

MIBI SCAN, BREAST – See Scintimammography.

NUCLEAR SCAN – Also called nuclear medicine scan, radioactive scan, radioisotope scan, scintigraphy, scintigram, scintiscan, gamma camera. General term for a diagnostic imaging procedure that uses small amounts of radioactive materials to examine internal organs. The patient is

Nuclear Imaging, ***continued***

Nuclear scan, continued
injected with a liquid that contains the radioactive substance, which collects in the part of the body to be imaged. A sophisticated instrument (scanner) detects the radioactive substance in the body and processes that information into an image. Each type of tissue that may be scanned (including bones, organs, glands, and blood vessels) uses a different radioactive compound as a tracer. Examples of isotopes include Iodine-131, gallium, technetium Tc 99m dextran, technetium Tc99m sulfur colloid, and technetium Tc 99m pertechnetate.

PANCREAS SCAN – Examination of the pancreas after administration by intravenous injection of a small amount of radioactive substance.

PAROTID or SALIVARY GLAND SCAN – Used to detect blockage of the salivary gland ducts and tumors of the major salivary glands.
Key words/possible involvement: area of increased uptake, hotspot, area of decreased uptake, cold spot, space occupying lesion, mass, enlargement, metastases
Other words/no involvement: no specific reference to visible abnormality, blockage or tumor, as well as references to calcifications, vascular abnormalities, congenital anomalies, and other benign conditions

PROSTASCINT SCAN – similar to bone scan, but ProstaScint radioisotope tracer material locates prostate cells throughout body thereby identifying metastases in lymph nodes or soft tissues.

SCAN – A general term for special types of imaging. See Scan in Other Imaging Techniques section.

SCINTIGRAPHY (SCINTIGRAM, SCINTISCAN) – See Nuclear Scan.

SCINTIMAMMOGRAM – Also called scintimammography, breast MIBI scan, Miraluma test, Sestamibi breast imaging, mammoscintigraphy. A nuclear breast imaging test used as an adjunct to an abnormal mammography. Not used in place of a mammogram or for screening, but to provide further evaluation of a tumor in the breast. Detects cancer cells in the breasts of some women who have had abnormal mammograms, or who have dense breast tissue. The woman receives an injection of a small amount of technetium 99, which is taken up by cancer cells, and a gamma camera is used to take pictures of the breasts.

SESTAMIBI BREAST IMAGING – See Scintimammogram.

SOMATOSTATIN RECEPTOR SCINTIGRAPHY (SRS) – Also known as OctreoScan. The patient receives an intravenous injection of a radioisotope conjugated to octreotide, which attaches to neuroendocrine tumor cells. Then the patient is scanned for areas where the radioactivity has accumulated in the body. SRS is useful in diagnosing pancreatic endocrine tumors.

THYROID SCAN – Also called radionuclide scan, I-131 or I-123 scan, technetium-99m pertechnetate scan. Nuclear scan of thyroid gland usually using radioactive iodine. A diagnostic thyroid scan will use less than 10 millicuries of radioactive iodine; in contrast, a therapeutic dose is 100 millicuries or more.
Key words/possible involvement: area of decreased uptake, cold spot, cold nodule, nonfunctioning nodule, area of decreased concentration, mass, nodule, space occupying lesion
Other words/no involvement: no specific reference to visible abnormality, normal function, size, shape, and position, as well as references to vascular abnormalities, benign adenomas, congenital anomalies, and other benign conditions

ULTRASOUND

ULTRASOUND – A non-invasive technique to locate abnormalities in the pelvis or other areas by recording the patterns of sound waves reflected by tissues. Also called ultrasonography, echography, echogram, sonography, sonogram, gynecologic sonogram. The report is sometimes called a scan.
Key words/possible involvement: density, mass effect, area of increased attenuation, abnormal density, abnormal echo, adnexal mass, cystic mass
Other words/no involvement: no specific reference to mass, density, metastasis, or lesion

ABDOMINAL ULTRASOUND – A non-invasive technique to locate abnormalities in the abdomen by recording the patterns of sound waves reflected by tissues. Also called: ultrasonography, echography, sonography, abdominal ultrasonography, sonogram. Report is sometimes called a scan.
Key words/possible involvement: density, mass effect, area of increased attenuation, abnormal density, abnormal echo, cystic mass
Other words/no involvement: no specific reference to mass, density, metastasis, or lesion

BREAST ULTRASOUND – A non-invasive technique to locate abnormalities in the breast by recording the patterns of sound waves reflected by tissues. May improve diagnosis of breast cancer when used in conjunction with mammogram, especially in women with dense breasts. Helps distinguish cysts from solid masses; not used for routine screening. Also called ultrasonography, echography, sonography, sonogram.
Key words/possible involvement: complex cyst, density, mass effect, abnormal density, abnormal echo, fibrous nodule, microcalcifications
Other words/no involvement: simple cyst, no specific reference to mass, density, metastasis, or lesion

COLOR DOPPLER ULTRASOUND – Measures blood flow within organ based on theory that tumors have more blood vessels than surrounding normal tissue. Under clinical investigation for prostate cancer.

ENDOBRONCHIAL ULTRASOUND (EUS) – See also Endoscopic Ultrasound. The scope and transducer are placed in the bronchus to evaluate lymph nodes and other structures in the mediastinum.

ENDORECTAL ULTRASOUND (ERUS) – See Transrectal Ultrasound.

ENDOSCOPIC ESOPHAGEAL ULTRASOUND – See also Endoscopic Ultrasound and Endobronchial Ultrasound. Evaluates mediastinal lymph nodes by placing the scope and transducer in the esophagus.

ENDOSCOPIC ULTRASOUND (EUS) – Combines endoscopy and ultrasound in order to obtain images and information about the digestive tract and the surrounding tissue and organs. A transducer is placed on the end of the scope. It allows visualization of the layers of the intestinal wall, lymph nodes, and blood vessels. Endoscopic ultrasound is the best way to diagnose pancreatic cancer and can be used to clinically stage GI or lung tumors. Lymph nodes can be biopsied (FNA) through organ wall.

PELVIC ULTRASOUND – Also called ultrasonography, echography, sonography, abdominal ultrasonography, transabdominal pelvic ultrasound, gynecologic ultrasound, sonogram. A non-invasive technique to visualize abnormalities in the pelvis by recording the patterns of sound waves reflected by tissues. The report is sometimes called a scan.

Ultrasound, *continued*

Pelvic ultrasound, continued
Key words/possible involvement: density, mass effect, area of increased attenuation, abnormal density, abnormal echo, cystic mass, adnexal mass
Other words/no involvement: no specific reference to mass, density, metastasis, or lesion

PROSTATIC ULTRASOUND – See Transrectal Ultrasound.

RENAL ULTRASOUND – A non-invasive technique to locate abnormalities in the kidney and renal pelvis by recording the patterns of sound waves reflected by tissues. Also called ultrasonography, echography, sonography, kidney ultrasound, sonogram. The report is sometimes called a scan.
Key words/possible involvement: density, mass effect, area of increased attenuation, abnormal density, abnormal echo, cystic mass
Other words/no involvement: no specific reference to mass, density, metastasis, or lesion

SONOGRAM – Also called ultrasound or scintigraphy. General term for the visualization of deep structures of the body by recording the reflection of ultrasonic (sound) waves directed into the tissues; a non-invasive technique to locate abnormalities in the pelvis or other areas.

THYROID SONOGRAM – Also called thyroid ultrasonography, thyroid scintigraphy. Differentiates cysts from solid tumors in the thyroid.
Key words/possible involvement: area of decreased uptake, cold spot, cold nodule, nonfunctioning nodule, area of decreased echoes, irregular echoes, mass, nodule, space occupying lesion
Other words/no involvement: no specific reference to visible abnormality, normal size, shape, and position, as well as references to benign adenomas, cysts, congenital anomalies, and other benign conditions

TRANSABDOMINAL ULTRASOUND – A procedure used to examine the organs in the abdomen. The ultrasound device is pressed firmly against the skin of the abdomen. Sound waves from the device bounce off tissues to create echoes, and a computer uses the echoes to make a sonogram.

TRANSRECTAL ULTRASOUND – A non-invasive technique to locate areas of abnormality (usually carcinoma) within the prostate, to assess whether the prostatic capsule is intact, and to guide the needle for biopsy core samples to be taken. A probe inserted into the rectum sends out high-energy sound waves that bounce off internal tissues or organs and make echoes. The echoes form a picture of body tissues called a sonogram. Not a screening tool but assists during the biopsy. Also called prostatic ultrasound, TRUS, endorectal ultrasound, ERUS, ultrasonography, echography, sonography. Procedure cannot assess lymph node size, but may be useful in guiding needle biopsies.
Key words/possible involvement: density, mass effect, area of increased attenuation, abnormal density, abnormal echo, hypoechoic
Other words/no involvement: no specific reference to mass, density, metastasis, or lesion

TRANSVAGINAL SONOGRAM – Also called transvaginal ultrasound, TVS. A procedure used to examine the vagina, uterus, fallopian tubes, ovaries, and bladder using an internal vaginal probe in combination with ultrasound for the detection of ovarian cancer and other gynecologic abnormalities. The vaginal probe can visualize the ovaries on an ultrasound screen better than the traditional external abdominal probe. An instrument is inserted into the vagina, and sound waves bounce off organs inside the pelvic area. These sound waves create echoes, which a computer uses to create the sonogram. See Transrectal Ultrasound for key words.

ULTRASOUND OF TESTES (Testicular ultrasound) – Also called ultrasonography, echography, sonography. A non-invasive technique to locate areas of carcinoma within the testes and to assess whether the testicular capsule is intact. See Transrectal Ultrasound for key words.

ENDOSCOPIES

TYPES OF ENDOSCOPIES
(not all are described below)

Ano – Anus and rectum
Broncho – Bronchial tree (lung)
Colono – Colon
Colpo – Cervix and vagina
Culdo – Pelvic cavity (rectovaginal pouch)
Cysto – Bladder
Cystourethro – Bladder and urethra
Duodeno – Duodenum
Esophago – Esophagus
Esophagogastroduodeno – Esophagus, stomach and duodenum
Gastro – Stomach
Gonio – Anterior chamber of eye
Hystero – Uterus
Laparo – Abdominal cavity
Laryngo – Larynx
Mediastino – Mediastinum
Nasopharyngo – Nasopharynx
Opthalamo – Eye
Oto – Ear
Peritoneo – Peritoneum
Pleuro – Pleura
Procto – Rectum and rectosigmoid
Proctosigmoido – Rectum, rectosigmoid and sigmoid
Rhino – Nose, nasal cavity
Sigmoido – Sigmoid colon
Thoraco – Chest cavity
Uretero – Ureter
Ureteropylo – Ureter and renal pelvis
Urethro – Urethra
Vagino – Vagina

ENDOSCOPY – General term for examination of the inside of an organ or body cavity using a fiberoptic instrument. Some endoscopic procedures can be accomplished through natural openings in the body. Others must be performed through incisions into the body. The report should describe the condition of the organ with reference to swelling, blockage, lesions, growths, and other abnormalities.
Key words/possible involvement: mass or lesion visualized in the opening, or if a biopsy via the endoscope yields a diagnosis of malignancy, fixation; stricture, polyp, adenoma, lesion, neoplasm, malignancy, ulcer
Other words/no involvement: no abnormalities visualized during the examination , no strictures or foreign bodies; inflammatory process, foreign bodies, abscess, infectious process, or other benign conditions
Key information: largest size of tumor, gross description of tumor, presence of multiple tumors, degree of induration of ureteric wall, extension outside of organ

ANOSCOPY – Examination of the rectum using an anoscope to see inside the rectum; a smaller version of the sigmoidoscope.

BREAST DUCT ENDOSCOPY – A method used to examine the lining of the breast ducts to look for abnormal tissue. A very thin, flexible, lighted tube attached to a camera is inserted through the nipple, and threaded into the breast ducts deep in the breast. Tissue and fluid samples may be removed during the procedure.

BRONCHOSCOPY – Endoscopic visualization of the trachea and mainstem and lobar bronchi to evaluate tumor invasion from lung or esophagus using a lighted tube inserted into the lungs through the mouth. Bronchoscopy cannot evaluate peripheral lesions in the lung.
Key words/possible involvement: mass or lesion visualized in the bronchial tree, or if a biopsy via the bronchoscope yields a diagnosis of malignancy
Other words/no involvement: no abnormalities visualized during the examination

Fluorescence bronchoscopy – Also known as autofluorescence bronchoscopy. The bronchoscope uses a special fluorescent light rather than a normal endoscopic light. Abnormal areas in

Endoscopies, *continued*

Bronchoscopy, continued

the bronchi show as color differences that may not be visible under normal light, allowing earlier detection of cancer.

Virtual bronchoscopy – Non-invasive diagnostic procedure that uses 3-dimensional images created by CT scans to visualize bronchi, including areas of the lung beyond tumor blockages. However, abnormal areas cannot be biopsied with this imaging technique.

CHOLANGIOSCOPY – A newer technique to visualize and biopsy bile duct tumors using a very thin fiberoptic tube passed through after ERCP or through a needle placed in a liver bile duct.

COLONOSCOPY – Examination of the large intestine using a fiberoptic instrument. The report should describe the condition of the colon in the cecum, ascending, hepatic flexure, transverse, splenic flexure, and descending portions of the colon, in addition to the sigmoid and rectum. Colonoscopy generally examines the colon to a level of about 150 cm. Virtual colonoscopy: see Computed Tomography Colography in Other Imaging Techniques section.
Key words/possible involvement: stricture, polyps, villous adenoma, lesion, neoplasm, malignancy, ulcer, obstruction, perforation, blockage
Other words/no involvement: diverticulosis, megacolon, ulcerative colitis, Crohn's disease, inflammatory process, foreign bodies, abscess, or infectious process, or other benign conditions

COLPOSCOPY – Examination of the vagina and cervix through a colposcope, an instrument containing a magnifying lens that is inserted into the vagina.
Key words/possible involvement: lesion, tumor, leukoplakia, whitish areas of epithelium, gray area, area of discoloration, bleeding, mosaic pattern, mosaic staining, Toluidine staining, Iodine staining, irregular blood vessels, infiltrated patches, atypical epithelium, abnormal epithelium, suspicious lesion, neoplasm, malignancy, ulceration, exophytic lesion, infiltration
Other words/no involvement: no abnormalities visualized during the examination

CULDOSCOPY – Visual examination of the female pelvic viscera by means of an endoscope introduced through the posterior vaginal wall into that part of the pelvic cavity known as the rectovaginal pouch or cul-de-sac. The cul-de-sac is also called the rectouterine pouch, an extension of the peritoneal cavity between the rectum and back wall of the uterus.

CYSTOSCOPY – Examination of the interior of the bladder and urethra using a fiberoptic instrument. May be performed for a fixed or highly invasive rectal tumor to assess involvement of bladder; usually not performed for colon tumors. May be done in the doctor's office.
Key words/possible involvement: bullous edema, lesion, tumor invasion, extrinsic mass, tumor infiltration, invasion of bladder mucosa, extension of tumor into bladder wall
Other words/no involvement: no reference to tumor or abnormality in the bladder

Fluorescence cystoscopy – The chemical porphyrin is instilled into the bladder via cystoscope and is taken up by cancer cells. The chemical fluoresces (glows) under a special light, identifying areas of cancer cells that may not be visible under normal light.

CYSTOURETHROSCOPY – Examination of the bladder and urethra using a fiberoptic instrument.

DUODENOSCOPY – Endoscopic visualization of the upper portion of the small intestine (duodenum) (see also esophagogastroduodenoscopy).

ERCP (ENDOSCOPIC RETROGRADE CHOLANGIOPANCREATOGRAPHY) – Evaluation of the gallbladder and pancreas using contrast material instilled in the duodenum or ampulla of Vater via an endoscope.

Endoscopies, *continued*

ERCP, continued
Key words/possible involvement: hypervascularity, stricture, extrinsic mass, lesion, neoplasm, malignancy, opacification, nonvisualization, stones, stenosis
Other words/no involvement: no specific reference to visible abnormality in the organ; inflammatory process, foreign bodies, or other benign conditions

ESOPHAGOGASTRODUODENOSCOPY (EGD) – Visualization of esophagus, stomach and small intestine (duodenum) as part of a single procedure.

ESOPHAGOSCOPY – Endoscopic visualization of the esophagus to evaluate invasion from a lung or stomach tumor.

GASTROSCOPY – Endoscopic visualization of the stomach to evaluate invasion from other organs.

HYSTEROSCOPY – Examination of the uterus using a fiberoptic instrument.
Key words/possible involvement: tumor, leukoplakia, whitish areas of epithelium, irregular blood vessels, infiltrated patches, atypical epithelium, abnormal epithelium, suspicious lesion, neoplasm, malignancy
Other words/no involvement: no abnormalities visualized during the examination

LAPAROSCOPY – Examination of the inside of the abdomen using a fiberoptic instrument. The report should describe the condition of organs in the abdomen with reference to swelling, blockage, lesions, growths, and other abnormalities.
Key words/possible involvement: mass, lesion, abnormal lymph nodes, seeding, salt and pepper, talcum powder appearance, nodules, caking, implants, encasement, frozen pelvis, matted organs
Other words/no involvement: no abnormalities visualized during the examination; adhesions

LARYNGOSCOPY – Endoscopic visualization of the larynx to evaluate for a head and neck primary tumor, to determine a cause for vocal cord paralysis other than recurrent laryngeal nerve paralysis due to involvement by lung cancer, or to determine invasion from esophagus.
Key words/possible involvement: evidence of inflammation, injury, strictures, tumors, signs of scar tissue, abnormal movement, or signs of paralysis
Other words/no involvement: foreign body in larynx, no abnormalities visualized during the examination

MEDIASTINOSCOPY – An invasive endoscopic procedure to biopsy the lymph nodes in the mediastinum by means of a bronchoscope inserted through an incision in the base of the neck.
Key words/possible involvement: mass, lesion, or abnormal lymph nodes visualized in the mediastinum, or if a biopsy of the mediastinum yields a diagnosis of malignancy
Other words/no involvement: no abnormalities visualized during the examination

NASOPHARYNGOSCOPY – Endoscopic visualization of the nasopharynx and pharynx to evaluate region for primary or secondary malignancy.

PANENDOSCOPY – See Triple Endoscopy.

PERITONEOSCOPY – Endoscopic examination of the peritoneum done via laparoscope.
Key words/possible involvement: mass, lesion, abnormal lymph nodes, nodules, encasement, frozen pelvis, matted organs
Other words/no involvement: no abnormalities visualized during the examination; adhesions

Endoscopies, *continued*

PROCTOSIGMOIDOSCOPY – Examination of the lower portion of the large intestine (sigmoid and rectum) using a fiberoptic instrument. Also called proctoscopy, sigmoidoscopy, rigid sigmoidoscopy. Proctosigmoidoscopy generally describes the condition of the lower colon to a level of 12 inches or 31 cm, or to 60 cm, depending on the instrument used.
Key words/possible involvement: stricture, polyps, villous adenoma, lesion, neoplasm, malignancy, invasion of rectal mucosa, extension of tumor into rectal wall
Other words/no involvement: diverticulosis, megacolon, ulcerative colitis, Crohn's disease, inflammatory process, foreign bodies, abscess, or infectious process, or other benign conditions

SIGMOIDOSCOPY – Also called proctoscopy, proctosigmoidoscopy, flexible sigmoidoscopy. Examination of the lower portion of the large intestine (sigmoid and rectum) using a fiberoptic instrument. Sigmoidoscopy generally describes the condition of the lower colon to a level of 12 inches or 31 cm, or to 60 cm, depending on the instrument used. See also Colonoscopy.
Key words/possible involvement: stricture, polyps, villous adenoma, lesion, neoplasm, malignancy
Other words/no involvement: diverticulosis, megacolon, ulcerative colitis, Crohn's disease, inflammatory process, foreign bodies, abscess, or infectious process, or other benign conditions

THORACOSCOPY – Also called pleural endoscopy. Endoscopic visualization of the thoracic cavity.

TRIPLE ENDOSCOPY (also called panendoscopy) – Combination procedure that examines the trachea, larynx, pharynx and esophagus via endoscopic visualization; used to investigate all mucosal surfaces of the upper respiratory tract and for second primaries.

URETEROSCOPY – Examination of the renal pelvis and ureters using a fiberoptic instrument (usually performed under general anesthesia).

VAGINOSCOPY – Examination of tissue of the vagina by use of a magnifying lens inserted into the vagina.

VIRTUAL COLONOSCOPY – See Computed Tomography Colography in Other Imaging Techniques section.

OPERATIVE PROCEDURES

Key information: exact location of tumor, especially helpful in colorectal cancer; surgeon's comments on involvement of adjacent organs and structures; fixation of tumor; invasion of major blood vessels; physical description of organ (hard, leathery, wine sack appearance); depth of organ cavity, for example, "sounding" of uterus; tumor encompassing nerves or blood vessels; fixed or matted lymph nodes; tissues or areas involved that are not included in the pathology specimen, names of organs or tissues removed; number, site, and involvement of lymph nodes removed; anatomic site and name of all involved lymph nodes not removed during the resection; site and description of any gross tumor not removed, any tumor on or in the liver that is not biopsied, appearance and size of organ, extent of involvement of other organs in same body cavity tumor implants, seeding, implants, talcum powder appearance, encasement, nodularity of viscera, frozen pelvis, which organs were removed, results of examination under anesthesia

OPERATIVE APPROACHES (The approach does not change the surgical treatment code.)
Open – an operation performed through an incision in the skin
Laparoscopic – also called minimally invasive surgery, "bandaid" surgery, pinhole surgery, or keyhole surgery; performing a surgery using lighted instruments inserted through small openings in

Operative Procedures, ***continued***

Operative approaches, continued
the abdominal wall rather than a large open incision; surgery performed via endoscopy—see also Endoscopies section of this chapter.
Robotic – minimally invasive surgery performed using robotic tools where the surgeon is viewing the surgical field on a video screen and manipulating the tools at a physical distance from the patient; nurses and surgical techs remain beside the patient to aid the surgeon. Robotic procedures can even be performed remotely (telesurgery) from miles away. The best known brand is DaVinci.

ANTERIOR MEDIASTINOTOMY – Also called Chamberlain procedure. A tube is inserted into the chest through an incision next to the sternum to view structures in the mediastinum between the sternum and heart and get tissue from the lymph nodes on the left side of the chest.

EXAMINATION UNDER ANESTHESIA – Also called EUA. Bimanual examination of the pelvis and external abdomen while patient is anesthetized, using one hand in the pelvis and the other hand to press on the organs externally. See also Bimanual Examination of Bladder in Physical Exam section.

EXPLORATORY LAPAROTOMY – Also called laparotomy. Evaluation of the contents of the abdomen for the purpose of determining the extent of disease. Exploratory laparotomy is performed through an incision in the abdomen.

INTRAOPERATIVE EVALUATION OF DIAPHRAGM – Visual and manual inspection of the diaphragm, particularly the right leaf, during laparotomy for treatment of ovarian cancer. Optimally, the intraoperative evaluation of the diaphragm should occur prior to any dissection of pelvic organs. Evaluation of the diaphragm is an important part of accurate staging of ovarian cancer.

MEDIASTINOTOMY – Examination of the area under the aorta (main artery leaving the heart). A small incision is made to the right or left of the sternum, and some rib cartilage is removed. The doctor can then view lymph nodes and remove for biopsy.

SECOND LOOK LAPAROTOMY – Also called second look operation, second look procedure, second look surgery. A surgical procedure in the abdomen performed for women with ovarian cancer and, on rare occasion, in other cancers and disorders. The surgery is done after a period of treatment to assess results and plan possible future treatment. May be done for diagnostic purposes, to evaluate treatment's effectiveness, and to determine if a tumor, which had been inoperable, has been sufficiently reduced by the treatment so that it can be removed. A second look operation for ovarian cancer is not coded as first course of treatment.

STAGING LAPAROTOMY – Evaluation of the contents of the abdomen for the purpose of determining the extent of disease. A staging laparotomy is not routinely done for Hodgkin lymphoma, unless the opportunity for obtaining better staging information exceeds the risk of operative morbidity. An adequate staging laparotomy includes abdominal exploration, wedge and needle biopsies of the liver, multiple lymph node biopsies, bone marrow biopsy, and splenectomy. Staging laparotomy is considered a diagnostic procedure rather than surgical treatment. The staging laparotomy is an opportunity to identify landmarks within the abdomen, such as unresectable large nodes or the splenic pedicle, which will affect the design of radiation treatment for the patient. Precise staging is important for Hodgkin lymphoma and to a lesser extent non-Hodgkin lymphoma.

STAGING PROCEDURES FOR OVARY – Adequate staging procedures during laparotomy should include evaluation of the undersurface of the diaphragm, pelvic and abdominal peritoneum biopsies, pelvic and paraaortic lymph node biopsies, peritoneal washings, and biopsies of any suspicious nodules or masses. The surgeon's report should reflect the results of these procedures.

Operative Procedures, ***continued***

SURGICAL STAGING OF TESTIS – Radical orchiectomy with laparotomy and removal of bilateral retroperitoneal lymph nodes (also called retroperitoneal lymphadenectomy) to determine the histologic cell type, remove the primary tumor, and evaluate the lymph nodes of the retroperitoneum. Surgical staging also provides debulking of tumor if lymph nodes are positive.

THORACOTOMY – Exploratory surgical procedure in which the chest is opened to inspect the heart, lungs, and mediastinal contents. Thoracotomy does not necessarily include removal of tissue.

VIDEO-ASSISTED THORACIC SURGERY (VATS) – Removal of small, early stage, peripheral lung cancers using a minimally invasive surgical technique consisting of three incisions, one for a video camera to visualize the surgical area on a monitor and two for the surgical instruments. Recovery is faster than for a thoracotomy with similar cure rates.

PATHOLOGY

See also Operative Procedures, which may yield tissue for pathologic examination

Key information from the pathology report: cell type and grade; behavior of tumor (in situ, microinvasive, invasive, infiltrating, malignant, cervical intraepithelial neoplasia); Gleason's grade or score for prostate, Bloom-Richardson score for breast, Fuhrman grade for kidney; location within organ, exact location within specimen; presence of multiple tumors in organ; number of microscopic foci (if tumor is occult); exact size of lesion (not the size of specimen); invasion of blood vessels and/or lymphatic channels within specimen; invasion of capsule; depth of invasion (mucosa, musculature, supporting tissues); involvement of surgical margins and serosal surface of organ; names of structures and organs removed; size and number of lymph nodes involved (ipsilateral or contralateral, including micrometastases); number and location of uninvolved lymph nodes; results of biopsies of possible metastatic sites; whether tumor arose in adenomatous polyp, villous adenoma or tubular adenoma; distance from tumor to edge of resected specimen (proximal, distal and radial margins); intraluminal extension (for example, extension along inner surface to contiguous segments of colon); location and number of lymph nodes positive and number of nodes pathologically examined; extension to adjacent tissues (peritoneum, serosa, omentum, mesentery adjacent fat, adjacent organs); depth of penetration of tumor through organ wall; involvement of other organs (surface vs parenchymal); biopsy results of any additional tumor sites noted during operation
Key words/possible involvement: any diagnosis of malignancy; evidence of tumor, lesion, mass, neoplastic tissue, atypical epithelium, gray, necrotic, or friable tissue, chunky material
Other words/no involvement: no reference to malignancy in the cells or tissues examined

ABDOMINAL WASHINGS – Instillation of approximately 200 ml. of saline solution into the abdomen during laparotomy. After the solution is allowed to contact surfaces in the abdomen for about five minutes, it is aspirated and sent for cytologic examination. This procedure is used to determine whether tumor is present in the abdomen in the absence of ascites.

ASPIRATION – Also called aspiration biopsy, aspiration cytology. Removal of fluid or a small sample of tissue cells for microscopic examination using a needle to suction fluid, cells, or tissue into a syringe. Biopsy of material (fluid, cells, or tissue) obtained by suction through a needle attached to syringe. See also Needle Aspiration and Biopsy.

AUTOPSY – Also called necropsy, post-mortem examination. Specimens from all the major organs and systems of a deceased patient are examined (gross and microscopic) unless the autopsy is restricted to certain organs.

Pathology, *continued*

BIOPSY – Includes aspiration, bone marrow, cone, core, core needle aspiration, curettage, excisional, fine needle aspiration, frozen section, incisional, percutaneous needle, permanent section, punch, sponge, stereotactic, suction, surface, surgical, total, transperineal, transrectal, wide core. General term for removal of a sample of live tissue for microscopic examination. A biopsy generally does not remove the gross tumor. An incisional biopsy removes only enough cancer tissue to confirm the diagnosis, leaving gross tumor in the patient's body. Removal and examination, gross and microscopic, of tissue or cells from the living body for the purpose of diagnosis.

BLADDER WASHINGS – Instillation of saline solution into the bladder during cystoscopy. After the solution is allowed to contact surfaces in the area for about five minutes, it is aspirated and sent for cytologic examination. This procedure is used to determine whether tumor is present in the absence of visible tumor.

BONE MARROW ASPIRATION – Also called bone tap. A procedure to remove cells from the bone marrow, usually before a bone marrow biopsy is taken, to determine involvement by tumor. After the skin is anesthetized, the aspirate needle is inserted into the bone, and a syringe is used to withdraw the liquid bone marrow. If this is performed, the needle will be removed and either repositioned, or another needle may be used for the biopsy. This procedure is optional in low stage lymphoma cases. Bilateral (may be done unilaterally) bone marrow biopsies and aspirations should be done for higher stage and symptomatic lymphoma cases. May also be diagnostic of bone metastases from carcinoma.

BONE MARROW BIOPSY – May also be called bone tap. Removal of tissue from bone marrow using a biopsy needle inserted into the bone. The core of the needle will then be removed, and the needle is pressed forward and rotated in both directions, forcing a tiny sample of the bone marrow into the needle. The needle is then removed, pressure is applied to the biopsy site to stop bleeding, and a bandage is applied.

Bone marrow histochemistry – Microscopic examination of the bone marrow using special staining techniques to determine subclassification of the leukemia. Histochemistry of the bone marrow is a laboratory study performed in addition to the standard histologic analysis of the specimen.

Bone marrow test – Examination of the bone marrow.

Bone marrow trephine – Examination of a circular disc of bone and bone marrow.

BRONCHIAL WASHINGS – Includes bronchial washings, aspirations, bronchial brushings obtained through a bronchoscope.

BRUSHINGS – Also called exfoliative cytology. Cells are obtained by passing a small brush through an endoscopy tube and scraping cells from the lesion. This tissue is analyzed cytologically.

CEREBROSPINAL FLUID (CSF) STUDIES – Cytologic analysis of cerebrospinal fluid for detection of bacteria, fungi, and malignant cells, as well as protein and glucose values.

CLOSED CHEST NEEDLE BIOPSY – Includes skinny-needle biopsy of chest, fine needle aspiration (FNA), CT scan guided biopsy. This procedure is performed by inserting a long needle through the surface of the chest to penetrate the lung cavity. Fluid suitable for cytologic analysis is drawn up into the needle, which is then withdrawn from the chest. Excludes any procedure requiring incision into chest cavity.

CONIZATION – Also called cone biopsy, surgical conization, cold knife conization. Procedure to remove a cone-shaped piece of tissue from the cervix and cervical canal. Conization may be used to diagnose or treat a cervical condition. See also Loop Electrocautery Excision Procedure.

Pathology, *continued*

CORE BIOPSY – Similar to needle biopsy, but a larger needle is used to remove a piece of tissue rather than a tiny sampling of cells. A sample of the tumor is removed, but not the whole tumor. Core biopsies include ultrasound-guided core biopsy and stereotactic biopsy.

CULDOCENTESIS – Procedure in which a doctor inserts a needle through the vaginal wall and removes fluid from the space surrounding the ovaries for microscopic examination.

CURETTAGE – Removal of growths or other material by scraping with a curette. See also Dilatation and Curettage.

CYTOGENETIC STUDIES – Also called chromosome studies. Cytogenetics involves the study of human chromosomes in health and disease and is a fusion science that joins cytology (the study of cells) with genetics (the study of inherited variation). Chromosome studies have traditionally been an important laboratory diagnostic procedure in prenatal diagnosis, in certain patients with mental retardation and multiple birth defects, in patients with abnormal sexual development, and in some cases of infertility or multiple miscarriages. Cytogenetic analysis is also useful in the study and treatment of patients with malignancies and hematologic disorders. Newer techniques allow for increased resolution of chromosome banding patterns, permitting differentiation of a greater number of abnormalities.

CYTOLOGY – Microscopic examination of body fluid for malignant cells; aspiration (fine or skinny needle) of a cyst or tumor, cells or fluid from a mass or lymph node; also pleural effusion (thoracentesis) or ascites (paracentesis); procedures include endoscopic brushings or washings of ulcerated areas, Pap smears; cytology of vaginal, cervical, endometrial and/or abdominal fluid.

CYTOREDUCTIVE SURGERY (Debulking) – Also called tumor reduction surgery. Surgical removal of as much macroscopic ovarian tumor as possible in the pelvis and abdomen to reduce the size of the largest residual tumor so that the effect of postoperative chemotherapy or radiation is maximized. Residual disease after debulking refers to the size of the largest tumor mass left in the pelvis and abdomen. Optimal debulking reduces the size of the largest individual residual tumor nodule to less than 1.0 cm in greatest dimension (also called minimal residual). So-called suboptimal debulking results in individual residual tumor nodule(s) more than 1.0 cm in size (also called macroscopic residual). The effectiveness of postoperative adjuvant radiation and chemotherapy is increased when the tumor burden is smallest. See also Omentectomy, a separate procedure.

DEBULKING – See Cytoreductive Surgery

DILATATION AND CURETTAGE (D & C) – Also called D and C. Dilation of the cervix and scraping or aspirating the contents for cytologic examination.

DUCTAL LAVAGE CYTOLOGY – A method used to collect cells from milk ducts in the breast. A hair-size catheter (tube) is inserted into the nipple, and a small amount of salt water is released into the duct. The water picks up breast cells, and is removed. The cells are checked under a microscope. Ductal lavage may be used in addition to clinical breast examination and mammography to detect breast cancer. Results of the test should not be used as absolute evidence for the presence or absence of breast carcinoma. The results of this test should only be as an adjunct to standard breast cancer detection methods including mammography and physical examination.

ENDOCERVICAL CURETTAGE – The scraping of the mucous membrane of the cervical canal using a spoon-shaped instrument called a curette. See also Fractional Curettage

Pathology, *continued*

ENDOMETRIAL or PELVIC WASHINGS – Instillation of saline solution into a body cavity to evaluate for occult tumor. After the solution is allowed to contact surfaces in the area for about five minutes, it is aspirated and sent for cytologic examination.

ENDOSCOPIC BIOPSY – Removal of tissue for microscopic examination by means of an endoscope (a fiberoptic cable for viewing inside the body), which is inserted into the body along with sampling instruments. The endoscope allows the physician to visualize the abnormality and guide the sampling.

EXCISIONAL BIOPSY – Also called surgical, total, or open biopsy. The purpose of an excisional biopsy is to attempt to remove the entire mass or a large portion of the mass for therapeutic as well as diagnostic purposes. The tissue that is removed is then sent to the pathologist for diagnosis. See also Biopsy. ***Note***: Read the body of the operative report carefully. Frequently surgeons will title the report "biopsy" but the report will describe an excisional biopsy and the intent of the procedure was to excise the entire lesion.

FISH (Fluorescent In Situ Hybridization) – See Fluorescent In Situ Hybridization in the Tumor Markers section.

FNA – See Needle Aspiration and Biopsy

FRACTIONAL CURETTAGE – Separate scraping of material from the endocervix and walls of uterus in a set order to determine which site may be the source of the malignancy. This is the preferred diagnostic procedure for endometrial cancer.

FROZEN SECTION – Also called FS. Biopsy specimens quickly frozen, thinly sliced, and examined to determine the presence or absence of cancer cells while the patient is still undergoing a procedure.

H&E (Hematoxylin and Eosin) – The standard stains applied to tumor cells; the most common pathology staining technique used to detect cancer cells. Also called routine stains or standard stains. Hematoxylin stains the nucleus of a cell blue, and eosin stains the cytoplasm pink. A pathologist can look at the proportion of nucleus to cytoplasm and make a determination about the cell's malignant potential.

HISTOLOGIC EXAMINATION – Also called tissue examination, histology. Microscopic examination of tissues removed from the site of a suspected cancer. The examination includes gross (description based on visual examination) microscopic (description based on histologic examination), and pathologic diagnosis (defining the disease).

IMMUNOHISTOCHEMISTRY (IHC) – A generic term for a pathologic examination technique that uses tumor specific antibodies linked to a dye. The antibodies react with antigens located on the surface of tumor cells and allow for detection of even single cells within a microscopic slide. This technique is used to examine regional lymph nodes of the breast that have been found to contain no tumor by standard stains (see H & E) but may contain isolated tumor cells or micrometastases. Other names for immunohistochemistry include immunocytochemistry, immunochemistry, keratin IHC staining, pankeratin, cytokeratin, A1/A3 or A1/3 (a specific stain), MNF116, and CAM 5.2.

INCISIONAL BIOPSY – Incomplete removal of living tissue for the purpose of diagnostic study. An incisional biopsy is different from an excisional biopsy because the surgeon does not attempt to remove the entire mass. The tissue is then examined under a microscope. See also Biopsy.

Pathology, *continued*

LARGE LOOP EXCISION OF THE TRANSFORMATION ZONE (LLETZ) – Procedure to obtain a cone biopsy of the transformation zone of the cervix using a loop of wire heated by electrical current. Similar to LEEP procedure below but targeting a different area of cervix. See also Conization.

LOOP ELECTROCAUTERY EXCISION PROCEDURE (LEEP) – Procedure to obtain a cone biopsy of the exocervix (cervical os) using a loop of wire heated by electrical current. Recovery tends to be faster than from a cold knife conization. See also Conization.

LUMBAR PUNCTURE – See Spinal Tap.

LYMPH NODE ASPIRATION – Biopsy procedure using a thin needle to take a sample of tissue or fluid from a lymph node. The procedure is also called fine needle aspiration. See also Needle Aspiration and Biopsy.

LYMPH NODE MAPPING – Also called lymphatic mapping, lymphoscintigraphy. The use of dyes and radioactive substances to identify lymph nodes that may contain tumor cells. See also Sentinel Lymph Node Biopsy.

LYMPHADENECTOMY – Surgical removal and examination of several lymph nodes to evaluate the extent of disease.

MICROSTAGING – A technique used to help determine the stage (extent) of melanoma and certain squamous cell cancers. A sample of skin that contains tumor tissue is examined under a microscope to find out how thick the tumor is and/or how deeply the tumor has grown into the skin or connective tissues. See also Mohs Surgery.

MOHS SURGERY – A microscopically controlled excision of a lesion where each bit of tissue removed is mapped and examined under the microscope to determine the site and extent of malignant cells before more tissue is removed. See also Microstaging.

NEEDLE ASPIRATION AND BIOPSY – Includes skinny-needle biopsy, fine needle aspiration (FNA), intraoperative fine needle aspiration (IOFNA), closed chest needle biopsy. This procedure is performed by inserting a needle through the surface into the questionable mass. Fluid suitable for cytologic analysis is drawn up into the needle, which is then withdrawn from the mass, and examined microscopically.

NEEDLE LOCALIZATION – Also called needle-localized biopsy, wire localization. A procedure that uses very thin needles or guide wires to mark the location of a small, suspicious area on the breast identified during mammography so that a biopsy can be performed. Needle localization is used when the doctor cannot feel the mass of abnormal tissue.

OMENTECTOMY – Surgical removal of the omentum, the fatty covering in the anterior abdomen, usually performed in the presence of ovarian cancer but may be done with uterine or GI cancers. The omentum can then be examined for nonpalpable metastases. This may be either a partial (infracolic) or complete omentectomy.

OPEN BIOPSY – A procedure in which a surgical incision (cut) is made through the skin to expose and remove tissues. The biopsy tissue is examined under a microscope by a pathologist. An open biopsy may be done in the doctor's office or in the hospital, and may use local anesthesia or general anesthesia. A lumpectomy to remove a breast tumor is a type of open biopsy. See also Biopsy.

Pathology, *continued*

PAP SMEAR – Also called Papanicolaou's smear. Aspiration, scraping or brushing of the cervix for cytologic evaluation. PAP smear is not a reliable method for ruling out endometrial cancer when used by itself, but can be diagnostic for cervical cancer.

PARACENTESIS – Also called peritoneocentesis. Removal of fluid from abdomen for cytologic analysis by inserting a long-needle syringe into the abdominal cavity. Surgical puncture of a cavity for aspiration of fluids, such as the abdominal cavity.

PELVIC LYMPHADENECTOMY – Also called staging lymphadenectomy, pelvic lymph node dissection. A procedure during which the lymph nodes of the pelvis are removed for evaluation. May also be performed via a laparoscope.

PERCUTANEOUS BIOPSY – A biopsy in which the needle goes through the skin. See also Biopsy.

PERITONEAL/PELVIC WASHINGS – Instillation of saline solution into a body cavity to evaluate for occult tumor. After the solution is allowed to contact surfaces in the area for about five minutes, it is aspirated and sent for cytologic examination.

PERMANENT SECTION – Preparation of tissue for microscopic examination. The tissue is soaked in formaldehyde, processed in various chemicals, surrounded by a block of wax, sliced very thin, attached to a microscope slide and stained. The process usually takes one to two days. Permanent sections provide a clear view of the tissue sample so that the presence or absence of cancer can be determined. See also Frozen Section.

PUNCH BIOPSY – Biopsy of material obtained from the body tissue usually a skin lesion) by a punch technique. See also Biopsy.

REVERSE TRANSCRIPTASE POLYMERASE CHAIN REACTION (RT-PCR) – A molecular biologic technique that produces millions of specific parts of a tissue's genetic code in order to detect abnormalities such as malignant transformation. See also Immunohistochemistry for a different method of detecting small amounts of malignant tumor.

SCRAPINGS – The procedure of scraping the lining of a structure with an instrument for the purpose of obtaining cells.

SENTINEL LYMPH NODE BIOPSY – Also called sentinel lymph node mapping, SLNB, sentinel node biopsy, lymphoscintigraphy. The use of dyes and radioactive substances to identify the first lymph node(s) to which cancer is likely to spread from the primary tumor. Cancer cells may appear first in the sentinel node before spreading to other lymph nodes and other places in the body. To identify the sentinel lymph node(s), the surgeon injects a radioactive substance, blue dye, or both near the tumor. The surgeon then uses a scanner to find the sentinel lymph node(s) containing the radioactive substance or looks for the lymph node(s) stained with dye. When a node is identified, it is removed and examined for cancer cells.

SHAVE BIOPSY – Removal of a small amount of skin to examine microscopically for cancer cells. If the biopsy is positive and all cancer has been removed, this can also be treatment. See also Biopsy.

SPINAL TAP – Also called lumbar puncture, L. P. Removal of a small amount of cerebrospinal fluid for microscopic examination for cancer cells or other conditions. A needle is put into the lower part of the spinal column to collect cerebrospinal fluid or to give anticancer drugs intrathecally.

Pathology, *continued*

SPLENECTOMY – Surgical removal of the spleen. Splenectomy may occur as part of a full staging laparotomy or occasionally as a separate procedure. Unsuspected Hodgkin lymphoma is found in about 25% of splenectomy specimens.

SPONGE BIOPSY – Removal of material (cells, particles of tissue, and tissue juices) by rubbing a sponge over a lesion or over a mucous membrane for examination. See also Biopsy.

SPUTUM CYTOLOGY – A specimen of lung secretions obtained by deep cough and spit out for cytologic examination.

STEREOTACTIC NEEDLE BIOPSY – Also called stereotactic percutaneous needle biopsy, stereotactic biopsy. A precise method of sampling a small region of brain tissue using three-dimensional image guidance and minimally invasive techniques. Through only a skin puncture and tiny bone opening, an instrument is accurately passed into a brain lesion in order to determine its nature. This approach is often used to diagnose brain tumors or other disorders. CT or MRI guidance is used.

SURFACE BIOPSY – Scraping of cells from surface epithelium, especially from the cervix, for microscopic examination. See also Biopsy.

THORACENTESIS – Also called chest tapping, pleural tap, paracentesis thoracic, paracentesis pulmonis. Removal of part of an abnormal collection of fluid from the pleural cavity for cytologic analysis by inserting a long needle-syringe instrument into the pleural cavity.

TRANSRECTAL/TRANSPERINEAL NEEDLE BIOPSY – Includes standard needle biopsy, core biopsy, skinny-needle biopsy, fine needle aspiration (FNA). Sometimes called a sextant biopsy because needle biopsies are taken from all regions of the prostate, but may include more than six cores of tissue. Excludes any procedure requiring incision or transurethral approach. This procedure is performed by inserting a needle through the perineum (external) or via the rectum through the rectal wall to penetrate areas of nodularity or induration of the prostate. Fluid or tissue suitable for pathologic analysis is drawn up into the needle, which is withdrawn from the prostate. Multiple random needle biopsies may be performed to determine if tumor is multifocal. TRUS for prostate is not a cytology report.

ULTRASOUND-GUIDED BIOPSY – A biopsy procedure that uses an ultrasound imaging device to find an abnormal area of tissue and guide its removal for examination under a microscope. See also Biopsy.

URINE CYTOLOGY – Cytologic examination of urinary sediment for malignant cells; fine needle aspiration of a cyst or tumor (detects 70% of bladder cancers).

VACUUM ASPIRATION – Also called endometrial aspiration, vaginal pool aspiration, aspiration curettage, vacuum curettage. Extraction of tissue from the uterine lining, by suction, for examination.

WASHINGS – Instillation of approximately 200 ml. of saline solution into the abdomen or pelvis during laparotomy. After the solution is allowed to contact surfaces in the area for about five minutes, it is aspirated and sent for cytologic examination. This procedure is used to determine whether tumor is present in the abdomen in the absence of ascites.

LABORATORY TESTS

LABORATORY TEST (Lab Test) – A general term for a medical procedure that involves testing a sample of blood, urine, or other substance from the body. Tests can help determine a diagnosis, plan treatment, check to see if treatment is working, or monitor the disease over time.
Key information: Any diagnosis of malignancy; record date and type of any positive or elevated lab tests pertinent to the primary site or assessment of metastases.

ALKALINE PHOSPHATASE – Also called alk phos, alk, ALP. May be included in blood chemistry screening panel. Normal range: 20-90 I.U./liter. Normal range may vary somewhat according to the brand of laboratory assay materials used.

BILIRUBIN – Part of liver function tests. Substance formed when red blood cells are broken down. Bilirubin is part of the bile, which is made in the liver and is stored in the gallbladder. The abnormal buildup of bilirubin causes jaundice. Elevated bilirubin is indicative of obstruction of the gallbladder or of hepatic disease that affects the function of the liver.

BUN (BLOOD UREA NITROGEN) – Chemistry study of blood serum to measure the level of urea in the blood, a sign of impaired kidney function or urinary obstruction. Normal range: 10-15 mg/100 ml.

CBC (COMPLETE BLOOD COUNT) WITH PLATELETS – Also called multichannel chemistry, blood test. CBC consists of several tests on blood serum to measure distribution of leukocyte cell types in circulating blood and check the number of red blood cells, white blood cells, and platelets in a sample of blood. Helps distinguish benign disease from leukemia. Non-specific; not usually diagnostic of leukemia without confirmation by examination of bone marrow specimen. The platelet count is usually ordered separately. The table that follows indicates the portions of the CBC relevant to malignancies.

Test	Normal Values
White Blood Count (WBC)	5,000-10,000 total WBC
Differential white cell count (Diff)	
Neutrophils PMNs, polys, segs)	60-70% total WBC
Eosinophils	1-4% total leukocyte count
Basophils	0.5-1% total leukocyte count
Monocytes	2-6% total leukocyte count
Lymphocytes	20-40% total leukocyte count
Red Blood Count (RBC)	3.6-5.0 million/cu.mm. (F) 4.2-5.4 million/cu.mm. (M)
Hematocrit (Hct)	37-47%
Hemoglobin (Hgb)	12-16 g/100 ml. (F) 14-18 g/100 ml. (M)
Red Blood Cell Indices	
Mean Corpuscular Volume (MCV)	87-103 cu.micrograms/red cell
Mean Corpuscular Hemoglobin (MCH)	27-32 picograms
Mean Corpuscular Hemoglobin Concentration (MCHC)	32-36%
Stained Red Cell Examination	Normocytic, normochromic
Platelet Count	150,000-300,000/cu.mm.

Lab Tests, *continued*

CHEMISTRY SCREENING PANEL – Also called blood chemistries, SMA-12, SMAC-6, ACA, MSSP, CP, and many other names, usually based on the piece of equipment in use. All are automatic blood analyzers that measure different chemistries. SMA is simultaneous multiple analysis. The blood chemistry panel consists of 12 to 20 tests:

Test	Normal Values
Total protein (TP)	6-8 g/dl
Albumin (Alb.)	4-4.5 g%
Calcium (CA+)	Total: 9-11 mg/dl
Inorganic phosphorus (Inor. Phos.)	2.5-4.8 mg/dl
Cholesterol (Chol)	150-330 mg/dl (age 40-59)
Glucose (Glu)	70-100 mg/dl (fasting serum)
Blood Urea Nitrogen (BUN)	10-15 mg/100 ml
Uric acid	2.2-7 mg/dl (F) 4.2-8 mg/100 ml (M)
Creatinine (Creat.)	0.6-1 mg/dl (F) 0.8-1.7 mg/100 ml (M)
Total Bilirubin (T. Bili.)	0.3-1.3 mg/dl
Alkaline Phosphatase (Alk. Phos)	20-90 I U/liter
Aspartate transaminase (AST or SGOT)	5-40 Sigma-Frankel u/ml OR 0-36 IU/ltr (lower in women)

Dx Tests

CHEMOSENSITIVITY ASSAY – A laboratory test that measures the number of tumor cells that are killed by a cancer drug. The test is done after the tumor cells are removed from the body. A chemosensitivity assay may help in choosing the best drug or drugs for the cancer being treated.

CHROMOSOME ABNORMALITIES (Chromosome Markers) – A group of identified chromosone rearrangements or aberrations that are consistently associated with certain cancers; specific characteristics on a chromosome that indicate a predisposition to a particular kind of cancer.

FECAL OCCULT BLOOD TEST – Also called FOBT, Guaiac, Hematest, Occultest, Hemoccult, Benzidine, or Orthotoluidine test. Identifies presence of blood in stool not grossly visible (from cancer, ulcers, hemorrhoids, etc.); reported as positive or negative.

Immunochemical fecal occult blood test (iFOBT) – Also called fecal immunochemical test (FIT). Tests for hemoglobin protein in blood; similar to FOBT but does not require drug or dietary restrictions prior to test.

Stool DNA – detects abnormal DNA (genetic mutations) shed from cancer or polyp cells into stool; more expensive than regular fecal tests

GENETIC TESTING – Analysis of a person's genes, chromosomes, and proteins (usually obtained from a blood sample) to determine whether the person is predisposed to develop a genetic or hereditary disease. More than 900 genetic tests are available for many different diseases, including breast, colon or ovarian cancer. The decision to undergo genetic testing should be accompanied by genetic counseling.

GUAIAC TEST – See Fecal Occult Blood Test.

HEMATOCRIT (Hct, 'crit') – The percentage of the volume of a blood sample occupied by cells, as determined by a centrifuge or device which separates the cells and other particulate elements of the blood from the plasma. The remaining fraction of the blood sample is called plasmocrit (blood plasma volume).

HEMOGLOBIN (Hgb) – The oxygen carrying protein found in red blood cells. A low concentration of hemoglobin in blood is called anemia.

Lab Tests, *continued*

HISTOCHEMISTRY OF BONE MARROW – Pathologic examination of bone marrow biopsy specimen using special staining techniques to determine subclassification of the leukemia. Histochemistry of the bone marrow is a laboratory study performed in addition to the standard histologic analysis of the specimen.

HLA TYPING (Human Leukocyte Antigen Typing, Human Lymphocyte Antigen Typing, HLA) – Immunodiagnostic study to determine which leukocyte antigens are present on human cells, permitting differential diagnosis of a variety of diseases. Provides histocompatibility typing for platelet transfusion. Not a diagnostic test; no normal or abnormal values. Done to anticipate problems matching blood for transfusions as part of treatment. An important part in the body's immune response to foreign substances.

I-131 UPTAKE TEST – Measures ability of thyroid gland to accumulate, concentrate and retain iodine; usually done at same time as a thyroid scan. Normal values: 1%-13% absorbed by thyroid after 2 hours; 2-25% absorbed after 6 hours; 15-45% absorbed after 24 hours. Used primarily to rule out a variety of benign conditions. This is not the same dosage as I-131 radioisotope treatment for thyroid cancer.

IMMUNOASSAY – A general term for a test of body fluids such as blood or urine for specific antigens, antibodies, and other biological substances; a test that uses the binding of antibodies to antigens to identify and measure certain substances. The presence of a high or low level of one of the substances could be a sign of cancer (or other diseases). Also, test results can provide information about a disease that may help in planning treatment (for example, when estrogen receptors are measured in breast cancer).

LIVER FUNCTION TESTS – A series of blood chemistry tests measuring enzymes excreted by the liver during abnormal functioning due to metastases, obstruction or other conditions. Also called liver panel, hepatic panel. A liver panel may contain any of the following tests. If any one of these tests is outside the normal range of values, the test should be reported as abnormal.

Test	Normal Values
Alkaline Phosphatase (Alk.Phos.)	20-90 IU/liter
Lactic Dehydrogenase (LDH)	100-190 u/L at 37 degrees
Transaminase	
SGOT (Serum glutamic oxalacetic transaminase, aspartate transaminase)	8-46 u/L (M) 4-35 u/L (F)
SGPT (Serum glutamate pyruvate transaminase, alanine transferase)	7-46 u/L (M) 4-35 u/L (F)
Leucine aminopeptidase (LAP)	80-200 Goldbarg-Rutenburg u/ml (M) 75-185 u/ml (F)
Bilirubin (total)	< 1.5 mg/dl

OCCULT BLOOD STOOL TEST – See Fecal Occult Blood Test.

ONCOTYPE DX® – a diagnostic test on breast cancer tissue that assesses the expression of certain gene patterns to determine the likelihood that the cancer will recur after treatment. The test results in a "Recurrence Score" that can be used to determine the type of postoperative treatment—hormones therapy alone, combination chemotherapy or some other option.

PERIPHERAL BLOOD SMEARS – Smears taken of the blood for microscopic examination.

Lab Tests, ***continued***

RENAL FUNCTION TESTS (Renal function panel) – Urine chemistry tests to measure the output of the kidneys.

Test	Normal Values
Albumin (protein)	2-8 mg/dl

SEROLOGY – The study of antigen-antibody reactions in vitro.

THYROGLOBULIN – See Thyroglobulin in Tumor Markers section.

URIC ACID – In any malignancy with rapid destruction of cells, uric acid may be elevated.

URINALYSIS – Also called UA, random specimen, clean catch, urine sediment test. Collection of urine to evaluate for blood, infection, or other urinary tract problems; analysis of the physical, chemical, or microscopic content of urine (including secretion of kidneys, passed through the ureters, stored in the bladder, and discharged through the urethra.)

TUMOR MARKERS

TUMOR MARKER (Biomarker, marker, serum tumor marker) – A substance sometimes found in the blood, other body fluids, or tissues. A high level of a biomarker may mean that a certain type of cancer is in the body.
Key information: For baseline and observation; to assess tumor burden and monitor levels of tumor and indicate a recurrence; prognosis (what treatment to use if the tumor should recur).

17-HYDROXYCORTICOSTEROIDS (17-OHCS) – A biomarker test that measures the amount of 17-OHCS in urine. Normal values are: male—4 to 14 mg/24 hr; female—2 to 12 mg/24 hr (milligrams per 24 hours). Measurement of 17-OHCS in the urine can be helpful in determining if the body is producing too much cortisol.

2IT-BAD MONOCLONAL ANTIBODY 170 – Normal range: < 16 mg/24 hr. Levels above 15 mg/24 hours indicate malignant carcinoid tumor (argentaffinoma) which may appear in the stomach, appendix, or lower intestine.

5-HIAA (5-Hydroxy-Indol Acetic Acid) – Quantitative analysis of urine levels for a specific excreted protein. Levels above 15 mg/24 hours indicate malignant carcinoid tumors (argentaffinomas), which may also appear in stomach, appendix, or lower intestine.

ACID PHOSPHATASE – Also called acid phos, acid ϕ, acid p'tase. A test of blood serum to detect a specific enzyme produced by several tissues, particularly the prostate. Acid phosphatase levels are elevated in 85% of cases with skeletal metastases, 60% of untreated cases, and 20% of localized cases. Usually ordered as a separate laboratory test. May also be ordered as prostatic acid phosphatase (PAP), a measure of acid phosphatase secreted by prostate gland cells specifically (rarely done anymore). *Note*: test results may be affected by recent prostatic massage or palpation; acid phosphatase level should be assayed before digital rectal examination. Normal range: varies according to method of processing the serum:

1.0 - 4	King Armstrong microns/dl
0.5 - 2	Bodansky or Gutman microns/dl
0 - 1.1	Shinowara microns/ml
0.1 - 0.73	Bessy Lowry microns/nk.
0.5 - 11.0	units/L

Tumor Markers, *continued*

ACTH (Adrenocorticotropic Hormone) – Elevated level found in paraneoplastic syndrome caused by small cell carcinoma. Non-diagnostic of lung cancer, but an indicator of metastases.

ALANINE AMINOPEPTIDASE (AAP) – Non-specific biomarker to detect damage to the kidneys; may be used to help diagnose certain kidney disorders. Found at high levels in the urine when there are kidney problems. Elevated levels found in paraneoplastic syndromes caused by small cell carcinoma.

ALKALINE PHOSPHATASE – Also called alk phos, alk ϕ, serum alkaline phosphatase, ALP. May be included in blood chemistry screening panel. Normal range: 20-90 I.U./liter. Normal range may vary somewhat according to the brand of laboratory assay materials used. Elevated levels found in osteoblastic skeletal metastases and liver tumors; specific isoenzymes within the total alkaline phosphatase indicate which organs are involved. Non-diagnostic; non-specific for malignancy or metastases.

ALLELIC LOSS OF 18Q/RER TYPING – Biomarker. Colorectal cancer patients having tumors with a deletion of the DCC (chromosome 18q) gene are far more likely to show tumor recurrence and have shorter disease-free survival than patients with tumors retaining both copies of the gene. An alternate pathway for tumor progression involves deficient DNA mismatch repair. Such replication error (RER+) tumors exhibit microsatellite instability and have a distinct clinical prognosis. See also Loss of Heterozygosity.

ALPHA-FETOPROTEIN – Also called FP, AFP, αFP, alpha-fetoglobulin. A serum test used as a tumor marker for hepatocellular cancer. Levels above 1000 ng/ml are diagnostic of primary hepatocellular carcinoma; higher results correlate with worse prognosis. Coded as CS Site-Specific Factor 1 for Liver. Elevated alpha-fetoprotein levels are also found in certain ovarian and teratocarcinoma or embryonal carcinoma of the testis. Coded as CS Site-Specific Factor 1 for Testis. Elevated alpha-fetoprotein levels are not found in other histologies of testicular cancer (pure seminoma or pure choriocarcinoma). Note: Observe the date of an alpha-fetoprotein study carefully. Record a pre-operative study only. Alpha-fetoprotein is also used as a marker postoperatively to monitor residual tumor. Normal range: Males and non-pregnant women: < 5.4 ng/ml. Also useful for detecting liver metastases from gastrointestinal and pancreatic tumors; also present in cirrhosis, hepatitis, hepatoblastoma, and hepatocellular carcinoma.

ANTI-CEA ANTIBODY – An antibody against carcinoembryonic antigen (CEA), a protein present on certain types of cancer cells.

B-2 MICROGLOBULIN – Also called Beta 2-M, β2-M. Elevated levels are present in lymphoproliferative disorders; non-specific to chronic lymphocytic leukemia.

BCL-2 ONCOGENE ANALYSIS – Differentiate B-cell and follicular types of lymphomas

BENCE-JONES PROTEIN (BJ) – Measures abnormal light chain immunoglobulins in urine. Presence of any level of Bence-Jones protein is diagnostic of multiple myeloma; absence of Bence-Jones protein does not rule out multiple myeloma. Bence-Jones protein also present in Waldenstrom's macroglobulinemia and low levels are occasionally present in benign monoclonal gammopathy.

BRCA1 and BRCA2 – A gene that normally helps to suppress cell growth. BRCA1 is found on chromosome 17; BRCA2 is found on chromosome 13. A person who inherits an altered version of either the BRCA1 or BRCA2 gene has a higher risk of developing breast, ovarian, or prostate cancer.

Tumor Markers, *continued*

BTA – A test for the bladder tumor-associated antigen (BTA) tumor marker in urine.

C219 – Presence of biomarker is associated with multidrug resistance.

CA-125 (Cancer Antigen-125) – A tumor marker useful for monitoring regression, stability of tumor and recurrence for ovarian cancer by measuring an antigen to epithelial neoplasms circulating in blood serum. Normal range: 0 - 35 U/mL. Normal range may vary somewhat according to institutional experience. Coded as CS Site-Specific Factor 1 for ovary. Levels above 35 suggest the presence of ovarian tumor. Useful in 90% of ovarian tumors (benign and malignant), but not specific to ovarian carcinoma. Elevated CA-125 can be caused by many conditions, such as peritonitis, pleuritis, menstruation, pregnancy, endometriosis, liver disease, benign ovarian growths, and by cancers of the uterine tubes, endometrium, lung, breast, and gastrointestinal tract.

CA 15-3 (Cancer Antigen 15-3) – Useful in monitoring the presence of metastatic breast cancer and the patient's response to chemotherapy; elevated in 76% of metastatic breast cancers. Not a screening procedure. The CA 15-3 assay value, regardless of level, should not be interpreted as absolute evidence for the presence or absence of malignant disease. The CA 15-3 assay value should be used in conjunction with information available from clinical evaluation and diagnostic procedure.

CA 195 (Carbohydrate Antigen 195) – Measures circulating antigen to gastrointestinal cancer. Monitors success of therapy and return of elevated level indicates recurrence. Useful as post-therapeutic monitor for upper gastrointestinal and pancreatic cancers for recurrence; non-specific to colorectal cancer.

CA 19-9 (Cancer Antigen 19-9) – Detects gastrointestinal cancers but cannot differentiate among primary sites; changing level indicates progression or regression of tumor load. Monitors post-therapeutic gastrointestinal cancer for recurrence; non-specific to stomach or colorectal cancer but used predominantly for pancreas cancer. Higher than normal amounts of CA 19-9 in the blood can be a sign of gallbladder or pancreatic cancer or other conditions. Normal range: 0-37.0 units/mL. CA 19-9 has been reported as positive in 70% to 80% of pancreatic carcinomas, 50% to 60% of gastric cancers, 60% of hepatobiliary cancer, 30% of colorectal cancer, and few lung, breast or prostate cancers. Test may also be positive in patients with non-neoplastic disease, particularly inflammatory disease of the bowel, cirrhosis, and autoimmune conditions including rheumatoid arthritis (33%), systemic lupus erythematosus (32%), and scleroderma (33%).

CA 27-29 (Carbohydrate Antigen 27-29) – Detects adenocarcinoma. Normal range: 0-38.6 units/mL. Non-specific; investigational; most effective in serial tests. A reduction in levels of this marker indicates a good response to treatment while increasing levels indicate resistance to therapy and progressive disease with an average lead time of 5.3 months before recurrence was clinically established.

CA 72-4 (Carbohydrate Antigen 72-4) – Measures overexpression of TAG-72 in gastrointestinal malignancies. Suggested use is as a complement to CEA.

CALCITONIN – Used to follow medullary thyroid cancer; elevated levels of this thyroid hormone occasionally occur with small cell lung cancer; increasing levels may indicate progression of disease.

CALCIUM (Serum Calcium) – Measures circulating calcium level; non-specific. Calcium circulates in the blood in equilibrium with the calcium in the bone. Normal: 8.5-10.5 mg/100 (slightly higher for children). Elevated in many malignancies as a sign of neuromuscular, endocrine and skeletal metastases. Non-diagnostic; test should be used in conjunction with other tests and site-specific markers.

Tumor Markers, ***continued***

CATECHOLAMINES – Measures urine or serum hormone levels in any of various amines (epinephrine, norepinephrine, and dopamine) that function as hormones or neurotransmitters or both. Fractional analysis helps distinguish tumor cell type; most useful in adrenal tumor. Elevated levels diagnostic of malignant pheochromocytoma of the adrenal medulla or sympathetic ganglia. Specific tests such as homovanillic acid and vanillylmandielic acid can differentiate pheochromoctyomas from other catecholamine-secreting tumors.

CATHEPSIN D – Distinguishes breast cancer node-negative patients who may recur (and therefore should receive adjuvant chemotherapy) from node-negative patients who probably will not recur. Elevation indicates a poorer prognosis.

CD4 CELL COUNT – CD4 is found on T helper cells (infection fighting lymphocytes) in the human immune system. When the patient is immunosuppressed as in HIV infection and AIDS, the CD4 cell count can monitor the health of the patient's immune system. CD4 count less than 200 is diagnostic of AIDS. This test is a prognostic marker for patients with Kaposi sarcoma.

CD20 (B-cell Pan) – Reacts with a membrane antigen that is present in B-cells. This antibody strongly recognizes Reed-Sternberg cells predominant in Hodgkin lymphoma. Since no staining of histiocytes or plasma cells has been observed and CD20 has not been detected in T-cell malignancies, it is a very strong marker of B-cell lymphomas.

C-ERB B-2 – See HER-2/neu.

CEA (Carcinoembryonic Antigen) – Also called oncofetal antigen, OFA, carcino-embryonic antigen. A blood test measuring the presence of an antigen in malignancies arising in entodermal (embryonic) or gastrointestinal tissue. The antigen is produced in the fetus but not in normal adult life. Code as CS Site-Specific Factor 1 for colon, rectosigmoid, and rectum. Persistent elevated levels indicate residual or recurrent metastatic carcinoma. CEA assay is not diagnostic of cancer and is non-specific for identifying a primary site (found in colorectal, breast, lung, liver, kidney and other primaries), but it does indicate the presence of malignancy. Smokers may have an elevated CEA without malignant disease; smoking may affect accuracy of CEA results. Normal range: < 2.5 ng/ml. Normal range may vary somewhat depending on the brand of assay used. Levels > 10 ng/ml suggest extensive disease and levels > 20 ng/ml suggest metastatic disease. Rising serum levels of CEA may indicate disease recurrence many months prior to clinical manifestations.

CHROMOGENIC IN SITU HYBRIDIZATION (CISH) – A type of genetic testing that uses special molecular probes that change color under the microscope when attached to the part of a chromosome that is their target. CISH identifies the same chromosome changes as less sophisticated cytogenetic testing, but can also be used on samples too small for standard testing. CISH technology is widely used in Canada instead of FISH, and is FDA approved for use in the United States. Its primary use is to detect over-expression of the HER2 protein (see below). A type of bright field in situ hybridization.

CHROMOGRANIN-A – A protein diagnostic of a neuroendocrine tumor, but cannot identify the source (organ) of involvement. Monitors tumor bulk in neuroblastoma, pancreatic endocrine tumors, pheochromocytoma; non-diagnostic of central nervous system tumor. Also called CGA, serum chromogranin A.

CHROMOSOME 6 AMPLIFICATION – Also called gain of chromosome 6p, multiplication of 6p, and overrepresentation of 6p. This genetic test indicates a more favorable prognosis for patients with melanoma of the choroid, ciliary body and iris. A portion (p25) of the short arm (p) of chromosome 6 is duplicated and added to chromosome 6. Amplification is the opposite of loss of heterozygosity (LOH), which is discussed below.

Tumor Markers, *continued*

CHROMOSOME 8 AMPLIFICATION – Also called gain of chromosome 8q, overrepresentation of 8q, multiple copies of chromosome 8q. This genetic test indicates a worse prognosis for patients with melanoma of the choroid, ciliary body and iris. A portion of the long arm of chromosome 8 is duplicated and added to chromosome 8. Amplification is the opposite of loss of heterozygosity (LOH), which is discussed below.

C-MYC DNA AMPLIFICATION – Elevated (amplified) in breast cancers in older women; juxtaposition of this chromosome with a heavy chain immunoglobulin occurs frequently in Burkitt lymphoma and other B-cell lymphomas, as well as acute lymphoblastic leukemia.

CREATININE – A tumor marker for liver cancer found in blood or urine that measures renal function associated with severe liver disease. Not the same as creatinine clearance. Creatinine is measured in different ways—milligrams per deciliter (mg/dL) in the US and micromoles per liter (µmoles/L) in Canada.

CYTOGENETICS – Examination of tumor cells for abnormal chromosomes (translocations, inversions, missing pieces of chromosome, too many or too few chromosomes). This type of test is used most commonly in lymphoma.

DNA STUDIES – Also called flow cytometry. Differentiates between tumors at high and low risk for recurrence. DNA studies are a prognostic tool for non-small cell lung and other solid tumors.

Ploidy Analysis—Aneuploid tumors correlate with more aggressive behavior and a greater risk of recurrence. Diploid tumors have a better prognosis than aneuploid or tetraploid tumors.

S-Phase (also called Cell Cycle Analysis)—Percentage of tumor cells synthesizing DNA; patients with high S-phase fraction have less favorable prognosis.

Proliferation Index—High rates indicate actively growing tumors and a greater risk of relapse.

EGFR (Epidermal Growth Factor Receptor) – Negative EGFR results correlate with better prognosis regardless of ER status in breast cancer. See also HER-2/neu.

ERYTHROCYTE SEDIMENTATION RATE (ESR) – A very old diagnostic test in which a special test tube is used to measure the rate of fall of red blood cells over time. An abnormal rate may be an indication of certain forms of cancer, such as multiple myeloma or Hodgkin lymphoma.

ESTROGEN RECEPTOR ASSAY (ERA) – Also called ER, estrogen receptor status, estradiol receptor, estrogen binding protein, estrogen receptor protein, hormone receptor status (with PRA). Code as CS Site-Specific Factor 1 for breast. Measures the amount of estrogen binding capacity of tumor specimen. Helps determine the responsiveness of a breast cancer to endocrine therapy or to removal of the ovaries. Tumors that are negative for estrogen receptors rarely respond to hormone manipulation; about 55% of ER positive tumors will respond to endocrine therapy. The unit of measurement is femtomoles (fmoles) per milligram of tumor. Test results—negative: 3 fmoles or less. ERA may not be performed if tumor is less than 1.0 cm in size or if tumor is completely in situ. Types of ERA: *Quantified* (measured in femtomoles or fmoles); *Immunohistochemical:* a *qualitative* measurement of the observed number of hormone responsive cells, reported as positive or negative.

FERRITIN – Measures iron storage protein in sialic acid; low levels suggest good prognosis in head and neck malignancies, although test is non-specific for head and neck cancer. Elevated levels are present in lymphoproliferative disease; may indicate Hodgkin lymphoma or leukemia. Monitors cause of disease in neuroblastoma; non-specific in neurogenic tumors.

Tumor Markers, *continued*

FIBROBLAST GROWTH FACTOR (FGF) – Heparin-binding mitogenic proteins that enhance proliferation of a wide variety of cell types under serum-free or serum-reduced conditions. Also used as a chemotactic or neurotrophic factor and to study wound healing, angiogenesis, and related processes.

FISH – See Fluorescent In Situ Hibridization.

FLOW CYTOMETRY – See DNA Studies.

FLUORESCENT IN SITU HYBRIDIZATION (FISH) – A type of genetic testing that uses highly specific DNA probes that fluoresce (glow) under the microscope when attached to the part of a chromosome that is their target. This technique is useful for identifying chromosomal abnormalities and gene mapping. FISH identifies the same chromosome changes as less sophisticated cytogenetic testing, but can also be used on samples too small for standard testing. FISH technology is commonly used to measure over-expression of the HER2 protein (see below), to diagnose chronic myelogenous leukemia, and other applications in evaluating abnormal chromosomes.

GASTRIN – Differentiates gastrin secreting non-beta islet cell tumors of pancreas; levels above 1000 pg/ml are diagnostic of gastrinoma; also found in some benign conditions

GENETIC ANALYSIS (Genetic Testing, Genotyping, Genetic Markers) – Analysis of a sample of DNA to look for mutations (changes) that may increase risk of disease risk of developing a specific disease or disorder or affect the way a person responds to treatment.

GLUCAGON – Differentiates alpha-cell tumors; levels above 900 are diagnostic of glucagonoma; also present in diabetes and other conditions

HE4 – A blood test for ovarian cancer used to monitor success of treatment in women who have a normal CA-125 level.

HER2 – Also called Her-2/Neu oncoprotein, HER-2, C-ERB B-2, neu oncoprotein) – An epidermal growth factor receptor (EFGR) protein product of the HER-2/*neu* oncogene. HER stands for Human Epidermal growth factor Receptor. Over-expression in a breast cancer is associated with larger sized tumors, shorter relapse time and lower survival rate. May indicate breast cancer that won't respond well to chemotherapy. HER-2/*neu* over-expression is also a predictor of response to certain breast cancer therapies, including targeted immunotherapies such as Herceptin (trastuzumab) and Tykerb (lapatinib).

HORMONE ASSAY (Hormone Receptor Test) – A test performed on cancer cells to determine if they are affected by hormones. See Estrogen Receptor Assay and Progesterone Receptor Assay.

HPV TEST – Also called human papillomavirus test, HPV hybrid capture test. The human papilloma virus is a common infection that is associated with anal, penile, cervical and head and neck cancers. HPV infection is a favorable prognostic factor for cancers of the oropharynx. The test looks identifies whether the patient has HPV and if so, which strain. HPV strains 16 and 18 are particularly high risk for cancer but over three dozen different strains have been identified.

HUMAN CHORIONIC GONADOTROPIN (hCG) (Alpha and Beta subunits) – Non-specific marker; both subunits present in trophoblastic tumors of the placenta, as well as other types of malignancies. Measures fetal hormone not present in normal adult female.
α-HCG (Alpha Subunit HCG) – A non-specific marker for pancreatic, pituitary, and placental tumors; elevated levels may be present in pancreatic cancer.

Tumor Markers, *continued*

Human chorionic gonadotropin, continued

Beta Subunit HCG A serum test used as a diagnostic tumor marker for choriocarcinoma (GTT/ gestational trophoblastic tumors) and for testicular carcinoma. Coded as CS Site-Specific Factor 2 in Testis. Normal reference range: < 10 mIU/ml. Beta-HCG levels are never found in normal men. When the presence of beta-HCG is detected in serum, it always indicates a malignancy. Also called: β-HCG, beta-HCG, beta chain HCG. Note: Observe the date of the beta-HCG study carefully. Record a pre-operative study only. Beta-HCG is also used as a marker postoperatively to monitor residual tumor and the effectiveness of therapy. In patients with choriocarcinoma who have had a hysterectomy and oophorectomy, the presence of beta-HCG will confirm the patient has residual cancer that requires further evaluation. In patients with testicular cancer who have had an orchiectomy, the presence of beta-HCG will confirm the patient has residual cancer that requires further treatment. However, when beta-HCG does not exist in the serum, the presence of active cancer cannot be excluded, especially in patients who have been previously treated.

HVA (Homovanillic Acid) – Elevated levels suggest catecholamine-secreting tumor such as neuroblastoma or ganglioneuroma; high levels rule out pheochromocytoma.

IMMUNOCYT – A trademarked urine test looking for carcinoembryonic antigen (CEA) and mucin associated with cancer cells.

IMMUNOELECTROPHORESIS (Protein electrophoresis, serum proteins, IEP) – Measures serum or urine for specific immunoglobulins. Elevated levels of specific immunoglobulins (IgA, IgG, etc.) diagnose multiple myeloma. Also diagnoses Waldenstrom's macroglobulinemia and some lymphomas.

IMMUNOHISTOCHEMISTRY (IHC) – A laboratory technique in which specific antigens are made visible by the use of fluorescent dye or enzyme markers; the process of detection of antigens in tissue using antibodies. See also Immunohistochemistry in Pathology section.

> **Immunohistochemical ERA, Immunohistochemical PRA** – Immunohistochemistry review of ERA and PRA results.
>
> **HER2 immunohistochemistry** – one of several methods to determine over-expression of HER2 (see above).

IMMUNOPHENOTYPING – A process used to identify cells, based on the types of antigens or markers on the surface of the cell. This process is used to diagnose specific types of leukemia and lymphoma by comparing the cancer cells to normal cells of the immune system.

INR FOR PRO TIME (International Normalized Ratio for Prothrombin Time) – Prothrombin time measures how quickly the blood clots, which is an indication of liver disease. The international normalized ratio (INR) is a calculation of the prothrombin time divided by the normal mean prothrombin time for the reagent used by the laboratory to perform the test. INR is of clinical value in the assessment of primary liver cancer.

INT-2 DNA AMPLIFICATION – Elevation (amplification) associated with recurrence of tumor.

JAK2 – A gene found in all humans; mutation of this enzyme is found in nearly all patients with polycythemia vera and about half of all patients with essential thrombocythemia and myelofibrosis. Identifying the JAK2 mutation helps diagnose a myeloproliferative neoplasms but does not indicate a specific type. The test looks for a mutation in a specific amino acid on the JAK2 gene (V617F) in the area of exon 14 or exon 12. JAK2 has future potential for development of targeted therapies for these diseases.

Tumor Markers, ***continued***

KI-67 LABELING INDEX – Also called MIB-1, Ki-67 proliferation marker, labeling index fraction, proliferative index, and other terms. The monoclonal antibody Ki-67 is found only in proliferating (dividing) human cells. A non-specific prognostic marker for brain, other central nervous system, and intracranial gland tumors, as well as lacrimal gland and conjunctiva cancers and lymphoma, Ki-67 can be measured on any tumor. A high level indicates that the tumor is actively growing (an unfavorable prognostic factor) and may respond to chemotherapy. Ki-67 must be tested on fresh tissue, while MIB-1 can also be used on formalin-fixed paraffin embedded tissue.

KIT GENE IMMUNOHISTOCHEMISTRY (IHC) – A special stain on a tissue sample indicating the presence of a gene that regulates cell growth and differentiation in gastrointestinal stromal tumors. The gene is mutated in 85-90% of GISTs and confirms the diagnosis of GIST. Patients who have the mutation are likely to respond to the drugs Gleevec or Sutent.

KIT GENE MUTATION – A more sophisticated test for the KIT gene than KIT gene IHC, this test looks for mutations of specific parts of the gene called exons, particularly exons 11 and 9, which if present indicate that the GIST tumor may have a better response to Gleevec and Sutent than a tumor without the mutation. This test is performed by only a few labs.

KRAS MUTATION ANALYSIS – A test to detect the presence of a mutation in the K-ras gene, which is present in 90% of pancreatic cancers, about 40% of colon cancers and 30% of non-small cell lung cancers. The mutation is associated with a low response rate to cetuximab (Erbitux), panitumomab (Vectibix), Erlotinib (Tarceva) and Gefitinib (Iressa), all of which are epidermal growth factor receptor (EGFR) inhibiting drugs. Patients with the KRAS (or K-ras) mutation should avoid treatment with EGFR inhibitors.

LASA (Lipid-Associated Sialic Acid) – A useful adjunct in the management of a variety of malignancies, generally used in conjunction with other tumor markers; non-specific, not a screening test. Normal range: 0-20 mg/dL. Elevated in several types of carcinoma, including breast cancer and occult pelvic malignancies. Elevated LASA levels have been reported in patients with breast, gastrointestinal, lung, and ovarian solid tumors, as well as leukemia, lymphoma, melanoma, sarcoma, and Hodgkin lymphoma. LASA levels can also be elevated in patients with certain benign diseases, including inflammatory disorders. LASA levels may be useful in monitoring the course of therapy and detecting disease recurrence in certain cancer patients.

LDH (Lactate Dehydrogenase, LD, lactic acid dehydrogenase, lactase dehydrogenase) – A blood chemistry study, usually part of a liver panel, useful in assessing liver and pulmonary disease; not a screening test; not diagnostic of cancer. Code as CS Site-Specific Factor 4 for malignant melanoma and CS Site-Specific Factor 3 for testis. All tumors produce LDH. Normal range: total LDH levels range from 48 to 115 IU/liter. Elevated LDH is an indirect indication of damage to an organ, such metastatic disease or a myocardial infarction. May be included in an organ function panel, such as a liver profile. Reference ranges vary widely by laboratory, patient age, and the units of measurement. There are five tissue-specific isoenzymes that can be identified and measured. The distribution of isoenzymes is as follows:

LDH1: 18.1% to 29% of the total (heart, red blood cells and kidneys)
LDH2: 29.4% to 37.5% of the total (heart, red blood cells and kidneys)
LDH3: 18.8% to 26% of the total (lungs)
LDH4: 9.2% to 16.5% of the total (liver and skeletal muscles)
LDH5: 5.3% to 13.4% of the total (liver and skeletal muscles)

LIVER FUNCTION TESTS (LFT) – See Liver Function Tests in Lab Tests section.

Tumor Markers, *continued*

LOSS OF HETEROZYGOSITY (LOH) – Heterozygosity is the normal presence of two complete copies of a chromosome in a cell. Loss of heterozygosity occurs when one of the two chromosomes in the pair is missing part of its genetic material. LOH means that tumor suppression is diminished, resulting in development or progression of the malignancy. Several types of LOH are important prognostic factors. Also called allelic loss, gene deletion.

1p LOH – In certain histologies of central nervous system tumors, this LOH indicates that the patient may be sensitive to lomustine, procarbazine and vincristine. 1p means that the short arm (p) of chromosome 1 is missing.

18q LOH – In colorectal cancer this LOH indicates that the tumor may be resistant to fluorouracil-based chemotherapy. 18q means that the long arm (q) of chromosome 18 is missing.

19q LOH – In certain histologies of central nervous system tumors, this LOH indicates that the patient may be sensitive to lomustine, procarbazine and vincristine. 19q means that the long arm (q) of chromosome 19 is missing.

Monosomy 3 – In ophthalmic melanomas (uvea, choroid, and ciliary body), loss of an entire copy of chromosome 3 is an important adverse prognostic factor.

MARROW ACID PHOSPHATASE – Used to detect early bone metastasis in patients with prostatic cancer. Elevated bone marrow acid phosphatase follows dissemination of prostatic cancer of the marrow space and contraindicates radical surgery in these patients.

METHYLATION OF MGMT – MGMT is O^6 methylguanine methyltransferase, an enzyme that repairs damaged DNA. When a brain tumor patient receives chemotherapy, MGMT repairs the damage caused by the chemotherapy, thereby making chemotherapy less effective. Methylation of MGMT reduces the level of DNA repair activity, allowing the chemotherapy to do a better job of killing tumor cells. The presence of highly methylated (hypermethylated) MGMT is an indicator that the patient is likely to respond to some of the few drugs that cross the blood-brain barrier, such as temozolomide and the nitrosoureas.

MIB-1 LABELING INDEX – See Ki-67 Labeling Index.

MICROARRAY ANALYSIS – Also called DNA 'chips', gene expression profiling, biochip, DNA microchip, gene array, genome chip. A way of studying how large numbers of genes interact with each other and how a cell's regulatory networks control vast batteries of genes simultaneously. Microarrays can be used to analyze the expression of genes of interest simultaneously in multiple tissue samples. Tissue microarrays consist of hundreds of individual tissue samples placed on slides ranging from 2 to 3 mm in diameter. Using conventional histochemical and molecular detection techniques, tissue microarrays are powerful tools to evaluate the expression of genes of interest in tissue samples, for example to determine target genes for the development of new drugs or to identify a specific subtype of a cancer. For ocular melanomas, gene expression profiling is the best way to predict metastatic spread.

MICROSATELLITE INSTABILITY (MSI) – A molecular marker that identifies differences in sections of DNA in tumor tissue from the lower GI tract; used as a marker for hereditary non-polyposis colorectal cancer (HNPCC or Lynch Syndrome). An elevated level of MSI (high or MSI-H) may indicate that the patient has this condition. Low-positive (MSI-L) or stable MSI (MSS) results indicate that it is unlikely that the cancer is a result of a hereditary condition.

MITOTIC COUNT – Also called mitotic rate, mitotic index. The number of tumor cells in the process of dividing is an indication of the potential aggressiveness of the tumor. Mitotic count is an important prognostic factor for gastrointestinal stromal tumors, neuroendocrine tumors, pancreatic cancer, melanoma, and other types of cancer. The pathologist looks for dividing cells in tumor tissue and counts the number in a number of high power fields, which varies according to the primary site.

Tumor Markers, *continued*

MOLECULAR RISK ASSESSMENT – A procedure in which biomarkers (for example, biological molecules or changes in tumor cell DNA) are used to estimate a person's risk for developing cancer. Specific biomarkers may be linked to particular types of cancer. See also Genetic Analysis in this section and Chromosomal Abnormalities in the Lab Tests section.

MONOCLONAL ANTIBODY (MC-Ab, MAB) – A laboratory-produced substance that can locate and bind to cancer cells wherever they are in the body. Many monoclonal antibodies are used in cancer detection or therapy; each one recognizes a different protein on certain cancer cells.

MONOCLONAL IMMUNOGLOBULINS (Monoclonal proteins, quantitative immunoglobulins) – Measures serum protein levels. Elevated levels help diagnose multiple myeloma. Non-diagnostic by itself; test should be used in conjunction with other multiple myeloma markers.

MONOSOMY 3 – See Loss of Heterozygosity.

NMP22 BladderChek – A trademarked urine test that looks for a specific protein (NMP22) found at higher levels in patients with bladder cancer.

NSE (Neuron Specific Enolase) – Elevated level indicates presence of small cell carcinoma of lung and neuroblastoma; of secondary use in testicular neoplasms; non-specific to central nervous system tumors. Reference range: 0 - 12.5 ng/mL. The test may have value in predicting response to therapy.

NUCLEAR NM23 STAINING – An immunohistochemistry test for a metastasis suppressor gene on the long arm of chromosome 17. Reduced NM23 expression is an indicator of poor prognosis and the likelihood of tumor progression in many solid tumors. Overexpression of NM23 in the nucleus of tumor cells suggests a better prognosis compare to tumor cells that are negative for the gene.

ONCOFETAL ANTIGEN – See Carcinoembryonic Antigen.

ONCOR TEST – The first gene-based test approved by the FDA for predicting whether a cancer will recur. The test measures the number of copies of the HER-2/neu gene in a patient with breast cancer. Five to ten copies per cell increases the risk of recurrence. Most people have two copies per cell. See also HER-2/neu Oncoprotein.

OVA1 – A blood test for ovarian tumors that measures four proteins and uses the information to place the patient into one of two categories, low risk (not likely to have cancer) and high risk (more likely to have ovarian cancer and needing exploratory surgery). Not a screening test; meant for use in women who have a known ovarian tumor but not yet confirmed as cancer.

P53 (p53) – A biomarker that plays multiple roles in cells. Expression of high levels of wild-type (but not mutant) p53 has two outcomes: cell cycle arrest or apoptosis. p53 acts as an "emergency brake" inducing either arrest or apoptosis, protecting the genome from accumulating excess mutations. Consistent with this notion, cells lacking p53 were shown to be genetically unstable and thus more prone to tumors.

PANCREATIC POLYPEPTIDE – Diagnoses pancreatic gamma cell tumors; elevated in APUD-omas, VIP-omas, PPomas, and MEN (Multiple Endocrine Neoplasia).

PARATHYROID HORMONE (Parathormone, PTH) – Biomarker that measures circulating polypeptide secreted by parathyroid gland. Detects neoplastic abnormalities of parathyroid glands. Abnormal parathyroid hormone secretion may be present in squamous cell carcinoma of the lung, renal, pancreatic or ovarian cancer.

Tumor Markers, *continued*

PDGFRA GENE MUTATION – The Platelet-Derived Growth Factor Receptor-Alpha (PDGFRA) gene mutation is mutually exclusive with the KIT gene mutation (see above) in gastrointestinal stromal tumors. In other words, no GIST has both gene mutations. The presence of the PDGFRA gene mutation is an indicator that the GIST tumor is likely to respond to the drugs Gleevec and Sutent.

PHILADELPHIA CHROMOSOME (Ph1, Ph[1]) – Detects presence of a specific abnormal chromosome in bone marrow; confirms diagnosis of chronic myelogenous leukemia; absence of Ph1 chromosome does not rule out CML. Also found in some cases of acute lymphoblastic leukemia. Chromosome abnormality is also described as BCR/ABL and t(9;22)(q34;q11).

PLAP (Placental Alkaline Phosphatase or PL-AP) – Differentiates the source of tumor among liver, bone, and germ cell origin; non-diagnostic by itself, it helps confirm malignancy in a small number of patients.

PLP (Parathyroid hormone-like Protein) – Elevated levels of this circulating hormone are found in squamous cell cancer and in breast cancer.

PROGESTERONE RECEPTOR ASSAY (PRA, PR, PgR, progesterone receptor status, hormone receptor status (with ERA)) – A laboratory test of breast cancer tissue to determine the responsiveness of the tumor to endocrine therapy or to removal of the ovaries. Code as CS Site-Specific Factor 2 for breast. Measures amount of progesterone binding capacity of breast cancer specimen. Progesterone receptor assay increases the reliability of estrogen receptor assay results: a positive progesterone receptor assay indicates greater likelihood that the patient will respond to hormone therapy. The unit of measurement is femtomoles (fmoles) per milligram of tumor. Test results: negative—5 fmoles or less. Test may not be performed if tumor is less than 1.0 cm in size or if tumor is completely in situ. Types of PRA: *Quantified* (measured in femtomoles or fmoles); *Immunohistochemical*—a *qualitative* measurement of the observed number of hormone responsive cells, reported as positive or negative. Patients with negative results seldom respond to endocrine therapy. Patients with elevated progesterone receptor levels in general have better survival rates and longer disease-free intervals.

PROINSULIN C-PEPTIDE – Differentiates cell type for endocrine-secreting tumors; elevated in insulinoma and islet cell tumors.

PROLACTIN – Measures circulating hormone. Normal range: < 100 ng/ml. Elevated levels (100-300 ng/ml) indicate benign or malignant pituitary tumor in patients with galactorrhea. Non-diagnostic for malignancy by itself.

PROSTATE ALKALINE PHOSPHATASE – An enzyme produced in liver and bone. Levels may be elevated in patients with liver and/or bone cancer or prostate cancer that has metastasized to the liver and/or bone as well as non-malignant conditions.

PROSTATE SPECIFIC ANTIGEN (PSA) – Not the same as prostatic acid phosphatase. Tumor marker assay (test) of blood serum for antigen released from cells in prostate tissue. Value may be elevated in benign prostatic hypertrophy; greatest elevation occurs in stage C and D prostate cancer. Code value in CS Site-specific Factor 1 for prostate and code physician's interpretation of value in CS Site-specific Factor 2 for prostate. PSA is a prognostic factor included in the TNM 7th edition stage grouping of prostate cancer. After radical prostatectomy or radiation therapy, rising levels of PSA indicate residual disease or recurrence. *Note*: test results may be affected by recent prostatic massage or palpation; PSA level should be assayed before digital rectal examination. Normal range:

Tumor Markers, *continued*

Prostate specific antigen, continued
0.1 - 1.8 ng/ml. Normal range may also vary depending on the brand of laboratory assay used, as well as age and race of patient.

Free PSA (percentage of PSA in blood without carrier protein) – If low indicates cancer, if high (above 25%) indicates benign lesion. Also called percent-free PSA, fPSA.
Complexed PSA – measures amount of PSA attached to other proteins (in other words, not free) rather than the total PSA and free PSA.
PSA velocity – tracks how fast PSA rises in sequential tests; not a separate method or technique for monitoring PSA.
PSA density (PSAD) – the ratio of the PSA number (test result) divided by the prostate gland volume (size). Higher PSAD indicates the man is more likely to have prostate cancer.

PROSTATIC ACID PHOSPHATASE (PAP) – Measures specific chemical released by prostate cancer. A measure of acid phosphatase secreted by prostate gland cells specifically. Elevated levels correlate strongly with metastatic prostate cancer (tumor that has spread beyond the prostate capsule). No sensitivity for early prostate cancer; not useful for screening or monitoring recurrence; less specific than Prostate Specific Antigen (PSA). Acid phosphatase level should be assayed before digital rectal examination. Also elevated in benign prostatic hypertrophy and prostatitis. Normal range varies according to method of processing the serum.

1.0 - 4 King Armstrong microns/dl
0.5 - 2 Bodansky or Gutman microns/dl
0 - 1.1 Shinowara microns/ml
0.1 - 0.73 Bessy Lowry microns/nk.
0.5 - 11.0 units/L

PROTEIN ELECTROPHORESIS – See Immunoelectrophoresis.

QUANTITATIVE IMMUNOGLOBULINS – See Monoclonal Immunoglobulins.

REED-STERNBERG CELL – Giant, abnormal cell with several nuclei ("owl's eyes") that appears in patients with Hodgkin lymphoma. The number of cells increases as the disease advances.

REVERSE TRANSCRIPTASE-POLYMERASE CHAIN REACTION – See same in Pathology section.

S100 PROTEIN — Measures cytoplasmic protein for melanoma. Differentiates between amelanotic melanoma and other poorly differentiated or anaplastic histologies. S100 protein is also present in nervous system tissue.

SERUM PROTEINS – See Immunoelectrophoresis.

SILVER IN SITU HYBRIDIZATION (SISH) – A type of genetic testing that uses metallic silver deposition to identify over-expression of HER2 (see HER2) in breast tumor cells. The deposited silver creates a dark mark on the tissue distinct from other types of staining. The SISH technique can be fully automated and delivers results in half a day rather than the longer times necessary for FISH and CISH. SISH is a type of bright field in situ hybridization.

SQUAMOUS CELL CARCINOMA (SCC) ANTIGEN — Monitors tumor burden after treatment for squamous cell carcinoma; usually used for advanced disease; primary application is head and neck cancer, secondarily for lung cancer; non-specific to cervical carcinoma but specific to squamous cell carcinoma

Tumor Markers, *continued*

STOOL GUIAC TEST – See Fecal Occult Blood Test.

T- AND B-CELL LYMPHOCYTE ANALYSIS – Distinguishes between types of hematopoietic disease. Elevated B-cell count: CLL, multiple myeloma, Waldenstrom's macrogloulinemia; decreased B-cell count: ALL. Elevated T-cell count: multiple myeloma, ALL; decreased T-cell count: AIDS, CLL, Waldenstrom's macroglobulinemia. Abnormal results suggest, but do not confirm, specific diseases.

TDT (Terminal Deoxynucleotidal Transferase) – Differentiates acute lymphocytic leukemia from acute non-lymphocytic leukemia; differentiates lymphoblastic lymphomas from other non-Hodgkin's lymphomas; TDT levels are absent in patients in remission

THYROGLOBULIN – Elevated levels of this serum hormone are found in follicular carcinoma and return to normal following treatment if all tumor is removed; useful for monitoring residual disease and recurrence of follicular carcinoma

TOTAL BILIRUBIN – A blood serum tumor marker that, if elevated, indicates damage to the liver including liver tumor, a blood disorder, or blockage of bile ducts. Total bilirubin is a combination of conjugated (direct), unconjugated (indirect), and delta (conjugated bilirubin bound to albumin) levels. This test provides clinical information about the severity of liver damage for patients with primary liver cancer. Total bilirubin is measured in different ways—milligrams per deciliter (mg/dL) in the US and micromoles per liter (µmoles/L) in Canada.

TPA (Tissue Polypeptide Antigen) — An antigen marker for cancers of gynecologic sites, bladder, and lung; non-specific to ovarian and cancer; elevated levels indicate presence of malignancy; also used to monitor bladder and lung cancer in males.

α-TSH (Alpha Subunit Thyroid Stimulating Hormone) – A marker that can differentiate pancreatic from other hormonal tumors; non-specific—also found in pituitary and placental tumors

TUMOR INFILTRATING LYMPHOCYTES (TIL) – A marker for Merkel cell carcinoma indicating the patient's response (immune reaction) to the cancer. TILs at the growth edges of the tumor are a favorable prognostic factor. TIL response is described as brisk, non-brisk, or absent.

URINARY 5-HIAA – See 5-HIAA.

UROVYSION – A trademarked test looking for chromosome changes in the urine that identify bladder cancer cells.

VASOINTESTINAL PEPTIDE (Vasoactive Intestinal Polypeptide, VIP) – Elevated levels suggest catecholamine-secreting tumor such as neuroblastoma or ganglioneuroma. High levels indicate pheochromoctyoma.

VMA (Vanillylmandelic Acid) elevated levels suggest catecholamine-secreting tumor such as neuroblastoma or ganglioneuroma; non-specific to VMA.

Page left blank.

THE LYMPHATIC SYSTEM

The lymphatic system is a specialized part of the body's circulatory system. It is often under-appreciated unless a cancer patient develops a nodal lymphoma or lymph node metastases from a solid organ. The lymphatic system serves several purposes:

- ***Returning water, proteins, fats and other substances from tissues*** back to the blood stream. During the exchange of oxygen and nutrients between the blood and body tissues, water from the capillaries enters the tissues and surrounds the cells. If this interstitial fluid is not properly drained, it builds up in the tissues and causes edema and decreased blood volume and blood pressure. To counteract this, the fluid and cellular waste that is not reabsorbed into the veins is drained from the tissues by the lymphatic vessels and is called lymph when it enters the lymphatic system. Figure 1 shows how the open-ended lymphatic capillaries intermingle with the arterioles and connecting venules to drain interstitial fluid from the tissues.

  Compared to the blood, lymph contains a greater water content, lower protein content, and no blood cells other than lymphocytes. The process of removing fluid from tissues helps maintain the fluid balance in the body.
- ***Transporting lipids*** (fats and fatty acids) in the form of chyle from the digestive tract to the circulatory system
- ***Defending against micro-organisms, infections, and disease***. As part of the immune system, the lymph nodes filter out foreign particles—including metastatic tumor cells—and the lymphocytes produced in the lymph nodes destroy the invading micro-organisms.

LYMPHATIC SYSTEM ELEMENTS

- **Lymph**—the clear fluid that flows throughout the body
- **Lymphatic vessels**—also called lymph channels, lymph vessels, or lymphatics. Lymphatic vessels are similar to veins but with thinner walls and run parallel to but separate from the veins. Small vessels within organs flow into larger vessels, then into either the right lymphatic duct or the thoracic duct, which empty the fluid back into the venous blood above the heart.
  - The ***thoracic duct*** is about 16 inches long and receives lymph from the entire left side of the body and the right side of the body below the diaphragm. It begins below the

Figure 1. Lymphatic Capillary Drainage of Interstitial Fluid

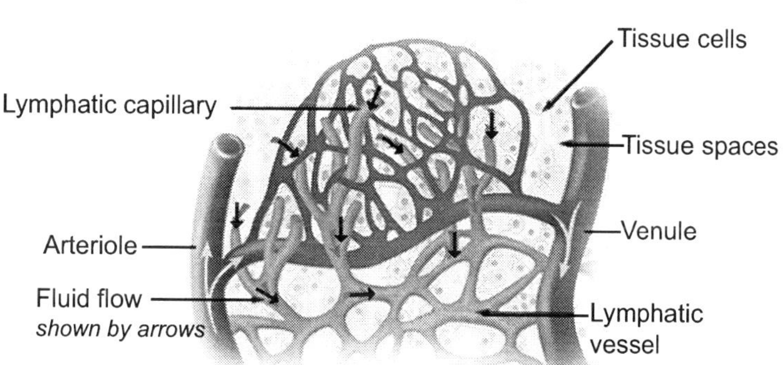

Image source: training.seer.cancer.gov. In the public domain.

Lymphatic System Elements, *continued*

diaphragm at the cysterna chyli and empties into the left subclavian vein just below the clavicle.

  - The ***right lymphatic duct*** receives lymph from only the right upper quadrant of the body—the right side of the head and neck, the right arm, and the right side of the thorax above the diaphragm. The right lymphatic duct empties into the right subclavian vein.
  - The fact that there are two drainage systems (Figure 2) in the upper half of the body helps explain why bilateral involvement of lymph nodes such as cervical or axillary nodes, is counted as two lymph node regions for staging of lymphoma—there are two routes for metastatic cells to circulate through the body.

Figure 2. Lymphatic System
Arrows mark boundaries of drainage systems

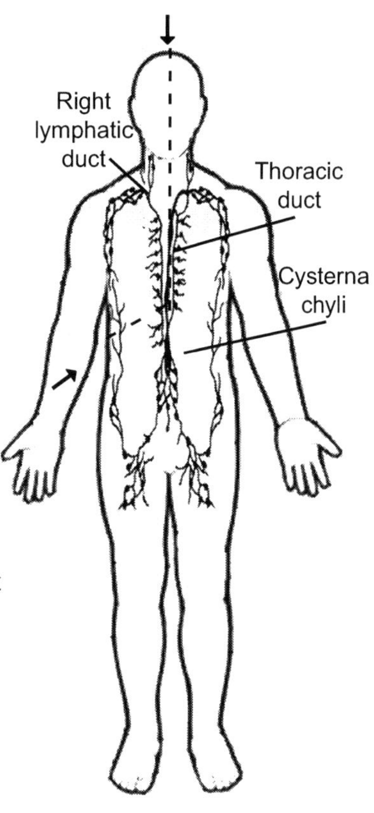

- **Lymph nodes**—oval or bean shaped encapsulated lymphoid tissue. Normal lymph nodes range from a few millimeters up to about 2 centimeters in size. There are about 500 lymph nodes in the body scattered along the lymphatic vessels in chains or clusters. The lymph nodes act as cleaners or filters for lymph fluid, removing foreign particles before the lymph is emptied back into the blood. Lymph must pass through at least two lymph nodes before it reaches the blood stream again. The lymph nodes also act as immune response centers, producing lymphocytes that defend against infection. Figure 3 is a schematic of the structure of a lymph node. The node receives lymph from two or more *afferent* lymphatic vessels from one or more organs or structures. After the lymph is filtered in the sinuses of the node, the fluid leaves through the *efferent* lymph vessels at the hilum of the node. Both the afferent and efferent vessels contain valves that prevent the lymph from flowing backwards—all lymph flows toward the heart. Functional areas of a lymph node include:
  - *Germinal center*—also known as follicle center; areas within lymph node where lymphocytes are produced; the site of follicular and Burkitt's lymphomas.
  - *Mantle zone*—area surrounding germinal center; also known as the corona; the site of mantle zone lymphomas.
  - *Capsule*—connective tissue covering the outside of the node
  - *Trabeculae*—extensions of the capsule that create septa to divide the inside of the node into chambers or spaces
  - *Cortex*—peripheral portion of node inside the capsule; contains many lymphocytes
  - *Medulla*—central portion of lymph node; contains few lymphocytes

Figure 3. Lymph Node
Schematic Illustration

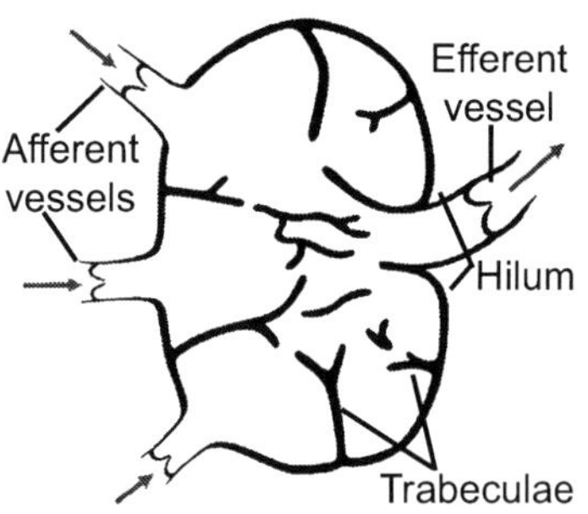

Image source: Webanatomy Image Database, University of Minnesota

- **Lymphatic organs**—larger areas of lymphoid tissue in various areas of the body that protect against infection and may be the site of lymphoid malignancies. The lymphatic organs generally have a surrounding capsule. The main lymphatic organs are:

Lymphatic System Elements, *continued*

- ◦ *Tonsils*—small masses of lymphatic tissue surrounding the opening of the pharynx. The tonsils protect against pathogens that enter the respiratory and digestive systems through the nose and mouth. There are three areas of tonsils in the pharynx:
  - *Palatine tonsils*—paired structures in the lateral walls of the oropharynx
  - *Lingual tonsil*—at the base of the tongue
  - *Pharyngeal tonsil* or *adenoids*—in the superior-posterior part of the nasopharynx
  - As a group, the tonsils are referred to as *Waldeyer's ring*, named after 19th century German anatomist Heinrich W.G. Waldeyer-Hartz, who first identified these structures as a defense against pathogens entering the upper aero-digestive tract.
- ◦ *Spleen*—the largest lymphoid organ in the body, located below the diaphragm on the left side. The spleen filters blood and also acts as a reservoir for blood.
- ◦ *Thymus*—located in the anterior mediastinum; receives lymphocyte precursors from the bone marrow and serves as their repository until they mature into T-cell lymphocytes. The thymus is large in an infant and atrophies after puberty.

- **Other lymphatic tissues**—smaller, unencapsulated aggregations of lymphoid tissue in various organs, such as:
  - ◦ *Peyer's patches* of the small intestine
  - ◦ *Lymphoid nodules* in the appendix
  - ◦ _____*-associated lymphoid tissues*—lymphoid nodules occurring within the lamina propria of the membranes that line the gastrointestinal, respiratory, reproductive and urinary tracts, specifically
    - MALT—mucosa-associated lymphoid tissue
    - GALT—gut-associated lymphoid tissue
    - BALT—bronchial-associated lymphoid tissue
    - SALT—skin-associated lymphoid tissue
  - ◦ *Bone marrow*—produces red and white blood cells (lymphocytes) and platelets
- **Extralymphatic sites**—even smaller areas of lymphoid tissue in solid organs that are responsible for immune responses to infections and are potential sites of malignant lymphoma. The most common extralymphatic sites are: stomach, small intestine, large intestine, bone, uterus, breast, and brain.

ABSTRACTING NOTES

- ***Regional lymph nodes*** are defined as the first lymph nodes to drain an organ. Within the regional lymph nodes, the ***sentinel lymph node***(s) are the first regional lymph node(s) potentially to receive and filter metastatic cancer cells. "Sentinel" is not the name of a specific lymph node in any chain.
- ***Juxtaregional lymph nodes*** are the next chain(s) to drain the regional lymph nodes. The TNM system uses the term juxtaregional (next to regional); in the Summary Staging system, juxtaregional nodes are defined as distant lymph nodes.
- The following organs and structures have no regional lymph nodes: brain, spinal cord, bone marrow, cartilage.
- In general, regional lymph nodes are specific to an organ. However, in large body systems such as the bone, soft tissues, skin (carcinoma and melanoma), soft tissue sarcoma, and even the segments of the colon, the lymph nodes in the area of the organ are defined as the regional lymph nodes. For example, the regional nodes for a melanoma of the scalp would be the cervical lymph nodes but not the axillary nodes.

Abstracting Notes, ***continued***

- The lymphatic system does not have a pump like the heart pumps blood through the circulatory system. Instead, movement of lymph through the lymphatic system occurs by contraction of skeletal muscles.
- As mentioned, lymph fluid flows one way, toward the heart through lymph vessels and nodes. Therefore, lymph fluid containing tumor cells cannot flow retrograde from a node to the organ it drains. Thus, an extralymphatic lymphoma starts in the organ and spreads to the regional lymph nodes, not vice versa. However, a lymphoma in lymph nodes may invade an adjacent organ by direct extension.

LYMPH NODE TERMINOLOGY

- *Visceral*—adjacent to an organ, or central within a body cavity
  Examples of visceral lymph chains: mediastinal, hilar, gastric, hepatic, mesenteric
- *Parietal*—near the walls of a body cavity
  Examples of parietal lymph chains: internal mammary, phrenic, aortic, iliac
- The *supraclavicular nodes* are defined as the transverse cervical chain with the lowest nodes of the upper deep jugular and spinal accessory chains.
- The *scalene nodes* are between the scalenus muscles at the base of the neck (supraclavicular).
- The *retroperitoneal nodes* are defined as the para-aortic, iliac and sacral lymph chains.
- The *retrocrural nodes* are posterior to the crus (plural = crura) of the diaphragm, the tendons that attach the diaphragm to the vertebral column. The retrocrural nodes are para-aortic (retroperitoneal) nodes at the level of the cisterna chyli.

On the following pages, Figure 4 shows the 36 major lymph node regions of the body. Figures 5–15 are more detailed looks at the lymph nodes in various body regions. At the end of this chapter are lists of nodes not shown in the figures and a final list of synonyms for various lymph nodes.

Detailed List of Lymph Nodes and Lymph Node Chains
Appendix C of the *2010 Hematopoietic and Lymphoid Neoplasm Case Reportability and Coding Manual* is an extensive listing of named lymph nodes and lymph node chains. This is an excellent resource for abstractors and serves several purposes beyond its use in the hematopoietic multiple primary rules. Lymph nodes are listed alphabetically, together with their ICD-O-3 code, the name of the ICD-O-3 lymph node region, and the AJCC lymph node region. The ICD-O-3 code information can be used for assigning the primary site for malignant lymphomas. The AJCC lymph node region information can be used to determine the lymphoma stage. Refer to Appendix C when there is any question whether two lymph node chains are in the same ICD-O-3 region or represent different regions for staging purposes.

Appendix C is part of the Hematopoietic Data Base and Coding Manual, which can be downloaded from seer.cancer.gov/tools/heme/index.html.

Figure 4. Major Lymph Node Chains

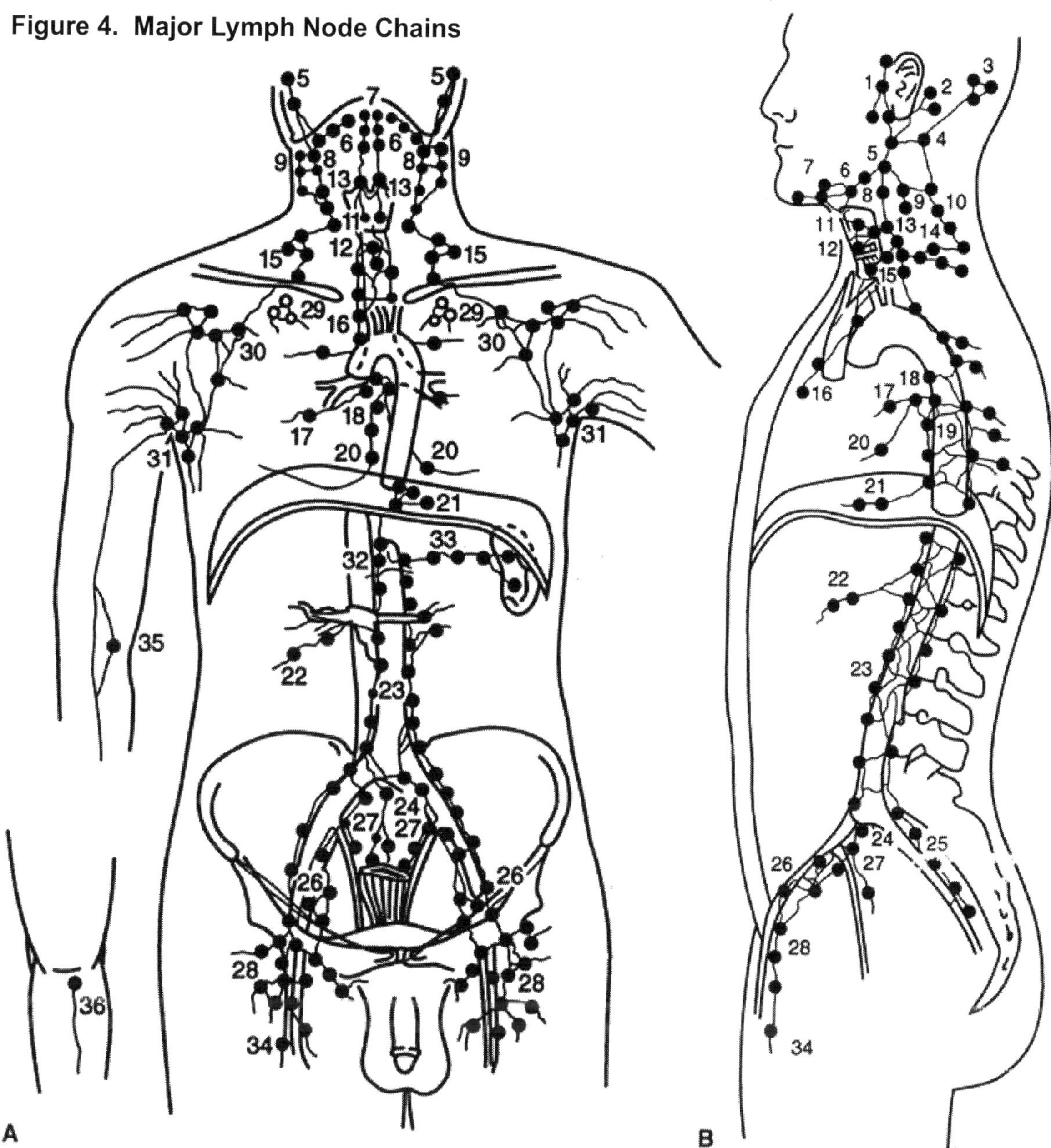

Image source: TNM Staging Atlas, P Rubin and JT Hansen. Wolters Kluwer, 2008. Used with permission; may not be reproduced without written consent from the original source.

1. Preauricular
2. Mastoid
3. Occipital
4. Upper cervical
5. Parotid
6. Submaxillary
7. Submental
8. Jugulo-digastric
9. Upper deep cervical
10. Spinal accessory chain
11. Infrahyoid
12. Pretracheal
13. Jugulo-omohyoid
14. Lower deep cervical
15. Supraclavicular
16. Mediastinal
17. Interlobar (hilar)
18. Intertracheal
19. Posterior mediastinal
20. Lateral pericardial
21. Diaphragmatic
22. Mesenteric
23. Para-aortic
24. Common iliac
25. Lateral sacral
26. External iliac
27. Hypogastric
28. Inguinal
29. Interpectoral
30. Axillary apex
31. Axillary
32. Cysterna chyli
33. Splenic
34. Femoral
35. Epitrochlear
36. Popliteal

KEY LN = lymph node • Not shown *Italics* = organs/areas drained by LN

Figures 5–7. Lymph Nodes of Head and Neck

SUPERFICIAL LYMPH NODES

Lymph node	Areas drained
1. Occipital LN	*scalp*
2. Mastoid (retroauricular) LN	*posterior external ear, auditory canal, scalp*
3. Superficial Parotid LN	*temporal area skin, anterior earlobe*
• Deep Parotid LN	*parotid gland, tympanic cavity, external auditory canal, temple, forehead, eyelids, root of nose, nasopharyngeal cavity*
• Preauricular	*parotid gland, eyelid, lacrimal gland, conjunctiva*
• Infraauricular	*parotid gland*
• Intraglandular parotid	*parotid gland*
4. Facial LN	*eyelids, nose, buccal mucosa, rest of face*
• Buccinator LN	
• Nasolabial LN	
• Mandibular LN	
• Anterior Cervical (Superficial) LN	*skin of frontal area of neck*
5. Superficial Cervical (Lateral) LN (external jugular)	*lower earlobe, lower parotid*

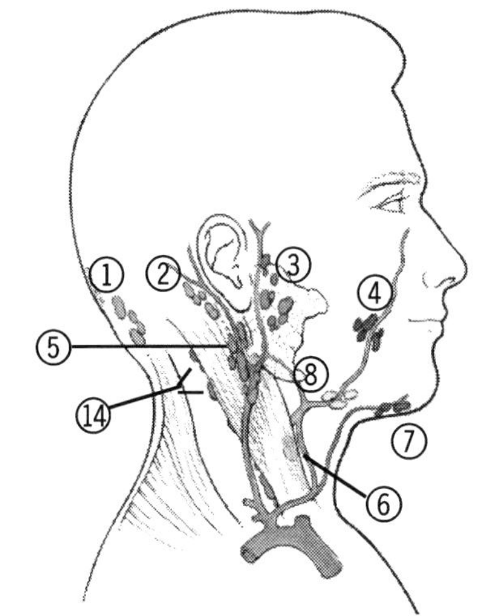

Figure 5. Superficial Lymph Nodes of Head and Neck

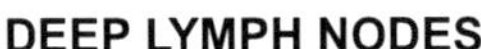

DEEP LYMPH NODES

Lymph node	Areas drained
6. Jugulo-omohyoid	*tongue, maxillary sinus, larynx, oral cavity, pharynx, lip, soft palate, uvula*
7. Submental LN	*central lower lip, floor of mouth, anterior 2/3 of tongue, oral cavity, soft palate, maxillary sinus, pharynx, larynx, uvula, base of tongue*
8. Submandibular (submaxillary) LN	*cheek, side of nose, eyelid, lacrimal gland, conjunctiva, upper lip, lateral lower lip, gums, frontal edge of tongue, inner canthus, larynx, submandibular salivary gland, maxillary sinus, base of tongue, uvula, pharynx, oral cavity, soft palate*
Anterior Cervical LN (Deep)	*thyroid gland*
9. Infrahyoid LN	*larynx, pyriform sinus, hypopharynx*
10. Prelaryngeal LN	*lower larynx*
11. Thyroid LN	*thyroid gland*
12. Pretracheal LN	*trachea, larynx, thyroid gland, lung*
13. Paratracheal LN	*trachea, larynx*
Lateral Deep Cervical LN	*all head and neck areas*
14. Superior Deep Cervical LN	*all head and neck areas*
15. Jugulodigastric LN	*oral cavity, uvula, larynx, lip, soft palate, pharynx, maxillary sinus, base of tongue, thyroid gland, submandibular salivary gland*
16. Inferior Deep Cervical LN	*all head and neck areas*
17. Supraclavicular (scalene) LN	*lung, cervical esophagus, breast*
18. Retropharyngeal LN	*thyroid gland*

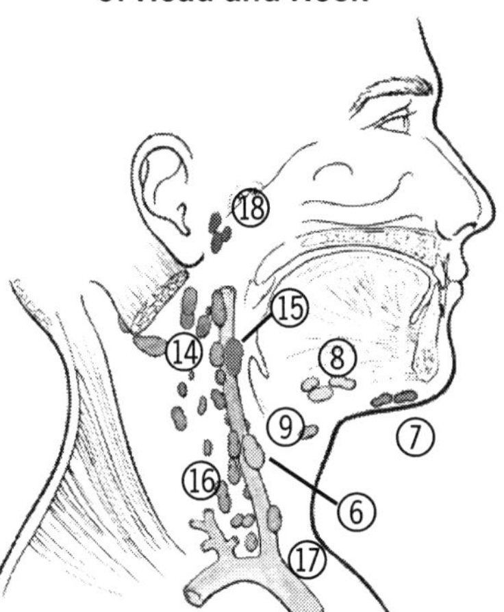

Figure 6. Deep Lymph Nodes of Head and Neck

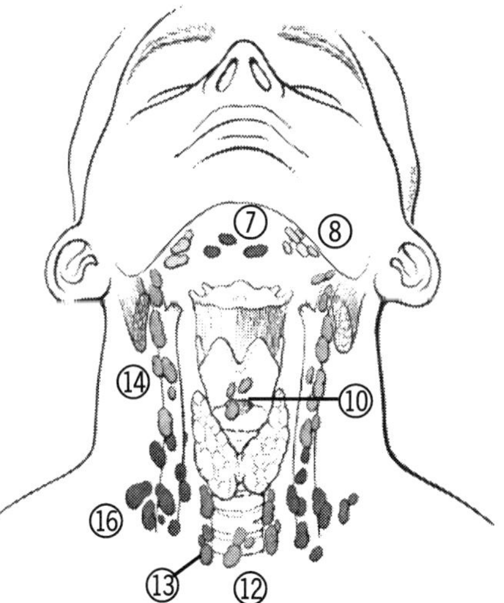

Figure 7. Lymph Nodes of Head and Neck — Anterior View

KEY	LN = lymph node	• Not shown	*Italics* = organs/areas drained by LN

Figure 8. Lymph Nodes of Breast and Upper Limb

Axillary LN *breast, upper arm*
1. Lateral (superficial) axillary LN (Level I, low axillary) *breast*
2. Interpectoral LN (Level II, Rotter's LN) *breast*
3. Apical axillary LN (Level III, deep, high axillary) *breast*
4. Infraclavicular LN *breast*
5. Supraclavicular LN *breast*
6. Paramammary LN (intramammary, Level I) *breast*

Other Regional LN of Breast

7. Internal Mammary (parasternal) LN *breast*

- Cubital LN *ulnar hand, fingers, forearm*
- Epitrochlear LN (elbow) *upper extremity*
- Brachial axillary LN *breast*

Figure 8. Lymph Nodes of Breast

Figures 9–10. Thoracic Lymph Nodes

THORACIC LYMPH NODE STATIONS

Superior Mediastinal LN *lung, upper and middle esophagus*

1	Superior mediastinal LN	
2R, 2L	Paratracheal (upper) LN	
3	Pretracheal, retrotracheal LN	
4R, 4L	Lower paratracheal LN	
Aortic LN		*lung*
5	Subaortic (aortic window) LN	
6	Para-aortic (ascending aorta or phrenic) LN	
Inferior Mediastinal LN		
7	Carinal LN	*lung*
7	Subcarinal LN	*lung*
8R, 8L	Paraesophageal (below carina) LN	*lung, esophagus*
9R, 9L	Pulmonary ligament LN	*lung*
Pulmonary LN (part of Posterior Mediastinal group)		
10R, 10L	Hilar LN	*lung, upper and middle esophagus*
11R, 11L	Intrapulmonic (interlobar) LN	*lung*
12R, 12L	Peribronchial (lobar) LN	*lung*
13R, 13L	Segmental LN	*lung*
14R, 14L	Subsegmental LN	*lung*

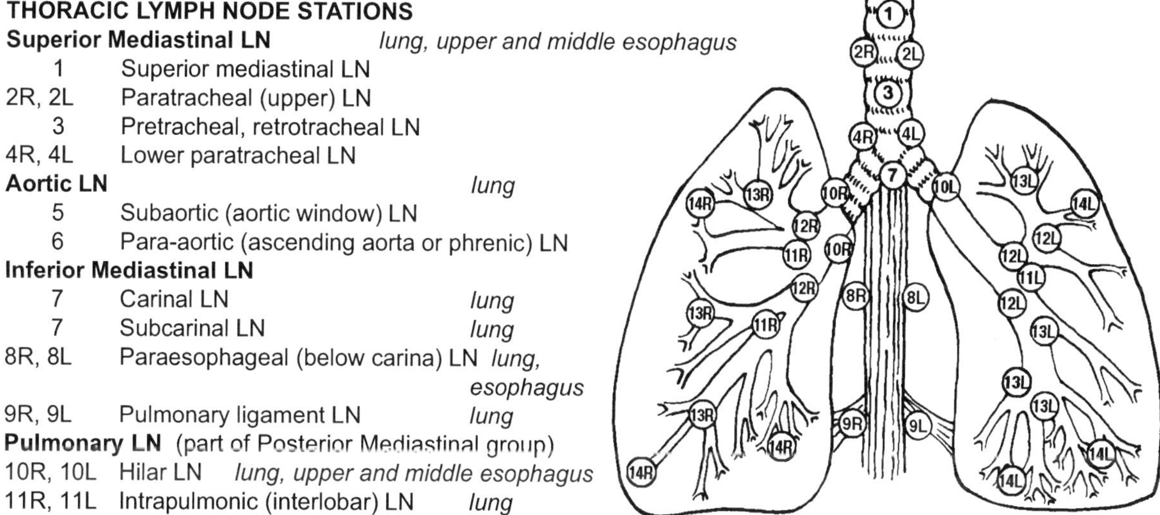

Figure 9. Thoracic Lymph Node Stations

PARIETAL LYMPH NODES OF THE THORAX

15. Prepericardial LN *sternum, anterior pericardium*
16. Lateral pericardial LN *pericardium*

OTHER LYMPH NODES OF THORAX

- Anterior mediastinal LN *lung, thyroid gland, thymus, pericardium*
- Node of ligamentum arteriosum
- Node of arch of azygos vein (part of posterior mediastinal group)
- Posterior Mediastinal LN *lungs, bronchi, trachea, esophagus, pericardium, diaphragm, superior region of liver*
- Intercostal LN *pleura, intercostal spaces*
- Paravertebral LN *surrounding area unless otherwise drained*
- Superior Phrenic LN *liver, diaphragm*

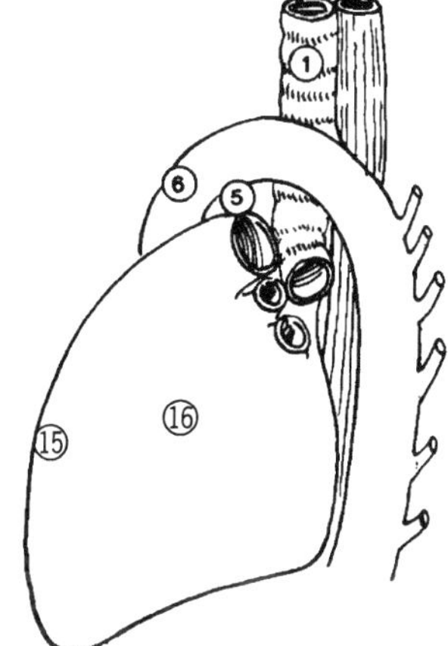

Figure 10. Pericardial Lymph Nodes

Figures 9 and 10 adapted from: Lung Cancer Lymph Node Staging, *AFIP Lung* fascicle by Colby, Koss and Travis.

Lymphatic Sys

KEY	LN = lymph node	• Not shown	*Italics* = organs/areas drained by LN

Figures 11–13. Abdominal Lymph Nodes

DEEP (PARIETAL) NODES OF ABDOMINAL CAVITY	
Para-aortic (Left Lumbar) LN	*adrenal glands, kidneys, renal pelvis, Wilms' tumor, ureter, testicles, ovary, fallopian tubes, fundus of uterus, abdominal wall*
1. Lateral aortic LN	*pancreas*
2. Preaortic LN	*see list above at para-aortic*
• Postaortic LN	
• Intermediate Lumbar LN	*adrenal glands, kidneys, ureter, testicles, ovary, fallopian tubes, fundus of uterus, abdominal wall*
Paracaval (Right Lumbar) LN	*adrenal glands, kidneys, renal pelvis, Wilms' tumor, ureter, testicles, ovary, fallopian tubes, fundus of uterus, abdominal wall*
3. Lateral caval LN	
• Precaval LN	
• Postcaval LN	
4. Inferior phrenic LN	*diaphragm, liver, adrenal gland*
VISCERAL NODES OF ABDOMINAL CAVITY	
5. Celiac LN	*pancreas (head), endocrine pancreas, gallbladder, stomach*
6. Hepatic LN	*liver, gallbladder, stomach*
7. Cystic LN	*gallbladder, endocrine pancreas*
8. Gastric (right and left) LN	*stomach, lower esophagus (left)*
• Cardioesophageal LN	*lower esophagus, stomach*
9. Gastroomental (right and left) LN (gastroepiploic)	*stomach (greater curvature)*
Pyloric LN	*stomach, Ampulla of Vater, pancreas, duodenum*
10. Suprapyloric LN	
11. Subpyloric LN	
• Retropyloric LN	
Pancreatic LN	*endocrine and exocrine pancreas, stomach, gallbladder*
12. Superior pancreatic LN	
13. Inferior pancreatic LN	
14. Splenic (Lienal) LN	*spleen, pancreas (body and tail), stomach*
Pancreaticoduodenal LN	*endocrine pancreas, pancreas, duodenum, ampulla of Vater*
15. Superior pancreaticoduodenal LN	
• Inferior pancreaticoduodenal LN	
16. Superior mesenteric LN	*secondary drainage from colon*
17. Mesenteric LN	*small intestine, colon, mesentery*

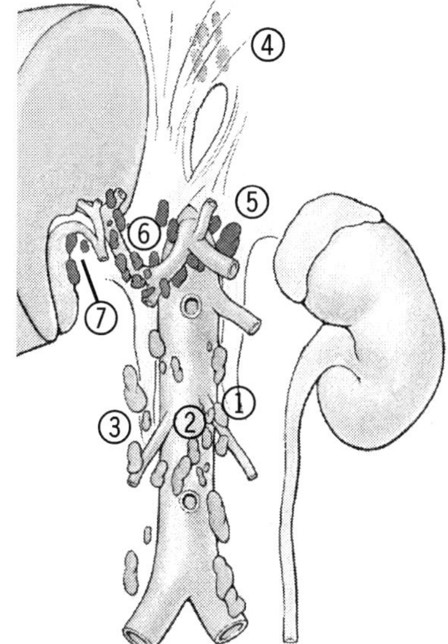

Figure 11. Para-aortic and Paracaval Lymph Nodes

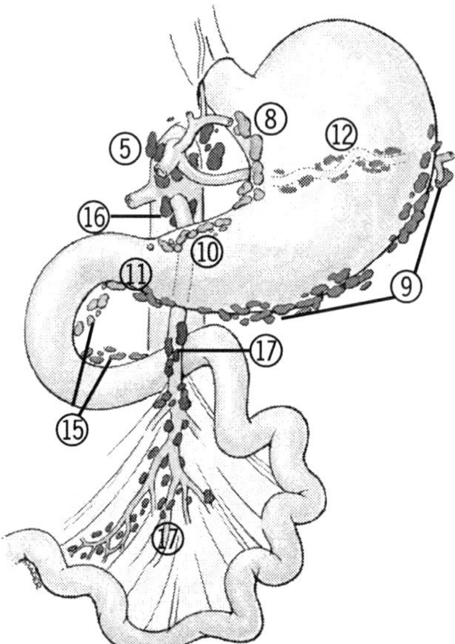

Figure 12. Lymph Nodes of Stomach, Pancreas, and Small Intestine

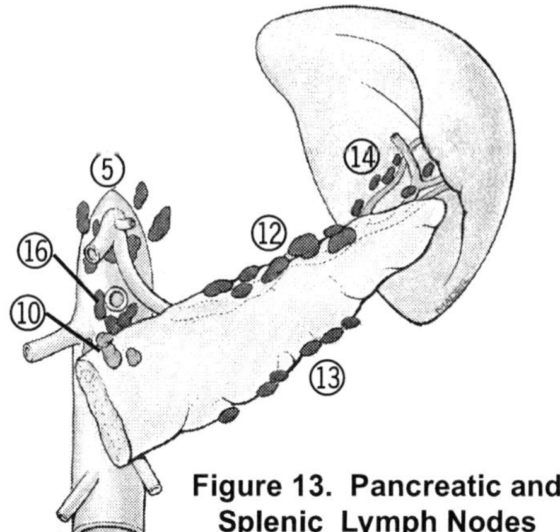

Figure 13. Pancreatic and Splenic Lymph Nodes

Except as noted, Figures 4–14 are adapted from MediClip (medical clip art), Williams and Wilkins, 1998.
Grant's Atlas Images 1: Thorax and Abdomen
Grant's Atlas Images 3: Perineum, Pelvis and Lower Limb
Grant's Atlas Images 4: Head, Neck and Cranial Nerves

KEY	LN = lymph node	• Not shown	*Italics* = organs/areas drained by LN

Figure 14. Lymph Nodes of Large Intestine and Lower Abdomen

Lymph Nodes of the Colon

1. Ileocolic LN	*appendix, cecum, ascending colon*
• Prececal LN	*cecum, appendix*
• Retrocecal LN	*appendix, cecum*
2. Appendicular LN	*appendix*
Mesocolic LN	
3. Paracolic LN	*all areas of large intestine*
4. Epicolic LN	*all areas of large intestine*
5. Left colic LN	*splenic flexure, rectosigmoid, rectum, descending colon*
6. Middle colic LN	*hepatic flexure, transverse colon, ascending colon, splenic flexure*
7. Right colic LN	*hepatic flexure, ascending colon, cecum, appendix*
8. Inferior mesenteric LN	*rectum, descending colon, splenic flexure, rectosigmoid, sigmoid*
9. Sigmoid LN	*descending colon, sigmoid, rectosigmoid, rectum*
10. Superior rectal LN	*sigmoid, rectosigmoid*

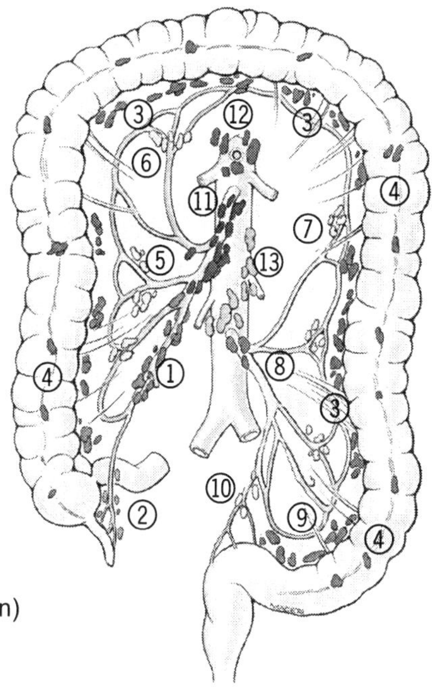

Figure 14. Lymph Nodes of Colon

Lymph Nodes of the Lower Abdomen (not staged as regional for colon)

11. Superior mesenteric LN	*endocrine pancreas, Ampulla of Vater, stomach, gallbladder*
12. Celiac LN	*pancreas (head), endocrine pancreas, gallbladder, stomach*
13. Para-aortic LN	*adrenal glands, kidneys, renal pelvis, Wilms' tumor, ureter, testicles, ovary, fallopian tubes, fundus of uterus, abdominal wall*

Figure 15. Lymph Nodes of Pelvis and Lower Limb

1. Common Iliac LN	*renal pelvis, vagina, urethra, cervix, corpus uteri, ureter, ovary*
2. External Iliac LN	*renal pelvis, vagina, vulva, cervix, corpus uteri, ovary, bladder, prostate, ureter, urethra*
3. Obturator (external iliac obturator) LN	*ovary, cervix, bladder, corpus uteri, prostate*
4. Internal Iliac (hypogastric) LN	*corpus uteri, vagina, bladder, renal pelvis, rectum, urethra, ureter, cervix, prostate, vulva, ovary, anal canal*
5. Superficial Inguinal LN	*penis, anal canal, prostate, vagina, vulva, ovary, testis, urethra*
6. Deep Inguinal LN	*penis*
7. Para-aortic LN	*see list above at 13*
8. Presacral LN	*cervix, bladder, prostate, anal canal, rectum, ovary, corpus uteri, pelvic wall, pelvic ureter, gluteal muscles*
9. Pararectal LN	*posteroinferior pelvic structures, inferior rectum*
• Popliteal LN (at knee)	*lower extremity*

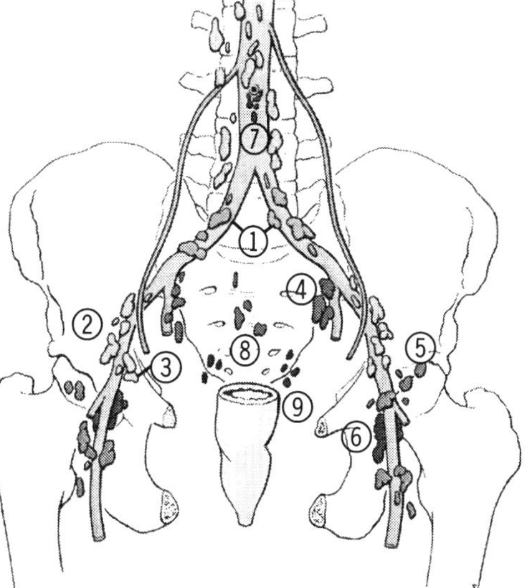

Figure 15. Lymph Nodes of Pelvis and Lower Extremity

ADDITIONAL LYMPH NODE CHAINS* NOT SHOWN IN ILLUSTRATIONS AND AREAS DRAINED

Anorectal LN	*anal canal*
Common bile duct LN	*pancreas, ampulla of Vater*
Delphian LN	*thyroid gland*
Femoral LN	*anal canal, vulva, vagina*
Gastrohepatic LN	*stomach*
Gastropancreatic LN	*stomach*
Infundibulopelvic LN	*corpus uteri*
Middle hemorrhoidal LN	*rectosigmoid*
Pancreaticolienal LN	*stomach, body and tail of pancreas*
Paracervical LN	*cervix*
Paraprostatic LN	*prostate*
Parauterine LN	*cervix, corpus uteri*
Pelvic LN, NOS	*prostate, bladder, penis*
Pericholedochal LN	*endocrine pancreas, gallbladder*
Periduodenal LN	*gallbladder, endocrine pancreas*
Perivesicular LN	*bladder, prostate*
Renal hilar LN	*renal pelvis, kidney, Wilms' tumor*
Suprahyoid LN	*thyroid gland*

* terminology used in *AJCC Cancer Staging Manual.*

EPONYMIC LYMPH NODES (named after someone)

Aselli's glands—nodes near the pancreas (Gasparo Aselli 1581–1626, Italian surgeon and anatomist)
Calot's node—hepatobiliary triangle; cystic duct (Jean-Francois Calot 1861–1944, French surgeon)
Cloquet's node—uppermost deep inguinal (Jules Germain Cloquet 1790–1883, French surgeon)
Delphian node—anterior to thyroid isthmus; prelaryngeal (mythical Oracle of Delphi)
Foramen of Winslow node—epiploic (omental) (Jacob Benignus Winslow 1669–1760, Danish-born French anatomist)
Gerota's node—sacral promontory (Dimitrie Gerota 1867–1939, Romanian anatomist and surgeon)
Rosenmüller's node—uppermost deep inguinal (Johann Christian Rosenmüller 1771–1820, German anatomist and surgeon)
Rosenmüller-Cloquet gland—uppermost deep inguinal (see Cloquet and Rosenmüller above)
Rotter's node—between pectoralis major and minor muscles (interpectoral) of the chest (Josef Rotter 1857–1924, German surgeon)
Rouvière's node—lateral retropharyngeal (Henri Rouvière 1875–1952, French anatomist)
Sister Mary Joseph's nodule—not a lymph node, but a metastatic nodule in the umbilical area (named after a Mayo Clinic surgical nurse who noted the nodule in patients with intra-abdominal malignancies usually from stomach or ovary)
Troisier's node—left supraclavicular (Charles Emile Troisier 1844–1919; French pathologist)
Virchow's node—supraclavicular (Rudolph Karl Ludwig Virchow 1821–1902, German pathologist)
Waldeyer's ring—lymphoid tissues (pharyngeal, palatine, and lingual) surrounding the throat (Heinrich W.G. Waldeyer-Hartz, 1836–1921, German Anatomist)

LYMPHATIC SYSTEM — GLOSSARY OF SYNONYMOUS TERMS

See also Eponymic Lymph Nodes on page 104.

Anorectal = Hemorrhoidal
Anorectal = Pararectal
Anterior cecal = Prececal
Anterior deep cervical = Laterotracheal
Anterior to thyroid isthmus = Delphian (thyroid)
Aortico-pulmonary window = Subaortic
Apical axillary = Level III axillary
Apical axillary = Subclavian
Ascending aortic = Phrenic
Aselli's glands = nodes near the pancreas
Axillary = Intramammary
Axillary = Paramammary
Axillary *see also Level I, Level II, Level III*
Azygos = Lower paratracheal

Brachial = Lateral axillary
Brachiocephalic = Innominate
Brachiocephalic = Thoracic
Bronchial = Tracheobronchial
Bronchopulmonary = Hilar
Buccal = Buccinator
Buccinator = Buccal

Calot's = Cystic duct
Carinal = Tracheal bifurcation
Cloquet's = Uppermost deep inguinal
Common bile duct = Pericholedochal
Cystic duct = Calot's

Deep inguinal (uppermost) = Cloquet's
Deep inguinal (uppermost) = Rosenmüller's
Deep axillary = Level III axillary
Deep inguinal = Subinguinal
Delphian (thyroid) = Anterior to thyroid isthmus

Epiploic = Foramen of Winslow node
Epiploic = Omental
Ewald's = Supraclavicular node enlarged due to abdominal tumor

Femoral = Superficial inguinal
Foramen of Winslow node = Epiploic (omental)

Gerota's = Sacral promontory
Gastroepiploic = Gastro-omental
Gastro-omental = Gastroepiploic

Hemorrhoidal = Anorectal
Hepatic = Portal; porta hepatis; hilar (liver)
Hilar = Pulmonary root
Hilar (liver) = Portal; porta hepatis; hepatic
Hilar (lung) = Bronchopulmonary
Hypogastric = Internal iliac
Hypogastric = Obturator

Inferior gastric = Right gastric
Infraclavicular = Subclavicular
Infrapyloric = Subpyloric
Infundibulopelvic = Utero-ovarian
Innominate = Brachiocephalic
Innominate = Thoracic
Internal iliac = Hypogastric
Internal iliac = Obturator
Internal mammary = Parasternal
Interpectoral = Level II
Interpectoral = Rotter's
Intramammary = Axillary
Intramammary = Paramammary

Jugulodigastric = Subdigastric
Jugulo-omohyoid = Supraomohyoid

Lateral aortic = Lumbar
Lateral aortic = Retroperitoneal
Lateral axillary = Brachial
Laterotracheal = Anterior deep cervical
Laterotracheal = Recurrent laryngeal nerve chain
Left gastric = Superior gastric
Left lumbar = Para-aortic
Level I axillary = Low axillary
Level I axillary = Superficial axillary
Level II = Interpectoral
Level II = Rotter's
Level III axillary = Apical axillary
Level III axillary = Deep axillary
Level III axillary = Subclavian
Lienal = Splenic
Low axillary = Level 1 axillary
Low axillary = Superficial axillary
Lower paratracheal = Azygos
Lumbar = Lateral aortic
Lumbar = Retroperitoneal

Lymph Node Synonyms, *continued*

Mastoid = Postauricular
Mastoid = Retroauricular

Obturator = Hypogastric
Obturator = Internal iliac
Omental = Epiploic
Omental = Foramen of Winslow node
Pancreaticolienal = Pancreaticosplenic
Pancreaticosplenic = Pancreaticolienal
Para-aortic = Left lumbar
Paracaval = Right lumbar
Paramammary = Axillary
Paramammary = Intramammary
Pararectal = Anorectal
Parasternal = Internal mammary
Pericholedochal = Common bile duct
Phrenic = Ascending aortic
Portal = Hepatic; porta hepatis
Portal = Hilar (liver)
Postauricular = Mastoid
Postauricular = Retroauricular
Posterior axillary = Subscapular
Posterior cecal = Retrocecal
Posterior cervical = Spinal accessory
Prececal = Anterior cecal
Pulmonary root = Hilar

Recurrent laryngeal nerve chain = Laterotracheal
Retroauricular = Mastoid
Retroauricular = Postauricular
Retrocecal = Posterior cecal
Retroperitoneal = Lateral aortic
Retroperitoneal = Lumbar
Retropharyngeal = Rouviere's node
Right gastric = Inferior gastric
Right lumbar = Paracaval
Rosenmüller's = Cloquet's
Rosenmüller's = Deep inguinal (uppermost)
Rotter's = Interpectoral
Rotter's = Level II
Rouviere's node = Retropharyngeal

Sacral promontory = Gerota's
Scalene = Cervical along scalenus muscle
Sister Mary Joseph's nodule *see page 96*
Splenic = Lienal
Spinal accessory = Posterior cervical
Subaortic = Aortico-pulmonary window
Subclavian = Apical axillary
Subclavian = Level III
Subclavicular = Infraclavicular
Subdigastric = Infraclavicular
Subinguinal = Deep inguinal
Submandibular = Submaxillary
Submaxillary = Submandibular
Subpyloric = Infrapyloric
Subscapular = Posterior axillary
Superficial axillary = Level I axillary
Superficial axillary = Low axillary
Superficial inguinal = Femoral
Superior gastric = Left gastric
Supraclavicular = Transverse cervical
Supraclavicular node enlarged due to abdominal tumor = Virchow's; Ewald's; Troisier's
Supraomohyoid = Jugulo-omohyoid

Thoracic = Brachiocephalic
Thoracic = Innominate
Tracheal bifurcation = Carinal
Tracheobronchial = Bronchial
Transverse cervical = Supraclavicular
Troisier's = Left supraclavicular; sentinel node for stomach or lung cancer

Upper deep cervical = Internal jugular
Utero-ovarian = Infundibulopelvic

Virchow's = Supraclavicular; sentinel node for stomach cancer

HEAD AND NECK CANCERS

Cancers of head and neck sites include a wide array of cell types, signs, symptoms, and prognoses, but they are generally diagnosed and treated in a similar fashion. Head and neck malignancies include primaries in both the respiratory system and the digestive system. This chapter discusses all head and neck sites with the exception of the malignancies of the central nervous system and the senses (eye and ear). For reporting purposes, head and neck cancers in ICD-O-3 code range C00.0 to C14.8 are often grouped together in the upper digestive system, while the paranasal sinuses, nasal cavity, and larynx are grouped with the respiratory organs, and thyroid gland is reported separately.

Head and neck cancer is relatively infrequent; over 50,000 cases were expected to be diagnosed in the U.S. in 2010—about 3.5% of all types of newly diagnosed cancers. Of these 50,000, about 41% will be in the oral cavity, 23% will be in the pharynx, and 22% will be in the larynx. In addition, over 44,670 thyroid cancers are expected to be diagnosed in 2010.

Unfortunately, these cancers are commonly found at higher stages when they are difficult to treat and cure.

ETIOLOGY AND NATURAL HISTORY

Abuse of tobacco products and excess consumption of alcohol are the two principal risk factors for head and neck cancers. About 80% of all head and neck cancers are related to the use of tobacco and alcohol. Tobacco users are at six times greater risk of developing cancers in the oral cavity and lip (particularly tobacco chewers and snuff dippers). Risks are 5–35 times greater for developing laryngeal cancer and nasopharyngeal cancer. Alcohol consumption has a synergistic (additive) effect in tobacco users, increasing risks even more than if a person used alcohol or tobacco individually.

Human Papillomavirus (HPV), which is also associated with cervical cancer, is responsible for between 15 and 35 percent of head and neck cancers in North America and up to 50 percent of squamous cell cancers of the tonsils and base of the tongue. Over the past three decades, the number of squamous cell cancers of the head and neck possibly related to HPV has been on the rise particularly in 30 to 50 year old Caucasians. It is believed that the presence of HPV may predict which people with squamous cell cancers of the head and neck are more likely to respond to treatment.

Other head and neck cancers are the result of a wide variety of risks, such as exposure to radiation, chemicals and dyes, sun exposure, occupational fumes, and poor oral hygiene. Men, particularly those over age 40, are twice as likely to develop head and neck cancers than women.

Head and neck cancers are prone to the so-called field effect or field defect (also called regional diathesis, field cancerization or condemned mucosa). This is a predisposition of the epithelium of a body system to develop more than one primary tumor. The mucosal surfaces of the head and neck have a propensity for multiple primaries, especially in people who smoke and drink. It is especially important that careful evaluation of all head and neck sites be conducted so as to identify and treat any additional cancers that may be the result of the field effect.

Table 1. ICD-O-3 Codes, Related Terms and Adjectives

Not a complete list of head and neck site codes. Other codes for substructures of these sites may apply.

C00.0 – C00.9	Lip	Labio-, labial; vermilion or vermillion border, vermilion or vermillion surface, external lip
C01.9	Base of tongue	Root of tongue, posterior tongue
C02.0 – C02.9	Tongue	Glosso-, lingual, lallio-
C02.3	Anterior 2/3 of tongue	Mobile tongue, anterior tongue (anterior border = tip)
C03.0 – C03.9	Gum	Gingiva, alveolus, alveolar mucosa, periodontal surface
C04.0 – C04.9	Floor of mouth	FOM
C05.0 – C05.9	Palate	Palato-; roof of mouth
C06.0	Cheek (inside)	Buccal; internal cheek, buccal mucosa
C06.1	Vestibule (of mouth)	Sulcus (upper and lower pocket or space between lip and gum), labial sulcus, alveolar sulcus
C06.2	Retromolar area	Retromolar angle, retromolar trigone
C06.9	Mouth	Oral cavity, oral mucosa, buccal cavity
	Pharynx	Pharyngeal, pharyngo-
C07.9–C08.9	Salivary glands	Sialo-
C07.9	Parotid gland	Paro-; Stenson's duct
C08.0	Submandibular gland	Submaxillary gland, Wharton's duct
C09.1	Tonsillar pillar	Palatoglossal arch, glossopalatal arch, faucial pillar
C09.9	Tonsil	Palatine tonsil, faucial tonsil
C10.0 – C10.9	Oropharynx	Oropharyngeal, mesopharynx, fauces
C11.0 – C11.9	Nasopharynx	Nasopharyngeal
C11.1	Adenoid	Pharyngeal tonsil, posterior wall of nasopharynx
C11.3	Anterior wall of nasopharynx	Pharyngeal fornix, choana, posterior wall of nasal septum, nasopharyngeal surface of soft palate
C13.0 – C13.9	Hypopharynx	Laryngopharynx
C13.0	Cricopharynx	Cricoid, postcricoid region, pharyngoesophagus
C32.0 – C32.9	Larynx	Laryngeal, laryngo-, glottic
C32.0	True vocal cord	Vocal cord, true cord, vocal fold
C32.1	False vocal cord	Vestibular fold
C32.1	Arytenoid epiglottis	Aryepiglottic
C32.1	Aryepiglottic fold	Arytenoid fold, arytenoid
C73.9	Thyroid	Thyro-, isthmus, isthm-

Regional lymph nodes: See lymph node tables at the front of this book for synonymous words.

ANATOMY OF THE HEAD AND NECK AND REGIONAL LYMPH NODES AS THEY RELATE TO STAGING

The anatomy of the head and neck is difficult for many registrars to understand because there are so many different structures. Respiratory, digestive, endocrine, and even nervous system organs are located within millimeters of each other. Sometimes, the front and back surfaces of a single structure have different names and are in different body systems. For example, the anterior surface of the epiglottis is part of the digestive system and the epiglottis itself is part of the larynx in the respiratory system. Many of the structures in the head and neck are known by more than one name, as shown in Table 1 above, and the synonymous terms are not always familiar to the registrar. Please review the anatomic diagrams that follow for details on organ structures and synonyms for organ names.

Anatomy, *continued*

None of the head and neck sites has a serosal surface. The muscularis propria forms the "wall" of the organ. Oral cavity and pharynx cancers described as *confined to mucosa* should be reviewed with a pathologist to determine whether the tumor has penetrated the basement membrane, or whether it remains in situ.

The gum and hard palate have neither a submucosa nor a muscularis propria, because they lie directly on bone. The equivalent structure to the submucosa for gum and hard palate is the mucoperiosteum.

The tongue is anatomically divided into two sections: the anterior two-thirds or mobile tongue is part of the oral cavity and the posterior one-third or base of tongue is part of the oropharynx. The anterior anatomic boundary on the dorsal surface of the tongue is the circumvallate papillae.

The soft palate is anatomically divided into two sections: the superior surface is part of the naso-pharynx (C11.3) and the remainder (oral surface) is part of the oropharynx (C05.1).

Paired organs include the parotid glands, other major salivary glands, maxillary and frontal sinuses, tonsils (including the tonsils themselves, tonsillar fossae and tonsillar pillars), the nasal cavities, and the middle ear. Involvement of the right and left of these paired organs are counted as separate primary sites unless it is stated in the medical record that one side is metastatic from the other. The Multiple Primary and Histology Coding Rules have identified additional sites to be counted as separate primaries: upper and lower lip, upper and lower gum, and nasal cavity and middle ear. All other sites are single or non-paired organs.

The major parts of the head and neck sites are the oral cavity, pharynx, larynx, accessory sinuses, salivary glands, and thyroid gland, each of which is defined and discussed in more detail below.

ORAL CAVITY

The **oral cavity** extends from the vermilion (reddish pigmented) border of the lips to the junction of the hard and soft palates in the roof of the mouth (posterior edge of the palatine bone), and to the circumvallate papillae on the tongue. The oral cavity consists of the lips, commissures, lingual tonsil, gums (alveolar ridge), floor of mouth, hard palate, buccal mucosa, retromolar trigone, and all surfaces (anterior 2/3 or oral, dorsal, ventral, border) of the tongue except the base of tongue (Figure 1).

PHARYNX

As shown on the right side of Figure 1, the pharynx consists of three regions: oropharynx (C10._), nasopharynx (C11._), and hypopharynx (C12.9, C13._). Each region is carefully defined for the purposes of staging and counting multiple primaries. Part of the digestive system, the pharynx is about 12 cm (5 inches) in length and extends from the base of the skull (superior nasopharynx) to about the C6 vertebra (inferior hypopharynx).

Oropharynx

The oropharynx or oral pharynx is the part of the pharynx that can be seen when the mouth is opened wide (Figure 1, left). The structures of the oropharynx are the base of tongue and vallecula inferiorly; underside of the soft palate and the uvula superiorly, posterior wall of oropharynx; and the lateral walls of the oropharynx, consisting of the tonsillar fossae and palatine tonsils, the glossotonsillar sulci, anterior and posterior tonsillar pillars (faucial arches); and the branchial cleft (as a possible site of neoplasm, not as an anatomical structure).

Figure 1. Anatomy of the Oral Cavity and Pharynx

1 Base of tongue
2 Anterior tongue
3 Gum (upper)
4 Lip
5 Commissure of lips
6 Retromolar trigone
7 Buccal mucosa
8 Hard palate
9 Soft palate
10 Uvula
11 Tonsil
12 Anterior tonsillar pillar
13 Posterior tonsillar pillar
14 Posterior wall of oropharynx
15 Epiglottis
16 Vallecula
17 Posterior wall of hypopharynx
18 Glottis (larynx)
19 Trachea
20 Esophagus
21 Nasal cavity

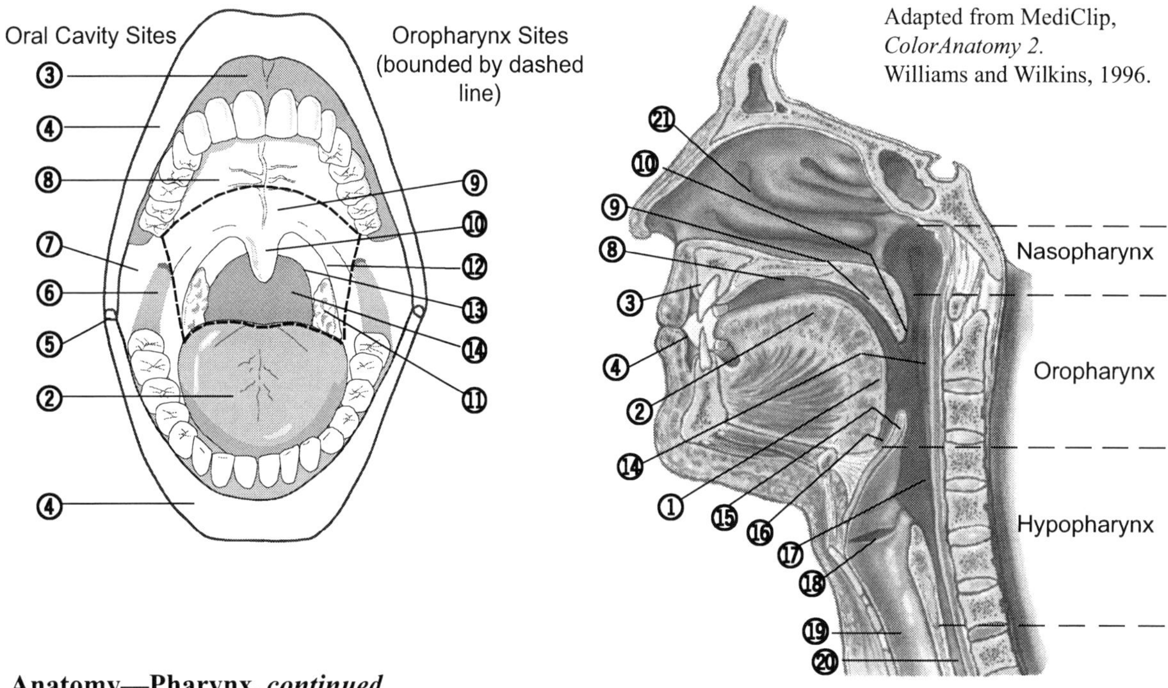

Anatomy—Pharynx, *continued*

The oropharynx extends from the roof of the mouth distally as far as the superior surface of the hyoid bone (at the same level as the lowest part of the vallecula, which is between the base of the tongue and the epiglottis). Anteriorly, the boundary is a plane created between the posterior edge of the palatine bone (where the hard palate ends and the soft palate begins) and the circumvallate papillae that form a dividing line between the anterior tongue and the base of the tongue.

There are two arches or tonsillar pillars surrounding the throat opening. The anterior pillar or palato-glossal arch is a fold of mucosa in front of the tonsillar fossa, extending from the base of the tongue to the soft palate. The posterior pillar or palatopharyngeal arch is a similar fold of mucosa extending from the soft palate to the posterior pharyngeal wall behind the tonsillar fossa. The tonsillar fossa itself is a recess or pocket in the mucosa in which the lymphatic tissue of the tonsil lies on either side of the oropharynx. The posterior wall of the oropharynx is the mucosa extending from the level of the soft palate to the tip of the epiglottis.

Nasopharynx

The structures of the nasopharynx cannot be seen directly by looking into the mouth because the soft palate (of the oropharynx) is suspended in front of them. The nasopharyngeal structures (Figure 2) are the four walls of the nasopharynx (anterior, superior {vault}, posterior, and lateral), the pharyngeal tonsils (adenoids), and the fossa of Rosenmuller, as well as the mucosa of the Eustachian tube orifice.

Figure 2. Nasopharyngeal Structures from Behind

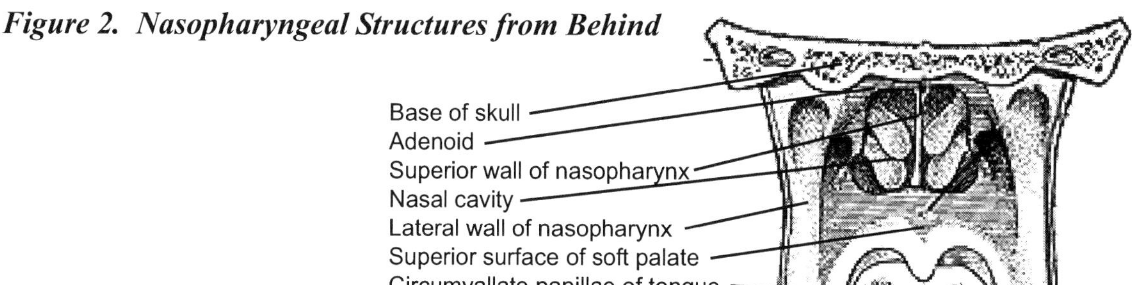

Anatomy—Pharynx, *continued*

The Eustachian tube is the passageway between the nasopharynx and middle ear that helps equalize air pressure in the middle ear.

The boundaries of the nasopharynx are the opening from the nasal cavity (choana) anteriorly and superiorly, and the superior surface of the soft palate inferiorly. The lateral and posterior walls enclose the nasopharynx. The fossa of Rosenmuller is a depression in the mucosa of the nasopharynx behind the opening of the Eustachian tube into the nasopharynx.

The choana of the nose and the posterior margin of nasal septum (C11.3) are not included in the nasopharynx TNM scheme; instead, they are included with the nasal cavity for staging purposes.

The area collectively referred to as the infratemporal fossa lies below the temporal bone and behind (internal to) the zygomatic arch and the muscles of the mandible. This area is contiguous with the nasal cavity and the nasopharynx. The infratemporal fossa contains the mandibular nerve, pterygoid and masseter muscles, masseteric artery and nerve, middle meningeal artery, maxillary artery and deep temporal arteries and nerves. Tumor extension into the soft tissues of the infratemporal fossa is classified as T4 in the nasopharynx and is difficult to access and to treat.

Hypopharynx

The structures of the hypopharynx are the pyriform sinus (C12.9), the hypopharyngeal aspect of the aryepiglottic fold, the posterior pharyngeal wall, and the postcricoid region. The hypopharynx extends from the floor of the vallecula (between the base of the tongue and the epiglottis—the lower boundary of the oropharynx) to the lower edge of the cricoid cartilage. The postcricoid region or pharyngo-esophageal junction is the lowermost region of the hypopharynx and comprises about 15% of all hypopharyngeal cancers.

About 70% of all hypopharyngeal malignancies arise in the pyriform sinuses, which are pear-shaped depressions or pockets extending from the pharyngoepiglottic fold to the upper edge of the esophagus on either side of the hypopharynx. Because there are few nerve endings in this area, pyriform sinus cancers can invade lymphatic channels and spread to lymph nodes before the primary tumor becomes symptomatic. Pyriform sinus cancers tend to present at an advanced stage, and their prognosis is the worst of all head and neck primary sites.

Waldeyer's Ring

Although Waldeyer's ring consists of lymphoid tissue rather than squamous epithelium, all of the structures are in the pharynx and considered part of it. Waldeyer's ring was first described by German anatomist Heinrich Waldeyer-Hartz in the late 19th century. He visualized the lymphoid tissues (palatine tonsils laterally, lingual tonsil inferiorly, and nasopharyngeal tonsils {adenoids} superiorly) as forming a ring around the opening of the throat to fight pathogens that might enter the respiratory system.

Figure 3. Regions and Structures of the Larynx

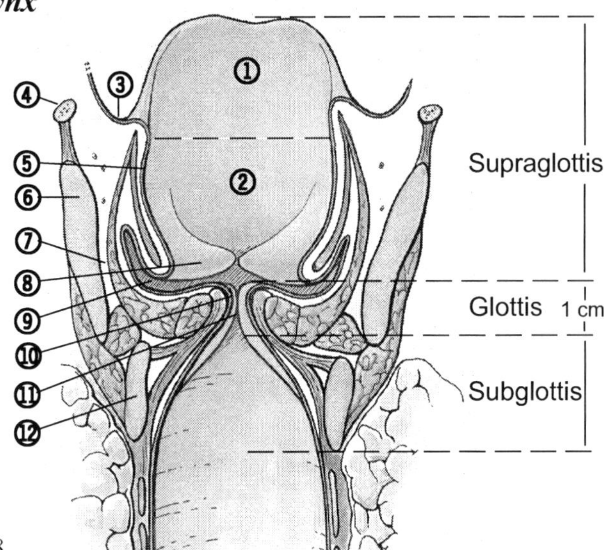

1 Epiglottis, suprahyoid
2 Epiglottis, infrahyoid
3 Pharyngo-epiglottic fold
4 Hyoid bone
5 Aryepiglottic fold
6 Thyroid cartilage
7 Pyriform sinus (hypopharynx)
8 False cords (ventricular bands)
9 Ventricle
10 True vocal cords
11 Glottis (space between cords)
12 Cricoid cartilage

Adapted from MediClip, *Grant's Atlas Images 4: Head, Neck and Cranial Nerves.* Williams and Wilkins, 1998.

Anatomy, *continued*

LARYNX

For staging purposes, the anatomic structures of the larynx are divided into three regions, glottis, supraglottis and subglottis (Figure 3). Each has its own definitions for the TNM T category and CS Extension. However, lymph node and distant metastases definitions are the same for all subsites.

Supraglottis

The supraglottic structures account for 25–40% of all laryngeal cancers. There are many structures in the supraglottis, all of which are coded to primary site C32.1: the epiglottis, false cords (also called ventricular bands), ventricles (space between the true and false cords), arytenoids, and the laryngeal aspect of the aryepiglottic (arytenoepiglottic) folds (Figures 3 and 4). The superior margin of the supraglottis is the tip of the epiglottis and the inferior margin is the floor of the ventricle.

Glottis

The majority of laryngeal cancers (50 to 75%) develop in the glottis, which consists of the true vocal cords and the anterior and posterior points at which the cords come together (commissures) (Figures 3 and 4). The glottis extends from the floor of the ventricle above the true cords to one centimeter below the edge of the true cords.

Figure 4. Glottis and Supraglottis (laryngoscopic view)

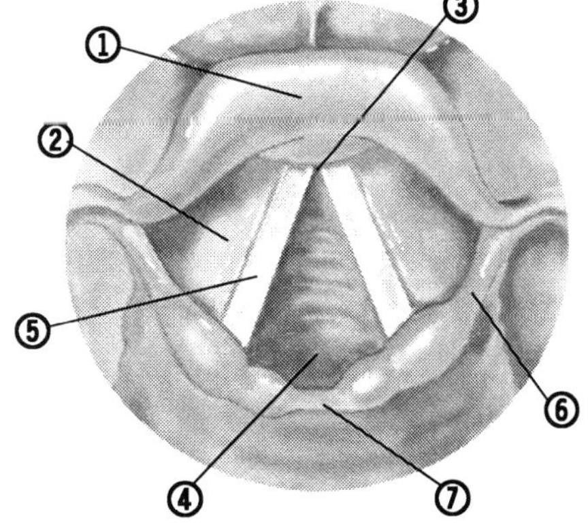

1 Epiglottis (supraglottis)
2 False cords (ventricular bands, supraglottis)
3 Anterior commissure (glottis)
4 Posterior commissure (glottis)
5 True cords (glottis)
6 Aryepiglottic fold (supraglottis)
7 Arytenoid (supraglottis)

Adapted from MediClip, *Grant's Atlas Images 4: Head, Neck and Cranial Nerves.* Williams and Wilkins, 1998.

Anatomy—Larynx, *continued*

Subglottis

Subglottic cancer is the least common (1 to 5%) but the most lethal of laryngeal cancers. There are no substructures in this area of the larynx, which begins 1 cm below the edge of the true vocal cord and extends to the first tracheal ring (inferior border of the cricoid cartilage).

OTHER HEAD AND NECK SITES

The **paranasal (or accessory) sinuses** include (in order of malignant frequency) the maxillary, ethmoid, sphenoid, and frontal sinuses (Figure 5). The *maxillary sinus* (antrum of Highmore) is divided into the infrastructure (anterior and inferior portion) and the suprastructure (superior and posterior) by Ohngren's line, a plane or imaginary line extending from the interior corner of the eye to the lower edge of the ear lobe. The ethmoid and sphenoid sinuses are on either side of the nose. The frontal sinuses are above the eyebrows. There is no staging system for the sphenoid and frontal sinuses.

Figure 5. Paranasal Sinuses

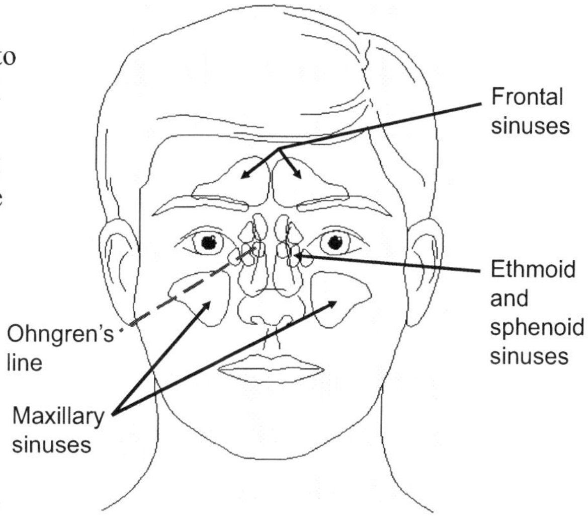

The **nasal cavity** or nasal fossa is divided into two chambers by the nasal septum. The nostrils are the external openings, the vestibule is immediately inside the nostrils, and the nasal cavity extends from the vestibule to the choana, the posterior opening into the nasopharynx. Each side of the nasal cavity contains three chonchae or turbinates, which direct secretions from the lacrimal ducts and sinuses toward the nose anteriorly or the nasopharynx posteriorly. All sinuses and the nasal cavity are paired sites. The TNM staging system for nasal cavity includes two structures coded in C11.3: the choana between the nasal cavity and nasopharynx and the posterior margin of nasal septum.

The **major salivary glands** (Figure 6) are the parotid (accounting for 90% of all salivary gland tumors), submandibular or submaxillary (about 10%), and sublingual glands (1%). Each of the major salivary glands is a paired site.

Minor salivary glands are located in many oral cavity structures, including the oral mucosa, palate, uvula, posterior tongue, retromolar trigone, paranasal sinuses, pharynx, larynx, peritonsillar area, and floor of mouth. Tumors of minor salivary glands are assigned the topography code of the site in which they arise; for example, a tumor of a minor salivary gland of the floor of the mouth is coded to floor of mouth. The most common site for minor salivary gland tumors is the palate.

Figure 6. Major Salivary Glands

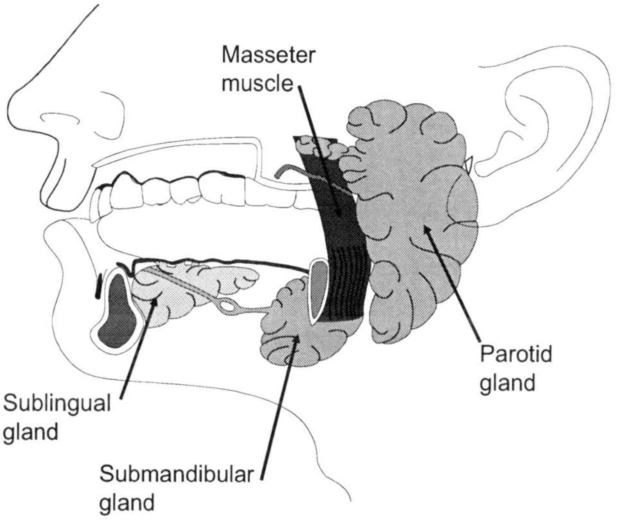

Anatomy, *continued*

The **thyroid gland** (Figure 7) consists of two lateral lobes joined by an isthmus. Sometimes a pyramidal lobe is also present, extending upward anterior to the thyroid cartilage. The thyroid is an endocrine gland; the regional lymph nodes are different from all other head and neck sites. The thyroid gland is not a paired site.

Figure 7. Thyroid Gland

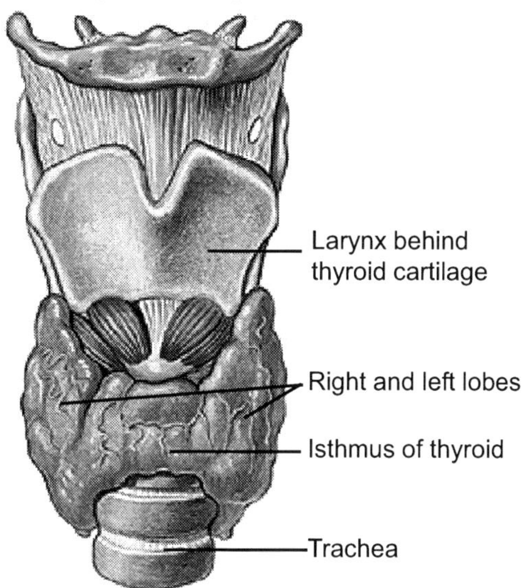

REGIONAL LYMPH NODES OF THE HEAD AND NECK

The regional lymph nodes of the head and neck may be described as cervical lymph nodes, NOS.

The major nodal chains are:

- Submental
- Submandibular
- Jugular (deep cervical)
- Superficial cervical
- Supraclavicular
- Prelaryngeal and paratracheal
- Retropharyngeal
- Parotid
- Buccal
- Retroauricular and occipital

These lymph node chains are frequently grouped into “levels” by head and neck specialists. The lymph node level descriptions have been standardized by the American Academy of Otolaryngology, Head and Neck Surgery.

Level I	Submandibular (submaxillary), submental
Level II	Jugulodigastric (subdigastric), upper deep cervical, upper jugular
Level III	Middle deep cervical, mid-jugular
Level IV	Jugulo-omohyoid (supraomohyoid), lower deep cervical, lower jugular
Level V	Posterior cervical, posterior triangle (spinal accessory and transverse cervical) (upper, middle, and lower, corresponding to the levels that define upper, middle, and lower jugular nodes). For descriptive purposes, Level V may be further subdivided into upper, middle, and lower levels corresponding to the superior and inferior planes that define Levels II, III, and IV.
Level VI	Anterior deep cervical, laterotracheal, paralaryngeal, paratracheal (cranial/suprathyroidal, caudal/infrathyroidal), prelaryngeal, pretracheal (Delphian–near thyroid isthmus), recurrent laryngeal (lateral tracheal)
Level VII	Upper (superior) mediastinal

Other lymph node chains in the head and neck that are not part of these levels are the facial (buccal or buccinator), parotid (intraparotid, superficial parotid, deep parotid {preauricular, infra-auricular, infraparotid, subparotid}), nasolabial, postauricular (retroauricular, posterior auricular {mastoid}), occipital (suboccipital), parapharyngeal, and retropharyngeal. The retropharyngeal lymph nodes (regional nodes primarily for nasopharynx) lie behind the pharyngeal wall at the level of the first cervical vertebra.

Figure 8. Lymph Nodes of Larynx and Pharynx

1 Submental
2 Submandibular
3 Upper jugular
4 Lower jugular
5 Pretracheal
6 Paratracheal
7 Prelaryngeal

Not shown:
Paralaryngeal
Retropharyngeal

Adapted from MediClip, *Grant's Atlas Images 4: Head, Neck and Cranial Nerves.* Williams and Wilkins, 1998.

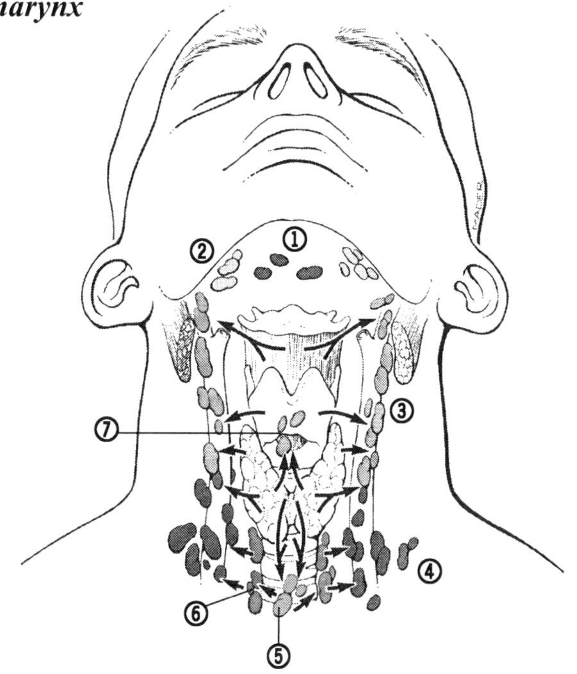

Regional Lymph Nodes, *continued*

Regional Lymph Nodes for Pharynx

The cervical lymph nodes are the regional nodes for the oropharynx and hypopharynx. See Figure 8. Both the *AJCC Cancer Staging Manual* and the Collaborative Stage Data Collection System (CS) coding instructions define specific lymph nodes for each region of the pharynx.

Nasopharynx	Oropharynx	Hypopharynx
Retropharyngeal	Upper jugular	Parapharyngeal
Upper jugular	Mid jugular	Paratracheal
Spinal accessory	Submandibular (submaxillary)	Mid jugular
	Submental	Lower jugular

These lymph node chains are in levels I, II, III, IV, and VI, but not level V (posterior triangle).

The regional lymph node categories for nasopharynx were revised in the fifth edition of the *AJCC Cancer Staging Manual* based on research from southeast Asia, where the incidence of nasopharyngeal cancer is the highest in the world. Those revised categories were carried forward into newer editions of TNM.

Other named regional lymph nodes for the pharynx include the internal jugular chain (jugulodigastric, jugulo-omohyoid, upper deep cervical, lower deep cervical), which is also divided into upper, mid- and lower jugular nodes. Lymph node involvement is common for all regions of the pharynx. Depending on the location of the primary site, the likelihood of regional lymph node metastases at the time of diagnoses ranges from 40% for the postcricoid region to more than 70% for nasopharynx, pyriform sinus, base of tongue and tonsil. Because of the midline location of the pharynx, contralateral and bilateral lymph node involvement is also common. The presence of positive regional lymph nodes is equivalent to at least Stage III disease for oropharyngeal and hypopharyngeal malignancies, and at least Stage IIB disease for nasopharyngeal cancers.

Regional Lymph Nodes, *continued*

Regional Lymph Nodes for Larynx

The cervical lymph nodes in general serve as the regional lymph nodes of the larynx. See Figure 8. TNM and CS both mention specific lymph node chains for each region of the larynx.

Supraglottis	Glottis	Subglottis
Submental	Prelaryngeal	Prelaryngeal
Submandibular	Pretracheal	Pretracheal
Retropharyngeal	Paralaryngeal	Paralaryngeal
Upper jugular	Paratracheal	Paratracheal
Mid jugular	Upper jugular	Mid jugular
	Mid jugular	Lower jugular
	Lower jugular	

These lymph node chains are in levels I, II, III, IV, and VI, but not level V (posterior triangle).

Lymph node involvement is common for supraglottic and subglottic primaries, but uncommon for glottic cancers. Because the larynx is midline in the neck, bilateral and contralateral lymph node involvement is also common. The presence of positive regional nodes is equivalent to at least Stage III disease.

Regional Lymph Nodes of Other Head and Neck Sites

Oral Cavity — Internal jugular (jugulodigastric, jugulo-omohyoid, upper deep cervical, lower deep cervical); parotid (preauricular, infraparotid, subparotid, posterior auricular); submandibular (submaxillary); submental; cervical, NOS

Maxillary Sinus — Internal jugular (jugulodigastric, jugulo-omohyoid, upper deep cervical, lower deep cervical); submandibular (submaxillary); submental; retropharyngeal; cervical, NOS

Salivary Glands — Parotid; submandibular (submaxillary); submental; deep cervical; cervical, NOS

Thyroid Gland — Jugular (upper, middle, lower); pretracheal (Delphian); lateral tracheal; tracheoe sophageal (posterior mediastinal); cervical, NOS; retropharyngeal; upper anterior mediastinal

Additional Lymph Nodes Notes

- Involved midline lymph nodes (submental and pretracheal) are defined as *ipsilateral* (on the same side of the body as the primary site).
- If cervical nodes are involved and laterality is not specified, assume nodes are ipsilateral.
- In descriptions of cervical lymph nodes, the terms *fixed* and *matted* are interpreted as involvement of the nodes. The terms *enlarged*, *palpable*, *lymphadenopathy*, and *shotty* are not considered to be involvement unless the physician makes an additional statement, such as "palpable cervical nodes suspicious for malignancy" or "patient has N2b lymphadenopathy".
- The supraclavicular fossa is described as the lymph node bearing triangular region of the shoulder defined by the superior edges of the clavicle (medial and lateral) and the junction of the neck and the shoulder.

COMMON METASTATIC SITES

Oral Cavity, pharynx, larynx Lungs, bone, liver, mediastinal lymph nodes

Maxillary Sinus Lungs, bone, distant lymph nodes

Salivary Glands Lungs

Thyroid Gland Lungs, bone

MULTIPLE PRIMARY RULES

Approximately 10-15% of head and neck cancers have a second primary diagnosed at the time of workup of the symptomatic primary site. Subclinical second primaries are most frequently diagnosed in the esophagus. Overall, 20-30% of head and neck patients develop a second primary at some point in their history.

The Multiple Primary and Histology Coding Rules for head and neck are fairly complex because of the wide range of primary sites. One of the principal difficulties in counting multiple primaries is identifying where the cancer(s) started. The site-specific rules for head and neck multiple primaries provide a detailed priority for determining the primary site. Remember that when the point of origin of a head and neck cancer cannot be determined, it is acceptable to use an overlapping site code (C_ _.8). There are a number of overlapping site codes within the three-character rubrics for individual organs. There are also three overlapping site codes that cover single tumors that extend into multiple organs:

- C02.8 Overlapping lesion of tongue
- C08.8 Overlapping lesion of major salivary glands
- C14.8 Overlapping lesion of lip, oral cavity, and pharynx

Unique Features of Head and Neck Rules

- 12 multiple primaries rules
- FIVE years between diagnoses
- Bilateral tumors are multiple primaries except if described as a metastasis
- A number of sites formerly grouped as single primaries in ICD-O first edition have been "ungrouped" and are now counted as multiple primaries
- Upper and lower lip, upper and lower gum recognized as separate primaries
- Histology coding rules in two sections (12 rules total)
  - 6 rules (H1 – H6) in Single Tumor module
  - 6 rules (H7 – H12) in Multiple Tumors Abstracted as a Single Primary
- Histology coding rules refer to a chart in the site-specific Terms and Definitions providing priorities for the most specific histology code

Summary of Multiple Primary Rules

This is only a summary of the multiple primary rules for head and neck. Details of the rules are provided in the official published documents available from www.seer.cancer.gov/tools/mphrules. Refer to the General Instructions for information about coding more specific terms, missing pathology or cytology reports, and other aspects of the rules for this and other sets of site-specific rules. **Always** refer to the site-specific rules themselves in your preferred format when determining how many abstracts to prepare or the correct histology code for an individual abstract. The published rules include more discussion, examples, and notes.

Multiple Primary Rules, ***continued***

The standard three modules of the multiple primaries rules are present: unknown if single or multiple tumors, single tumor, and multiple tumors.

- Count only macroscopic, non-metastatic tumors when deciding which module applies.

The first module, unknown if single or multiple tumors, is the same as for all other site-specific sets of rules:

M1. Number of tumors (single or multiple) can't be determined = single

The head and neck rules are similar to most other site-specific rules in that there is only one rule for single tumors:

M2. Single tumor = single

The priority of the multiple tumors rules is as follows:

M3. Tumors on both sides = multiple
- Paired sites include major salivary glands, tonsils, nasal cavity, accessory sinuses, middle ear.

M4. Upper and lower lip = multiple
M5. Upper and lower gum = multiple
M6. Nasal cavity and middle ear = multiple
M7. Topography code different at 2nd or 3rd character = multiple
M8. Invasive carcinoma after in situ more than 60 days = multiple
M9. Diagnosis dates more than 5 years apart = multiple
M10. Nonspecific and specific histology codes = single
M11. Histology different at first, second, or third digit = multiple
M12. All other scenarios = single

HISTOLOGIC CELL TYPES OF HEAD AND NECK CANCERS

The majority of head and neck malignancies (85-95%) are squamous cell cancers.

Subcategories of squamous cell carcinoma include
Papillary carcinomas (morphology codes 8050, 8051, 8052)
Squamous cell subtypes (8070, 8071, 8072, 8073, 8074, 8075, 8078)
Lymphoepithelioma (Schminke tumor) and variants (8082, 8083, 8084)

Other histologies include
Adenocarcinoma: adenocarcinoma with mixed subtypes, mucoepidermoid carcinoma, adenocystic carcinoma, acinar carcinoma
Adenosquamous carcinoma

Histologies for thyroid cancer

Papillary adenocarcinoma (1-2%) (8260/3) Papillary carcinoma of the thyroid is coded the same as papillary adenocarcinoma of the thyroid.
Papillary microcarcinoma is defined as a tumor 10 mm or smaller; it has its own histology code (8341/3)
Papillary-follicular adenocarcinoma (60%)
Follicular adenocarcinoma (20%)
Hurthle cell carcinoma, also called follicular carcinoma, oxyphilic type
Undifferentiated carcinoma (small cell or giant cell carcinoma) (10-15%)
Medullary carcinoma (5-6%)
Other: sarcoma, lymphoma, epidermoid carcinoma, and teratoma

ICD-O Morphology Codes, *continued*

Synonyms for in situ carcinoma: confined to epithelium, noninfiltrating, intraepithelial, intrasquamous, involvement up to but not including the basement membrane, noninvasive, no stromal involvement, papillary noninfiltrating, Stage 0 or Tis in the TNM system.

OTHER HISTOLOGIES

Nasopharynx lymphomas, adenocarcinoma, adenoid cystic carcinoma, melanoma

Oropharynx adenocarcinoma (minor salivary glands), lymphoma

Hypopharynx minor salivary gland tumors

Larynx fibrosarcoma, chondrosarcoma, paraganglioma, rhabdomyosarcoma

Salivary glands Tumors are malignant in 20-25% of parotid gland masses, 35-40% of submandibular gland, 50% of palate, and 95-100% of sublingual gland. Less common tumors of the salivary glands include acinic cell tumors, mucoepidermoid carcinoma, adenocarcinoma, malignant mixed tumors, and adenoid cystic carcinoma.

Paranasal sinuses and nasal cavity squamous cell carcinoma (80%); adenocarcinoma (up to 20%). The maxillary sinuses tend to develop squamous cell carcinoma, while the ethmoid sinuses tend to develop adenocarcinoma. Other rare tumors include esthesioneuroepithelioma, chondro- and osteo-sarcomas, soft tissue sarcomas, melanoma and lymphoma.

Melanoma
Mucosal melanoma of head and neck sites is rare but extremely aggressive. In the seventh edition of the *AJCC Cancer Staging Manual* and CS version 2, mucosal melanomas of head and neck sites have separate staging and coding systems.

HISTOLOGY CODING RULES

For head and neck sites, there are two modules based on number of tumors. Make sure you are looking at the rules in the correct section. The first few rules may seem repetitive, but this is so that each module is self-contained and avoids having the reader jump from one place to another in the rules.

The Histology Coding Rules include two important new concepts.

1. A rule has been added that, when a tumor has both an invasive histology and a different in situ histology, the invasive histology should be coded. Pathologists generally agree that it is the invasive part of the tumor that has the potential to do the most harm to the patient; thus the in situ component should be disregarded and the histology of the invasive component should be assigned to the case.
2. A chart of prioritized histologic terms is included in the Equivalent Terms and Definitions in the head and neck rules. Use this chart to determine the most specific diagnostic term and code. Less specific terms are at the top of the chart; more specific terms are toward the bottom of the chart.

Note: In the nonspecific/specific coding rules (H5 and H11), the following terms indicate a more specific type:

- Invasive cancers: type, subtype, predominantly, with features of, major, with [something] differentiation
- In situ cancers: pattern, architecture, type,subtype, predominantly, with features of, major, with [something] differentiation

Histology Coding Rules, *continued*

Single Tumor

- H1. If no pathology/cytology report available, code the histology stated by the clinician.
- H2. Code histology from a metastatic site if there is no tissue or cells from the primary site.
- H3. If only one histology is stated, code that.
  - Another way of saying this is if you can find a single histology code that covers all of the terms in the pathologic diagnosis, use that code.
- H4. Code the invasive histology when both invasive and in situ tumor is present.
- H5. Code the more specific histology when one term is NOS and the other is more specific.
  - NOS terms: cancer, NOS; carcinoma, NOS; adenocarcinoma, NOS; squamous cell carcinoma, NOS; melanoma, NOS; sarcoma, NOS
- H6. If no other rule applies, use the numerically higher ICD-O-3 code as a last priority.

Multiple Tumors Abstracted as a Single Primary

- H7. If no pathology/cytology report available, code the histology stated by the clinician. This is the same rule as H1 but applies to multiple tumors abstracted as a single primary.
- H8. Code histology from a metastatic site if there is no tissue or cells from the primary site.
- H9. If only one histology is stated, code that.
- H10. Code the histology of the most invasive tumor (see staging guidelines later in this chapter).
- H11. Code the more specific histology when one term is NOS and the other is more specific.
  - NOS terms: cancer, NOS; carcinoma, NOS; adenocarcinoma, NOS; squamous cell carcinoma, NOS; melanoma, NOS; sarcoma, NOS
- H12. If no other rule applies, use the numerically higher ICD-O-3 code as a last priority.

HEAD AND NECK CANCER ABSTRACTING GUIDELINES

DETERMINING THE PRIMARY SITE

Head and neck cancers commonly involve adjacent sites, so one of the great challenges of abstracting head and neck cancers is determining the primary site. The primary site is the basis for assigning the topography code, as well as bringing up the correct Collaborative Staging schema and surgery codes. Be aware that the biopsy site is not necessarily the primary site of the cancer. If multiple biopsies have been performed and the primary site is still not clear, the Multiple Primary and Histology Coding Rules list the following priorities for determining the primary site:

1. Tumor Board discussion, either specialty or general
2. Staging physician's statement on TNM staging form or in medical record
   Note: This may be problematic as staging forms are no longer required. If a staging form is still used, it may have been placed on the medical record by the cancer registrar.
3. If total or complete resection of tumor performed, surgeon's statement in operative report or final diagnosis on pathology report.
4. If no resection, documentation from:
   a. Endoscopy (physical exam with scope)
   b. Radiation oncologist
   c. Diagnosing physician
   d. Primary care physician
   e. Other physician
   f. Radiologist impression from diagnostic imaging
   g. Physician statement based on physical exam (clinical impression)

HISTORY

The signs and symptoms that bring the patient to a doctor are a valuable part of the diagnostic work-up for head and neck cancer, as the symptoms may help to localize the cancer to a specific organ. A careful history is important to establish both the type and duration of symptoms. General symptoms of head and neck cancer include a mass, ulcer, referred or localized pain, neurologic defects, hoarseness, or swelling in the neck (involved lymph nodes). Many head and neck cancers are "silent," meaning that they have no pain or other symptoms until in an advanced stage.

In addition, many primary sites in the head and neck have specific symptoms:

Pharynx

Nasopharynx—nasal obstruction, epistaxis, tinnitus, sore throat, headache, diminished hearing, facial pain
Oropharynx—pain, sore throat, dysphagia, pain radiating to the ear; asymptomatic mass in neck
Hypopharynx—odynophagia, referred otalgia, dysphagia; hoarseness; occasionally excessive salivation

Larynx

Supraglottis—sore throat, painful swallowing (odynophagia), difficulty swallowing (dysphagia), ear pain (otalgia)
Glottis and subglottis—hoarseness
Subglottis—neck mass

Parotid gland—asymptomatic swelling; occasionally painful mass

Paranasal sinuses and nasal cavity—early stages are asymptomatic; advanced stages develop dull face or tooth pain, loose teeth, nasal obstruction, rhinorrhea, nosebleeds, and other symptoms

Thyroid—cold nodule in thyroid; firm or hard nodule in base of neck. Sudden development of pain, hoarseness, or dysphagia may indicate a highly invasive thyroid cancer.

- Medullary carcinoma is asociated with multiple endocrine neoplasia (MEN) syndrome (types IIA and IIB) in about 20% of cases. A diagnosis of medullary carcinoma of the thyroid requires a more thorough workup, including genetic studies, CT scans, and detailed family history.

Where to look in the patient's record

- History and physical exam report
- Consultation report(s)
- Physician's progress notes

What information to select and record (record all dates)

- History of any previous malignancy(ies) or pre-malignant conditions
- Type of symptom: hoarseness, pain, ringing in ears, other
- Signs of advanced disease (neck masses, skin involvement, bone pain, other signs)

Other information to note (but does not document location, tumor size, or extent of disease)

- Tobacco and alcohol usage, sun exposure, other risk factors
- How the head and neck abnormality was detected (patient, family member, physician)
- Duration and intensity of symptoms

PHYSICAL EXAM

The physician should visually inspect and palpate the patient's head and neck looking for masses, lesions, asymmetry between right and left sides, and abnormal-appearing areas. The visual inspection can be either direct or using a mirror. Even though the primary site may be obvious, the physician should perform a careful examination to identify any additional primary sites. The neck lymph nodes, including the supraclavicular lymph nodes, should be examined by the physician to feel for abnormalities. Involvement of lymph nodes occurs in up to 75% of cases even though no abnormal nodes may be palpated.

Where to look in the patient's record

- History and physical exam report
- Consultation report(s)
- Physician's progress notes

What information to select and record

Pertinent findings as to *what the physician sees and feels* when examining the patient

- Use "evidence of" and "no evidence of" statements
- Document both positive and negative findings

Findings to look for:

- Obvious lesions on the skin or mucosa
- Ulceration, bleeding
- Size and location (especially if tumor crosses midline) of primary tumor(s)
- Swelling
- Location of any masses or enlarged organs (organomegaly; hepatomegaly; splenomegaly)
- Fixation of mass
- Invasion/erosion of bone
- Mobility of vocal cords (hoarseness) and/or tongue or other movable structures
- Laterality, size and number of palpable lymph nodes, especially cervical or supraclavicular
- Evaluation of cranial nerves (nasopharyngeal lesions), facial nerves (salivary gland tumors)

Descriptive terminology

- Leukoplakia—a white patch on the mucosa of the oral cavity that does not rub off and cannot be characterized as any other disease. Leukoplakia could be an early invasive lesion, hyperkeratosis, lichen planus, or another benign disease.
- Erythroplakia—red, velvety plaque arising on the mucosa of the oral cavity that cannot be identified as any other condition. Erythroplakia is one of the earliest signs of oral cavity cancer.

VISUAL EXAMINATION (also called indirect or mirror examination) visualization of clinically accessible areas of the head and neck by viewing them in a mirror or through an endoscope (see also Endoscopy).

DIAGNOSTIC PROCEDURES OVERVIEW

Malignancies in some head and neck sites are more effectively diagnosed using certain procedures. Table 2 shows the most effective diagnostic procedures for tumors of head and neck sites.

Table 2. Recommended Diagnostic Procedures for Head and Neck Cancers

SITE	PHYS EXAM	BIOPSY	INDIRECT EXAM	ENDOSCOPY	CT	MRI
Oral Cavity	X	X				
Nasopharynx	X		X	X	X	X
Oropharynx	X	X, FN	X	X	X	X
Hypopharynx	X	FN	X	X	X	
Larynx	X		X	X	X	X
Salivary glands	X	FN*			X	
Paranasal sinuses and nasal cavity				X		
Thyroid	X	FN	X		X	

* FN = fine needle aspiration

Note: Other diagnostic evaluations for thyroid malignancies include thyroid function test, sonogram, serum thyrocalcitonin (medullary carcinoma)

IMAGING *(For more information on these procedures, see the chapter on diagnostic tests)*

Radiology, ultrasound, and computer imaging studies may be used to determine the location and extent of head and neck cancers, as well as the involvement of cervical lymph nodes. Tests may be performed on an outpatient basis both pre- and post-admission.

Common imaging tests for head and neck cancers (refer to Diagnostic Tests chapter in this book)

- **Plain X-rays**
- **CT Imaging**
- **Magnetic Resonance Imaging (MRI)**
- **Positron Emission Tomography (PET Scan)**
- **Esophagogram**
- **Cine-pharyngoesophagram**
- **Barium swallow or Upper GI Series**
- **Tomograms**
- **Parotid or Salivary Gland Scan**
- **Sialography** (salivary gland imaging)
- **Bronchogram**
- **Thyroid Scan and/or Sonogram**
- **Imaging for mets: chest, bone, brain**

Imaging, ***continued***

What information to select and record (record all dates)

Pertinent findings as stated by the radiologist from each study including:

- Name of study and area of the body being examined (for example, CT neck, nasopharyngeal tomograms)
- Tumor location, including subsite(s)
- Laterality
- Tumor size and extent of tumor
- Relationship of tumor to other tissues, such as impingement/compression of or extension to another tissue (another organ, skin, muscle, bone, cartilage)
- Constriction of airway or food pathway
- Lymph node status—laterality, number and size; fixed or matted nodes
- Statements regarding regional or distant spread, including location and number of metastatic lesions

LABORATORY TESTS AND TUMOR MARKERS *(see also Diagnostic Tests and Tumor Markers chapter)*

Tumor markers taken at the time of diagnosis (baseline) and during follow-up help to assess tumor burden and monitor for recurrence. Some tests help to identify the cell type of the tumor. Laboratory tests are usually not useful for head and neck cancers, with the exception of thyroid cancer.

- **Squamous Cell Carcinoma (SCC) Antigen**—monitors tumor burden after treatment for squamous cell carcinoma; usually used for advanced disease; primary application is head and neck cancer, secondarily for lung cancer
- **Ferritin**—measures iron storage protein in sialic acid; low levels suggest good prognosis in head and neck malignancies, although test is nonspecific for head and neck cancer
- **PLP (Parathyroid hormone-like Protein)**—elevated levels of this circulating hormone are found in squamous cell cancer and in breast cancer
- **Other tumor markers**
    - **CEA (Carcinoembryonic Antigen)**—persistent elevated levels indicate residual or recurrent metastatic carcinoma; smoking may affect accuracy of CEA results
    - **Calcitonin** (primarily for medullary thyroid cancer)—elevated levels of this thyroid hormone occasionally occur with small cell lung cancer; increasing levels may indicate progression of disease. If calcitonin is normal, patient may undergo pentagastrin challenge.
    - **Thyroglobulin** (for thyroid cancer)—elevated levels of this serum hormone are found in follicular carcinoma and return to normal following treatment if all tumor is removed; useful for monitoring residual disease and recurrence of follicular carcinoma
- **I-131 Uptake test**—measures ability of thyroid gland to accumulate, concentrate and retain iodine; usually done at same time as a thyroid scan. Normal values: 1%-13% absorbed by thyroid after 2 hours; 2-25% absorbed after 6 hours; 15-45% absorbed after 24 hours. Used primarily to rule out a variety of benign conditions.

What information to select and record (record all dates)

- Test type
- Test result
- Normal test value/range

ENDOSCOPY (Scopes)

Endoscopy allows access to areas of the head and neck that cannot be seen directly or palpated easily, such as the nasopharynx, hypopharynx, and larynx. A thorough endoscopic examination of the head and neck is necessary to rule out concurrent primaries. Endoscopic instruments can be either rigid or flexible, depending on the area being accessed.

Common endoscopic procedures for head and neck cancers (refer to Diagnostic Tests chapter in this book for more information)

- **Laryngoscopy**—examination of the larynx
- **Bronchoscopy**—examination of the trachea and bronchi
- **Esophagoscopy**—examination of the esophagus
- **Nasopharyngoscopy**—examination of the nasopharynx and upper oropharynx
- **Triple Endoscopy** (also called panendoscopy)—combination procedure that examines the trachea, larynx, pharynx and esophagus via endoscopic visualization; used to investigate all mucosal surfaces of the upper respiratory tract for second primaries

What information to select and record (record all dates)

- Name of procedure
- Record both positive and negative findings
- Pertinent findings as described by the physician
    - Mass or lesion visualized
    - Extent of tumor (other structures involved)
    - Size of the tumor
    - Fixation of vocal cords, impairment of vocal cord movement
    - Mention of obstruction or stricture
    - Location of any biopsies

OPERATIVE FINDINGS

In addition to the pathology report of the tissues removed during a procedure, the operative report from diagnostic exploratory procedures and/or cancer directed definitive treatment can provide valuable information about the precise location of the primary tumor, any tumor or nodes left behind, as well as clinical information that might affect the staging or histologic diagnosis.

What information to select and record (record all dates)

Pertinent findings as described by the surgeon

- Tumor location including site(s)
- Organs and tissues removed—removal of just the tumor or removal of entire primary site
- Involved tissues or areas not included in pathology specimen
- Size of tumor/involved area before removal
- Tumor encompassing nerves or blood vessels; fixation to or invasion of skin, muscle or bone
- Status of regional lymph nodes, including anatomic name/level, size, laterality and number
- Fixed or matted lymph nodes
- If no findings are documented, document as "findings not recorded"
- Reason if no cancer-directed surgery was performed

DIAGNOSTIC PROCEDURES

CYTOLOGY REPORTS

The following procedures yield tumor cells that can confirm the diagnosis of head and neck cancer.

- **Fine needle aspiration (FNA),** fine needle aspiration cytology (**FNAC**), fine needle aspiration biopsy (**FNAB**)—FNA is used extensively in the diagnosis of malignant head and neck lesions and cervical lymph nodes. A thin needle is inserted into the lesion or suspicious area to remove fluid and/or cells. FNAs are frequently equivocal or show abnormal cells without a diagnosis of cancer. A benign cystic mass will disappear after aspiration; a persistent residual mass may require an excisional biopsy. FNA may be guided by ultrasound or computerized tomography when direct visualization of the lesion is not possible.
- **Brushings**—Cells are obtained by passing a small brush through an endoscopy tube and scraping cells from the lesion. The brush contents are analyzed cytologically. Sometimes called exfoliative cytology (see below).
- **Exfoliative cytology**—scraping a suspicious area and putting the scrapings on a slide for review under the microscope. If cancer cells are seen, the area can be biopsied.
- **Lymph node aspiration**—Biopsy procedure using a thin needle to take a sample of tissue or fluid from a lymph node. The procedure is also called fine needle aspiration.

What information to select and record (record all dates)

- Test type and tissue biopsied
- Positive or negative findings
- Cell type, if given

HISTOLOGY

The following procedures yield pieces of tumor that confirm the diagnosis of cancer and can be used to determine the extent of tumor and further treatment.

- **Incisional biopsy**—A diagnostic procedure in which surgeon cuts out a sample of tissue from the lesion or suspicious area. Incisional biopsy cuts through tumor; it is performed when complete removal is unnecessary or not possible. Incisional biopsy may also be performed to establish a diagnosis when cancer is suspected or possible and neoadjuvant (preoperative) treatment is being planned.
- **Excisional biopsy**—Also called surgical, total, or open biopsy. The purpose of an excisional biopsy is to attempt to remove the entire mass or a large portion of the mass for therapeutic as well as diagnostic purposes. The tissue that is removed is then sent to the pathologist for diagnosis. **Note**: Read the body of the operative report carefully. Frequently surgeons will title the report "biopsy" but the report will describe an excisional biopsy and the intent of the procedure was to excise the entire lesion.
- **Endoscopic biopsy**—Removal of tissue for microscopic examination by means of an endoscope (a fiberoptic cable for viewing inside the body) that is inserted into the body along with sampling instruments. The endoscope allows the physician to visualize the abnormality and guide the sampling.

PATHOLOGY REPORTS

Pathologic evaluation of any resected tissue not only establishes a diagnosis, but also provides important staging (and therefore prognostic) information. All parts of the pathology report—the gross examination of the specimen, the microscopic examination, the final diagnosis and comments—should be reviewed for staging, grade, and histology information, but only the final diagnosis should be used to code the histology.

If a CAP checklist (outline format provided by the College of American Pathologists) is provided, the information may be easier to find in that section of the pathology report than in the gross and microscopic narrative sections. The CAP checklist is also called a synoptic report or CAP protocol. An example of a CAP protocol is shown in Table 3.

What information to select and record (record all dates)

Final Diagnosis

- Histology (cell type and subtype)—Follow the histology coding rules for using this information. Remember that for head and neck cancers the histology is taken only from the final diagnosis.
- Behavior and grade
- Information about mixed histologies

Gross

- Location of tumor (area of head and neck) and location of tumor within resected specimen
- Aggregate size of tumor, if provided by pathologist
- Size of largest focus of tumor
- Size of invasive component of the tumor
- Presence of multiple tumors

Microscopic (primary tumor)

- Depth of invasion (mucosa, musculature, supporting tissues)
- Invasion of capsule (salivary glands and thyroid)
- Extent of disease: adjacent tissues, skin/dermis, muscle, cartilage or bone invasion
- Status of surgical margins
- Lymphovascular invasion (invasion of blood vessels and/or lymphatic channels within specimen)

Microscopic (regional lymph nodes)

- Location, number and size of involved nodes—lymph node level(s) or names of lymph node chain(s), ipsilateral or contralateral; (include all nodes aspirated, incised, and excised)
- Total number and location of regional nodes examined (include all nodes aspirated, incised, and excised)
- Size of metastasis in involved lymph nodes (not size of node)
- Involvement of node capsule (extracapsular extension)
- Fixed/matted lymph nodes
- Presence of nodules in axillary fat

Other Information

- Stage as stated by pathologist
- Results of biopsies of possible metastatic sites

Table 3. Example of College of American Pathologists (CAP) Head and Neck Cancer Protocol

Oropharynx CAP Protocol

Microscopic Diagnosis
Right tonsillectomy with right radical neck dissection
Moderate to poorly differentiated squamous cell carcinoma, 1.5 x 1.1 x 0.9 cm (please see tumor details below).
Six out of twenty-four (6/24) lymph nodes with metastatic squamous cell carcinoma.
Submandibular gland, no tumor present.
Segment of jugular vein with fibrous adhesion, no tumor present.
Skeletal muscle (omohyoid), no tumor present.

Tumor Details
Tumor site: Palatine tonsil
Tumor laterality: Right
Tumor focality: Unifocal
Tumor size: 1.5 cm
Histologic type: Squamous cell carcinoma
Histologic grade: G3, poorly differentiated

Number of lymph nodes examined: 24
Number of lymph nodes positive: 6, with largest lymph node measuring 4.0 x 3.0 x 2.5 cm
Level I (0/1)
Level II (4/7) with extranodal extension
Level III (2/9) with extranodal extension
Level IV (0/3)
Level VI (0/1)

Distant metastasis: Not assessed
TNM designation:
pT1
pN2
pM not applicable

Margins: Focally involved by invasive carcinoma
Lymph-vascular invasion: Not identified
Perineural invasion: Not identified

HEAD AND NECK CANCER DISEASE MANAGEMENT

OVERVIEW

Table 4 on the following page provides a short summary of preferred treatment modalities by site. More details of site-specific treatment are listed in the "'Usual' Treatment by Stage" section which follows.

Oral cavity Low stage lesions are highly curable by surgery alone, radiation therapy alone, or a combination. The choice of modality depends on the location of the tumor, the potential cosmetic defect, and the functional result of the treatment. The treatment decision must be made in consultation with the surgeon, radiation oncologist, and medical oncologist, as well as rehabilitation specialists. For more advanced cancers, treatment with surgery and postoperative radiation is appropriate, with or without neoadjuvant chemotherapy.

Oropharynx Treatment options are similar to those for oral cavity.

Hypopharynx Surgery (laryngopharyngectomy) followed by high dose radiation therapy to primary site and neck is the treatment of choice. Neoadjuvant chemotherapy (given prior to other modalities) is under clinical investigation.

Larynx In general, the preferred treatment for early stage laryngeal cancers should be external beam radiation because the results are good while preserving the voice, and retaining the possibility of salvage surgery if there is local recurrence. For small superficial tumors, laser excision is an option, along with radiation or surgery. Laryngectomy can be a subsequent treatment for patients who have persistent disease following radiation or who have less than a 50% response rate to chemotherapy. More advanced laryngeal cancers can be treated with combination radiation and surgery. Induction therapy with cisplatin and 5-FU followed by radiation therapy may be tried before total laryngectomy.

Paranasal sinuses and nasal cavity The treatment of choice is a combination of radiation and surgery. Sequence of treatment depends on the stage of the tumor at diagnosis.

Salivary glands Surgery is the preferred treatment for low-grade, low-stage tumors. Lymph node dissection should be included as part of the definitive treatment if nodes are involved. Radiation therapy may be added when lymph nodes are involved, or when the possible cosmetic result from surgery is unfavorable.

Thyroid gland Surgery is the treatment of choice for localized lesions, followed by TSH-suppressing doses of exogenous thyroid hormone (thyroxine) to decrease the likelihood of recurrence. In some cases of advanced stage papillary and follicular cancers, external beam radiation is an option after surgery.

Treatments under clinical evaluation for higher stages of many head and neck cancers include a variety of radiation therapy fractionation schemes, which reduce toxicities to normal tissue and improve tumor control rates, and clinical trials of chemotherapy preoperatively, before radiation therapy, as adjuvant therapy after surgery, or as part of combined modality therapy.

Table 4. Common Treatment Methods for Head and Neck Cancers

(from *Manual of Clinical Oncology)*

Early lesions are commonly T1 and T2 with negative nodes; advanced lesions are T3 and T4, or any tumor with positive regional lymph nodes.

KEY S = Surgery R = Radiation Therapy C = Chemotherapy ± = with or without
/ = a choice of treatments (preferred modality is first) ( ) = a lesser therapeutic alternative

Primary	Early	Advanced
Lip	R/S	R
Oral Cavity		
Oral tongue	S/R	R or S+R
Floor of mouth	S/R	R or S+R
Gingiva	S	S+R
Hard Palate	S	S+R
Buccal mucosa	S/R	S+R
Retromolar trigone	S	S+R
Oropharynx		
Soft palate	R	R
Tonsillar fossa	S/R	S+R
Anterior tonsillar pillar	S/R	S+R
Pharyngeal tongue	S/R	R
Pharyngeal wall	R	S+R
Hypopharynx		
Pyriform sinus	S/R	R or S+R
Posterior pharynx	R	R

Primary	Early	Advanced
Larynx		
Glottic (vocal cord)	R/(S)	S+R
Supraglottic	R/(S)	S+R
Subglottic	S/R	S+R
Nasopharynx	R	R
Paranasal sinuses		
Nasal cavity	S/R	S+R
Nasal vestibule	R/(S)	R
Ethmoid sinus	S+R	S+R
Frontal and sphenoid sinuses	R	R
Maxillary antrum	S	S+R±C
Salivary glands		
Parotid gland	S±R	S±R
Submandibular gland	S,S+R	S+R
Thyroid gland	S	S+R (ablation)

SURGERY

Laser surgery is becoming more commonly used for excisional biopsies, debulking, and some types of resections (small tumors and vocal cord lesions). Cryosurgery is another method of removing oral cancers: the tumor is frozen, after which it becomes necrotic and sloughs off. Endoscopic photodynamic therapy is another option in which the patient is given a radiosensitizer that concentrates in the tumor, then a concentrated light beam activates the radiosensitizer, which heats the tumor and kills the cancer cells.

Considerations for reconstruction should be included in the planning process for surgical resections of head and neck cancers, particularly for oral cavity, lip, sinus, and other visible sites. Preservation of facial nerve function is important when planning treatment for salivary gland cancers.

Oral Cavity The decision to perform surgery for oral cavity cancer depends on the location of the lesion and the functional deficit that results. Because surgical access is good, local excision of the lesion is the treatment of choice for early stage mouth cancers, while more extensive surgery and postoperative radiation is better for higher stage cancers.

- **Glossectomy**—removal of all or part of the tongue; also called lingulectomy
- **Partial glossectomy** (FORDS surgery code 30)—removal of part of the tongue, usually less than half of the tongue, such as a wedge resection with clear margins
- **Hemiglossectomy** (FORDS surgery code 30)—removal of one lateral half of the tongue or sometimes the front (anterior) half of the tongue

Surgery–Oral Cavity, *continued*

- **Total** or **radical glossectomy** (FORDS surgery codes 41-43)—removal of the entire tongue (base and anterior two-thirds), resulting in significant defects in swallowing and speaking and requiring reconstruction. A radical glossectomy includes resection of the mandible and may include total laryngectomy.

Pharynx Surgical procedures of the pharynx are usually for lesions in the oropharynx or hypopharynx. The usefulness of cancer-directed surgery in nasopharyngeal cancer is limited. The decision to perform surgery for pharyngeal cancer depends on the location of the lesion and the functional deficit that results. For example, surgery is preferred for a tonsillar pillar cancer, but radiation is preferred for base of tongue tumors where surgery could cause deficits in speech and/or swallowing.

- **Pharyngectomy** (FORDS surgery codes 30-32)—removal of all or part of the oropharynx and/or hypopharynx
  - **Limited** or **partial pharyngectomy** (FORDS surgery code 31)—removal of part of the pharynx, usually the hypopharynx, or a portion of the oropharynx or hypopharynx such as the posterior pharyngeal wall
  - **Tonsillectomy**, **bilateral tonsillectomy** (FORDS surgery code 31)—removal of one or both tonsils
  - **Total pharyngectomy** (FORDS surgery code 32)—removal of the entire pharynx only; sometimes called larynx-preserving pharyngectomy
- **Laryngopharyngectomy** (FORDS surgery code 41)—removal of all or part of the pharynx and larynx, with or without removal of adjacent bone and may also involve removal of part of the esophagus. Partial laryngopharyngectomy can be performed for pyriform sinus lesions. Other procedures include hemi- and supra-cricoid laryngopharyngectomy.
- **Radical pharyngectomy** (FORDS surgery codes 50-52) includes total removal of the mandible with or without laryngectomy and with or without partial esophagectomy

Larynx As previously noted, radiation therapy is usually attempted first for laryngeal cancers to preserve speech function. Cordectomy is an option for low stage vocal cord lesions. Partial or hemilaryngectomy can be performed to retain some voice function. Full or total laryngectomy is usually reserved for extensive disease at the time of diagnosis or as a salvage procedure when laryngeal cancer progresses.

- **Laser excision** (FORDS surgery code 25)—endoscopic removal of early stage vocal cord cancer using a CO2 (carbon dioxide) laser
- **Vocal cord stripping** (FORDS surgery code 28)—removal of the top cell layer of the vocal cord and any surface lesion, polyp, or early stage carcinoma
- **Cordectomy** (FORDS surgery code 30)—removal of one vocal cord
- **Hemilaryngectomy** (FORDS surgery code 30)—removal of the anterior soft parts of the larynx in continuity with the underlying thyroid cartilage; also called vertical partial laryngectomy
- **Vertical laryngectomy** (FORDS surgery code 31)—removal of involved true vocal cord, ipsilateral false vocal cord, ventricle, ipsilateral thyroid and may include removal of the arytenoids
- **Anterior commissure laryngectomy** (FORDS surgery code 32)—removal of the involved true vocal cord, the anterior commissure, and part of the healthy true vocal cord; also called fronto-lateral partial laryngectomy. Anterior commissure lesions may also be treated with vertical partial laryngectomy (see hemilaryngectomy above).
- **Supraglottic laryngectomy** (FORDS surgery code 33)—conservative surgery intended to preserve laryngeal function. Procedure removes supraglottic larynx (epiglottis, false vocal cords, aryepiglottic folds, arytenoid cartilages, ventricle), upper one third of thyroid cartilage, thyroid membrane. The true vocal cords and arytenoids remain in place to allow

Surgery–Larynx, ***continued***

vocalization and swallowing. If part of the hypopharynx is removed with the cancer, this additional procedure is called a partial pharyngectomy.

- **Supracricoid laryngectomy** (FORDS surgery code 33)—a type of horizontal partial laryngectomy that removes the entire supraglottis, the false and true vocal cords, and the thyroid cartilage including the paraglottic and preepiglottic spaces.

- **Total laryngectomy** (FORDS surgery code 41)—removal of the entire larynx. A person can no longer speak normally after a total laryngectomy because the vocal cords have been removed. During this operation, a tracheostomy stoma is created in the front of the neck to allow the person to breathe.
- **Radical laryngectomy** (FORDS surgery code 42)—removal of entire larynx and surrounding tissues including thyroid gland, cartilages, part of trachea, and cervical lymph nodes. If all or part of the pharynx is removed, the procedure is a pharyngolaryngectomy.
- **Pharyngolaryngectomy**, also called **laryngopharyngectomy** (FORDS surgery code 50)—removal of the larynx and part or all of the pharynx requiring reconstruction of the pharynx using skin flaps or a segment of the intestine. A person can no longer speak normally and may also have difficulty swallowing after laryngopharyngectomy.

Parotid gland The parotid gland extends from in front of the ear down onto the mandible. The facial (7th cranial) nerve and its branches run through the substance of the parotid gland, dividing it into the superficial and deep "lobes". Eighty percent of the parotid gland is superficial to the facial nerve. Surgical removal of the parotid gland requires careful dissection around the facial nerve so as not to damage it ("nerve sparing"). If the facial nerve must be removed ("nerve sacrificed") due to the extent of the tumor, the patient is left with limited ability to close the eye, wrinkle the nose or move the lip on that side of the face.

- **Partial** or **less than total parotidectomy** (FORDS surgery codes 30-38)—removal of part of the parotid gland or a single lobe (superficial, codes 33-35; deep, codes 36-38; or unspecified, codes 30-32).
- **Total parotidectomy** (FORDS surgery codes 40-42)—removal of the entire parotid gland
- **Radical parotidectomy** (FORDS surgery codes 50-53)—removal of the entire parotid gland and adjacent structures such as temporal bone and overlying skin, requiring reconstruction of the area

Thyroid Lobectomy can be performed for thyroid cancer, but about 10% of cases will have a recurrence in the thyroid. Total thyroidectomy is the preferred treatment, although a small amount of thyroid and parathyroid tissue may be left behind. In most cases, the surgeon will attempt to identify and dissect around the parathyroid glands, which are on the thyroid gland surface or may be imbedded in the thyroid, leaving the parathyroid glands in place to control calcium levels in the body.

- **Lobectomy** (FORDS surgery code 21)—removal of the right or left lobe of the thyroid; used to treat localized papillary cancers smaller than 1 cm (papillary microcarcinomas); also called hemithyroidectomy, unilateral thyroidectomy or partial thyroidectomy
- **Isthmusectomy** (FORDS surgery code 22)—removal of only the thyroid tissue between the two larger glands (isthmus)
- **Removal of a lobe and partial removal of the contralateral lobe** (FORDS surgery code 30)—includes resection of one lobe, isthmusectomy and partial resection of opposite lobe; also called Harley Dunhill procedure
- **Subtotal** or **near-total thyroidectomy** (FORDS surgery code 40)—removal of up to 95% of thyroid tissue. A bilateral subtotal thyroidectomy removes the front part of each lobe and leaves 1-5 grams of thyroid tissue in place on each side. A near-total thyroidectomy removes one entire lobe, the isthmus, and most of the opposite lobe, leaving a small amount of thyroid tissue on only one side.

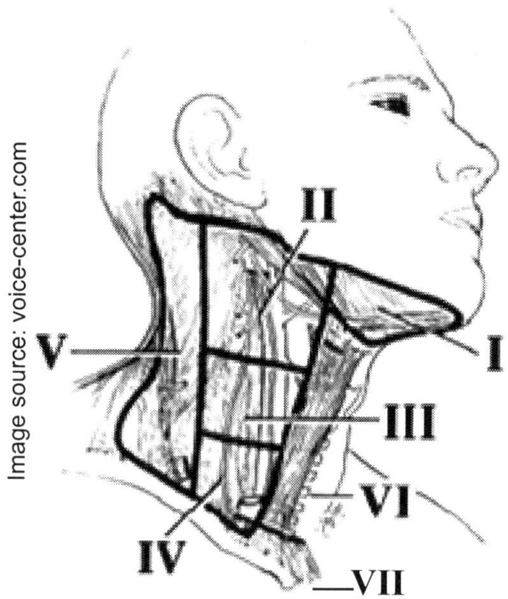

Figure 9. Lymph Node Levels

Level I	Submental, submaxillary
Level II	Upper jugular
Level III	Mid-jugular
Level IV	Lower jugular
Level V	Posterior triangle
Level VI	Anterior central compartment
Level VII	Superior mediastinal

Surgery, ***continued***

- **Total thyroidectomy** (FORDS surgery code 50)—removal of all thyroid tissue, resulting in hypothyroidism requiring replacement hormones for the remainder of the patient's life

Other Surgical Procedures of Head and Neck Sites

- *Mohs technique*—a shave excision procedure removing thin layers of skin tumor to assure that all signs of malignancy have been removed from the base of the tumor
- *Caldwell-Luc procedure*—opening the maxillary sinus by way of an incision into the supradental fossa opposite the premolar teeth
- *Maxillary exenteration*—removal of entire contents of maxillary antrum
- *Composite resection* (also called "commando" procedure)—en bloc resection of primary tumor, cervical nodes, and part of mandible if tumor lies close to bone

Treatment Options for Regional Lymph Nodes

In the head and neck, the lymphatic system is very rich but there are relatively few nerves in underlying tissue that can signal pain from a growing mass or other symptoms. Consequently, many pharyngeal cancers involve regional lymph nodes at the time of diagnosis. The following table shows the likelihood of regional node metastases at diagnosis.

Table 5. Likelihood of Regional Lymph Node Involvement at Time of Diagnosis

20%	Paranasal sinus
30-65%	Soft palate, pharyngeal wall, postcricoid area, posterior hypopharynx, medullary carcinoma of thyroid
70% or higher	Base of tongue, tonsil, pyriform sinus, nasopharynx

For other head and neck sites, the risk of metastases to lymph nodes increases with high-grade histology, large lesions, and deeply invasive lesions. Patients with Stage III and higher head and neck cancers should have elective lymph node radiation therapy or node dissection. In general, either radiation or a neck dissection is effective therapy for the following TNM Node categories: N1 (single

Surgery—Regional Lymph Nodes, *continued*

involved node up to 2 cm in size) and N2b (multiple involved nodes, all of which are smaller than 2 cm). Single or multiple lymph nodes larger than 2 cm should be considered for a combined surgical and radiation therapy approach. Surgery with postoperative radiation therapy is indicated for patients with multiple positive nodes, contralateral subclinical metastases, bilateral metastases, or extracapsular extension of tumor in the lymph node. Preoperative radiation therapy is indicated for large fixed nodes.

Radical neck dissection (cervical lymphadenectomy) is an option as part of definitive therapy, as a diagnostic procedure when the size of the primary indicates a possibility of nodal metastases, or as a secondary procedure if irradiated cervical nodes persist in size or recur. There are many techniques for removing cervical nodes, and the American Academy of Otolaryngology, Head and Neck Surgery has developed standardized descriptions not only of the lymph node levels that can be removed, but also of the structures affected by the neck dissection.

Figure 9 shows the locations of possible cervical lymph node involvement. A modification of this figure will be shown in the Collaborative Staging section of this chapter, because it is an important part of coding the site-specific factors for head and neck cancers. Table 6 is a summary of the various named neck dissection procedures indicating which levels of lymph nodes and other structures are removed. All lymph node procedures are coded in Scope of Regional Lymph Node Surgery based on the number of lymph nodes removed. In addition, the lymph node procedures in Table 6 are consid-

Table 6. Classification of Neck Dissections

Name of Procedure	Nodal Levels Dissected	Structures* Preserved	Additional Comments
Radical neck dissection (ND)	I–V plus LN around tail of parotid	None	Standard basic cervical lymphadenectomy procedure
Modified radical ND	I–V	1 or more	
• Type 1	I–V	SAN	
• Type 2	I–V	SAN, SCM	
• Type 3	I–V	All	
Comprehensive ND	I–V	Varies	Nonstandard term referring to any dissection removing node levels I-V
Selective neck dissections	Varies	All	General term for removal of certain LN groups and preservation of others
• Supraomohyoid ND	I–III (selective), sometimes IV	All	
• Lateral (jugular) ND	II–IV		
• Anterolateral ND	I–IV	All	
• Anterior Compartment ND	VI (selective)	All	Usually bilateral, may be unilateral
• Posterolateral	II–V plus suboccipital and postauricular	All	Used for cutaneous scalp malignancies

* Specific non-lymphatic structures are the spinal accessory (11th cranial) nerve (SAN), internal jugular vein (IJV), and sternocleidomastoid muscle (SCM)

Surgery—Regional Lymph Nodes, ***continued***

ered dissections for the purposes of coding Regional Lymph Nodes Examined; use code 97 in this field if the number of lymph nodes removed and examined is not counted or unknown. If lymph nodes are described as matted and cannot be counted individually, the procedure that removed them should be coded as a lymph node dissection.

By definition, a radical neck dissection removes all fibrofatty tissue on the same side of the neck as the primary tumor from mandible to clavicle, from anterior border of trapezius muscle to midline strap muscles, in the plane of the deep cervical fascia, including accessory nerve, internal jugular vein, and sternocleidomastoid muscle; severe disfigurement results. An extended neck dissection refers to any type of dissection listed in the table, but involves the removal of additional lymph node groups or nonlymphatic structures beyond what is normally included, for example an extended selective anterior compartment neck dissection. A selective neck dissection preserves one or more lymph node groups and/or neck structures that would otherwise be removed in a radical neck dissection; ordinarily six or more nodes are removed in a selective, or limited, neck dissection. Various types of neck dissections are described in Table 6.

RADIATION THERAPY

Clinically accessible oral cavity cancers may be treated with interstitial radiation therapy, external beam, or a combination of both. Interstitial treatments (brachytherapy) may include radioactive needles (radium 226, cesium 137), wires (iridium 192), or seeds (iridium 192).

High dose radiation therapy to the primary site and regional lymph nodes is the treatment of choice for cancer of the nasopharynx. High dose radiation therapy is necessary to treat cancers of the paranasal sinuses and nasal cavity, which frequently invade adjacent bony structures.

Radiation therapy for salivary gland tumors is usually reserved for tumors that are inoperable, unresectable or recurrent. However, neutron beam radiation has been proven to be effective for salivary gland cancers in clinical trials.

Radiation therapy alone is a treatment option for low stage laryngeal cancers, to preserve the voice.

Hyperfractionated and other novel fractionation radiation therapy techniques are under clinical investigation for many head and neck sites. Radiation modifiers, such as chemosensitizers, are under clinical investigation for treatment of large or bulky lesions.

Iodine isotope (iodine 131) is used in thyroid cancer cases to decrease the recurrence rate for follicular and papillary carcinomas.

SYSTEMIC THERAPY

Chemotherapy/Immunotherapy/Other Therapy
What information to record

- Start and stop date (if available)
- Statement that treatment was given pre-operatively or post-operatively
- Names of agents or regimens administered
- Number of courses

CHEMOTHERAPY

Chemotherapy for head and neck cancer serves two purposes: to improve locoregional control in conjunction with surgery and/or radiation therapy and to treat systemic metastases. Chemotherapy is generally not administered for early stage, localized disease. For more extensive tumors, chemotherapy can be given before, concurrent with, or after other modalities.

- ***Neoadjuvant chemotherapy***—chemotherapy administered prior to surgery or radiation therapy, intended to shrink tumor mass and make it more treatable by another modality; also called induction chemotherapy
- ***Chemoradiation***—treatment with chemotherapy and radiation therapy concurrently or in a rapid alternating sequence for surgically unresectable, locally advanced tumor. Adding chemotherapy enhances the effectiveness of radiation and the combination is superior to radiation therapy alone; however, the best drug(s) to use and the most effective way to integrate the two modalities are still unresolved.
- ***Adjuvant chemotherapy***—chemotherapy administered after surgery with the intent to destroy any remaining subclinical (microscopic) disease

Chemotherapy agents used alone or in combinations:

Cisplatin (Platinol), Carboplatin (Paraplatin)
5-FU (5-Fluorouracil)
Methotrexate
Taxotere (docetaxel), Taxol (paclitaxel)
Cetuximab (Erbitux)

Less commonly used drugs
Navelbine (vinorelbine)
Bleomycin
Adriamycin (doxorubicin)
Cytoxan (cyclophosphamide)
Ifosfamide (Ifos)

Combination chemotherapy is more effective than single agent chemotherapy, and recently, three-drug combinations (adding cetuximab) have been shown to be more effective than the commonly used two drug regimens such as Cisplatin and 5-FU. Examples of combination chemotherapy regimens include:

TPF (docetaxel [Taxotere], cisplatin [Platinol], 5-FU) and TPFL (TPF plus leucovorin)
PFLI (cisplatin, 5-FU, leucovorin, and interferon), an intense induction regimen

Under clinical investigation for treatment of various head and neck cancers is Isoretinoin (Retin-A, 13-cis-retinoic acid). Used daily for a year, it may prevent development of subsequent primaries in the respiratory and digestive tracts of the head and neck.

HORMONE THERAPY

Hormone therapy is not effective for head and neck cancer.

IMMUNOTHERAPY

Interferon and interleukin, as well as newer biological response modifiers, have been used as single agent treatment of head and neck cancer.

'USUAL' TREATMENT BY PRIMARY SITE AND STAGE GROUP (from NCI PDQ)

Lip and Oral Cavity Cancer Treatment Options

LIP

Stage I

- Surgery or radiation therapy as determined by anticipated cosmetic and functional results

Stage II

- Surgery for smaller T2 lesions on the lower lip if there is an acceptable cosmetic result
- Radiation (external beam or interstitial as appropriate) if reconstructive surgery is anticipated

Stage III and IV

- Surgery or radiation therapy (external beam or brachytherapy) depending on the size and location of the lesion and the needs for reconstruction
- Clinical trials of chemotherapy preoperatively, before radiation therapy, as adjuvant therapy after surgery, or as part of combined modality therapy
- Superfractionated radiation therapy

ANTERIOR TONGUE

Stage I

- Wide local excision for small lesions that can be resected transorally
- For larger lesions, either surgery or radiation therapy, interstitial implantation alone or with external-beam radiation therapy

Stage II

- Radiation therapy for T2 lesions with minimal infiltration to preserve speech and swallowing
- Surgery is reserved for radiation treatment failures
- Neck dissection may be considered when primary brachytherapy is used
- Surgery, radiation therapy, or a combination of both for deeply infiltrative lesions

Stage III

- External-beam radiation with or without interstitial implant for minimally infiltrative lesions
- Surgery with postoperative radiation therapy for deeply infiltrative lesions

Stage IV

- Combined surgery (such as total glossectomy, sometimes requiring laryngectomy) with postoperative radiation therapy in selected patients
- Palliative radiation therapy for very advanced lesions

BUCCAL MUCOSA

Stage I

- Surgery alone for lesions < 1 cm if the commissure is not involved. If the commissure is involved, consider adding radiation therapy (including brachytherapy)
- Surgical excision with split-thickness skin graft or radiation therapy for larger T1 lesions

Stage II

- Radiation therapy for lesions ≤ 3 cm or if tumor involves commissure
- Surgery, radiation therapy, or a combination for lesion > 3 cm
- Surgery if tumor invades the mandible or maxilla

Stage III and IV

- Radical surgical resection alone
- Radiation therapy alone
- Surgical resection plus radiation therapy, usually postoperative
- Clinical trials for chemotherapy preoperatively, before radiation therapy, as adjuvant therapy after surgery, or as part of combined modality therapy

'Usual' Treatment by Stage, *continued*

FLOOR OF MOUTH

Stage I

- Surgery or radiation therapy for T1 lesions. For lesions < 0.5 cm, excision alone if there is a margin of normal mucosa between the lesion and the gingiva. For larger lesions, surgery if lesion involves periosteum, or radiation if lesion involves tongue

Stage II

- Surgery for lesions ≤3 cm if lesion is attached to periosteum, or radiation if the lesion involves tongue
- For large T2 lesions (>3 cm), surgery and radiation therapy are alternatives; the choice depends primarily on the expected extent of disability from surgery.
- Postoperative external beam radiation therapy with or without interstitial radiation therapy should be considered for larger lesions

Stage III

- Rim resection or partial mandibulectomy plus neck dissection as appropriate
- External beam radiation therapy (EBRT) alone or EBRT plus an interstitial implant
- Clinical trials using novel radiation therapy fractionation schemas
- Clinical trials of chemotherapy preoperatively, before radiation therapy, as adjuvant therapy after surgery, or as part of combined modality therapy

Stage IV

- Combination surgery and radiation therapy, generally postoperative
- For fixed nodes (≥ 5 cm), preoperative radiation therapy

RETROMOLAR TRIGONE

Stage I and II

- Limited resection of the mandible for early lesions without detectable bone invasion
- Radiation therapy (with possible salvage surgery) if limited resection is not feasible

Stage III and IV

- Surgical composite resection that may be followed by postoperative radiation therapy
- Clinical trials of chemotherapy preoperatively, before radiation therapy, as adjuvant therapy after surgery, or as part of combined modality therapy
- Clinical trials using novel radiation therapy fractionation schemas

LOWER GINGIVA

Stage I and II

- Intraoral resection with or without a rim resection of bone and repaired with a split-thickness skin graft for small lesions
- Radiation therapy for small lesions but results are generally better after surgery alone

Stage III

- Combined radiation therapy (pre- or postoperative) and radical resection or by radical resection alone for extensive lesions with moderate bone destruction and/or nodal metastases

Stage IV

- Far-advanced tumors with extensive destruction of the mandible and with nodal metastases are poorly controlled by surgery, radiation therapy, or a combination of both.

UPPER GINGIVA AND HARD PALATE

Stage I and II

- Surgical resection with postoperative radiation therapy as appropriate

Stage III

- Radiation therapy alone for superficial lesions with extensive involvement of gingiva, hard palate, or soft palate
- Combined surgery and radiation for deeply invasive lesions involving bone

'Usual' Treatment by Stage—Upper Gingiva and Hard Palate, *continued*

Stage IV

- Combined surgery and radiation therapy

Pharynx Cancer Treatment Options

OROPHARYNX

Stage I and II

- Surgery or radiation are equally successful
  Radiation is preferred when the functional deficit will be great, such as the tongue base
  Surgery is preferred when the functional deficit will be minimal, such as tonsil pillar

Stage III

- Combined surgery and postoperative radiation therapy or postoperative chemoradiation
- Aggressive radiation therapy alone for tonsil or base of tongue
- External beam radiation augmented with interstitial implants
- Hyperfractionation
- Chemoradiation
- Neoadjuvant chemotherapy or radiation clinical trials

Stage IVA (resectable); Stage IVB and IVC (unresectable)

- Surgery and postoperative radiation therapy plus chemotherapy
- Radiation therapy or chemoradiation therapy
- Radiation alone for stage IVA tonsillar cancer
- Chemotherapy clinical trials
  Neoadjuvant chemotherapy
  Chemotherapy with radiation as well as with radiosensitizers
- Radiation clinical trials; hyperfractionation and/or brachytherapy
  Simultaneous chemotherapy and hyperfractionated radiation therapy
  Particle-beam radiation therapy
  Hyperthermia combined with radiation therapy

NASOPHARYNX

Stage I and II

- High-dose radiation therapy to primary site and prophylactic radiation to regional nodes
- Chemoradiation for Stage II cancers

Stage III and IV

- Chemoradiation
- High-dose or superfractionated radiation therapy to primary site and clinically positive bilateral neck nodes
- Neck dissection for persistent or recurrent nodes if the primary site is controlled
- Intensity-modulated radiation therapy (IMRT) and other newer radiation techniques
- Chemotherapy for patients with stage IVC disease
- Clinical trials of neoadjuvant chemotherapy and adjuvant chemotherapy after radiation

HYPOPHARYNX

Stage I and II

- Laryngopharyngectomy and neck dissection
- Partial laryngopharyngectomy for selected pyriform sinus cancers
- Postoperative radiation to both sides of neck, retropharyngeal and lateral cervical nodes
- Radiation therapy alone for rare T1 or T2 N0 tumors
- Neoadjuvant chemotherapy for Stage II cases

'Usual' Treatment by Stage—Hypopharynx, *continued*

Stage III and IVA (resectable)

- Newer surgical techniques for resection and reconstruction, such as gastric pull-up or free jejunal transfer
- Postoperative radiation therapy or chemoradiation
- Neoadjuvant chemotherapy

Stage IVB and IVC (unresectable)

- Radiation therapy or chemoradiation
- Clinical trials of radiation hyperfractionation schedules with chemotherapy

Larynx Cancer Treatment Options

SUPRAGLOTTIS

Stage I

- External-beam radiation therapy alone, reserving surgery for radiation failure
- Supraglottic laryngectomy
- Total laryngectomy in certain situations

Stage II

- External-beam radiation therapy alone for smaller lesions
- Postoperative radiation therapy for positive or close surgical margins
- Supraglottic laryngectomy or total laryngectomy, depending on location of the lesion, clinical status of the patient, and surgical expertise
- Hyperfractionated radiation therapy

Stage III

- Surgery with or without postoperative radiation therapy
- Definitive radiation therapy with surgery for salvage of radiation failures
- Concurrent chemoradiation
- Clinical trials of chemotherapy, radiosensitizers, or particle-beam radiation therapy

Stage IV

- Total laryngectomy with postoperative radiation therapy
- Definitive radiation therapy with surgery for salvage of radiation failures
- Hyperfractionalted radiation therapy
- Concurrent chemoradiation

Stage II–IV

- Clinical trial of isotretinoin as a preventative of subsequent tumors

GLOTTIS

Stage I and II

- Radiation therapy
- Cordectomy for carefully selected patients with limited and superficial T1 lesions
- Partial or hemilaryngectomy or total laryngectomy, depending on anatomic considerations
- Laser excision or microsurgery in selected patients
- Hyperfractionated radiation therapy

Stage III and IV

- Surgery with or without (Stage III) or with (Stage IV) postoperative radiation therapy
- Definitive radiation therapy with surgery for salvage of radiation failures
- Concurrent chemoradiation
- Clinical trials exploring chemotherapy, radiosensitizers, or particle beam radiation therapy

Sage II–IV

- Clinical trial of isotretinoin as a preventative of subsequent tumors

'Usual' Treatment by Stage—Larynx, *continued*

SUBGLOTTIS

Stage I and II

- Radiation therapy alone with preservation of normal voice, reserving surgery for radiation failure

Stage III

- Laryngectomy plus isolated thyroidectomy and tracheoesophageal node dissection usually followed by radiation therapy
- Radiation therapy alone for patients who are not surgical candidates
- Clinical trials exploring chemotherapy, radiosensitizers, or particle-beam radiation therapy

Stage IV

- Laryngectomy plus total thyroidectomy and bilateral tracheoesophageal node dissection usually followed by postoperative radiation therapy
- Radiation therapy alone is indicated for patients who are not surgical candidates
- Clinical trials of simultaneous chemotherapy and hyperfractionated radiation therapy
- Clinical trials exploring chemotherapy, radiosensitizers, or particle-beam radiation therapy

Stage II–IV

- Clinical trial of isotretinoin as a preventative of subsequent tumors

Nasal Cavity and Paranasal Sinuses Cancer Treatment Options

MAXILLARY SINUS

Stage I (small lesions of the infrastructure)

- Surgical resection
- Postoperative radiation therapy for close margins (particularly in tumors of the suprastructure).

Stage II and III

- Surgical resection with high-dose preoperative or postoperative radiation therapy
- Superfractionated preoperative or postoperative radiation therapy for Stage III is under clinical evaluation
- Neoadjuvant or adjuvant chemotherapy is under clinical evaluation for Stage III

Stage IV

- High-dose radiation therapy with localized drainage of the sinus(es)

ETHMOID SINUS

Stage I and II

- External-beam radiation therapy alone for unresectable lesions
- Resection of well-localized lesions, including resection of the ethmoids, maxilla, and orbit
- Postoperative radiation therapy even with clear surgical margins

Stage III

- Craniofacial resection with postoperative radiation therapy
- Neoadjuvant or adjuvant chemotherapy is under clinical evaluation

Stage IV

- Craniofacial resection in combination with preoperative or postoperative radiation therapy
- Concomitant chemotherapy and radiation therapy for inoperable tumors

SPHENOID SINUS

All stages

- Treatment is the same as for nasopharynx (see above)
- Chemoradiation for stages II and higher

'Usual' Treatment by Stage, *continued*

NASAL CAVITY (squamous cell carcinomas)

Stage I and II

- Surgery for tumors of the septum
- Radiation therapy for tumors of the lateral and superior walls
- Surgery plus radiation therapy for tumors of the septal and lateral walls

Stage III and IV

- Combined surgery and postoperative radiation therapy
- Surgery alone or radiation therapy alone
- Neoadjuvant or adjuvant chemotherapy is under clinical evaluation
- Chemoradiation

NASAL VESTIBULE

Stage I and II

- Surgery for small lesions when no deformity is expected and reconstruction is not anticipated
- Radiation therapy for other small lesions

Stage III and IV

- Radiation to minimize deformity
- External beam (photons or electrons) and/or interstitial implantation
- Neoadjuvant or adjuvant chemotherapy is under clinical evaluation
- Surgery for salvage

Major Salivary Gland Cancer Treatment Options

Low-grade Carcinomas (acinic cell ca, basal cell adenoca, clear cell ca, cystadenocarcinoma, epithelial-myoepithelial ca, mucinous adenoca, polymorphous low grade adenoca, and some cases of adenoca, mucoepidermoid ca, and squamous cell ca)

Stage I

- Surgery alone
- Postoperative radiation therapy when resection margins are positive
- Radiation therapy when resection involves a significant cosmetic or functional deficit

Stage II

- Surgery alone or with postoperative radiation therapy, if indicated
- Chemotherapy in special circumstances, such as when other modalities are refused

Stage III

- Surgery alone or with postoperative radiation therapy when indicated
- Chemotherapy in special circumstances, such as when other modalities are refused or when tumors are recurrent or nonresponsive to other modalities
- Neutron-beam therapy for tumor spread to lymph nodes
- Clinical trials of fast neutron-beam radiation and adjuvant chemotherapy

Stage IV

- Fast neutron-beam radiation or accelerated hyperfractionated photon beam therapy
- Conventional x ray therapy for inoperable, unresectable, or recurrent tumors
- Clinical trials of combined chemotherapy and radiation

High-grade Carcinomas (anaplastic small cell ca, carcinosarcoma, large cell undifferentiated ca, small cell undifferentiated ca, salivary duct ca, myoepithelial carcinoma, and some cases of adenoca, mucoepidermoid ca, and squamous cell ca)

Stage I

- Radical surgery alone for localized tumors confined to gland of origin
- Postoperative radiation for high-grade tumors, positive margins, or perineural invasion
- Clinical trials exploring newer methods of local control, including adjuvant chemotherapy

'Usual' Treatment by Stage, *continued*

Stage II and III

- Radical surgery alone for localized tumors confined to gland of origin
- Postoperative radiation for high-grade tumors, positive margins, or perineural invasion
- Primary radiation therapy, such as fast neutron-beam radiation, for inoperable, unresectable, or recurrent tumors
- Primary conventional x-ray radiation therapy as palliation for unresectable tumors
- For regional lymph node involvement, resection of the primary tumor and the involved lymph nodes, with or without radiation therapy
- Clinical trials exploring newer methods of local control, including adjuvant chemotherapy, radiation therapy and/or radiosensitizers

Stage IV

- Fast neutron-beam radiation or accelerated hyperfractionated photon beam therapy
- Clinical trials with chemotherapy and radiation

Thyroid Cancer Treatment Options

PAPILLARY AND FOLLICULAR CARCINOMA

Stage I and II

- Surgery is the therapy of choice for all primary lesions (see definitions of surgical procedures under Head and Neck Cancer Disease Management)
  Total thyroidectomy *Advantages:* handles high incidence of multicentric, bilateral involvement and virtually eliminates the possibility of dedifferentiation of any residual tumor to anaplastic cell type. *Disadvantages:* associated with a higher incidence of hypo-parathyroidism, but this may be reduced when a small amount of tissue is left on the contralateral side (near-total thyroidectomy); facilitates follow-up thyroid scanning since nearly all thyroid tissue is removed.
  Lobectomy *Advantages:* associated with a lower incidence of complications. *Disadvantages:* may miss microcarcinoma in contralateral lobe; 5% to 10% of patients will have a recurrence in the thyroid following lobectomy. Also, use of I-131 ablative therapy is compromised because the isotope will concentrate in the thyroid, not in metastatic sites.
- Biopsies of abnormal lymph nodes at the time of surgery and removal of involved nodes, most often by selective node dissection; radical neck dissection is usually not required
- Postoperative therapeutic (ablative) doses of I-131, especially for follicular carcinoma, to treat subclinical metastases and reduce likelihood of recurrent cancer
- Exogenous (replacement) thyroid hormone therapy to suppress production of thyroid stimulating hormone (TSH) and reduce likelihood of recurrent cancer

Stage III

- Total thyroidectomy plus removal of involved lymph nodes or other sites of extrathyroid disease
- I-131 ablation following total thyroidectomy if tumor demonstrates uptake of this isotope
- External beam radiation therapy if I-131 uptake is minimal

Stage IV

- Ablation of metastases with therapeutic doses of I-131
- External-beam radiation therapy for localized lesions unresponsive to I-131
- Resection of limited metastases when the tumor has no uptake of I-131
- Thyroid-stimulating hormone suppression with thyroxine for lesions not sensitive to I-131
- Clinical trials evaluating new treatment approaches, including adjuvant chemotherapy

'Usual' Treatment by Stage—Thyroid, *continued*

MEDULLARY THYROID CARCINOMA

- Total thyroidectomy, unless there is evidence of distant metastasis. Medullary carcinoma has a high incidence (75%) of microscopically involved nodes.
- Routine central and bilateral modified neck dissections
- External beam radiation therapy for palliation of locally recurrent tumors
- **Note:** Radioactive iodine is not effective for medullary thyroid carcinoma
- Palliative chemotherapy for patients with metastatic disease

ANAPLASTIC THYROID CARCINOMA

- Total thyroidectomy for the infrequent localized anaplastic carcinoma; tracheostomy is frequently necessary
- External beam radiation therapy for patients who are not surgical candidates or who have unresectable tumor
- Chemotherapy with doxorubicin and cisplatin
- **Note:** Anaplastic thyroid carcinoma is not responsive to I-131 therapy
- Clinical trials of combined chemotherapy and radiation therapy following complete resection

COLLABORATIVE STAGE DATA COLLECTION SYSTEM (CS)

Review the medical record for the diagnostic and staging procedures listed previously in this chapter under Cancer Abstracting Guidelines. Look for information (positive and negative) that describes the tumor location, depth of invasion into the mucosa or muscularis propria, tumor size, histologic grade, lymph node involvement, extension to adjacent organs and structures, or metastasis to distant sites or organs. All of this information can be coded in CS.

Make sure that your CS manual is complete by downloading any replacement pages from www.cancerstaging.org/cstage/manuals/index.html. Review carefully the notes preceding each table of the appropriate head and neck schema in the Collaborative Stage Data Collection System Coding Instructions version 02.03.02. Use the notes and comments in this section to supplement the information in the CS documentation. Remember that all of the general rules in Part I of the CS documentation apply to the site schema.

With minor exceptions, Collaborative Staging for head and neck uses the following common or standard tables. They will not be discussed in detail here, although you should read them carefully:

CS TS/Ext Eval
CS Reg Nodes Eval
Reg LN Pos
Reg LN Exam
CS Mets Eval

Collaborative Staging for head and neck (except thyroid) uses either nine or all ten Site-Specific Factors, which will be discussed in detail below.

CS Tumor Size

Although CS Tumor Size uses the common table for all sites, for many of the head and neck sites, tumor size is more important than CS Extension for determining the mapping of the AJCC T category. In fact, CS Tumor Size takes priority for mapping to T1, T2 and T3 tumors in the following Collaborative Staging schemas:

Tumor Size, ***continued***

- Lip (upper, lower, other)
- Tongue (base, anterior two-thirds)
- Gum (upper, lower, other)
- Salivary Glands* (parotid, submandibular, other)
- Tonsil (lingual, palatine)
- Pharynx (oropharynx, hypopharynx*, pyriform sinus*, laryngopharynx*)
- Floor of Mouth
- Palate (hard, soft) and Uvula
- Other mouth
- Buccal Mucosa
- Retromolar Area
- Thyroid*
- Mucosal melanomas of all sites except salivary glands

* For these sites, T category definitions include additional anatomic or symptom descriptions

These are "accessible" sites, meaning that the tumor can be directly visualized or palpated and measured clinically. Precise coding of tumor size is important for these primary sites, because TNM's T category represents a range of tumor sizes: T1 is tumor ≤ 2 cm; T2 is tumor > 2 cm and ≤ 4 cm; and T3 is tumor > 4 cm. T4 is direct extension into adjacent structures, which vary by site.

For all other sites in the head and neck, the amount of extension is more important than tumor size, but a sincere effort to identify and code the tumor size should be made.
To determine whether Tumor Size or Extension takes priority when the CS TS/Ext Eval code is assigned, look at the CS Extension table for the site being abstracted. If there is a carat (^) in the TNM7 Map column or an asterisk (*) in the TNM6 Map column of the Extension code, this is an indication that the tumor size is needed to assign the T category and that the Eval code should be based on how the tumor size was determined.

Head-Neck

CS Extension
In general, the structures in the head and neck, except the tongue, salivary glands, tonsils, middle ear, and thyroid, are the surfaces of body cavities or hollow organs in the upper digestive and upper respiratory systems. For most sites, therefore, the numerically lower codes refer to levels or layers of the organ, while higher codes refer to adjacent structures. For inaccessible sites, such as hypopharynx, subglottic larynx, nasal cavity, and middle ear, the numerically lower codes may refer to structures within the organ while higher codes refer to structure beyond the organ of origin.

For head and neck sites, CS Extension generally follows the following pattern:

000	In situ
100–290	Lamina propria/submucosa or structures within the organ (T1-T2)
300	Localized, NOS
400–590	Adjacent structures (T3, site specific)
600–690	Mixed T3-T4 (site specific)
700–850	Adjacent structures (T4a—moderately advanced; T4b—very advanced)
950	No evidence of primary tumor (T0)

The localized, NOS category is always included in CS Extension for those cases where the information about the tumor is not specific but the tumor is known to be confined to the organ of origin. Read the descriptions of the various codes carefully. Keep in mind that, for some sites, there are numerically higher combination codes that may apply to the case. Continue reading down the list of descriptions until you are assured that the tumor has not directly extended that far. What you are trying to do is document the structure or organ that is farthest away from the primary site and is involved by direct extension of tumor.

- In situ extension of a tumor onto an adjacent site or structure is not sufficient involvement to assign a higher CS Extension code. In other words, if spread to an adjacent site or structure is superficial or limited to the mucosa, do not assign a code in the T4a–T4b equivalent range —use a lower extension code. T category mapping is based on the size of the primary tumor.

Figure 10. Examples of CS Extension Codes for Head and Neck Primary Sites

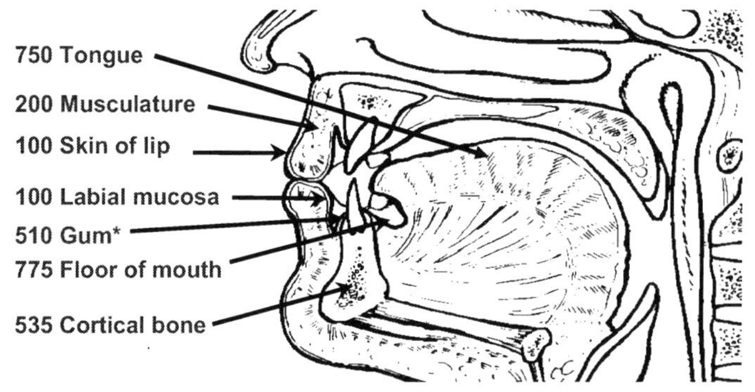

Figure 10A. Lip (upper, lower, other)
For codes 100–515, tumor size takes priority.

* Lower gum from lower lip; lower gum from upper lip is 780

Figure 10B. Base of Tongue and Lingual Tonsil
For codes 100–645, tumor size takes priority.

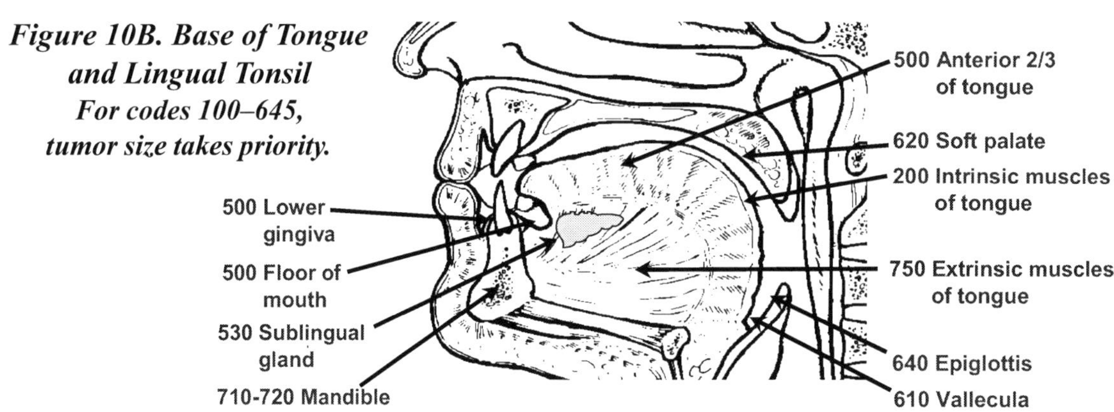

Figure 10C. Mobile Tongue (Anterior 2/3) and Tongue, NOS
For codes 100–545, tumor size takes priority.

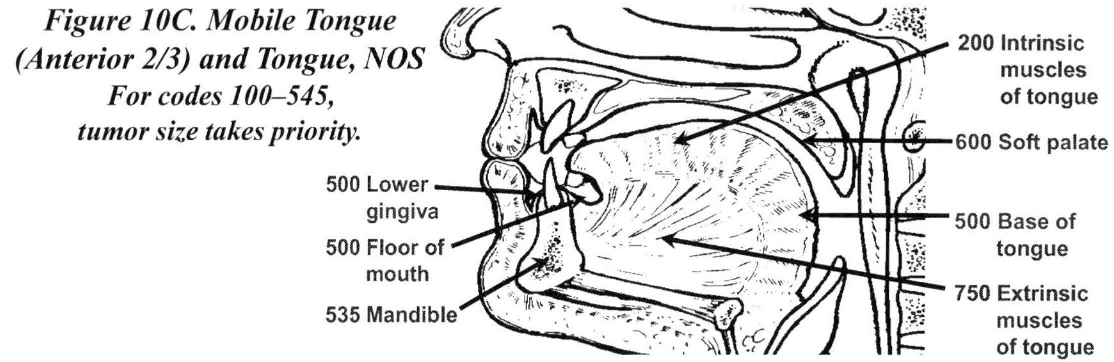

Figure 10D. Gum/Gingiva (upper, lower, other) and Retromolar Trigone
For codes 100–650, tumor size takes priority.

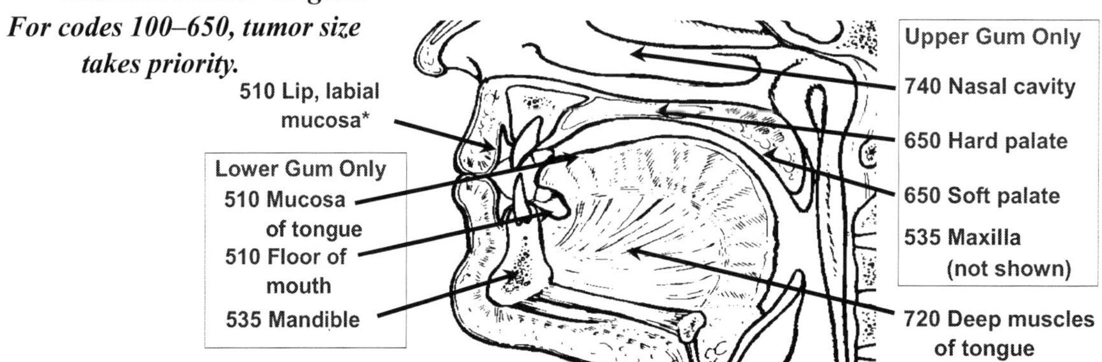

Not shown: 100 Mucoperiosteum (stroma)

* Upper lip from upper gum; lower lip from upper gum is 780

Figure 10, continued. Examples of CS Extension Codes for Head and Neck Primary Sites

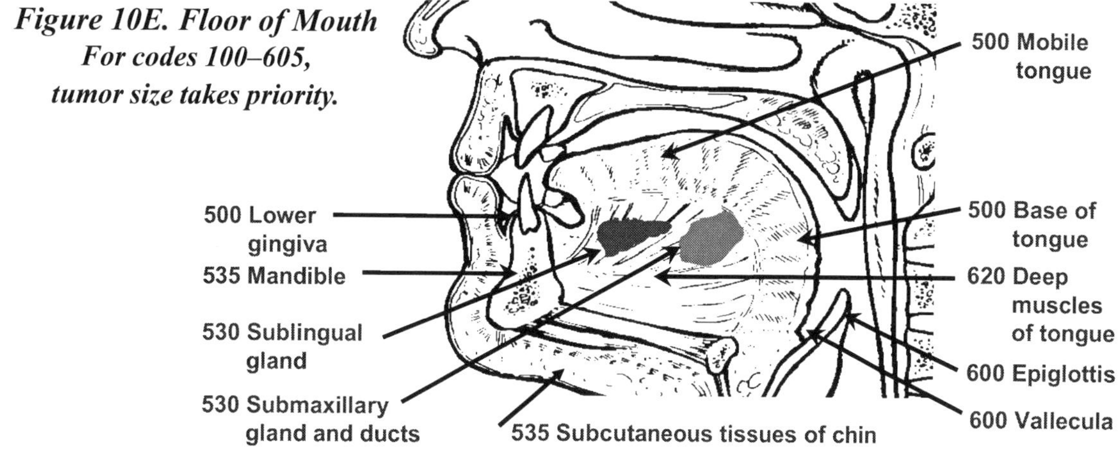

Figure 10E. Floor of Mouth
For codes 100–605, tumor size takes priority.

Figure 10F. Hard Palate, Soft Palate and Uvula
For codes 100–535 in Hard Palate, tumor size takes priority.
For codes 100–640 in Soft Palate and Uvula, tumor size takes priority.

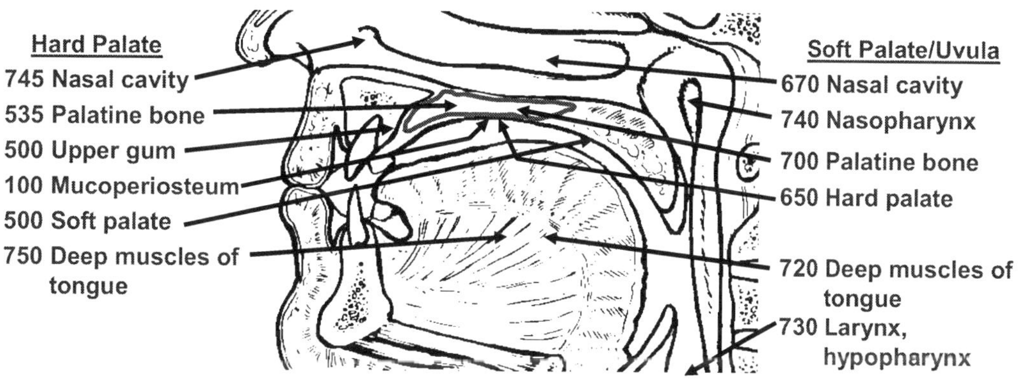

Figure 10G. Major Salivary Glands
For codes 100–350, tumor size takes priority.

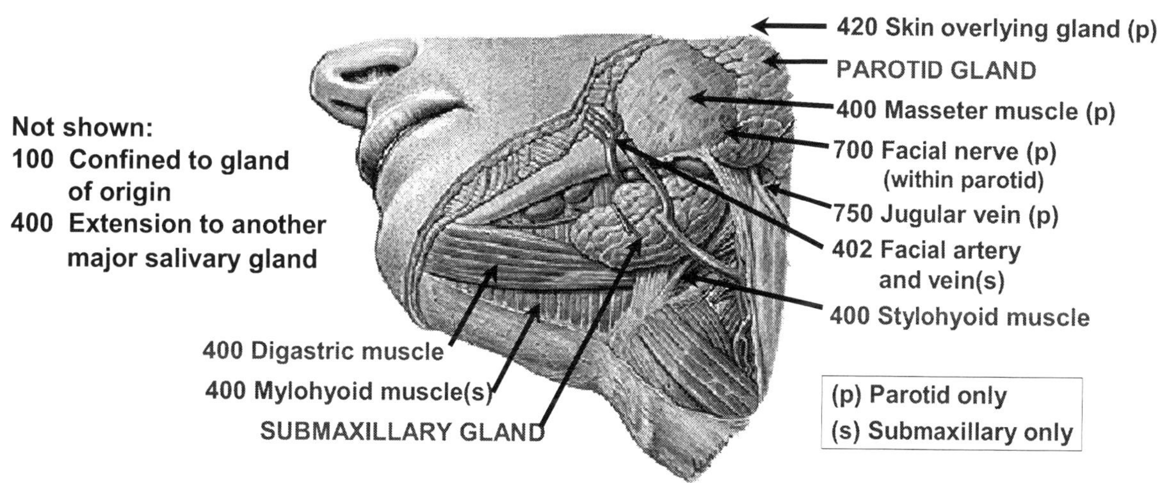

Figure 10, continued. Examples of CS Extension Codes for Head and Neck Primary Sites

Figure 10H. Oropharynx and Palatine Tonsil

For codes 100–540, tumor size takes priority.

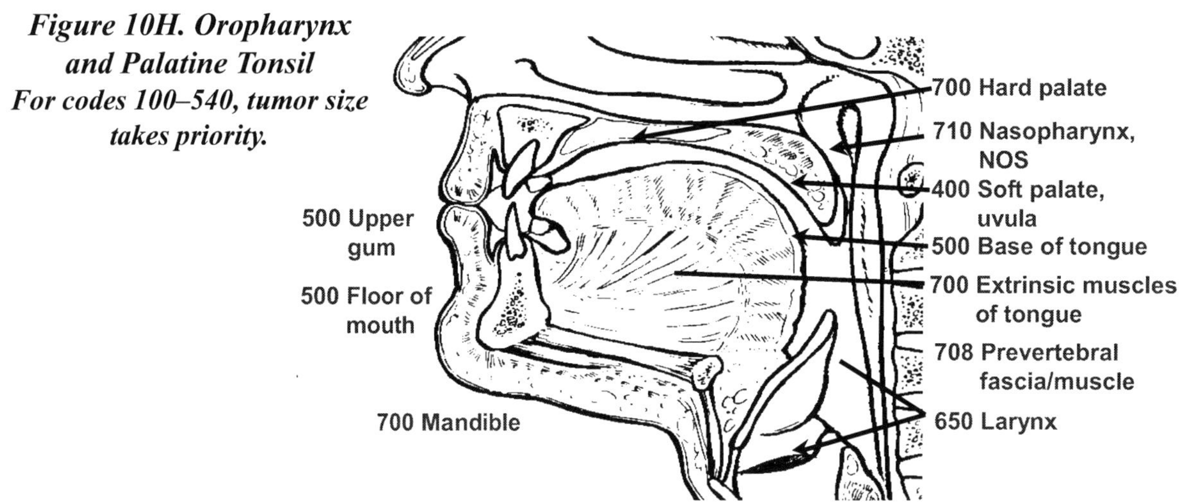

Figure 10I. Nasopharynx

Not shown:
105 Confined to one subsite
205 Involving two or more subsites

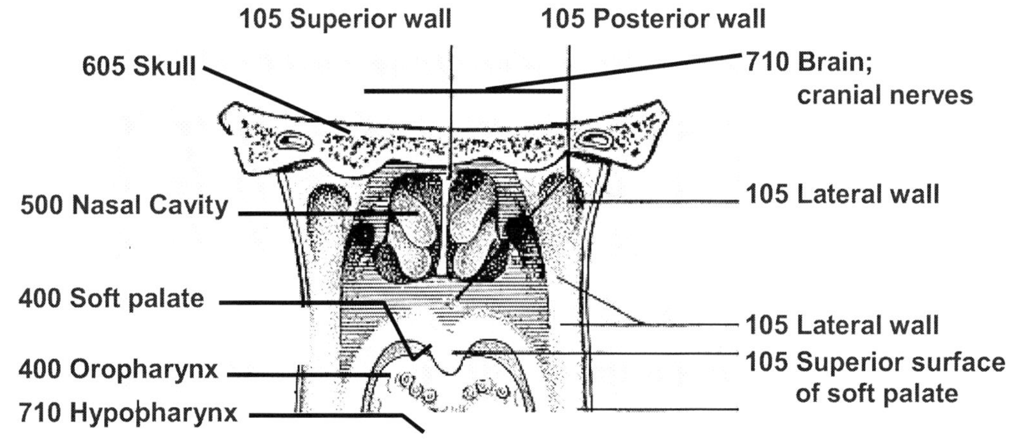

Figure 10J. Hypopharynx and Pyriform Sinus

For codes 100–565, tumor size takes priority.

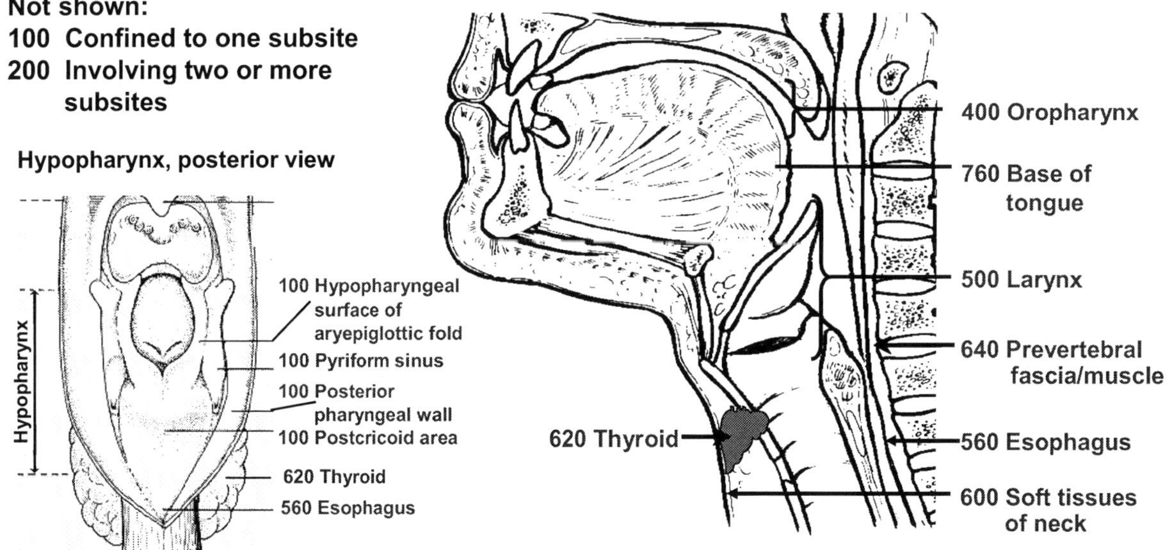

Figure 10, continued. Examples of CS Extension Codes for Head and Neck Primary Sites

Figure 10K. Supraglottic Larynx

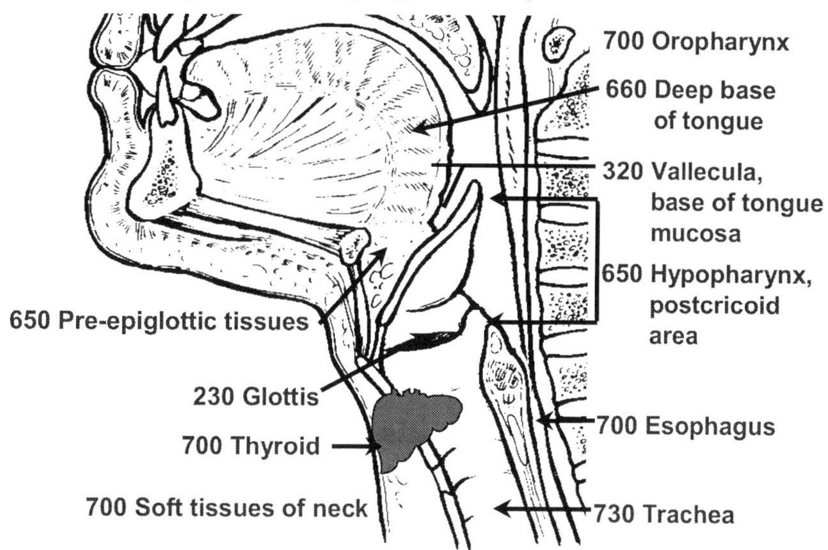

Figure 10L. Laryngoscopic View of Glottic and Supraglottic Larynx

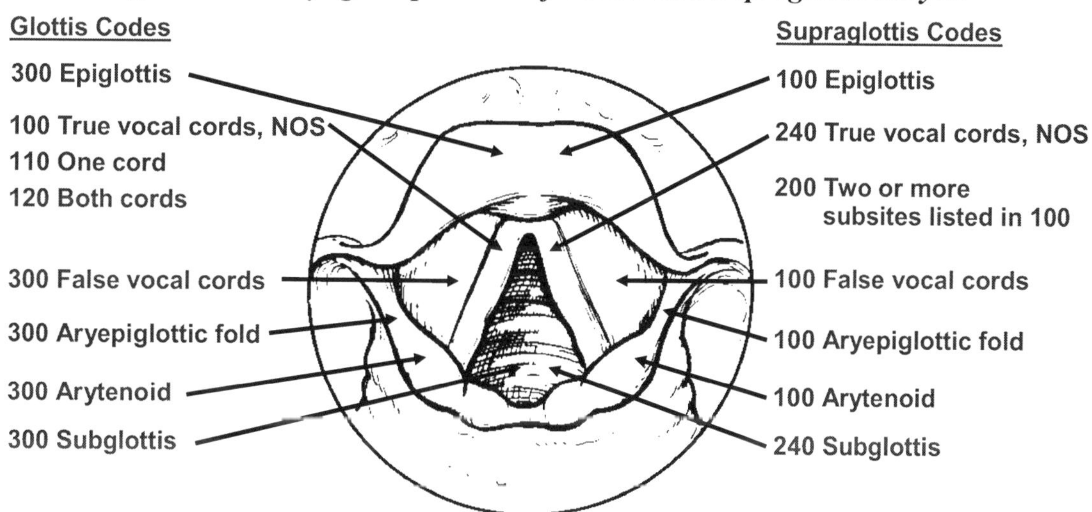

Figure 10M. Glottic and Subglottic Larynx

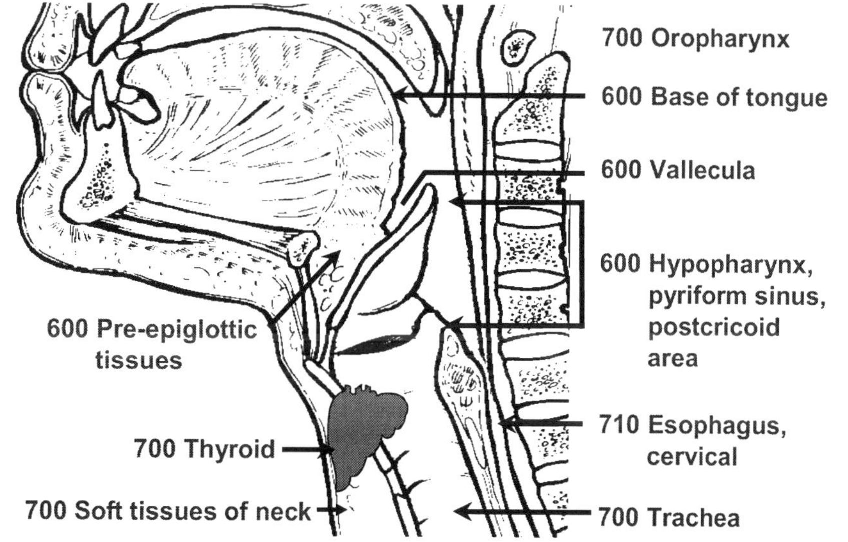

CS Extension, *continued*

- Codes in the T4a–T4b equivalent range (range varies by schema) require deep invasion of adjacent structures. Invasion can be vertical or horizontal, but must involve muscle, bone, or other deep structures in order to be coded in the T4 range.
- The two types of muscles in the tongue have very different sets of codes, which are equivalent to different T values. The muscles of the tongue shape the mouth for speech, chewing and swallowing.
- The intrinsic or lingual muscles have no bony attachment and are the muscles that curl the sides of the tongue upward. When involved, the intrinsic muscles are coded in the 200 range for the sites where they are listed; they are not equivalent to T4 involvement.
- The extrinsic muscles anchor the tongue to the mandible, hyoid bone, styloid process of the temporal bone or the palate. With the exception of floor of mouth and submandibular gland primary sites, extrinsic muscle involvement is coded in the 700-750 range and is equivalent to T4a involvement.
- As with most staging issues, when the record says muscles are involved but does not specify whether they are intrinsic or extrinsic, use the lower or less involved category and code to intrinsic muscles.
- For thyroid, the number of individual tumors or foci is a factor in coding CS Extension.
- Figure 10 shows examples of CS Extension codes for many of the head and neck sites.

CS Mets at DX

- CS Mets at Dx is fairly standard across all head and neck sites.
- Code 10 is involved distant lymph nodes.
- Supraclavicular (transverse cervical) lymph nodes are regional lymph nodes (usually in code 12 in CS Lymph Nodes), rather than distant lymph nodes.
- Code 40 is distant metastasis (a discontinuous tumor trail from the point of origin to the distant site). A few head and neck sites have additional codes in the 40-49 range.
- Code 50 is combined distant lymph nodes and other distant metastases.

CODING LYMPH NODES FOR HEAD AND NECK SITES

Regional lymph node information is coded in CS Lymph Nodes and Site-Specific Factors 1, 3–6, 7, and 8–9. All nine fields must be coded in order that the computer algorithm can correctly output the N value for TNM stage grouping.

- CS Lymph Nodes captures which nodes are involved, how many are involved, and whether they are ipsi- or contralateral.
- Site-specific factors 1 and 8–9 capture the size of the involved lymph nodes and whether there is extracapsular extension.
- Site-specific factors 3 through 6 capture the presence or absence of involvement in seven specific levels of regional nodes (specific, standardized terminology) and other groups of regional nodes defined by the AJCC.
- Site-specific factor 7 documents whether the involved lymph nodes are above or below the cricoid cartilage. Involved nodes below the cricoid cartilage have a worse prognosis.
- Thyroid gland is the exception: CS Lymph Nodes is different and only one site-specific factor is used to describe a solitary or multifocal primary.

CS Lymph Nodes

The code ranges for CS Lymph Nodes vary by primary site, mainly because there are differences in how certain lymph node chains map to Summary Stage 1977 and Summary Stage 2000. Record the highest applicable code for clinical or pathologic involvement, whichever is greater.

- The major categories are:

Codes 100–120	Single, positive ipsilateral node involved
Codes 200–220	Multiple ipsilateral nodes involved
Codes 300–320	Positive regional nodes, NOS (number not stated)
Codes 400–420	Bilateral or contralateral nodes involved
Codes 500–520	Positive nodes, laterality and number not stated

- If laterality is not specified, assume the lymph nodes are ipsilateral (on the same side as the primary tumor). Midline nodes are also defined as ipsilateral.
- There are long lists of specific lymph nodes in codes 100–120. Higher codes refer to those lists but do not repeat them. For example, code 300 refers to the lymph nodes listed in code 100. Use code 300 when you know that more than one of the nodes listed in code 100, say Level II or upper jugular nodes, is involved but you do not know how many nodes are positive.

Note: Remember that the higher codes exist—many registrars are unintentionally tripped up when they find the involved lymph nodes listed in codes 100–120 that they forget to include the information about laterality and number involved described in the higher codes.

- In the 200–520 range, use the highest code that applies. For example, if multiple nodes are involved, including two listed in code 100 and a single node listed in code 120, assign code 220. In other words, think of codes 210–220, 310–320, 410–420, and 510–520 as saying "multiple nodes *any of which is* listed in code 110 or 120, respectively." Use the higher code even if just a single involved node is in the higher category.
- The terms *fixed* and *matted* are to be interpreted as clinically involved lymph nodes. Terms such as *lymphadenopathy*, *enlarged*, and *palpable*, are not considered involvement, unless accompanied by a more definite statement of involvement by the clinician.
- In addition to the specifics of location, number and laterality, codes referring to clinician descriptions based on the N category have been included for those situations where the specific information is missing from the medical record but the clinician or staging form has included a reference to the N category.

Code 180	Stated as N1, no other information
Code 190	Stated as N2a, no other information
Code 290	Stated as N2b, no other information
Code 490	Stated as N2c, no other information
Code 600	Stated as N2, no other information
Code 700	Stated as N3, no other information

- A note explains that "Supraclavicular" is a nonspecific description of lymph nodes that can be coded to either Level IV (deep to the sternocleidomastoid muscle or in the lower jugular chain) or Level V (in the posterior triangle, inferior to the transverse cervical artery). Try to determine whether the reference to supraclavicular refers to Level IV or Level V nodes and code appropriately. If all the information you have is "supraclavicular," code to Level V. Nasopharynx and Thyroid are the only exceptions to this new note. As a clarification, "Supraclavicular, NOS" has been added to Code 120 in all schemas except Nasopharynx and Thyroid, where it is covered in other codes.

Figure 11. Lymph Node Levels and Lymph Node Chains

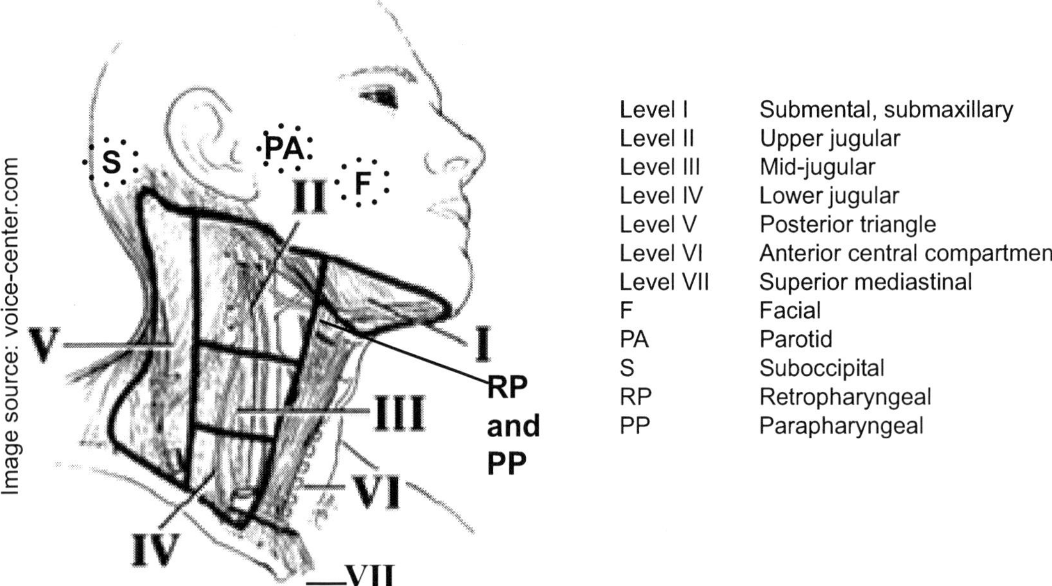

HEAD AND NECK SITE-SPECIFIC FACTORS 1 – 11

Note: Part I Section 2 of the CS Coding Manual Version 02.03 includes extensive discussion of the site-specific factors for every schema. Rather than rewrite those coding instructions for inclusion in this CASEbook chapter, refer to Part I Section 2 if questions arise. The discussion that follows provides more rationale for why those site-specific factors were included in the head and neck schemas. Except as noted below, all head and neck schemas use the same site-specific factors.

SSF1—Size of Lymph Nodes

- Code only from involved regional lymph nodes, not distant lymph nodes.
- Code the size of the largest involved lymph node. This is the size of the entire node, not just the size of the metastasis. The extent of the perinodal or extracapsular extension (see Site-Specific Factor 2 below) should be considered when the size of the lymph node or lymph node mass is measured.
- The code structure is almost the same as for CS Tumor Size. There are two additional codes—996 for size less than 6 cm and 997 for size more than 6 cm.

SSF2—Extracapsular Extension

- Site-specific factor 2 was made obsolete in CS version 2 and was split into SSFs 8 and 9 because clinical information about extracapsular extension had to be distinguished from pathologic information for correct mapping of the N category in TNM seventh edition.

SSFs 3 through 6

SSFs 3–6 can be discussed as a group, because they refer to the various "levels" of lymph nodes as defined by head and neck specialists, surgeons and pathologists. Review the discussion of head and neck lymph node levels in Part I Section 2 of the CS Coding Instructions; it will make more sense now.

- The lymph node levels relate to various planes and anatomical compartments in the neck where lymph nodes are clustered. The concept of describing lymph node levels is relatively new in the registry community (with the sixth edition of TNM), but head and neck surgeons

Site-Specific Factors, *continued*

and pathologists have been using them for years. Figure 11 is an illustration of which nodes are at what level. This list is also included in the CS Coding Instructions and on pages 23–25 in the TNM manual seventh edition. The seventh edition illustration also shows how levels I, II and V have been subclassified.

- To make these four site-specific factors easier to understand, treat each of them as three separate fields. Each of the levels noted in the illustration above has its own location in the matrix, as follows:

Site-Specific Factor 3	(Levels I, II, III)	I	II	III
Site-Specific Factor 4	(Levels IV, V, retropharyngeal nodes)	IV	V	RP
Site-Specific Factor 5	(Levels VI, VII, facial nodes)	VI	VII	F
Site-Specific Factor 6	(ParaPharyngeal, PArotid, Suboccipital)	PP	PA	S

- Note that the retropharyngeal (RP) and parapharyngeal (PP) lymph nodes are not part of Level III, but are behind the larynx and pharynx or lateral to the pharynx deep in the neck.
- Coding for each of these "sub-fields" is simply yes–involved (1) or not involved (0), not how many lymph nodes are involved at each level.

Example: A patient with positive (involved) Level I, Level VI and retropharyngeal nodes would be coded as follows:

SSF 3	1	0	0
SSF 4	0	0	1
SSF 5	1	0	0
SSF 6	0	0	0

This may seem overwhelming at first, but if you break the lymph nodes down to their individual digits, it makes more sense.

SSF7—Upper and Lower Cervical Node Levels

- As mentioned previously, lymph node involvement below the level of the cricoid cartilage has a worse prognosis that lymph node involvement above the level of the cricoid cartilage. The cricoid cartilage is at approximately the level of the lower edge of the thyroid gland. Most regional lymph nodes for head and neck primaries are above this level. Those that are not include supraclavicular, scalene, Level IV (lower deep cervical), Level VB (lower posterior triangle), and Level VII (superior mediastinal—thyroid only).
- The table notes indicate whether the various lymph node levels are above or below the cricoid cartilage. In addition, there is a long table of head and neck lymph nodes in Part I Section 2 of the CS Coding Instructions. Refer to this table if you are unsure whether the involved lymph nodes are upper cervical (code 010), lower cervical (code 020), or both above and below the cricoid cartilage (code 030).
- Use code 000 when no lymph nodes are involved clinically or pathologically. Use code 040 when the level of the involved lymph nodes cannot be determined or when the involved lymph nodes are described as "mid neck."

Site-Specific Factors, *continued*

SSF8— Extracapsular Extension—Clinical
SSF9—Extracapsular Extension—Pathologic

- These two site-specific factors collect clinical (SSF8) and pathologic (SSF9) information about extracapsular extension of regional lymph nodes. Extracapsular extension is tumor that has broken through the capsule of a lymph node and has extended into the soft tissues around the node or into an adjacent node. This is a sign of aggressive tumor and indicates a poor prognosis. Extracapsular extension is also called ECS (extracapsular spread).
- In either field, use code 000 for when no lymph nodes are involved and code 010 when lymph nodes are involved but there is no extracapsular extension.
- A description of "fixed" or matted lymph nodes is evidence of clinical extracapsular extension and is coded in site-specific factor 8. Extracapsular extension may be seen on imaging studies but may not be palpable. The imaging report may use such phrases as amorphous spiculated margins on lymph nodes, involvement of internodal fat, or loss of the normal round or oval shape of the node(s). Code 020 is used for lymph node involvement described clinically (such as matted or fixed) but without microscopic examination. Use code 030 if lymph nodes are involved clinically but whether there is extracapsular extension is unknown.
- Lymph nodes that have been removed and found to have extracapsular extension pathologically are coded as 020 (microscopic) or 030 (macroscopic) in site-specific factor 9.
- If lymph nodes are involved and extracapsular extension is not mentioned in either the clinical assessment or the pathology report, code as 999, not documented. Do not assume there is no extracapsular extension if it is not mentioned.

SSF10—Human Papilloma Virus (HPV) Status

- HPV has a role in the pathogenesis of head and neck and some other squamous cell cancers. Interestingly, patients with HPV infection may have a better prognosis that patient who are not infected. This site-specific factor codes the results of HPV testing for various high-risk and low-risk strains, in particular strains 16 and 18 that are also associated with cervical cancer.
- Read the codes and definitions carefully—there are many to choose from. Code information from pathologic specimens, not blood or serum tests. If no pathology specimen was available, use code 998. If no information about HPV testing is available at all, use code 999.

SSF11—Measured Thickness (Depth)

- This site-specific factor is not used for carcinomas of the pharynx or larynx, nor for salivary gland tumors. Thickness or depth of tumor is coded from a pathology report in tenths of millimeters. It is usually the third measurement of a specimen. For example, on a specimen measuring 1.3 cm x 0.8 cm x 0.3 cm, code 003 in this field.
- If there is no surgical specimen, or if there was neoadjuvant treatment, use code 998. If the tumor thickness is not stated, use code 999.

Thyroid SSF1—Solitary vs Multifocal Tumor

- The thyroid schema uses only one site-specific factor to identify whether the tumor is single (code 010) or multiple (code 020). This provides supplemental information for the seventh edition of TNM, allowing researchers to identify the T categories as solitary (s) or multifocal (m), such as T2(s).

OTHER STAGING SYSTEMS

AJCC TNM STAGING

Consult the ***AJCC Cancer Staging Manual, seventh edition*** for detailed descriptions of the components and other staging guidelines. For "accessible" sites, T1 through T3 are based on the size of the primary tumor. For "inaccessible" sites, T1 through T3 describe increasing involvement of adjacent structures and tissues and/or symptoms such as hoarseness. T4 for head and neck sites is subdivided into T4a moderately advanced local disease and T4b very advanced local disease. Wherever possible, stage head and neck cancers both clinically and pathologically.

All head and neck sites with the exception of thyroid use the same classification system for regional lymph nodes.

N1	Metastasis in a single ipsilateral lymph node 3 cm or less in greatest dimension	
N2	N2a	Metastasis in a single ipsilateral lymph node more than 3 cm but not more than 6 cm in greatest dimension
	N2b	Metastases in multiple ipsilateral lymph nodes, none more than 6 cm in greatest dimension
	N2c	Metastases in bilateral or contralateral lymph nodes, none more than 6 cm in greatest dimension
N3	Metastases in a lymph node more than 6 cm in greatest dimension	

TNM STAGING GUIDELINES

- The size of the primary tumor must be recorded in order to determine the T (tumor) classification mapping in the TNM staging system for
  - Oral cavity sites (lip, buccal mucosa, alveolar ridge(s), retromolar trigone, floor of mouth, hard palate, and oral tongue)
  - Oropharynx sites (anterior wall of oropharynx, vallecula, base of tongue, tonsil, tonsillar fossa, faucial pillars, posterior wall of oropharynx, soft palate, and uvula)
  - Hypopharynx sites (hypopharynx, pharyngo-esophageal junction (postcricoid area), pyriform sinus, and posterior pharyngeal wall)
  - Major salivary glands
  - Thyroid
- In situ extension of the tumor into an adjacent site or structure is not sufficient involvement to assign a higher T category. In other words, if spread to an adjacent site or structure is superficial or limited to the mucosa, do not classify the tumor in the T3-T4 range.
- T4 requires deep invasion of adjacent structures. Invasion can be vertical or horizontal, but must involve muscle, bone, or other deep structures in order to be coded as T4.
- Assign the T classification based on the structures involved, not a statement by the physician that the tumor is "unresectable." AT3 or T4a lesion may prove to be technically unresectable, and a T4b lesion may prove to be resectable after neoadjuvant treatment.
- The two types of tongue muscles have different sets of codes that are equivalent to different T values. The muscles of the tongue shape the mouth for speech, chewing and swallowing.
- The intrinsic or lingual muscles have no bony attachment and are the muscles that curl the sides of the tongue upward. When involved, the intrinsic muscles are classified according to where they are listed in the TNM staging chapter; however, they are not equivalent to T4 involvement.

TNM Guidelines, *continued*

- The extrinsic muscles anchor the tongue to the mandible, hyoid bone, styloid process of the temporal bone or the palate. With the exception of floor of mouth and submandibular gland primary sites, extrinsic muscle involvement is classified as T4 involvement.
- As with most staging issues, when the record says muscles are involved but does not specify whether they are intrinsic or extrinsic, use the lower or less involved category and code to intrinsic muscles.
- All primary sites of the nasopharynx are coded to C11 in ICD-O-3. All primary sites of the hypopharynx are coded to either C12 or C13. For purposes of TNM staging, the oropharynx includes sites in C09 and C10, as well as the inferior surface of the soft palate (C05.1), base of tongue (C01.9) and uvula (C05.2). The lingual tonsil is also considered part of the oropharynx in the seventh edition of the *AJCC Cancer Staging Manual.*
- Various research and reporting agencies group anatomic subsites of the head and neck in different ways for coding and staging purposes. The following variances are noted:
    - AJCC/TNM includes inferior surface of the soft palate (C05.1), base of tongue (C01.9) and uvula (C05.2) with oropharynx (C10._) for staging purposes.
    - AJCC/TNM includes lingual (anterior) surface of epiglottis (C10.1) with larynx (C32._).
    - Soft palate excludes the nasopharyngeal (superior surface) of soft palate (C11.3).
    - The retromolar area (C06.2) is included with gum (C03._).
    - ICD-O code C06._ for buccal mucosa includes the membrane lining of the cheeks but not of the lips. AJCC/TNM includes labial mucosa with buccal mucosa.
- For thyroid, the number of individual tumors or foci is a factor in assigning the T category.
- Fixation of the larynx (supraglottic T3, glottic T3, subglottic T3) or hemilarynx (hypopharynx T3) is defined as immobility of the arytenoid noted on endoscopy. Other terms for fixation of the hemilarynx are direct extension of tumor from the hypopharynx into the larynx, paralysis of the vocal cord, and deviation of the larynx to the affected (fixed) side. Diagnostic manipulations that do not indicate fixation of the larynx are normal larynx mobility on laryngoscopy and normal phonation.
    - Fixation of the larynx can be determined by laryngoscopy. Any case with fixation of the hemilarynx is at least T3 regardless of the size of tumor or the number of hypopharynx subsites involved.
- Impaired cord mobility (glottic T2, subglottic T2) may be described as impairment of vocal cord motion, or vocal cord paresis. Pathologically, impaired vocal cord mobility is defined as tumor invasion more than 5 mm into the cord.
- According to the *TNM Supplement, third edition,* a lesion involving more than one anatomical site in the head and neck or in the pharynx is classified according to the TNM scheme for the site in which the majority of the tumor is situated. For example, a tumor that is two-thirds in the base of tongue and one-third in the hypopharynx or mobile tongue would be classified as a base of tongue primary and oropharynx definitions of T would apply.
- The classification of a tumor in the oropharynx extending to the oral cavity, nasopharynx or hypopharynx is based on the clinical size of the tumor only, unless there is deep extension to muscle or bone in addition to the mucosal involvement.
- Parapharyngeal extension is tumor infiltration beyond the pharyngobasilar fascia posterior and lateral to the nasopharynx. The pharyngobasilar fascia is the uppermost part of the pharyngeal wall (above the pharyngeal muscles) that attaches the pharynx to the base of skull.
- The deep muscles of the tongue (oropharynx T4) are the *extrinsic* muscles that move the tongue: the hyoglossus, styloglossus, genioglossus and palatoglossus muscles. Involvement of the *intrinsic* muscles of the tongue (the longitudinalis superior and inferior, transversus linguae and verticalis linguae) is not a criterion for T4 of the oropharynx.

BRIEF SUMMARIES OF 7th EDITION T CATEGORIES

For most sites, T4a = moderately advanced and T4b = very advanced tumor extension

LIP AND ORAL CAVITY (C00, C02-C06)

T1 ≤ 2 cm
T2 > 2 to 4 cm
T3 > 4 cm
T4a, b Invades adjacent structures

PHARYNX (C01, C05.1, C09, C10.0, C10.2, C10.3, C11-C13)

Oropharynx

T1 ≤ 2 cm
T2 > 2 to 4 cm
T3 > 4 cm
T4a, b Invades adjacent structures

Hypopharynx

T1 ≤ 2 cm and limited to one subsite
T2 > 2 to 4 cm or more than one subsite
T3 > 4 cm or with hemilarynx fixation
T4a, b Invades adjacent structures

Nasopharynx

T1 Nasopharynx, oropharynx, or nasal cavity
T2 Parapharyngeal extension
T3 Invades bony structures and/or paranasal sinuses
T4 Intracranial extension, cranial nerves, orbit, hypopharynx, infratemporal fossa, hypopharynx, orbit, masticator space

SALIVARY GLANDS (C07, C08)

T1 ≤ 2 cm without extraparenchymal extension
T2 > 2 to 4 cm, without extraparenchymal extension
T3 Extraparenchymal extension, and/or > 4 cm
T4a, b Further adjacent extension

THYROID GLAND (C73)

Papillary, follicular and medullary carcinoma

T1 ≤ 2 cm, intrathyroidal
T2 > 2 to 4 cm, intrathyroidal
T3 > 4 cm, minimal extrathyroidal extension
T4a, b Extends beyond gland

Anaplastic/undifferentiated carcinoma

T4a Tumor limited to thyroid
T4b Tumor beyond thyroid capsule

LARYNX (C32.0, C32.1, C32.2, C10.1)

Supraglottis

T1 One subsite, normal mobility
T2 Involving mucosa of > one adjacent subsite of supraglottis or glottis or adjacent region outside the supraglottis; no fixation
T3 Vocal cord fixation or invades postcricoid area, pre-epiglottic tissues, paraglottic space, thyroid cartilage erosion
T4a, b Extends beyond larynx

Glottis

T1 Limited to vocal cord(s), normal mobility
T2 Supraglottis, subglottis, impaired cord mobility
T3 Cord fixation, paraglottic space, thyroid cartilage erosion
T4a, b Extends beyond larynx

Subglottis

T1 Limited to subglottis
T2 Extends to vocal cord(s) with normal/ impaired mobility
T3 Cord fixation
T4a, b Extends beyond larynx

NASAL CAVITY AND PARANASAL SINUSES (C30.0, C31.0, C31.1)

Maxillary Sinus

T1 Antral mucosa
T2 Bone erosion/destruction, hard palate, middle nasal meatus
T3 Posterior wall maxillary sinus, subcutaneous tissues, floor/medial wall of orbit, pterygoid fossa, ethmoid sinus(es)
T4a, b Further adjacent extension

Nasal Cavity and Ethmoid Sinus

T1 One subsite
T2 Two subsites or adjacent nasoethmoidal site
T3 Medial wall/floor orbit, maxillary sinus, palate, cribriform plate
T4a, b Further adjacent extension

TNM Guidelines, *continued*

- In the oropharynx and hypopharynx, the difference between T1–3 and T4 is a distinction between mucosal and deep extension of the tumor into adjacent structure(s). Mucosal extension is defined as superficial involvement of the contiguous structure's mucosa and is classified T1, T2, or T3 by the size of the tumor for oropharynx and by the size of tumor and number of subsites involved for hypopharynx.
  - An example would be a 3.5 cm hypopharyngeal tumor extending onto the mucosal surface of the base of tongue (T2) or the same tumor involving the surface of the posterior tongue and the styloglossus muscle of the tongue (T4).
- T4 extension to adjacent structures is defined as direct vertical tumor extension through the cartilage or bone surrounding the pharynx and into other organs outside the pharynx, such as the esophagus, thyroid or larynx or cranial nerves. Deep extension may also be defined as involvement of a contiguous structure extending deeper than the mucosa in that structure.
  - An example of this type of extension would be a hypopharyngeal tumor extending submucosally into the esophagus and involving the muscularis of the esophagus.
- In the supraglottis, the difference between a T2 and T4 is a distinction between superficial and deep extension of the tumor into adjacent structure(s). Superficial extension is defined as involvement only of the contiguous structure's mucosa and is classified as T2. Deep extension (T4) is defined as direct vertical tumor extension through the cartilage surrounding the larynx and into muscle, bone or other organs outside the larynx, such as the esophagus, trachea or pharynx. Deep extension may also be defined as involvement of a contiguous structure extending deeper than the mucosa in that structure. An example of this type of deep extension would be a supraglottic tumor extending into the base of tongue (oropharynx) and involving both the mucosa and the deep muscles of the tongue.
- In the supraglottis, the epiglottis is considered two subsites for the purpose of assigning the T category. The suprahyoid epiglottis is that part with the freely movable edge above the level of the hyoid bone (visible on imaging), and the infrahyoid epiglottis is that part below the level of the hyoid bone (less movable). A tumor covering both the suprahyoid and infrahyoid portions of the epiglottis would be at least T2 in the supraglottic T category.

SUMMARY STAGE

There are 23 individual summary staging schemas in the *SEER Summary Staging Manual 2000*—too many to discuss in detail in this chapter. Most of the staging concepts for these primary sites have been carried forward into the Collaborative Staging System and have been discussed elsewhere in this chapter. If you are unfamiliar with summary staging, take a few moments to review the contents of the manual and note the following points:

- The SEER Summary staging system for head and neck cancers is classified according to the primary site. That's why it is so important for a cancer registrar to accurately identify the tumor's site of origin in order to identify the appropriate staging scheme for that site.
- The boundaries of the individual organs in the oral cavity, pharynx and major salivary glands are defined on pages 16–19 in the *Summary Staging Manual 2000*. Anatomical boundaries of the subsites of the larynx are defined on page 131.
- Many anatomical illustrations are included in the Summary Staging Manual 2000, although some are several pages away from the staging schemas. You can find the illustrations on pages 22–24, 46–47, 52–53, 119, 123, and 130.
- Page 20 is a table of the anatomic structures of the lip, oral cavity, and oropharynx showing which organs have a mucosa, submucosa, and muscularis propria. None of these sites has a serosal surface.

Summary Stage, *continued*

- Page 21 discusses how to distinguish in situ and localized stages when the tumor is described as "confined to mucosa." This information is not included in either the TNM manual or Collaborative Staging.
- For most sites within the oral cavity and pharynx, Localized stage lists terms like mucosa, muscularis, lamina propria, and so forth, indicating that information about the depth of invasion into the organ is necessary for staging. Regional stage usually refers to other adjacent organs.
- For sites within the nasal cavity, sinuses and larynx, Localized stage lists individual structures within these sites. Regional stage usually refers to adjacent organs and their structures.

EPIDEMIOLOGY AND ETIOLOGY

- Oral cavity cancer is the eleventh most common cancer worldwide
  - Two-thirds of new cases occur in the less developed world
  - One-third of all cases occur in the Indian subcontinent
  - Highest rates in areas where betel quid is chewed—south and southeast Asia, Taiwan, China
  - Associated with low socioeconomic status
- Highest rates of laryngeal cancer are in south central Asia and southern and eastern Europe
- Highest rates of nasopharyngeal cancer are in China, where the incidence rate in the Cantonese population is 40 times that of white males in the United States.

General Head and Neck Risk Factors

- More common in men than women
- More common in blacks than whites
- Age (90% over age 45)
- Tobacco (smoking, chewing, dipping snuff)—primary risk factor
- Alcohol (ethanol)
- Alcohol and tobacco together are much worse than either one individually
- Asbestos, nickel, and polyvinyl chloride exposure
- Mustard gas exposure
- Bartenders, waitresses and waiters, leather workers, paper manufacturers, electronics workers, farmers, outdoor workers
- Poor oral hygiene (ill-fitting bridgework, broken teeth, sharp or jagged teeth irritating mucosa)
- In the less developed world, chewing betel nut products for its many properties: stimulant, antiseptic, breath-freshener, aphrodisiac. It is said to cure headaches, arthritis and joint pain, toothache, indigestion, constipation, decongestant, and aid lactation. Betel nuts and leaves are also extremely carcinogenic.

Lip Risk Factors

- Sun exposure
- Chronic irritation
- Direct contact with tobacco

Epidemiology and Etiology, *continued*

Nasopharynx Risk Factors

- Chinese/Asian ancestry
- Epstein-Barr virus exposure
- Familial clusters

Salivary Glands Risk Factors

- Prior radiation to the head and neck

Thyroid Gland Risk Factors

- More common in women than men
- Most common between ages 25 and 65
- Prior radiation to head and neck in infancy or childhood
- Familial association for medullary carcinoma

Related Conditions

Plummer-Vinson syndrome —(achlorhydria, sideropenic anemia, atrophy of the mucous membranes of the mouth, pharynx, and esophagus)—associated with oral cavity and hypopharynx cancers

Multiple endocrine neoplasia (MEN) syndrome—multiple benign or malignant tumors of endocrine organs, pheochromocytoma of adrenal gland, secretion of calcitonin—associated with familial medullary carcinoma of the thyroid

Abstracting, Staging, and Coding Exercises

This section includes eighteen single-page head and neck cancer cases to be coded in ICD-O-3, Summary Stage 2000, TNM seventh edition (clinical and pathologic), and CS version 0203.

NOTE: For the purposes of these brief cases, assume that all other tests not mentioned in the case are negative for malignancy.

- Identify the primary site and schema.
- Assign the codes for primary site, histology, behavior, and grade.
- Assign codes to all applicable CS fields.
- Assume that your facility does offer a test and that the standards setters for your facility require the data field. In other words, avoid using code 988 (not applicable).
- 20XX is the diagnosis year, and where applicable, 20YY is the following year
- Identify the TNM region (oral cavity, pharynx, supraglottis, etc.) for the schema used for the case.
- Assign the clinical and pathologic T, N, M, and Stage Group.
- Cases 1-5 are lip and oral cavity
- Cases 6-10 are pharynx
- Cases 11-15 are larynx
- Cases 16-18 are other head and neck sites

CASE 1

HISTORY AND PHYSICAL EXAM

4-16-20XX Tobacco chewer for 50 years. Large (3.5 cm) fungating tumor of right floor of mouth involving retromolar trigone and lower alveolar ridge. No palpable nodes or masses.

X-RAYS AND SCANS

4-17-20XX CXR: Negative

LABORATORY REPORTS Not significant.

ENDOSCOPIC PROCEDURES

4-21-20XX Triple Endoscopy: No additional lesions visualized in pharynx, larynx, esophagus or bronchi.

PRE-OPERATIVE TREATMENT

5-6-20XX to 6-20-20XX 5400 centiGray to right retromolar trigone and lower alveolar ridge

OPERATIVE REPORTS

7-10-20XX Extensive leukoplakia, healing ulcer right floor of mouth.

PATHOLOGY REPORTS

7-10-20XX Resection of tongue, mandible and floor of mouth, right radical neck dissection: Residual 2.8 cm moderately differentiated squamous cell carcinoma, right floor of mouth. No metastases to 35 lymph nodes in levels I through IV. Mandible and submandibular gland: radiation reaction, no tumor.

Site Code ___ ___ ___.___	cT ___ cN ___ cM ___	SSF1 Size of LN ___ ___ ___
Histology/Behavior/Grade ___ ___ ___ ___/___ ___	Clin Stage Group _____	SSF2 OBSOLETE 988
Grade Path Value ___	pT ___ pN ___ M ___	SSF3 LN Levels I-III ___ ___ ___
Grade Path System ___	Path Stage Group _____	SSF4 LN Levels IV-V, RP ___ ___ ___
Lymph Vascular Invasion ___	CS Tumor Size ___ ___ ___	SSF5 LN Levels VI-VII, Facial ___ ___ ___
Ambiguous Terminol ___	CS Extension ___ ___ ___	SSF6 LN levels PP, PA, Occ ___ ___ ___
Date Conclusive Terminol ___ ___ ___ ___ ___ ___ ___ ___	CS TS/Ext Eval ___	SSF7 Upper/Lower Cerv LN Levels ___ ___ ___
Date Conclus Dx Flag ___ ___	CS LN ___ ___ ___	SSF8 Extracaps Exten Clinical ___ ___ ___
Multiplicity Counter ___ ___	CS Reg Nodes Eval ___	SSF9 Extracaps Exten Pathologic ___ ___ ___
Date Mult Tumors ___ ___ ___ ___ ___ ___ ___ ___	Reg LN Pos ___ ___	SSF10 HPV Status ___ ___ ___
Date Mult Tumors Flag ___ ___	Reg LN Exam ___ ___	SSF11 Measured Thickness Depth ___ ___ ___
Mult Tum Reported as One Prim ___ ___	CS Mets at Dx ___ ___	
Summary Stage 2000 _____	CS Mets at Dx - Bone ___ Brain ___ Liver ___ Lung ___	
	CS Mets Eval ___	

CASE 2

HISTORY AND PHYSICAL EXAM

11-1-20XX 1.5 cm blister-like lesion on upper right buccal mucosa. Hard bump on cheek, most likely an involved facial node.

X-RAYS AND SCANS

11-3-20XX CXR: Negative

LABORATORY REPORTS None.

ENDOSCOPIC PROCEDURES

11-3-20XX Panendoscopy: Thorough search for additional primaries was negative. No cervical adenopathy.

OPERATIVE REPORTS

11-22-20XX Excision of buccal lesion and buccal lymph node: No additional findings.

PATHOLOGY REPORTS

11-22-20XX Excision of buccal lesion and lymph node: 2.1 cm well differentiated squamous cell carcinoma associated with extensive in situ squamous carcinoma, right buccal mucosa. Tumor infiltrates deeply into buccal musculature. Metastatic squamous carcinoma present in right buccal lymph node showing extracapsular extension. Node size less than 3 cm.

Head-Neck

Site Code ___ ___ ___.___	cT ___ cN ___ cM ___	SSF1 Size of LN ___ ___ ___
Histology/Behavior/Grade ___ ___ ___ ___/___ ___	Clin Stage Group _____	SSF2 OBSOLETE 988
Grade Path Value ___	pT ___ pN ___ M ___	SSF3 LN Levels I-III ___ ___ ___
Grade Path System ___	Path Stage Group _____	SSF4 LN Levels IV-V, RP ___ ___ ___
Lymph Vascular Invasion ___	CS Tumor Size ___ ___ ___	SSF5 LN Levels VI-VII, Facial ___ ___ ___
Ambiguous Terminol ___	CS Extension ___ ___ ___	SSF6 LN levels PP, PA, Occ ___ ___ ___
Date Conclusive Terminol ___ ___ ___ ___ ___ ___ ___ ___	CS TS/Ext Eval ___	SSF7 Upper/Lower Cerv LN Levels ___ ___ ___
Date Conclus Dx Flag ___ ___	CS LN ___ ___ ___	SSF8 Extracaps Exten Clinical ___ ___ ___
Multiplicity Counter ___ ___	CS Reg Nodes Eval ___	SSF9 Extracaps Exten Pathologic ___ ___ ___
Date Mult Tumors ___ ___ ___ ___ ___ ___ ___ ___	Reg LN Pos ___ ___	SSF10 HPV Status ___ ___ ___
Date Mult Tumors Flag ___ ___	Reg LN Exam ___ ___	SSF11 Measured Thickness Depth ___ ___ ___
Mult Tum Reported as One Prim ___ ___	CS Mets at Dx ___ ___	
Summary Stage 2000 ___	CS Mets at Dx - Bone ___ Brain ___ Liver ___ Lung ___	
	CS Mets Eval ___	

CASE 3

HISTORY AND PHYSICAL EXAM

4-3-20XX ENT: 1.5 cm ulcerated lesion, midline, on undersurface of tongue lateral to frenulum. Cordlike submucosal extension to smaller ulcerated lesion in anterolateral floor of mouth opposing tongue lesion when tongue is at rest. Soft right submandibular lymph node palpable.

X-RAYS AND SCANS

4-3-20XX CT chest: Negative for abnormalities.

LABORATORY REPORTS None.

ENDOSCOPIC PROCEDURES

Non-contributory.

OPERATIVE REPORTS

No unusual findings.

PATHOLOGY REPORTS

4-23-20XX Adenoid cystic carcinoma, moderately differentiated, undersurface of lateral tongue and lateral floor of mouth. Metastases to two submandibular lymph nodes.

TREATMENT

4-23-20XX Wide resection, floor of mouth and anterior tongue. Excision, submandibular lymph nodes.
4000 rads to bilateral cervical lymph nodes.

Site Code ___ ___ ___.___
Histology/Behavior/Grade ___ ___ ___ ___ / ___ ___
Grade Path Value ___
Grade Path System ___
Lymph Vascular Invasion ___
Ambiguous Terminol ___
Date Conclusive Terminol ___ ___ ___ ___ ___ ___ ___ ___
Date Conclus Dx Flag ___ ___
Multiplicity Counter ___ ___
Date Mult Tumors ___ ___ ___ ___ ___ ___ ___ ___
Date Mult Tumors Flag ___ ___
Mult Tum Reported as One Prim ___ ___
Summary Stage 2000 ___

cT ___ cN ___ cM ___
Clin Stage Group ___
pT ___ pN ___ M ___
Path Stage Group ___
CS Tumor Size ___ ___ ___
CS Extension ___ ___ ___
CS TS/Ext Eval ___
CS LN ___ ___ ___
CS Reg Nodes Eval ___
Reg LN Pos ___ ___
Reg LN Exam ___ ___
CS Mets at Dx ___ ___
CS Mets at Dx - Bone ___ Brain ___ Liver ___ Lung ___
CS Mets Eval ___

SSF1 Size of LN ___ ___ ___
SSF2 OBSOLETE 988
SSF3 LN Levels I-III ___ ___ ___
SSF4 LN Levels IV-V, RP ___ ___ ___
SSF5 LN Levels VI-VII, Facial ___ ___ ___
SSF6 LN levels PP, PA, Occ ___ ___ ___
SSF7 Upper/Lower Cerv LN Levels ___ ___ ___
SSF8 Extracaps Exten Clinical ___ ___ ___
SSF9 Extracaps Exten Pathologic ___ ___ ___
SSF10 HPV Status ___ ___ ___
SSF11 Measured Thickness Depth ___ ___ ___

CASE 4

HISTORY AND PHYSICAL EXAM

4-8-20XX HEENT: 2 cm ulcerating lesion, buccal mucosa opposite 1st molar which is broken. No nodes palpable.

X-RAYS AND SCANS

All within normal limits.

LABORATORY REPORTS

Not significant.

ENDOSCOPIC PROCEDURES

4-14-20XX Triple endoscopy: Negative except for noted buccal lesion.

OPERATIVE REPORTS

Not reported.

PATHOLOGY REPORTS

4-25-20XX Infiltrating poorly differentiated squamous carcinoma, buccal mucosa, within margins of resection.

TREATMENT

4-25-20XX Excisional biopsy, buccal mucosa.

Site Code ___ ___ ___.___

Histology/Behavior/Grade ___ ___ ___ ___/___ ___

Grade Path Value ___

Grade Path System ___

Lymph Vascular Invasion ___

Ambiguous Terminol ___

Date Conclusive Terminol ___ ___ ___ ___ ___ ___ ___ ___

Date Conclus Dx Flag ___ ___

Multiplicity Counter ___ ___

Date Mult Tumors ___ ___ ___ ___ ___ ___ ___ ___

Date Mult Tumors Flag ___ ___

Mult Tum Reported as One Prim ___ ___

Summary Stage 2000 ___

cT ___ cN ___ cM ___

Clin Stage Group _____

pT ___ pN ___ M ___

Path Stage Group _____

CS Tumor Size ___ ___ ___

CS Extension ___ ___ ___

CS TS/Ext Eval ___

CS LN ___ ___ ___

CS Reg Nodes Eval ___

Reg LN Pos ___ ___

Reg LN Exam ___ ___

CS Mets at Dx ___ ___

CS Mets at Dx - Bone ___ Brain ___ Liver ___ Lung ___

CS Mets Eval ___

SSF1 Size of LN ___ ___ ___

SSF2 OBSOLETE 988

SSF3 LN Levels I-III ___ ___ ___

SSF4 LN Levels IV-V, RP ___ ___ ___

SSF5 LN Levels VI-VII, Facial ___ ___ ___

SSF6 LN levels PP, PA, Occ ___ ___ ___

SSF7 Upper/Lower Cerv LN Levels ___ ___ ___

SSF8 Extracaps Exten Clinical ___ ___ ___

SSF9 Extracaps Exten Pathologic ___ ___ ___

SSF10 HPV Status ___ ___ ___

SSF11 Measured Thickness Depth ___ ___ ___

CASE 5

HISTORY AND PHYSICAL EXAMINATION

57 year old man complaining of a sore throat for 6 months.

9-29-20XX PE: 3 x 2 cm superficial ulcer in the lateral margin, right side of his tongue, just anterior to junction of mobile tongue and base of tongue. It does not extend into the tonsillar sulcus. It does not extend into the base of the tongue.

X-RAYS AND SCANS

10-5-20XX MRI: No gross extension beyond tongue. The MRI visualized levels 1, 2, and 3 lymph nodes with no evidence of nodal metastases.

10-5-20XX CXR: Negative for metastatic disease or abnormal mediastinal lymph nodes.

OPERATIVE REPORTS

10-25-20XX Hemiglossectomy with a right functional neck dissection. Reconstruction with a mini-plate for the osteotomy and radial forearm flap. Right selective neck dissection, levels 2 through 4. Left selective neck dissection, level 1.

PATHOLOGY REPORTS

10-1-20XX Tongue (biopsy): Squamous carcinoma, invasive, moderately well differentiated, incompletely excised.

10-25-20XX Hemiglossectomy: Confirmed invasive squamous cell carcinoma with squamous dysplasia. In fact, there is evidence of tumor invading the muscle in one section. LVI present. Right selective neck dissection: one of eight level 2 nodes positive, with evidence of extracapsular extension. Total size: 2.8 cm. An additional 20 lymph nodes from the right-sided neck dissection were negative, including 0 of 11 level 3 and 0 of 9 level 4. Left level 1 nodes negative (9).

- Site Code ___ ___ ___.___
- Histology/Behavior/Grade ___ ___ ___ ___/___ ___
- Grade Path Value ___
- Grade Path System ___
- Lymph Vascular Invasion ___
- Ambiguous Terminol ___
- Date Conclusive Terminol ___ ___ ___ ___ ___ ___ ___ ___
- Date Conclus Dx Flag ___ ___
- Multiplicity Counter ___ ___
- Date Mult Tumors ___ ___ ___ ___ ___ ___ ___ ___
- Date Mult Tumors Flag ___ ___
- Mult Tum Reported as One Prim ___ ___
- Summary Stage 2000 ___

- cT ___ cN ___ cM ___
- Clin Stage Group ___
- pT ___ pN ___ M ___
- Path Stage Group ___
- CS Tumor Size ___ ___ ___
- CS Extension ___ ___ ___
- CS TS/Ext Eval ___
- CS LN ___ ___ ___
- CS Reg Nodes Eval ___
- Reg LN Pos ___ ___
- Reg LN Exam ___ ___
- CS Mets at Dx ___ ___
- CS Mets at Dx - Bone ___ Brain ___ Liver ___ Lung ___
- CS Mets Eval ___

- SSF1 Size of LN ___ ___ ___
- SSF2 OBSOLETE 988
- SSF3 LN Levels I-III ___ ___ ___
- SSF4 LN Levels IV-V, RP ___ ___ ___
- SSF5 LN Levels VI-VII, Facial ___ ___ ___
- SSF6 LN levels PP, PA, Occ ___ ___ ___
- SSF7 Upper/Lower Cerv LN Levels ___ ___ ___
- SSF8 Extracaps Exten Clinical ___ ___ ___
- SSF9 Extracaps Exten Pathologic ___ ___ ___
- SSF10 HPV Status ___ ___ ___
- SSF11 Measured Thickness Depth ___ ___ ___

CASE 6

HISTORY AND PHYSICAL EXAMINATION

11-9-20XX Patient was noted to have a 1.5 cm lesion on the posterior surface of the root of the tongue. The sublingual area, vallecula, and side walls of the throat were palpated and no nodes were clinically involved. Remainder of physical exam within normal limits.

X-RAYS AND SCANS

11-15-20XX CT scan of the neck showed tumor invasion of the palatoglossus muscle beyond the base of tongue.

OPERATIVE REPORTS

11-22-20XX Wide excision of lesion of the root of tongue.

PATHOLOGY REPORTS

11-22-20XX Pathology positive for squamous cell carcinoma of the root of tongue with invasion of the musculature.

Site Code ___ ___ ___.___	cT ___ cN ___ cM ___	SSF1 Size of LN ___ ___ ___
Histology/Behavior/Grade ___ ___ ___ ___/___ ___	Clin Stage Group _____	SSF2 OBSOLETE 988
Grade Path Value ___	pT ___ pN ___ M ___	SSF3 LN Levels I-III ___ ___ ___
Grade Path System ___	Path Stage Group _____	SSF4 LN Levels IV-V, RP ___ ___ ___
Lymph Vascular Invasion ___	CS Tumor Size ___ ___ ___	SSF5 LN Levels VI-VII, Facial ___ ___ ___
Ambiguous Terminol ___	CS Extension ___ ___ ___	SSF6 LN levels PP, PA, Occ ___ ___ ___
Date Conclusive Terminol ___ ___ ___ ___ ___ ___ ___ ___	CS TS/Ext Eval ___	SSF7 Upper/Lower Cerv LN Levels ___ ___ ___
Date Conclus Dx Flag ___ ___	CS LN ___ ___ ___	SSF8 Extracaps Exten Clinical ___ ___ ___
Multiplicity Counter ___ ___	CS Reg Nodes Eval ___	SSF9 Extracaps Exten Pathologic ___ ___ ___
Date Mult Tumors ___ ___ ___ ___ ___ ___ ___ ___	Reg LN Pos ___ ___	SSF10 HPV Status ___ ___ ___
Date Mult Tumors Flag ___ ___	Reg LN Exam ___ ___	SSF11 Measured Thickness Depth ___ ___ ___
Mult Tum Reported as One Prim ___ ___	CS Mets at Dx ___ ___	
Summary Stage 2000 ___	CS Mets at Dx - Bone ___ Brain ___ Liver ___ Lung ___	
	CS Mets Eval ___	

Head-Neck

CASE 7

HISTORY AND PHYSICAL EXAMINATION

12-9-20XX Patient presented with an ulcerative exophytic lesion of the left tonsillar fossa measuring more than 5 cm. A 3.5 x 2 cm node was noted to be firm and mobile in the left neck.

X-RAYS AND SCANS

12-14-20XX CT scan: Extension of the lesion with mucosal spread into the hard palate and extending into the base of the skull and also to the lateral pharyngeal wall down to the level of the pharyngoepiglottic fold.

12-16-20XX CXR: Negative for metastases.

LABORATORY REPORTS None.

OPERATIVE REPORTS

12-16-20XX Biopsy (incisional) of the ulcerative lesion and core needle biopsy of the node in the neck.

PATHOLOGY REPORTS

12-16-20XX Both biopsies were positive for a poorly differentiated squamous cell carcinoma.

Site Code ___ ___ ___.___	cT ___ cN ___ cM ___	SSF1 Size of LN ___ ___ ___
Histology/Behavior/Grade ___ ___ ___ ___/___ ___	Clin Stage Group _____	SSF2 OBSOLETE 988
Grade Path Value ___	pT ___ pN ___ M ___	SSF3 LN Levels I-III ___ ___ ___
Grade Path System ___	Path Stage Group _____	SSF4 LN Levels IV-V, RP ___ ___ ___
Lymph Vascular Invasion ___	CS Tumor Size ___ ___ ___	SSF5 LN Levels VI-VII, Facial ___ ___ ___
Ambiguous Terminol ___	CS Extension ___ ___ ___	SSF6 LN levels PP, PA, Occ ___ ___ ___
Date Conclusive Terminol ___ ___ ___ ___ ___ ___ ___ ___	CS TS/Ext Eval ___	SSF7 Upper/Lower Cerv LN Levels ___ ___ ___
Date Conclus Dx Flag ___ ___	CS LN ___ ___ ___	SSF8 Extracaps Exten Clinical ___ ___ ___
Multiplicity Counter ___ ___	CS Reg Nodes Eval ___	SSF9 Extracaps Exten Pathologic ___ ___ ___
Date Mult Tumors ___ ___ ___ ___ ___ ___ ___ ___	Reg LN Pos ___ ___	SSF10 HPV Status ___ ___ ___
Date Mult Tumors Flag ___ ___	Reg LN Exam ___ ___	SSF11 Measured Thickness Depth ___ ___ ___
Mult Tum Reported as One Prim ___ ___	CS Mets at Dx ___ ___	
Summary Stage 2000 _____	CS Mets at Dx - Bone ___ Brain ___ Liver ___ Lung ___	
	CS Mets Eval ___	

CASE 8

HISTORY AND PHYSICAL EXAM
9-8-20XX 4 cm lesion on left base of tongue. Palpable cervical lymph node on the left side. No other abnormal findings reported.

X-RAYS AND SCANS
9-14-20XX CXR: Negative.

LABORATORY REPORTS None.

ENDOSCOPIC PROCEDURES
9-12-20XX Laryngoscopy: Negative.

OPERATIVE REPORTS
9-15-20XX Resection of left base of tongue lesion and left radical neck dissection.

PATHOLOGY REPORTS
9-15-20XX Base of tongue: moderately differentiated non-keratinizing squamous cell carcinoma, completely resected. Tumor size: 3x2 cm. No muscle invasion. Metastatic squamous cell carcinoma in 2 (size 2 cm) of 8 Level I lymph nodes and 0 of 12 Level II lymph nodes.

Site Code ___ ___ ___.___	cT ___ cN ___ cM ___	SSF1 Size of LN ___ ___ ___
Histology/Behavior/Grade ___ ___ ___ ___ / ___ ___	Clin Stage Group _____	SSF2 OBSOLETE 988
Grade Path Value ___	pT ___ pN ___ M ___	SSF3 LN Levels I-III ___ ___ ___
Grade Path System ___	Path Stage Group _____	SSF4 LN Levels IV-V, RP ___ ___ ___
Lymph Vascular Invasion ___	CS Tumor Size ___ ___ ___	SSF5 LN Levels VI-VII, Facial ___ ___ ___
Ambiguous Terminol ___	CS Extension ___ ___ ___	SSF6 LN levels PP, PA, Occ ___ ___ ___
Date Conclusive Terminol ___ ___ ___ ___ ___ ___ ___ ___	CS TS/Ext Eval ___	SSF7 Upper/Lower Cerv LN Levels ___ ___ ___
Date Conclus Dx Flag ___ ___	CS LN ___ ___ ___	SSF8 Extracaps Exten Clinical ___ ___ ___
Multiplicity Counter ___ ___	CS Reg Nodes Eval ___	SSF9 Extracaps Exten Pathologic ___ ___ ___
Date Mult Tumors ___ ___ ___ ___ ___ ___ ___ ___	Reg LN Pos ___ ___	SSF10 HPV Status ___ ___ ___
Date Mult Tumors Flag ___ ___	Reg LN Exam ___ ___	SSF11 Measured Thickness Depth ___ ___ ___
Mult Tum Reported as One Prim ___ ___	CS Mets at Dx ___ ___	
Summary Stage 2000 ___	CS Mets at Dx - Bone ___ Brain ___ Liver ___ Lung ___	
	CS Mets Eval ___	

Head-Neck

CASE 9

HISTORY AND PHYSICAL EXAM

2-4-20XX ENT: Oropharynx showed presence of granular lesion involving lateral aspect of uvula creeping towards edge of soft palate and onto posterior pillar on the left side. No palpable nodes in the neck or supraclavicular area.

X-RAYS AND SCANS

2-5-20XX CXR: Question of nodule in right lower lobe.

LABORATORY REPORTS None.

ENDOSCOPIC PROCEDURES

2-4-20XX Direct laryngoscopy with biopsy of soft palate and uvula. Findings: granular lesion of soft palate appears to be involving uvula.

OPERATIVE REPORTS

2-10-20XX Excision of palatal carcinoma, tonsillectomy, palatal pharyngoplasty. Findings: Palatal carcinoma involving uvula extending along left edge of soft palate onto anterior and posterior pillar with no direct infiltration of tonsil.

PATHOLOGY REPORTS

2-10-20XX Micro: Infiltrating moderately to poorly differentiated focally keratinizing squamous cell carcinoma arising from epithelium of uvula. No vascular invasion. Deep margins free. Epithelial margins show one margin negative and the opposite involved microscopically by malignant process. Tumor size 1.0 cm.

Site Code ___ ___ ___.___

Histology/Behavior/Grade ___ ___ ___ ___/___ ___

Grade Path Value ___

Grade Path System ___

Lymph Vascular Invasion ___

Ambiguous Terminol ___

Date Conclusive Terminol ___ ___ ___ ___ ___ ___ ___ ___

Date Conclus Dx Flag ___ ___

Multiplicity Counter ___ ___

Date Mult Tumors ___ ___ ___ ___ ___ ___ ___ ___

Date Mult Tumors Flag ___ ___

Mult Tum Reported as One Prim ___ ___

Summary Stage 2000 ___

cT ___ cN ___ cM ___

Clin Stage Group _____

pT ___ pN ___ M ___

Path Stage Group _____

CS Tumor Size ___ ___ ___

CS Extension ___ ___ ___

CS TS/Ext Eval ___

CS LN ___ ___ ___

CS Reg Nodes Eval ___

Reg LN Pos ___ ___

Reg LN Exam ___ ___

CS Mets at Dx ___ ___

CS Mets at Dx - Bone ___ Brain ___ Liver ___ Lung ___

CS Mets Eval ___

SSF1 Size of LN ___ ___ ___

SSF2 OBSOLETE 988

SSF3 LN Levels I-III ___ ___ ___

SSF4 LN Levels IV-V, RP ___ ___ ___

SSF5 LN Levels VI-VII, Facial ___ ___ ___

SSF6 LN levels PP, PA, Occ ___ ___ ___

SSF7 Upper/Lower Cerv LN Levels ___ ___ ___

SSF8 Extracaps Exten Clinical ___ ___ ___

SSF9 Extracaps Exten Pathologic ___ ___ ___

SSF10 HPV Status ___ ___ ___

SSF11 Measured Thickness Depth ___ ___ ___

CASE 10

HISTORY AND PHYSICAL EXAMINATION

1-12-20XX HEENT: Patient presented with an exophytic tumor eroding the hypopharyngeal aspect of the right aryepiglottic fold. There was fixation of the hemilarynx. Physical exam: otherwise within normal limits

X-RAYS AND SCANS

1-15-20XX CT scan: Lesion extending to the right arytenoid cartilage, medial and anterior wall and right pyriform sinus. No lymph nodes visualized.

LABORATORY REPORTS None.

ENDOSCOPIC PROCEDURES

None.

OPERATIVE REPORTS

1-22-20XX Partial pharyngectomy and total laryngectomy with right node dissection.

PATHOLOGY REPORTS

1-22-20XX Pathology was positive for squamous cell carcinoma extending into the right pyriform sinus, right arytenoid cartilage and medial and anterior walls. All nodes were negative.

Site Code ___ ___ ___.___

Histology/Behavior/Grade ___ ___ ___ ___/___ ___

Grade Path Value ___

Grade Path System ___

Lymph Vascular Invasion ___

Ambiguous Terminol ___

Date Conclusive Terminol ___ ___ ___ ___ ___ ___ ___ ___

Date Conclus Dx Flag ___ ___

Multiplicity Counter ___ ___

Date Mult Tumors ___ ___ ___ ___ ___ ___ ___ ___

Date Mult Tumors Flag ___ ___

Mult Tum Reported as One Prim ___ ___

Summary Stage 2000 ___

cT ___ cN ___ cM ___

Clin Stage Group ___

pT ___ pN ___ M ___

Path Stage Group ___

CS Tumor Size ___ ___ ___

CS Extension ___ ___ ___

CS TS/Ext Eval ___

CS LN ___ ___ ___

CS Reg Nodes Eval ___

Reg LN Pos ___ ___

Reg LN Exam ___ ___

CS Mets at Dx ___ ___

CS Mets at Dx - Bone ___ Brain ___ Liver ___ Lung ___

CS Mets Eval ___

SSF1 Size of LN ___ ___ ___

SSF2 OBSOLETE 988

SSF3 LN Levels I-III ___ ___ ___

SSF4 LN Levels IV-V, RP ___ ___ ___

SSF5 LN Levels VI-VII, Facial ___ ___ ___

SSF6 LN levels PP, PA, Occ ___ ___ ___

SSF7 Upper/Lower Cerv LN Levels ___ ___ ___

SSF8 Extracaps Exten Clinical ___ ___ ___

SSF9 Extracaps Exten Pathologic ___ ___ ___

SSF10 HPV Status ___ ___ ___

SSF11 Measured Thickness Depth ___ ___ ___

CASE 11

HISTORY AND PHYSICAL EXAM

8-22-20XX 48 year old male smoker complaining of hoarseness. 2 cm firm lymph node in left upper jugular region.

X-RAYS AND SCANS

9-5-20XX Chest X-ray: Negative.

LABORATORY REPORTS

Not significant.

ENDOSCOPIC PROCEDURES

8-22-20XX Laryngoscopy: Lesion of left false cord visualized. Vocal cords fixed.

OPERATIVE REPORTS

9-7-20XX Supraglottic laryngectomy and left radical node dissection

PATHOLOGY REPORTS

9-7-20XX Squamous cell carcinoma of the supraglottic larynx. Tumor size, 2.5 cm. Metastases present in 2 of 5 Level VI lymph nodes, 1 of 7 parapharyngeal nodes and 1 of 3 middle deep cervical nodes. Largest node measures 5.3 cm. None of the involved lymph nodes demonstrate evidence of extracapsular extension.

Site Code ___ ___ ___.___
Histology/Behavior/Grade ___ ___ ___ ___/___ ___
Grade Path Value ___
Grade Path System ___
Lymph Vascular Invasion ___
Ambiguous Terminol ___
Date Conclusive Terminol ___ ___ ___ ___ ___ ___ ___ ___
Date Conclus Dx Flag ___ ___
Multiplicity Counter ___ ___
Date Mult Tumors ___ ___ ___ ___ ___ ___ ___ ___
Date Mult Tumors Flag ___ ___
Mult Tum Reported as One Prim ___ ___
Summary Stage 2000 ___

cT ___ cN ___ cM ___
Clin Stage Group ___
pT ___ pN ___ M ___
Path Stage Group ___
CS Tumor Size ___ ___ ___
CS Extension ___ ___ ___
CS TS/Ext Eval ___
CS LN ___ ___ ___
CS Reg Nodes Eval ___
Reg LN Pos ___ ___
Reg LN Exam ___ ___
CS Mets at Dx ___ ___
CS Mets at Dx - Bone ___ Brain ___ Liver ___ Lung ___
CS Mets Eval ___

SSF1 Size of LN ___ ___ ___
SSF2 OBSOLETE 988
SSF3 LN Levels I-III ___ ___ ___
SSF4 LN Levels IV-V, RP ___ ___ ___
SSF5 LN Levels VI-VII, Facial ___ ___ ___
SSF6 LN levels PP, PA, Occ ___ ___ ___
SSF7 Upper/Lower Cerv LN Levels ___ ___ ___
SSF8 Extracaps Exten Clinical ___ ___ ___
SSF9 Extracaps Exten Pathologic ___ ___ ___
SSF10 HPV Status ___ ___ ___
SSF11 Measured Thickness Depth ___ ___ ___

CASE 12

HISTORY AND PHYSICAL EXAM

1-28-20XX Right vocal cord covered with a fungating lesion. Lesion does not extend beyond true vocal cord.
Neck: supple. No nodes palpable.

X-RAYS AND SCANS None.

LABORATORY REPORTS None.

ENDOSCOPIC PROCEDURES

See Operative Reports.

OPERATIVE REPORTS

2-5-20XX Direct laryngoscopy and biopsy. Findings: Entire surface of right true vocal cord covered with a fungating mass. Mass extended partially into ventricle and approximately 2 mm over the free margin onto inferior border of the vocal cord.

PATHOLOGY REPORTS

2-5-20XX Biopsy of larynx: Invasive moderately differentiated keratinizing squamous cell carcinoma.

TREATMENT

2-14-20XX to 3-28-20XX 6480 cGy to glottis at staff physician's office.

Site Code ___ ___ ___.___
Histology/Behavior/Grade ___ ___ ___ ___ / ___ ___
Grade Path Value ___
Grade Path System ___
Lymph Vascular Invasion ___
Ambiguous Terminol ___
Date Conclusive Terminol ___ ___ ___ ___ ___ ___ ___ ___
Date Conclus Dx Flag ___ ___
Multiplicity Counter ___ ___
Date Mult Tumors ___ ___ ___ ___ ___ ___ ___ ___
Date Mult Tumors Flag ___ ___
Mult Tum Reported as One Prim ___ ___
Summary Stage 2000 ___

cT ___ cN ___ cM ___
Clin Stage Group ___
pT ___ pN ___ M ___
Path Stage Group ___
CS Tumor Size ___ ___ ___
CS Extension ___ ___ ___
CS TS/Ext Eval ___
CS LN ___ ___ ___
CS Reg Nodes Eval ___
Reg LN Pos ___ ___
Reg LN Exam ___ ___
CS Mets at Dx ___ ___
CS Mets at Dx - Bone ___ Brain ___ Liver ___ Lung ___
CS Mets Eval ___

SSF1 Size of LN ___ ___ ___
SSF2 OBSOLETE 988
SSF3 LN Levels I-III ___ ___ ___
SSF4 LN Levels IV-V, RP ___ ___ ___
SSF5 LN Levels VI-VII, Facial ___ ___ ___
SSF6 LN levels PP, PA, Occ ___ ___ ___
SSF7 Upper/Lower Cerv LN Levels ___ ___ ___
SSF8 Extracaps Exten Clinical ___ ___ ___
SSF9 Extracaps Exten Pathologic ___ ___ ___
SSF10 HPV Status ___ ___ ___
SSF11 Measured Thickness Depth ___ ___ ___

CASE 13

HISTORY AND PHYSICAL EXAM

A 65 year old white female presented with neck mass. She was referred to the ENT Surgeon.

10-10-20XX Physical examination: 2x3cm fixed matted immobile mass in the left neck.

X-RAYS AND SCANS

10-15-20XX CT Neck: 2cm x 1.5cm left jugular-digastric lymph node.

10-15-20XX CT Brain: WNL.

ENDOSCOPIC PROCEDURES

10-10-20XX Laryngoscopy: fixed mass left true cord extending upward to left false vocal cord with left cord paralysis. Incisional biopsy of the mass was taken.

OPERATIVE REPORTS

11-6-20XX Lesion involved the entire left aryepiglottic fold, false vocal cord, true vocal cord, and extended into the wall of the pyriform sinus.

PATHOLOGY REPORTS

10-10-20XX Biopsy of left true vocal cord was positive for invasive carcinoma.

11-6-20XX Surgical Pathology: Total laryngectomy, left mod rad neck dissect: Glottic squamous cell carcinoma 2.4 cm tumor size, involving aryepiglottic fold and pyriform recess. Positive angio-lymphatic invasion, no perineural invasion. 1 of 4 Level 2 lymph node with metastatic squamous cell carcinoma; 3 of 8 Level 3 lymph nodes; 0 of 4 Level 4 lymph nodes; 0 of 4 Level 5 lymph nodes. Total 4 of 20 regional lymph nodes involved.

TREATMENT

11-6-20XX Total laryngectomy and left modified radical neck dissection.

1-7-20YY to 2-13-20YY External beam radiation to upper neck, supraclavicular region with boost dose to right and left posterior neck and anterior neck.

Site Code ___ ___ ___.___

Histology/Behavior/Grade ___ ___ ___ ___/___ ___

Grade Path Value ___

Grade Path System ___

Lymph Vascular Invasion ___

Ambiguous Terminol ___

Date Conclusive Terminol ___ ___ ___ ___ ___ ___ ___ ___

Date Conclus Dx Flag ___ ___

Multiplicity Counter ___ ___

Date Mult Tumors ___ ___ ___ ___ ___ ___ ___ ___

Date Mult Tumors Flag ___ ___

Mult Tum Reported as One Prim ___ ___

Summary Stage 2000 ___

cT ___ **cN** ___ **cM** ___

Clin Stage Group ___

pT ___ **pN** ___ **M** ___

Path Stage Group ___

CS Tumor Size ___ ___ ___

CS Extension ___ ___ ___

CS TS/Ext Eval ___

CS LN ___ ___ ___

CS Reg Nodes Eval ___

Reg LN Pos ___ ___

Reg LN Exam ___ ___

CS Mets at Dx ___ ___

CS Mets at Dx -
Bone ___ **Brain** ___
Liver ___ **Lung** ___

CS Mets Eval ___

SSF1 Size of LN ___ ___ ___

SSF2 OBSOLETE 988

SSF3 LN Levels I-III ___ ___ ___

SSF4 LN Levels IV-V, RP ___ ___ ___

SSF5 LN Levels VI-VII, Facial ___ ___ ___

SSF6 LN levels PP, PA, Occ ___ ___ ___

SSF7 Upper/Lower Cerv LN Levels ___ ___ ___

SSF8 Extracaps Exten Clinical ___ ___ ___

SSF9 Extracaps Exten Pathologic ___ ___ ___

SSF10 HPV Status ___ ___ ___

SSF11 Measured Thickness Depth ___ ___ ___

CASE 14

HISTORY AND PHYSICAL EXAMINATION

9-5-20XX Hoarseness; difficulty breathing for two weeks. No palpable lymphadenopathy.

X-RAYS AND SCANS

9-6-20XX Upper GI: Apparent mass high in esophagus.
9-6-20XX CXR: negative.

ENDOSCOPIC PROCEDURES

See Operative Reports.

OPERATIVE REPORTS

9-7-20XX Direct laryngoscopy, esophagoscopy, biopsies and debulking of laryngeal mass. Findings: fungating mass on posterior wall of larynx beginning about 2 cm below vocal cords and extending nearly to inferior edge of cricoid cartilage. Smaller, 1 cm lesion on anterior wall of esophagus; apparent extension completely through laryngoesophageal wall.

PATHOLOGY REPORTS

9-7-20XX Endoscopic biopsies: P-d squamous carcinoma in subglottis and esophagus.

Site Code ___ ___ ___.___
Histology/Behavior/Grade ___ ___ ___ ___/___ ___
Grade Path Value ___
Grade Path System ___
Lymph Vascular Invasion ___
Ambiguous Terminol ___
Date Conclusive Terminol ___ ___ ___ ___ ___ ___ ___ ___
Date Conclus Dx Flag ___ ___
Multiplicity Counter ___ ___
Date Mult Tumors ___ ___ ___ ___ ___ ___ ___ ___
Date Mult Tumors Flag ___ ___
Mult Tum Reported as One Prim ___ ___
Summary Stage 2000 ___

cT ___ cN ___ cM ___
Clin Stage Group ___
pT ___ pN ___ M ___
Path Stage Group ___
CS Tumor Size ___ ___ ___
CS Extension ___ ___ ___
CS TS/Ext Eval ___
CS LN ___ ___ ___
CS Reg Nodes Eval ___
Reg LN Pos ___ ___
Reg LN Exam ___ ___
CS Mets at Dx ___ ___
CS Mets at Dx - Bone ___ Brain ___ Liver ___ Lung ___
CS Mets Eval ___

SSF1 Size of LN ___ ___ ___
SSF2 OBSOLETE 988
SSF3 LN Levels I-III ___ ___ ___
SSF4 LN Levels IV-V, RP ___ ___ ___
SSF5 LN Levels VI-VII, Facial ___ ___ ___
SSF6 LN levels PP, PA, Occ ___ ___ ___
SSF7 Upper/Lower Cerv LN Levels ___ ___ ___
SSF8 Extracaps Exten Clinical ___ ___ ___
SSF9 Extracaps Exten Pathologic ___ ___ ___
SSF10 HPV Status ___ ___ ___
SSF11 Measured Thickness Depth ___ ___ ___

CASE 15

HISTORY AND PHYSICAL EXAMINATION

7-9-20XX Patient presented with an ulcerative tumor of the laryngeal aspect of the left aryepiglottic fold extending into the pharyngo-epiglottic fold.
Physical exam noted no adenopathy.

X-RAYS AND SCANS

7-11-20XX CXR: within normal limits.

OPERATIVE REPORTS

7-23-20XX Partial laryngectomy and radical node dissections.

PATHOLOGY REPORTS

7-23-20XX Specimen positive for moderately differentiated squamous cell carcinoma in multiple areas of the supraglottis. Two left neck nodes at Level III both less than 3 cm were positive for metastatic squamous cell carcinoma.

Site Code ___ ___ ___.___	cT ___ cN ___ cM ___	SSF1 Size of LN ___ ___ ___
Histology/Behavior/Grade ___ ___ ___ ___/___ ___	Clin Stage Group _____	SSF2 OBSOLETE 988
Grade Path Value ___	pT ___ pN ___ M ___	SSF3 LN Levels I-III ___ ___ ___
Grade Path System ___	Path Stage Group _____	SSF4 LN Levels IV-V, RP ___ ___ ___
Lymph Vascular Invasion ___	CS Tumor Size ___ ___ ___	SSF5 LN Levels VI-VII, Facial ___ ___ ___
Ambiguous Terminol ___	CS Extension ___ ___ ___	SSF6 LN levels PP, PA, Occ ___ ___ ___
Date Conclusive Terminol ___ ___ ___ ___ ___ ___ ___ ___	CS TS/Ext Eval ___	SSF7 Upper/Lower Cerv LN Levels ___ ___ ___
Date Conclus Dx Flag ___ ___	CS LN ___ ___ ___	SSF8 Extracaps Exten Clinical ___ ___ ___
Multiplicity Counter ___ ___	CS Reg Nodes Eval ___	SSF9 Extracaps Exten Pathologic ___ ___ ___
Date Mult Tumors ___ ___ ___ ___ ___ ___ ___ ___	Reg LN Pos ___ ___	SSF10 HPV Status ___ ___ ___
Date Mult Tumors Flag ___ ___	Reg LN Exam ___ ___	SSF11 Measured Thickness Depth ___ ___ ___
Mult Tum Reported as One Prim ___ ___	CS Mets at Dx ___ ___	
Summary Stage 2000 _____	CS Mets at Dx - Bone ___ Brain ___ Liver ___ Lung ___	
	CS Mets Eval ___	

CASE 16

HISTORY AND PHYSICAL EXAM

2-14-20XX 50 year old executive in for routine physical. Left neck firm with a non-tender 3.0 cm mass just lateral to the thyroid, most likely matted lymph nodes.

X-RAYS AND SCANS

2-16-20XX Chest X-ray: negative.
2-16-20XX CT Chest: Lungs negative.

LABORATORY REPORTS

None.

OPERATIVE REPORTS

2-28-20XX Thyroidectomy with left neck dissection

PATHOLOGY REPORTS

2-28-20XX Thyroid Gland: Poorly differentiated papillary carcinoma of the thyroid, multifocal, bilateral. Largest tumor size is 2.3 cm left lobe. 20 of 27 left cervical lymph nodes positive for metastatic papillary carcinoma. Largest node is 5 cm.

Site Code __ __ __.__	cT __ cN __ cM __	SSF1 Size of LN __ __ __
Histology/Behavior/Grade __ __ __ __/__ __	Clin Stage Group ____	SSF2 OBSOLETE 988
Grade Path Value __	pT __ pN __ M __	SSF3 LN Levels I-III __ __ __
Grade Path System __	Path Stage Group ____	SSF4 LN Levels IV-V, RP __ __ __
Lymph Vascular Invasion __	CS Tumor Size __ __ __	SSF5 LN Levels VI-VII, Facial __ __ __
Ambiguous Terminol __	CS Extension __ __ __	SSF6 LN levels PP, PA, Occ __ __ __
Date Conclusive Terminol __ __ __ __ __ __ __ __	CS TS/Ext Eval __	SSF7 Upper/Lower Cerv LN Levels __ __ __
Date Conclus Dx Flag __ __	CS LN __ __ __	SSF8 Extracaps Exten Clinical __ __ __
Multiplicity Counter __ __	CS Reg Nodes Eval __	SSF9 Extracaps Exten Pathologic __ __ __
Date Mult Tumors __ __ __ __ __ __ __ __	Reg LN Pos __ __	SSF10 HPV Status __ __ __
Date Mult Tumors Flag __ __	Reg LN Exam __ __	SSF11 Measured Thickness Depth __ __ __
Mult Tum Reported as One Prim __ __	CS Mets at Dx __ __	
Summary Stage 2000 __	CS Mets at Dx - Bone __ Brain __ Liver __ Lung __	
	CS Mets Eval __	

CASE 17

HISTORY AND PHYSICAL EXAM
A 61 year old white female presented with a chief complaint of soreness in the periauricular region. Remainder of physical examination normal.

X-RAYS AND SCANS
1-10-20XX CT: Parotid: 2cm left parotid gland mass.
1-15-20XX CXR: WNL.

ENDOSCOPIC PROCEDURES
None.

OPERATIVE REPORTS
2-12-20XX Left parotidectomy: No significant findings.

PATHOLOGY REPORTS
1-15-20XX FNA of left parotid gland was positive for poorly differentiated carcinoma.
2-12-20XX Surgical Pathology: Left parotid gland excision: 5 x 4 x 2.8 cm tumor consistent with high grade mucoepidermoid carcinoma, infiltrating the skeletal muscle and adipose tissue, with microscopic positive inked surgical margin.

TREATMENT
2-12-20XX Surgery: Left parotidectomy.
2-26-20XX to 4-17-20XX External beam radiation therapy given to left parotid gland region and adjacent neck 7072 cGy in 34 fractions over 49 days.

Site Code ___ ___ ___.___
Histology/Behavior/Grade ___ ___ ___ ___/___ ___
Grade Path Value ___
Grade Path System ___
Lymph Vascular Invasion ___
Ambiguous Terminol ___
Date Conclusive Terminol ___ ___ ___ ___ ___ ___ ___ ___
Date Conclus Dx Flag ___ ___
Multiplicity Counter ___ ___
Date Mult Tumors ___ ___ ___ ___ ___ ___ ___ ___
Date Mult Tumors Flag ___ ___
Mult Tum Reported as One Prim ___ ___
Summary Stage 2000 ___

cT ___ **cN** ___ **cM** ___
Clin Stage Group ___
pT ___ **pN** ___ **M** ___
Path Stage Group ___
CS Tumor Size ___ ___ ___
CS Extension ___ ___ ___
CS TS/Ext Eval ___
CS LN ___ ___ ___
CS Reg Nodes Eval ___
Reg LN Pos ___ ___
Reg LN Exam ___ ___
CS Mets at Dx ___ ___
CS Mets at Dx - **Bone** ___ **Brain** ___ **Liver** ___ **Lung** ___
CS Mets Eval ___

SSF1 Size of LN ___ ___ ___
SSF2 OBSOLETE 988
SSF3 LN Levels I-III ___ ___ ___
SSF4 LN Levels IV-V, RP ___ ___ ___
SSF5 LN Levels VI-VII, Facial ___ ___ ___
SSF6 LN levels PP, PA, Occ ___ ___ ___
SSF7 Upper/Lower Cerv LN Levels ___ ___ ___
SSF8 Extracaps Exten Clinical ___ ___ ___
SSF9 Extracaps Exten Pathologic ___ ___ ___

CASE 18

HISTORY AND PHYSICAL EXAM

5-18-20XX PE: Rt eye with 2 mm proptosis and marked enlargement pushing medial canthus consistent with naso-orbital tumor. No palpable lymphadenopathy in head or neck.

X-RAYS AND SCANS

5-11-20XX MRI: Lesion in right anterior ethmoid sinus extending to right frontal sinus with associated mass effect on right orbit and proptosis compatible with malignant process such as carcinoma or lymphoma. No other lesions identified in head or neck.

5-11-20XX CXR: Negative.

LABORATORY REPORTS None significant.

OPERATIVE REPORTS

5-18-20XX Partial debulking of right ethmoid tumor: Tumor mass in right sinus which had eroded partially through orbital wall

PATHOLOGY REPORTS

5-18-20XX Rt ethmoid tumor: Undifferentiated non-keratinizing carcinoma. No further pathologic description. Final diagnosis: Carcinoma, right ethmoid sinus

TREATMENT

5-18-20XX Partial debulking of right ethmoid tumor

6-XX-20XX Chemotherapy and radiation therapy started

Site Code ___ ___ ___.___	cT ___ cN ___ cM ___	SSF1 Size of LN ___ ___ ___
Histology/Behavior/Grade ___ ___ ___ ___ / ___ ___	Clin Stage Group _____	SSF2 OBSOLETE 988
Grade Path Value ___	pT ___ pN ___ M ___	SSF3 LN Levels I-III ___ ___ ___
Grade Path System ___	Path Stage Group _____	SSF4 LN Levels IV-V, RP ___ ___ ___
Lymph Vascular Invasion ___	CS Tumor Size ___ ___ ___	SSF5 LN Levels VI-VII, Facial ___ ___ ___
Ambiguous Terminol ___	CS Extension ___ ___ ___	SSF6 LN levels PP, PA, Occ ___ ___ ___
Date Conclusive Terminol ___ ___ ___ ___ ___ ___ ___ ___	CS TS/Ext Eval ___	SSF7 Upper/Lower Cerv LN Levels ___ ___ ___
Date Conclus Dx Flag ___ ___	CS LN ___ ___ ___	SSF8 Extracaps Exten Clinical ___ ___ ___
Multiplicity Counter ___ ___	CS Reg Nodes Eval ___	SSF9 Extracaps Exten Pathologic ___ ___ ___
Date Mult Tumors ___ ___ ___ ___ ___ ___ ___ ___	Reg LN Pos ___ ___	SSF10 HPV Status ___ ___ ___
Date Mult Tumors Flag ___ ___	Reg LN Exam ___ ___	SSF11 Measured Thickness Depth ___ ___ ___
Mult Tum Reported as One Prim ___ ___	CS Mets at Dx ___ ___	
Summary Stage 2000 ___	CS Mets at Dx - Bone ___ Brain ___ Liver ___ Lung ___	
	CS Mets Eval ___	

ANSWERS TO HEAD AND NECK CANCER CASE EXERCISES

—— CASE 1 ——

Site Code	C04.1	Lateral floor of mouth (near retromolar trigone)
Histology	8070/32	Moderately differentiated squamous cell carcinoma
Grade Path Value	Blank	Does not apply
Grade Path System	Blank	Does not apply
Lymph Vascular Invasion	9	Lymph-vascular invasion not mentioned in path report
Ambiguous Terminology	0	Conclusive terminology
Date Conclusive Terminol	Blank	Diagnosis made by conclusive terminology
Date Conclus Dx Flag	11	Not applicable
Multiplicity Counter	01	One tumor only
Date Multiple Tumors	Blank	Not applicable
Date Mult Tumors Flag	15	Single tumor only (multiplicity counter is coded 01)
Type Mult Tum as 1 Prim	00	Single tumor
Summary Stage	2	Regional direct extension only

Region	Lip and oral cavity			
CLINICAL	T 2	N 0	M 0	Stage Group II
PATHOLOGIC	yT 2	yN 0	cM 0	Stage Group II

Collaborative Staging Schema used: FloorMouth (Floor of Mouth)

CS Tumor Size	035	3.5 cm tumor on physical examination pre-treatment
CS Extension	500	Lower alveolar ridge (retromolar trigone is the part of the lower gum at the angle of the jaw)
CS TS/Ext Eval	5	Clinical information prior to radiation therapy
CS Lymph Nodes	000	No palpable nodes on physical exam
CS Reg Nodes Eval	5	Based on physical exam prior to radiation therapy
Reg LN Pos	00	No metastases in lymph nodes
Reg LN Exam	35	35 lymph nodes examined
CS Mets at Dx	00	Chest x-ray negative
CS Mets at Dx–Bone	0	No bone metastases
CS Mets at Dx–Brain	0	No brain metastases
CS Mets at Dx–Liver	0	No liver metastases
CS Mets at Dx–Lung	0	No lung metastases
CS Mets Eval	0	Based on imaging
SSF1 Size of LN	000	No involved lymph nodes
SSF2 OBSOLETE	988	Not applicable; information not collected
SSF3 LN levels I-III	000	No level I, II or III nodes involved
SSF4 LN levels IV, V, RP	000	No level IV, V or retropharyngeal nodes involved
SSF5 LN levels VI, VII, FA	000	No level VI, VII or facial nodes involved
SSF6 LN levels PP, PA, Occ	000	No parapharyngeal, parotid, or suboccipital nodes involved
SSF7 Upper/Lower Cerv LN	000	No regional lymph nodes involved
SSF8 Extracaps Exten Clin	000	No regional lymph nodes involved clinically
SSF9 Extracaps Exten Path	000	No regional lymph nodes involved pathologically
SSF10 HPV Status	999	HPV status not documented
SSF11 Thickness/Depth	999	Thickness/depth not stated

Case 1, continued

This case will map to cT2 cN0 cM0 Stage Group II (clinical stage prior to radiation therapy)

—— CASE 2 ——

Site Code	C06.0	Buccal (cheek) mucosa
Histology	8070/31	Squamous cell carcinoma, well differentiated
Grade Path Value	Blank	Does not apply
Grade Path System	Blank	Does not apply
Lymph Vascular Invasion	9	Lymph-vascular invasion not mentioned in path report
Ambiguous Terminology	0	Conclusive terminology
Date Conclusive Terminol	Blank	Diagnosis made by conclusive terminology
Date Conclus Dx Flag	11	Not applicable
Multiplicity Counter	01	One tumor only
Date Multiple Tumors	Blank	Not applicable
Date Mult Tumors Flag	15	Single tumor only (multiplicity counter is coded 01)
Type Mult Tum as 1 Prim	00	Single tumor
Summary Stage	3	Regional lymph nodes involved only

Region	Lip and oral cavity			
CLINICAL	T 1	N 1	M 0	Stage Group III
PATHOLOGIC	T 2	N 1	cM 0	Stage Group III

Collaborative Staging Schema used: BuccalMucosa (Buccal or cheek mucosa)

CS Tumor Size	021	2.1 cm lesion per pathology report
CS Extension	200	Buccal musculature infiltrated
CS TS/Ext Eval	3	Based on resection
CS Lymph Nodes	100	Buccinator lymph node is in facial group
CS Reg Nodes Eval	3	Based on neck dissection
Reg LN Pos	01	One facial lymph node involved
Reg LN Exam	01	One lymph node examined
CS Mets at Dx	00	Chest x-ray negative
CS Mets at Dx–Bone	0	No bone metastases
CS Mets at Dx–Brain	0	No brain metastases
CS Mets at Dx–Liver	0	No liver metastases
CS Mets at Dx–Lung	0	No lung metastases
CS Mets Eval	0	Based on imaging
SSF1 Size of LN	993	Lymph node described as less than 3 cm in size
SSF2 OBSOLETE	988	Not applicable; information not collected
SSF3 LN levels I-III	000	No level I, II or III nodes involved
SSF4 LN levels IV, V, RP	000	No level IV, V or retropharyngeal nodes involved
SSF5 LN levels VI, VII, FA	001	Only facial node involved
SSF6 LN levels PP, PA, Occ	000	No parapharyngeal, parotid, or suboccipital nodes involved
SSF7 Upper/Lower Cerv LN	010	Facial (buccal) nod involved (Note 2)
SSF8 Extracaps Exten Clin	030	No extracapsular extension clinically (Note 4)
SSF9 Extracaps Exten Path	040	Extracapsular extension pathologically, NOS (Note 5)
SSF10 HPV Status	999	HPV status not documented
SSF11 Thickness/Depth	999	Thickness/depth not stated

This case will map to pT2 pN1 cM0 Stage Group III

—— CASE 3 ——

Site Code	C02.2	Underside (ventral surface) of tongue
Histology	8200/32	Moderately differentiated adenoid cystic carcinoma
Grade Path Value	Blank	Does not apply
Grade Path System	Blank	Does not apply
Lymph Vascular Invasion	9	Lymph-vascular invasion not mentioned in path report
Ambiguous Terminology	0	Conclusive terminology
Date Conclusive Terminol	Blank	Diagnosis made by conclusive terminology
Date Conclus Dx Flag	11	Not applicable
Multiplicity Counter	01	One tumor only
Date Multiple Tumors	Blank	Not applicable
Date Mult Tumors Flag	15	Single tumor only (multiplicity counter is coded 01)
Type Mult Tum as 1 Prim	00	Single tumor
Summary Stage	4	Regional direct extension (submucosal extension to lesion in floor of mouth) and regional lymph nodes

Region	Lip and oral cavity			
CLINICAL	T 1	N 0	M 0	Stage Group I
PATHOLOGIC	T 1	N 2b	M 0	Stage Group IVA

The physical exam describes direct submucosal extension between the undersurface of the tongue and the floor of mouth lesion. Even though no pathologic size is given, the involved lymph nodes determine the pathologic stage group as IVA.

Collaborative Staging Schema used: TongueAnterior (Anterior 2/3 of tongue—ventral surface)

CS Tumor Size	015	Tumor size 1.5 cm per physical examination
CS Extension	500	Extension to floor of mouth
CS TS/Ext-Eval	0	Based on physical examination
CS Lymph Nodes	200	Multiple (2) positive submandibular lymph nodes
CS Reg Nodes Eval	3	Based on pathology report
Reg LN Pos	02	Two lymph nodes positive
Reg LN Exam	96	"Excision" (sampling) of lymph nodes, number removed not stated
CS Mets at DX	00	No distant metastases
CS Mets at Dx–Bone	0	No bone metastases
CS Mets at Dx–Brain	0	No brain metastases
CS Mets at Dx–Liver	0	No liver metastases
CS Mets at Dx–Lung	0	No lung metastases
CS Mets Eval	0	Based on negative CT chest
SSF1 Size of LN	999	Size of metastasis in lymph nodes not stated
SSF2 OBSOLETE	988	Not applicable; information not collected
SSF3 LN levels I-III	100	Level I nodes involved; no level II or III nodes involved
SSF4 LN levels IV, V, RP	000	No level IV, V or retropharyngeal nodes involved
SSF5 LN levels VI, VII, FA	000	No level VI, VII or facial nodes involved
SSF6 LN levels PP, PA, Occ	000	No parapharyngeal, parotid, or suboccipital nodes involved
SSF7 Upper/Lower Cerv LN	010	Submandibular nodes involved (Note 2)
SSF8 Extracaps Exten Clin	000	No regional nodes involved clinically
SSF9 Extracaps Exten Path	010	No extracapsular extension pathologically (Note 3)
SSF10 HPV Status	999	HPV status not documented
SSF11 Thickness/Depth	999	Thickness/depth not stated

Case 3, continued

This case will map to cT1 pN2b cM0 Stage Group IVA

This appears to be a "bookleaf" or "kissing" tumor in which tumor cells involved another structure by direct contact when the tongue is at rest. There is also evidence of direct tumor extension under the mucosal surface between the two obvious lesions. The only size given is 1.5 cm which may or may not represent the entire tumor size (tongue and floor of mouth) but it's the best information available for staging.

—— CASE 4 ——

Site Code	C06.0	Buccal mucosa
Histology	8070/33	Poorly differentiated squamous cell carcinoma
Grade Path Value	Blank	Does not apply
Grade Path System	Blank	Does not apply
Lymph Vascular Invasion	9	Lymph-vascular invasion not mentioned in path report
Ambiguous Terminology	0	Conclusive terminology
Date Conclusive Terminol	Blank	Diagnosis made by conclusive terminology
Date Conclus Dx Flag	11	Not applicable
Multiplicity Counter	01	One tumor only
Date Multiple Tumors	Blank	Not applicable
Date Mult Tumors Flag	15	Single tumor only (multiplicity counter is coded 01)
Type Mult Tum as 1 Prim	00	Single tumor
Summary Stage	1	Localized

Region Lip and oral cavity
CLINICAL T 1 N 0 M 0 Stage Group I

PATHOLOGIC T X N X cM 0 Stage Group Unstageable

Collaborative Staging Schema used: BuccalMucosa (Buccal or cheek mucosa)

CS Tumor Size	020	Tumor size 2.0 cm per physical exam
CS Extension	300	Localized, NOS (confined to buccal mucosa, NOS)
CS TS/Ext-Eval	0	Tumor size (on which T mapping is calculated) based on physical exam
CS Lymph Nodes	000	No nodes palpable
CS Reg Nodes Eval	0	Based on physical examination
Reg LN Pos	98	No nodes removed
Reg LN Exam	00	No nodes removed
CS Mets at DX	00	All x-rays and scans within normal limits
CS Mets at Dx–Bone	0	No bone metastases
CS Mets at Dx–Brain	0	No brain metastases
CS Mets at Dx–Liver	0	No liver metastases
CS Mets at Dx–Lung	0	No lung metastases
CS Mets Eval	0	Based on imaging
SSF1 Size of LN	000	No involved regional nodes
SSF2 OBSOLETE	988	Not applicable; information not collected
SSF3 LN levels I-III	000	No level I, II or III nodes involved
SSF4 LN levels IV, V, RP	000	No level IV, V or retropharyngeal nodes involved
SSF5 LN levels VI, VII, FA	000	No level VI, VII or facial nodes involved
SSF6 LN levels PP, PA, Occ	000	No parapharyngeal, parotid, or suboccipital nodes involved
SSF7 Upper/Lower Cerv LN	000	No regional lymph nodes involved (PE and scans negative)
SSF8 Extracaps Exten Clin	000	No regional lymph nodes involved clinically

Case 4, continued

SSF9 Extracaps Exten Path	998	No histopathologic examination of regional nodes
SSF10 HPV Status	999	HPV status not documented
SSF11 Thickness/Depth	999	Thickness/depth not stated

This case will map to cT1 cN0 cM0 Stage Group I

—— CASE 5 ——

Site Code	C02.3	Anterior 2/3 of tongue
Histology	8070/32	Moderately [well] differentiated squamous cell carcinoma
Grade Path Value	Blank	Does not apply
Grade Path System	Blank	Does not apply
Lymph Vascular Invasion	1	Lymph-vascular invasion present per path report
Ambiguous Terminology	0	Conclusive terminology
Date Conclusive Terminol	Blank	Diagnosis made by conclusive terminology
Date Conclus Dx Flag	11	Not applicable
Multiplicity Counter	01	One tumor only
Date Multiple Tumors	Blank	Not applicable
Date Mult Tumors Flag	15	Single tumor only (multiplicity counter is coded 01)
Type Mult Tum as 1 Prim	00	Single tumor
Summary Stage	3	Regional lymph nodes involved only

Region	Lip and oral cavity			
CLINICAL	T 2	N 0	M 0	Stage Group II
PATHOLOGIC	T X	N 1	cM 0	Stage Group III *see note*

TNM Note: Technically this case cannot be pathologically stage-grouped because there is no pathologic tumor size for the primary. However, the stage group is at least Stage III because of the positive lymph node, and there is evidence that the tumor has extended into the deep muscles of the tongue, which would make it Stage IVA.

Collaborative Staging Schema used: TongueAnterior (Anterior 2/3 of tongue)

CS Tumor Size	030	Tumor size 3.0 cm per physical examination
CS Extension	200	Muscle involved, NOS
CS TS/Ext-Eval	3	Based on pathology report
CS Lymph Nodes	100	One positive Level II lymph node involved
CS Reg Nodes Eval	3	Based on pathology report
Reg LN Pos	01	One lymph node positive
Reg LN Exam	37	8 Level II + 11 Level III + 9 Level IV on right; 9 Level I on left
CS Mets at DX	00	No distant metastasis
CS Mets at Dx–Bone	0	No bone metastases
CS Mets at Dx–Brain	0	No brain metastases
CS Mets at Dx–Liver	0	No liver metastases
CS Mets at Dx–Lung	0	No lung metastases
CS Mets Eval	0	Based on CXR
SSF1 Size of LN	028	Size of metastasis in lymph nodes stated as 2.8 cm
SSF2 OBSOLETE	988	Not applicable; information not collected
SSF3 LN levels I-III	010	Level II node involved; no level I or III nodes involved
SSF4 LN levels IV, V, RP	000	No level IV, V or retropharyngeal nodes involved
SSF5 LN levels VI, VII, FA	000	No level VI, VII or facial nodes involved

Case 5, continued

SSF6 LN levels PP, PA, Occ	000	No parapharyngeal, parotid, or suboccipital nodes involved
SSF7 Upper/Lower Cerv LN	000	No regional nodes involved (scans all negative)
SSF8 Extracaps Exten Clin	000	No regional nodes involved clinically
SSF9 Extracaps Exten Path	040	Extracapsular extension pathologically, NOS (Note 5)
SSF10 HPV Status	999	HPV status not documented
SSF11 Thickness/Depth	999	Thickness/depth not stated

This case will map to cT1 pN1 cM0 Stage Group III

—— CASE 6 ——

Site Code	C01.9	Base (root) of tongue
Histology	8070/39	Squamous cell carcinoma
Grade Path Value	Blank	Does not apply
Grade Path System	Blank	Does not apply
Lymph Vascular Invasion	9	Lymph-vascular invasion not mentioned in path report
Ambiguous Terminology	0	Conclusive terminology
Date Conclusive Terminol	Blank	Diagnosis made by conclusive terminology
Date Conclus Dx Flag	11	Not applicable
Multiplicity Counter	01	One tumor only
Date Multiple Tumors	Blank	Not applicable
Date Mult Tumors Flag	15	Single tumor only (multiplicity counter is coded 01)
Type Mult Tum as 1 Prim	00	Single tumor

Summary Stage	7	Distant site (extrinsic muscle of tongue)

Region	Oropharynx			
CLINICAL	T 4a	N 0	M 0	Stage Group IVA
PATHOLOGIC	T X	N X	cM 0	Stage Group Unstageable

Collaborative Staging Schema used: TongueBase (Base of tongue)

CS Tumor Size	015	Tumor size 1.5 cm per physical examination
CS Extension	750	Invasion of palatoglossus muscle
CS TS/Ext-Eval	0	Based on imaging
CS Lymph Nodes	000	No regional lymph nodes involved
CS Reg Nodes Eval	0	Based on physical exam
Reg LN Pos	98	No lymph nodes examined
Reg LN Exam	00	No lymph nodes examined
CS Mets at DX	00	No distant mets described
CS Mets at Dx–Bone	0	No bone metastases
CS Mets at Dx–Brain	0	No brain metastases
CS Mets at Dx–Liver	0	No liver metastases
CS Mets at Dx–Lung	0	No lung metastases
CS Mets Eval	0	Based on physical exam
SSF1 Size of LN	000	No lymph nodes involved
SSF2 OBSOLETE	988	Not applicable; information not collected
SSF3 LN levels I-III	000	No level I, II or III nodes involved
SSF4 LN levels IV, V, RP	000	No level IV, V or retropharyngeal nodes involved
SSF5 LN levels VI, VII, FA	000	No level VI, VII or facial nodes involved
SSF6 LN levels PP, PA, Occ	000	No parapharyngeal, parotid, or suboccipital nodes involved
SSF7 Upper/Lower Cerv LN	000	No regional nodes involved per physical exam
SSF8 Extracaps Exten Clin	000	No regional nodes involved clinically

Case 6, continued

SSF9 Extracaps Exten Path	998	No histopathologic examination of regional nodes
SSF10 HPV Status	999	HPV status not documented
SSF11 Thickness/Depth	999	Thickness/depth not stated

This case will map to cT4a cN0 cM0 Stage Group IVA

The palatoglossus muscle is one of the deep (extrinsic) muscles of the tongue and makes the case Extension 750 and T4a, which is Stage IVA.

—— CASE 7 ——

Site Code	C09.0	Tonsillar fossa
Histology	8070/33	Poorly-differentiated squamous cell carcinoma
Grade Path Value	Blank	Does not apply
Grade Path System	Blank	Does not apply
Lymph Vascular Invasion	9	Lymph-vascular invasion not mentioned in path report
Ambiguous Terminology	0	Conclusive terminology
Date Conclusive Terminol	Blank	Diagnosis made by conclusive terminology
Date Conclus Dx Flag	11	Not applicable
Multiplicity Counter	01	One tumor only
Date Multiple Tumors	Blank	Not applicable
Date Mult Tumors Flag	15	Single tumor only (multiplicity counter is coded 01)
Type Mult Tum as 1 Prim	00	Single tumor
Summary Stage	7	Distant site (bone–base of skull)

Region	Oropharynx			
CLINICAL	T 4b	N 2a	M 0	Stage Group IVB
PATHOLOGIC	T X	N X	cM 0	Stage Group Unstageable

Collaborative Staging Schema used: Oropharynx (Tonsil, Oropharynx—Tonsillar fossa)

CS Tumor Size	051	Tumor size "more than 5 cm" per physical examination; no better way to code size
CS Extension	750	Tumor extension to base of skull
CS TS/Ext-Eval	0	Based on CT imaging
CS Lymph Nodes	100	Lymph node, NOS
CS Reg Nodes Eval	1	Based on biopsy of neck node
Reg LN Pos	95	Biopsy of one node
Reg LN Exam	95	Biopsy (not stated as excision) of node
CS Mets at DX	00	No distant metastasis
CS Mets at Dx–Bone	0	No bone metastases
CS Mets at Dx–Brain	0	No brain metastases
CS Mets at Dx–Liver	0	No liver metastases
CS Mets at Dx–Lung	0	No lung metastases
CS Mets Eval	0	Based on imaging
SSF1 Size of LN	035	3.5 cm per physical exam
SSF2 OBSOLETE	988	Not applicable information not collected
SSF3 LN levels I-III	999	Unknown if Level I, level II or III nodes involved
SSF4 LN levels IV, V, RP	999	Unknown if level IV, V or retropharyngeal nodes involved
SSF5 LN levels VI, VII, FA	999	Unknown if level VI, VII or facial nodes involved
SSF6 LN levels PP, PA, Occ	999	Unknown if parapharyngeal, parotid, or suboccipital nodes involved

Case 7, continued

SSF7 Upper/Lower Cerv LN	040	Left neck node involved, unknown level
SSF8 Extracaps Exten Clin	030	Node(s) involved clinically, unknown if extracapsular extension
SSF9 Extracaps Exten Path	090	Node(s) involved pathologically, unknown if extracapsular extension
SSF10 HPV Status	999	HPV status not documented
SSF11 Thickness/Depth	999	Thickness/depth not stated

This case will map to cT4b cN2a cM0 Stage Group IVB

The Stage Group is IVB based on the T category (very advanced tumor extension).

—— CASE 8 ——

Site Code	C01.9	Base (root) of tongue
Histology	8072/32	Moderately differentiated non-keratinizing squamous cell carcinoma
Grade Path Value	Blank	Does not apply
Grade Path System	Blank	Does not apply
Lymph Vascular Invasion	9	Lymph-vascular invasion not mentioned in path report
Ambiguous Terminology	0	Conclusive terminology
Date Conclusive Terminol	Blank	Diagnosis made by conclusive terminology
Date Conclus Dx Flag	11	Not applicable
Multiplicity Counter	01	One tumor only
Date Multiple Tumors	Blank	Not applicable
Date Mult Tumors Flag	15	Single tumor only (multiplicity counter is coded 01)
Type Mult Tum as 1 Prim	00	Single tumor
Summary Stage	3	Regional lymph nodes involved only

Region	Oropharynx			
CLINICAL	T 2	N 0	M 0	Stage Group II
PATHOLOGIC	T 2	N 2b	cM 0	Stage Group IVA

Collaborative Staging Schema used: TongueBase (Base of tongue and lingual tonsil)

CS Tumor Size	030	3 x 2 cm per pathology report
CS Extension	100	Stated as completely resected, no muscle invasion
CS TS/Ext Eval	3	Based on resection
CS Lymph Nodes	200	Level I nodes are listed in code 10; MULTIPLE Level I nodes is code 20
CS Reg Nodes Eval	3	Based on neck dissection
Reg LN Pos	02	Two Level I nodes involved
Reg LN Exam	20	Twenty lymph nodes examined
CS Mets at Dx	00	Chest x-ray negative
CS Mets at Dx–Bone	0	No bone metastases
CS Mets at Dx–Brain	0	No brain metastases
CS Mets at Dx–Liver	0	No liver metastases
CS Mets at Dx–Lung	0	No lung metastases
CS Mets Eval	0	Based on imaging
SSF1 Size of LN	020	Lymph node size 2 cm per pathology report
SSF2 OBSOLETE	988	Not applicable; information not collected
SSF3 LN levels I-III	100	Only Level I nodes involved

Case 8, continued

SSF4 LN levels IV, V, RP	000	No level IV, V or retropharyngeal nodes involved
SSF5 LN levels VI, VII, FA	000	No level VI, VII or facial nodes involved
SSF6 LN levels PP, PA, Occ	000	No parapharyngeal, parotid, or suboccipital nodes involved
SSF7 Upper/Lower Cerv LN	010	Upper level (Level I) nodes involved
SSF8 Extracaps Exten Clin	030	No regional nodes involved clinically
SSF9 Extracaps Exten Path	090	No extracapsular extension pathologically (Note 3)
SSF10 HPV Status	999	HPV status not documented
SSF11 Thickness/Depth	999	Thickness/depth not stated

This case will map to pT2 pN2b cM0 Stage Group IVA.

—— CASE 9 ——

Site Code	C05.2	Uvula
Histology	8070/33	Poorly-differentiated squamous cell carcinoma; disregard "focally keratinizing"
Grade Path Value	Blank	Does not apply
Grade Path System	Blank	Does not apply
Lymph Vascular Invasion	0	No vascular invasion per path report
Ambiguous Terminology	0	Conclusive terminology
Date Conclusive Terminol	Blank	Diagnosis made by conclusive terminology
Date Conclus Dx Flag	11	Not applicable
Multiplicity Counter	01	One tumor only
Date Multiple Tumors	Blank	Not applicable
Date Mult Tumors Flag	15	Single tumor only (multiplicity counter is coded 01)
Type Mult Tum as 1 Prim	00	Single tumor
Summary Stage	2	Regional direct extension only

Region	Oropharynx			
CLINICAL	T X	N 0	M 0	Stage Group Unstageable
PATHOLOGIC	T 1	N X	cM 0	Stage Group Unstageable

TNM Note: The tumor size was not measured clinically, so the case cannot be clinically stage-grouped. No lymph nodes were removed, so the case cannot be pathologically stage-grouped.

Collaborative Staging Schema used: PalateSoft (Uvula)

CS Tumor Size	010	Tumor size 1.0 cm per path report
CS Extension	600	Tumor involves tonsillar pillar
CS TS/Ext-Eval	3	Based on pathology report
CS Lymph Nodes	000	No involved neck or supraclavicular nodes
CS Reg Nodes Eval	0	Based on physical examination
Reg LN Pos	98	No nodes removed
Reg LN Exam	00	No nodes removed
CS Mets at DX	00	Chest x-ray negative (disregard questionable nodule because they proceeded with surgery to primary site)
CS Mets at Dx–Bone	0	No bone metastases
CS Mets at Dx–Brain	0	No brain metastases
CS Mets at Dx–Liver	0	No liver metastases
CS Mets at Dx–Lung	0	No lung metastases
CS Mets Eval	0	Based on imaging
SSF1 Size of LN	000	No involved regional nodes

Case 9, continued

SSF2 OBSOLETE	988	Not applicable; information not collected
SSF3 LN levels I-III	000	No level I, II or III nodes involved
SSF4 LN levels IV, V, RP	000	No level IV, V or retropharyngeal nodes involved
SSF5 LN levels VI, VII, FA	000	No level VI, VII or facial nodes involved
SSF6 LN levels PP, PA, Occ	000	No parapharyngeal, parotid, or suboccipital nodes involved
SSF7 Upper/Lower Cerv LN	000	No regional nodes involved (PE negative)
SSF8 Extracaps Exten Clin	000	No regional nodes involved clinically
SSF9 Extracaps Exten Path	998	No histopathologic examination of regional nodes
SSF10 HPV Status	999	HPV status not documented
SSF11 Thickness/Depth	999	Thickness/depth not stated

This case will map to pT1 cN0 cM0 Stage Group I

—— CASE 10 ——

Site Code	C13.1	Hypopharyngeal aspect of aryepiglottic fold
Histology	8070/39	Squamous cell carcinoma
Grade Path Value	Blank	Does not apply
Grade Path System	Blank	Does not apply
Lymph Vascular Invasion	9	Lymph-vascular invasion not mentioned in path report
Ambiguous Terminology	0	Conclusive terminology
Date Conclusive Terminol	Blank	Diagnosis made by conclusive terminology
Date Conclus Dx Flag	11	Not applicable
Multiplicity Counter	01	One tumor only
Date Multiple Tumors	Blank	Not applicable
Date Mult Tumors Flag	15	Single tumor only (multiplicity counter is coded 01)
Type Mult Tum as 1 Prim	00	Single tumor

Summary Stage 2 Regional direct extension only

Region	Hypopharynx			
CLINICAL	T 3	N 0	M 0	Stage Group III
PATHOLOGIC	T 3	N 0	cM 0	Stage Group III

TNM Note: Pathologic staging includes clinical information (fixation of hemilarynx).

Collaborative Staging Schema used: Hypopharynx (Pyriform sinus, Hypopharynx, Laryngopharynx—hypopharyngeal aspect of aryepiglottic fold)

CS Tumor Size	999	No tumor size stated
CS Extension	550	Fixation of hemilarynx
CS TS/Ext-Eval	3	Based on pathology report
CS Lymph Nodes	000	No regional lymph nodes involved
CS Reg Nodes Eval	3	Based on pathology report
Reg LN Pos	00	No lymph nodes positive
Reg LN Exam	97	"Dissection" of lymph nodes, number removed not stated
CS Mets at DX	00	Inaccessible sites rule
CS Mets at Dx–Bone	0	No bone metastases
CS Mets at Dx–Brain	0	No brain metastases
CS Mets at Dx–Liver	0	No liver metastases
CS Mets at Dx–Lung	0	No lung metastases
CS Mets Eval	0	Based on clinical assessment
SSF1 Size of LN	000	No involved regional lymph nodes

Case 10, continued

SSF2 OBSOLETE	988	Not applicable; information not collected
SSF3 LN levels I-III	000	No level I, II or III nodes involved
SSF4 LN levels IV, V, RP	000	No level IV, V or retropharyngeal nodes involved
SSF5 LN levels VI, VII, FA	000	No level VI, VII or facial nodes involved
SSF6 LN levels PP, PA, Occ	000	No parapharyngeal, parotid, or suboccipital nodes involved
SSF7 Upper/Lower Cerv LN	000	No regional nodes involved (PE negative)
SSF8 Extracaps Exten Clin	000	No regional nodes involved clinically
SSF9 Extracaps Exten Path	000	No regional nodes involved pathologically
SSF10 HPV Status	999	HPV status not documented
SSF11 Thickness/Depth	999	Thickness/depth not stated

This case will map to pT3 pN0 cM0 Stage Group III

—— CASE 11 ——

Site Code	C32.1	False cord
Histology	8070/39	Squamous cell carcinoma
Grade Path Value	Blank	Does not apply
Grade Path System	Blank	Does not apply
Lymph Vascular Invasion	9	Lymph-vascular invasion not mentioned in path report
Ambiguous Terminology	0	Conclusive terminology
Date Conclusive Terminol	Blank	Diagnosis made by conclusive terminology
Date Conclus Dx Flag	11	Not applicable
Multiplicity Counter	01	One tumor only
Date Multiple Tumors	Blank	Not applicable
Date Mult Tumors Flag	15	Single tumor only (multiplicity counter is coded 01)
Type Mult Tum as 1 Prim	00	Single tumor
Summary Stage	3	Regional lymph nodes involved only

Region	Supraglottic larynx			
CLINICAL	T 3	N 1	M 0	Stage Group III
PATHOLOGIC	T 3	N 2b	cM 0	Stage Group IVA

Collaborative Staging Schema used: LarynxSupraglottic (Supraglottic larynx)

CS Tumor Size	025	2.5 cm tumor per pathology report
CS Extension	400	Limited to larynx (supraglottis) with vocal cord fixation per laryngoscopy
CS TS/Ext Eval	3	Based on laryngectomy
CS Lymph Nodes	220	MULTIPLE nodes, at least one of which is listed in code 12
CS Reg Nodes Eval	3	Based on pathology report
Reg LN Pos	04	2 + 1 + 1 lymph nodes positive
Reg LN Exam	15	5 + 7 + 3 lymph nodes examined
CS Mets at Dx	00	Chest x-ray and CT negative
CS Mets at Dx–Bone	0	No bone metastases
CS Mets at Dx–Brain	0	No brain metastases
CS Mets at Dx–Liver	0	No liver metastases
CS Mets at Dx–Lung	0	No lung metastases
CS Mets Eval	0	Based on imaging
SSF1 Size of LN	053	Largest lymph node measures 5.3 cm
SSF2 OBSOLETE	988	Not applicable; information not collected
SSF3 LN levels I-III	000	No level IV, V or retropharyngeal nodes involved

Case 11, continued

SSF4 LN levels IV, V, RP	001	Middle deep cervical are Level III nodes
SSF5 LN levels VI, VII, FA	100	Only Level VI nodes involved
SSF6 LN levels PP, PA, Occ	100	Only parapharyngeal nodes involved
SSF7 Upper/Lower Cerv LN	040	Unknown level of Level VI node(s)
SSF8 Extracaps Exten Clin	000	No regional lymph nodes involved clinically
SSF9 Extracaps Exten Path	010	No extracapsular extension pathologically
SSF10 HPV Status	999	HPV status not documented
SSF11 Thickness/Depth	999	Thickness/depth not stated

This case will map to pT3 pN2b cM0 Stage Group IVA

The vocal cord fixation (a clinical symptom) was seen on endoscopy, it would not have been evident on the surgical resection, and the surgical resection meets the criteria for pathologic staging.

—— CASE 12 ——

Site Code	C32.0	True vocal cord
Histology	8071/32	Moderately-differentiated keratinizing squamous cell carcinoma
Grade Path Value	Blank	Does not apply
Grade Path System	Blank	Does not apply
Lymph Vascular Invasion	9	Lymph-vascular invasion not mentioned in path report
Ambiguous Terminology	0	Conclusive terminology
Date Conclusive Terminol	Blank	Diagnosis made by conclusive terminology
Date Conclus Dx Flag	11	Not applicable
Multiplicity Counter	01	One tumor only
Date Multiple Tumors	Blank	Not applicable
Date Mult Tumors Flag	15	Single tumor only (multiplicity counter is coded 01)
Type Mult Tum as 1 Prim	00	Single tumor

Summary Stage	1	Localized

Region	Glottic larynx			
CLINICAL	T 2	N 0	M 0	Stage Group II
PATHOLOGIC	T X	N X	cM 0	Stage Group Unstageable

Collaborative Staging Schema used: LarynxGlottic (True vocal cord)

CS Tumor Size	999	No size stated
CS Extension	300	Tumor involves supraglottis (ventricle)
CS TS/Ext-Eval	1	Based on endoscopy
CS Lymph Nodes	000	No nodes palpable
CS Reg Nodes Eval	0	Based on physical examination
Reg LN Pos	98	No nodes removed
Reg LN Exam	00	No nodes removed
CS Mets at DX	00	No mention of mets, patient received standard treatment
CS Mets at Dx–Bone	0	No bone metastases
CS Mets at Dx–Brain	0	No brain metastases
CS Mets at Dx–Liver	0	No liver metastases
CS Mets at Dx–Lung	0	No lung metastases
CS Mets Eval	0	Based on clinical assessment
SSF1 Size of LN	000	No involved regional nodes
SSF2 OBSOLETE	988	Not applicable; information not collected

Case 12, continued

SSF3 LN levels I-III	000	No level I, II or III nodes involved
SSF4 LN levels IV, V, RP	000	No level IV, V or retropharyngeal nodes involved
SSF5 LN levels VI, VII, FA	000	No level VI, VII or facial nodes involved
SSF6 LN levels PP, PA, Occ	000	No parapharyngeal, parotid, or suboccipital nodes involved
SSF7 Upper/Lower Cerv LN	000	No regional nodes involved (PE negative)
SSF8 Extracaps Exten Clin	000	No regional nodes involved clinically
SSF9 Extracaps Exten Path	998	No histopathologic examination of regional nodes
SSF10 HPV Status	999	HPV status not documented
SSF11 Thickness/Depth	999	Thickness/depth not stated

This case will map to cT2 cN0 cM0 Stage Group II

—— CASE 13 ——

Site Code	C32.0	True vocal cord
Histology	8070/39	Squamous cell carcinoma, grade not stated
Grade Path Value	Blank	Does not apply
Grade Path System	Blank	Does not apply
Lymph Vascular Invasion	1	Positive angio-lymphatic invasion per path report
Ambiguous Terminology	0	Conclusive terminology
Date Conclusive Terminol	Blank	Diagnosis made by conclusive terminology
Date Conclus Dx Flag	11	Not applicable
Multiplicity Counter	01	One tumor only
Date Multiple Tumors	Blank	Not applicable
Date Mult Tumors Flag	15	Single tumor only (multiplicity counter is coded 01)
Type Mult Tum as 1 Prim	00	Single tumor
Summary Stage	4	Regional both direct extension and lymph nodes

Region	Glottic larynx			
CLINICAL	T 4a	N 1	M 0	Stage Group IVA
PATHOLOGIC	T 4a	N 2b	cM 0	Stage Group IVA

Collaborative Staging Schema used: LarynxGlottic (True vocal cord)

CS Tumor Size	024	Tumor size stated as 2.4 cm in pathology report
CS Extension	600	Extension into pyriform sinus
CS TS/Ext-Eval	3	Based on pathology report
CS Lymph Nodes	200	Multiple (4) regional nodes involved as listed in code 10
CS Reg Nodes Eval	3	Based on pathology report
Reg LN Pos	04	Four lymph nodes positive (1 Level II and 3 Level III)
Reg LN Exam	20	4 Level II + 8 Level III + 4 Level IV + 4 Level V
CS Mets at DX	00	No distant metastasis
CS Mets at Dx–Bone	0	No bone metastases
CS Mets at Dx–Brain	0	No brain metastases
CS Mets at Dx–Liver	0	No liver metastases
CS Mets at Dx–Lung	0	No lung metastases
CS Mets Eval	0	Based on CT of brain
SSF1 Size of LN	020	Largest size of involved regional node 2.0 cm per CT scan
SSF2 OBSOLETE	988	Not applicable; information not collected
SSF3 LN levels I-III	011	No level I nodes involved; Level II and III nodes involved
SSF4 LN levels IV, V, RP	000	No level IV, V or retropharyngeal nodes involved
SSF5 LN levels VI, VII, FA	000	No level VI, VII or facial nodes involved

Case 13, continued

SSF6 LN levels PP, PA, Occ	000	No parapharyngeal, parotid, or suboccipital nodes involved
SSF7 Upper/Lower Cerv LN	010	Level II and III nodes are above the cricoid cartilage (upper)
SSF8 Extracaps Exten Clin	020	Jugular-digastric node described as "fixed"
SSF9 Extracaps Exten Path	010	Nodes involved; extracapsular extension not mentioned (Note 3)
SSF10 HPV Status	999	HPV status not documented
SSF11 Thickness/Depth	999	Thickness/depth not stated

This case will map to pT4a pN2b cM0 Stage Group IVA

—— CASE 14 ——

Site Code	C32.2	Subglottis		
Histology	8070/33	Poorly-differentiated squamous cell carcinoma		
Grade Path Value	Blank	Does not apply		
Grade Path System	Blank	Does not apply		
Lymph Vascular Invasion	9	Lymph-vascular invasion not mentioned in path report		
Ambiguous Terminology	0	Conclusive terminology		
Date Conclusive Terminol	Blank	Diagnosis made by conclusive terminology		
Date Conclus Dx Flag	11	Not applicable		
Multiplicity Counter	01	One tumor only		
Date Multiple Tumors	Blank	Not applicable		
Date Mult Tumors Flag	15	Single tumor only (multiplicity counter is coded 01)		
Type Mult Tum as 1 Prim	00	Single tumor		
Summary Stage	7	Distant site (esophagus)		
Region	Subglottic larynx			
CLINICAL	T 4a	N 0	M 0	Stage Group IVA
PATHOLOGIC	T X	N X	cM 0	Stage Group Unstageable

Collaborative Staging Schema used: LarynxSubglottic (Subglottis)

CS Tumor Size	999	No tumor size stated
CS Extension	700	Direct extension to esophagus
CS TS/Ext-Eval	1	Based on endoscopy *see note*
CS Lymph Nodes	000	No regional lymph nodes involved (no adenopathy)
CS Reg Nodes Eval	0	Based on physical exam
Reg LN Pos	98	No lymph nodes examined
Reg LN Exam	00	No lymph nodes examined
CS Mets at DX	00	No distant metastasis
CS Mets at Dx–Bone	0	No bone metastases
CS Mets at Dx–Brain	0	No brain metastases
CS Mets at Dx–Liver	0	No liver metastases
CS Mets at Dx–Lung	0	No lung metastases
CS Mets Eval	0	Based on CXR
SSF1 Size of LN	000	No lymph nodes involved
SSF2 OBSOLETE	988	Not applicable; information not collected
SSF3 LN levels I-III	000	No level I, II or III nodes involved
SSF4 LN levels IV, V, RP	000	No level IV, V or retropharyngeal nodes involved
SSF5 LN levels VI, VII, FA	000	No level VI, VII or facial nodes involved
SSF6 LN levels PP, PA, Occ	000	No parapharyngeal, parotid, or suboccipital nodes involved
SSF7 Upper/Lower Cerv LN	000	No regional nodes involved (PE negative)

Head-Neck

Case 14, continued

SSF8 Extracaps Exten Clin	000	No regional nodes involved clinically
SSF9 Extracaps Exten Path	998	No histopathologic examination of regional nodes
SSF10 HPV Status	999	HPV status not documented
SSF11 Thickness/Depth	999	Thickness/depth not stated

This case will map to cT4a cN0 cM0 Stage Group IVA

Endoscopic debulking of the laryngeal lesion does not meet the pathologic staging criteria of surgical resection of the primary site. Based on the endoscopy findings and lack of any lymph node biopsy or resection, this is a clinical stage IVA.

—— CASE 15 ——

Site Code	C32.1	Laryngeal aspect of aryepiglottic fold
Histology	8070/32	Moderately differentiated squamous cell carcinoma
Grade Path Value	Blank	Does not apply
Grade Path System	Blank	Does not apply
Lymph Vascular Invasion	9	Lymph-vascular invasion not mentioned in path report
Ambiguous Terminology	0	Conclusive terminology
Date Conclusive Terminol	Blank	Diagnosis made by conclusive terminology
Date Conclus Dx Flag	11	Not applicable
Multiplicity Counter	01	One tumor only
Date Multiple Tumors	Blank	Not applicable
Date Mult Tumors Flag	15	Single tumor only (multiplicity counter is coded 01)
Type Mult Tum as 1 Prim	00	Single tumor
Summary Stage	3	Regional lymph nodes involved only

Region	Supraglottic larynx			
CLINICAL	T 2	N 0	M 0	Stage Group II
PATHOLOGIC	T 2	N 2b	cM 0	Stage Group IVA

Collaborative Staging Schema used: LarynxSupraglottic (Supraglottis—left aryepiglottic fold)

CS Tumor Size	999	No tumor size stated
CS Extension	200	Stated as multiple areas of supraglottis involved
CS TS/Ext-Eval	3	Based on pathology report of resection
CS Lymph Nodes	210	Multiple (2) positive Level III lymph nodes
CS Reg Nodes Eval	3	Based on pathology report
Reg LN Pos	02	Two lymph nodes positive
Reg LN Exam	97	"Dissection" of lymph nodes, number removed not stated
CS Mets at DX	00	No distant metastasis
CS Mets at Dx–Bone	0	No bone metastases
CS Mets at Dx–Brain	0	No brain metastases
CS Mets at Dx Liver	0	No liver metastases
CS Mets at Dx–Lung	0	No lung metastases
CS Mets Eval	0	Based on imaging
SSF1 Size of LN	993	Size of metastasis in lymph nodes stated as less than 3 cm
SSF2 OBSOLETE	988	Not applicable; information not collected
SSF3 LN levels I-III	001	No level I or II nodes involved; Level III nodes involved
SSF4 LN levels IV, V, RP	000	No level IV, V or retropharyngeal nodes involved
SSF5 LN levels VI, VII, FA	000	No level VI, VII or facial nodes involved
SSF6 LN levels PP, PA, Occ	000	No parapharyngeal, parotid, or suboccipital nodes involved
SSF7 Upper/Lower Cerv LN	010	Level III nodes are upper cervical

Case 15, continued

SSF8 Extracaps Exten Clin	000	No regional nodes involved clinically
SSF9 Extracaps Exten Path	010	No extracapsular extension pathologically (Note 3)
SSF10 HPV Status	999	HPV status not documented
SSF11 Thickness/Depth	999	Thickness/depth not stated

This case will map to pT2 pN2b cM0 Stage Group IVA

—— CASE 16 ——

Site Code	C73.9	Thyroid gland
Histology	8260/33	Poorly differentiated papillary adenocarcinoma. Papillary carcinoma of the thyroid is coded to 8260 according to rule H14 of the "Other Sites" histology coding rules.
Grade Path Value	Blank	Does not apply
Grade Path System	Blank	Does not apply
Lymph Vascular Invasion	9	Lymph-vascular invasion not mentioned in path report
Ambiguous Terminology	0	Conclusive terminology
Date Conclusive Terminol	Blank	Diagnosis made by conclusive terminology
Date Conclus Dx Flag	11	Not applicable
Multiplicity Counter	99	Multifocal
Date Multiple Tumors	20XX0228	Date of diagnosis
Date Mult Tumors Flag	Blank	Valid date provided
Type Mult Tum as 1 Prim	40	Multiple invasive tumors
Summary Stage	3	Regional lymph nodes involved only

Region	Thyroid			
CLINICAL	T X	N 1a	M 0	Stage Group Unstageable
PATHOLOGIC	T 2b	N 1b	cM 0	Stage Group IVA

TNM Note: This case cannot be clinically staged because no tumor size is stated. (A full medical record would likely have a tumor size noted by a clinician.) The size of the largest tumor removed is 2.3 cm (T2) and there were multiple tumors (add "(m)" on the T category). Because so many lymph cervical nodes (N1b) are involved, the case is pathologic Stage IVA.

Collaborative Staging Schema used: Thyroid (Thyroid gland)

CS Tumor Size	023	Largest tumor nodule is 2.3 cm per pathology report
CS Extension	200	Multiple foci confined to thyroid
CS TS/Ext Eval	3	Based on thyroidectomy
CS Lymph Nodes	135	Cervical lymph nodes involved
CS Reg Nodes Eval	3	Based on pathology report
Reg LN Pos	20	Twenty lymph nodes involved
Reg LN Exam	27	27 lymph nodes examined
CS Mets at Dx	00	Chest x-ray and CT negative
CS Mets at Dx–Bone	0	No bone metastases
CS Mets at Dx–Brain	0	No brain metastases
CS Mets at Dx–Liver	0	No liver metastases
CS Mets at Dx–Lung	0	No lung metastases
CS Mets Eval	0	Based on imaging
SSF1 Size of LN	020	Multiple tumor nodules (thyroid SSFs are different from all other head and neck sites)

This case will map to pT2a pN1b cM0 Stage Group IVA (papillary tumor; patient over 45 years of age).

—— CASE 17 ——

Site Code	C07.9	Parotid gland
Histology	8430/34	High grade mucoepidermoid carcinoma. "High grade" is ICD-O 6th digit differentiation code 4, although not all pathologists agree.
Grade Path Value	Blank	Does not apply
Grade Path System	Blank	Does not apply
Lymph Vascular Invasion	9	Lymph-vascular invasion not mentioned in path report
Ambiguous Terminology	0	Conclusive terminology
Date Conclusive Terminol	Blank	Diagnosis made by conclusive terminology
Date Conclus Dx Flag	11	Not applicable
Multiplicity Counter	01	One tumor only
Date Multiple Tumors	Blank	Not applicable
Date Mult Tumors Flag	15	Single tumor only (multiplicity counter is coded 01)
Type Mult Tum as 1 Prim	00	Single tumor

Summary Stage	2	Regional direct extension only

Region Major salivary glands (parotid)

CLINICAL	T 1	N 0	M 0	Stage Group I
PATHOLOGIC	T 3	N X	cM 0	Stage Group Unstageable

Collaborative Staging Schema used: ParotidGland

CS Tumor Size	050	Size stated on pathology report
CS Extension	400	Involving skeletal muscle
CS TS/Ext Eval	3	Based on parotidectomy
CS Lymph Nodes	000	Stated as "remainder of physical examination normal"
CS Reg Nodes Eval	0	Based on physical examination
Reg LN Pos	98	No lymph nodes removed for examination
Reg LN Exam	00	No lymph nodes examined
CS Mets at Dx	00	No distant metastases
CS Mets at Dx–Bone	0	No bone metastases
CS Mets at Dx–Brain	0	No brain metastases
CS Mets at Dx–Liver	0	No liver metastases
CS Mets at Dx–Lung	0	No lung metastases
CS Mets Eval	0	Based on chest x-ray and physical exam
SSF1 Size of LN	000	No regional lymph nodes involved
SSF2 OBSOLETE	988	Not applicable; information not collected
SSF3 LN levels I-III	000	No level I, II or III nodes involved
SSF4 LN levels IV, V, RP	000	No level IV, V or retropharyngeal nodes involved
SSF5 LN levels VI, VII, FA	000	No level VI, VII or facial nodes involved
SSF6 LN levels PP, PA, Occ	000	No parapharyngeal, parotid, or suboccipital nodes involved
SSF7 Upper/Lower Cerv LN	000	No regional nodes involved (PE normal)
SSF8 Extracaps Exten Clin	000	No regional nodes involved clinically
SSF9 Extracaps Exten Path	998	No histopathological examination of regional nodes

This case will map to pT3 cN0 cM0 Stage Group III.

—— CASE 18 ——

Site Code	C31.1	Ethmoid sinus
Histology	8010/34	Undifferentiated carcinoma
Grade Path Value	Blank	Does not apply
Grade Path System	Blank	Does not apply
Lymph Vascular Invasion	9	Lymph-vascular invasion not mentioned in path report
Ambiguous Terminology	0	Conclusive terminology
Date Conclusive Terminol	Blank	Diagnosis made by conclusive terminology
Date Conclus Dx Flag	11	Not applicable
Multiplicity Counter	01	One tumor only
Date Multiple Tumors	Blank	Not applicable
Date Mult Tumors Flag	15	Single tumor only (multiplicity counter is coded 01)
Type Mult Tum as 1 Prim	00	Single tumor

Summary Stage	2	Regional direct extension only

Region Nasal cavity and paranasal sinuses (ethmoid sinus)

CLINICAL	T 4a	N 0	M 0	Stage Group IVA
PATHOLOGIC	T 3	N X	cM 0	Stage Group Unstageable

TNM Note: Involvement of frontal sinus (T4a) was determined clinically. Surgical findings confirmed involvement of orbital wall (T3), but without biopsy of lymph nodes, case cannot be pathologically staged.

Collaborative Staging Schema used: SinusEthmoid (Ethmoid sinus)

CS Tumor Size	999	No tumor size stated
CS Extension	700	Frontal sinus involved
CS TS/Ext-Eval	0	Based on MRI
CS Lymph Nodes	000	No regional lymph nodes involved
CS Reg Nodes Eval	0	Based on physical exam and MRI
Reg LN Pos	98	No lymph nodes removed for examination
Reg LN Exam	00	No lymph nodes examined
CS Mets at DX	00	No distant metastasis
CS Mets at Dx–Bone	0	No bone metastases
CS Mets at Dx–Brain	0	No brain metastases
CS Mets at Dx–Liver	0	No liver metastases
CS Mets at Dx–Lung	0	No lung metastases
CS Mets Eval	0	Based on physical exam and chest x-ray
SSF1 Size of LN	000	No involved regional nodes
SSF2 OBSOLETE	988	Not applicable; information not collected
SSF3 LN levels I-III	000	No level I, II or III nodes involved
SSF4 LN levels IV, V, RP	000	No level IV, V or retropharyngeal nodes involved
SSF5 LN levels VI, VII, FA	000	No level VI, VII or facial nodes involved
SSF6 LN levels PP, PA, Occ	000	No parapharyngeal, parotid, or suboccipital nodes involved
SSF7 Upper/Lower Cerv LN	000	No regional nodes involved (PE normal)
SSF8 Extracaps Exten Clin	000	No regional nodes involved clinically
SSF9 Extracaps Exten Path	998	No histopathologic examination of regional nodes
SSF10 HPV Status	999	HPV status not documented
SSF11 Thickness/Depth	999	Thickness/depth not stated

This case will map to cT4a cN0 cM0 Stage Group IVA

Page left blank.

CANCERS OF THE UTERUS: CORPUS AND CERVIX

Cancers of the female reproductive tract include primaries in the cervix uteri, corpus uteri (endometrium), ovaries, fallopian tubes, and other parts of the female genital system. This chapter concentrates on cancers of the uterus: corpus uteri and cervix uteri. Another chapter in this book will discuss ovary, fallopian tubes and placenta.

Corpus uteri cancer is the most common cancer of the female genital system. The ACS estimates 43,470 new cases were diagnosed in 2010; more than 95% of them are cancers of the lining of the corpus, the endometrium. Incidence rates for corpus cancer have been declining in the past decade.

The American Cancer Society estimates that there were over 12,200 cases of invasive cervical cancer diagnosed in the United States during 2010. Incidence rates for cervical cancer have been declining in the past decade. Carcinoma in situ (CIS) of the cervix is not reportable to the national population based cancer registries, but can be collected in state registries if required and as a reportable-by-agreement cancer in medical facilities if there is sufficient interest among researchers to use the data. CIS is estimated to be three to four times more common than invasive cancer. Estimates are that more than 39,000 non-invasive cervical cancer cases are diagnosed each year. Cervical cancer was once one of the deadliest cancers among women—and still is in some underdeveloped countries, but the death rate has declined significantly since the Pap test was developed in the mid-1930s. Cervical cancer that is caught early is very curable.

There is a great deal of similarity in the anatomy, abstracting, staging, and treatment of these two primary sites. Because corpus cancer is more common, it will be discussed first in each section to make it easier for the reader to find the information. When the information is the same for both, they will be referred to collectively as uterine cancers.

ETIOLOGY AND NATURAL HISTORY

Each of the cancers of the female genital system has its own set of risk factors and symptoms. Endometrial or corpus uteri cancer is strongly related to the presence or use of estrogen during the woman's life. Early onset of menstruation (early menarche, before age 12) and late menopause (after age 52) contribute to a long period of hormonal activity in the uterus. The total duration of fertility, and thus continued exposure to estrogens, may be a more important factor than early menarche or late menopause. Thus most endometrial cancer is diagnosed in women between 50 and 69, and it is uncommon in women under age 40. Infertility (estrogen exposure not counterbalanced by the progesterones present during pregnancy) is a risk factor.

The use of estrogen replacement therapy to treat hot flashes and other symptoms of menopause increases the risk of developing corpus cancer. An anti-estrogen called Tamoxifen or Nolvadex given to women as treatment for breast cancer has been shown to increase the risk of endometrial changes and endometrial cancer. However, its benefits in preventing a second breast cancer and reducing the recurrence rate for an initial breast cancer far outweigh the risks of developing a cancer in the uterus.

Etiology and Natural History, *continued*

Obesity is also a risk factor for endometrial cancer, because fat tissue can convert other hormones into estrogens. A diet high in animal fat has been linked to endometrial cancer and contributes to obesity. Diabetes, also associated with obesity, is also believed to be a risk factor for endometrial cancer. A family history of colon cancer or a personal history of hereditary non-polyposis colorectal cancer (HNPCC) or of breast or ovarian cancer are also known risk factors.

Cervical cancer is primarily a disease of women in their 30s to 50s. The development of cervical cancer is related to sexual intercourse. Infection with the human papilloma virus (HPV) is perhaps the most important risk factor. Other risk factors include early onset of sexual activity, sexually transmitted diseases, many partners during her lifetime, and multiparity (several children) before her mid-20s. Smoking doubles a woman's risk of developing cervical cancer. The incidence of cervical cancer is higher in African-Americans, Hispanics, and women of low socioeconomic status.

Cervical cancer is also described as an AIDS-defining condition; in other words, the presence of cervical cancer in a woman infected with HIV is a clear sign that full-blown AIDS has developed.

ANATOMY OF THE UTERUS AND REGIONAL LYMPH NODES AS THEY RELATE TO STAGING

The female genital system consists of the vulva, vagina, cervix uteri, corpus uteri, two fallopian tubes, two ovaries, placenta, supporting ligaments, and miscellaneous small glands (Figures 1 and 2). These organs are situated in the true pelvis along with the bladder, lower ureters, urethra and rectum.

The organs of the female genital system have a variety of names and word roots both individually and in groups.

- Word roots that may refer to the uterus as a whole are utero-, metra-, and hyster-. These may also be specific to the corpus uteri.
- The cervix is also called the uterine cervix, cervix uteri, and cervical canal. The common word root is cervico-, less common is trachel-.
- The corpus is also called the corpus uteri, uterus, and uterine body. Word roots referring to the corpus include utero-, endometrio-, and uterine.
- The ovaries are also called the female gonads. Adjectives referring to the ovary are ovarian and the word root oophor-.
- The fallopian tubes are also called the oviducts, uterine tubes, or just tubes. Word roots referring to the fallopian tubes are salpingo- and tubo-.
- The fallopian tubes, ovaries and the supporting ligaments of the internal genitalia are referred to collectively as the adnexa.

Parts of the Uterus

The largest organ of the female genital system is the ***uterus*** (Figure 3), a hollow organ about 7 cm long, located in the pelvis between the bladder and the rectum. The normal uterus is about the size and shape of a medium-sized pear and actually has two separate functions.

The upper two-thirds of the uterus comprise the ***body*** or ***corpus***. The lower boundary of the corpus is the level of the internal os.

The ***isthmus***, or ***lower uterine segment***, is the narrow, distal part of the corpus, which joins with the cervical canal and during pregnancy expands to become the lower part of the uterine cavity.

Figure 1. Anatomy of Internal Female Genital Organs (*partial cutaway anterior view*)

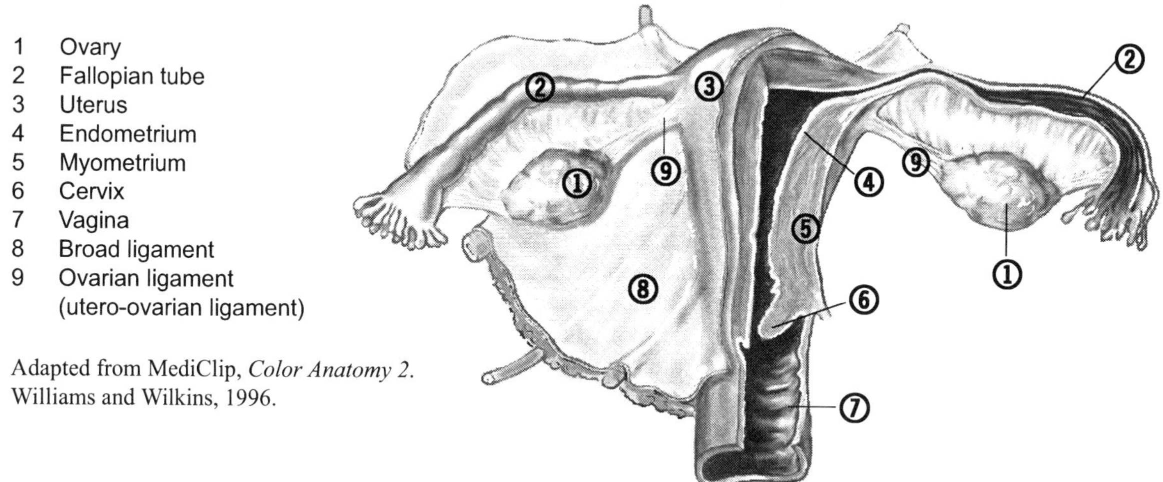

1 Ovary
2 Fallopian tube
3 Uterus
4 Endometrium
5 Myometrium
6 Cervix
7 Vagina
8 Broad ligament
9 Ovarian ligament (utero-ovarian ligament)

Adapted from MediClip, *Color Anatomy 2.* Williams and Wilkins, 1996.

Figure 2. Anatomy of Female Genital and Pelvic Organs (*sagittal view*)

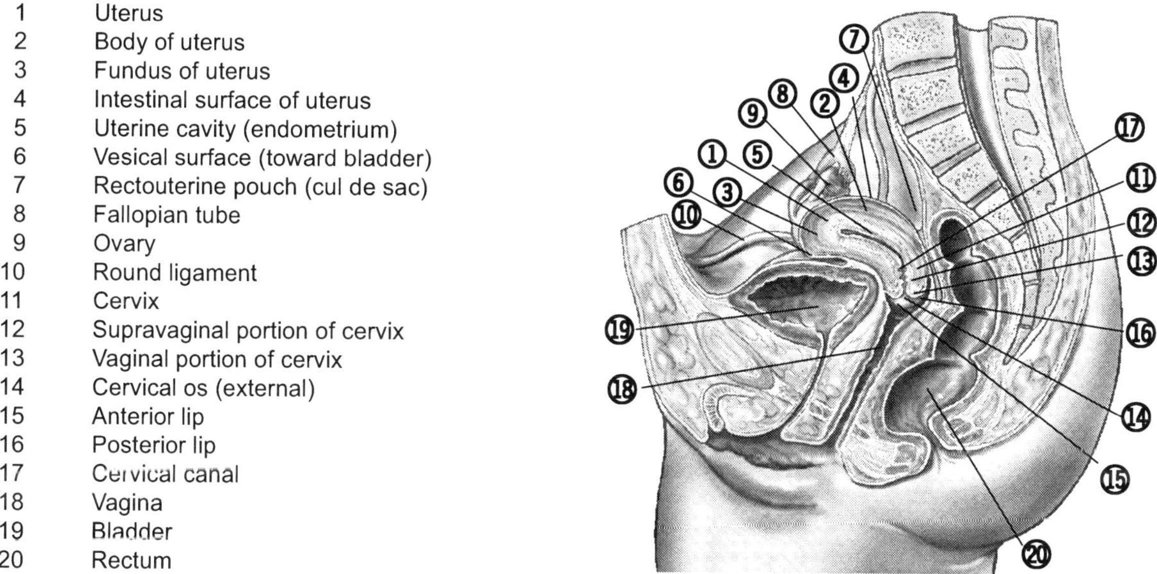

1 Uterus
2 Body of uterus
3 Fundus of uterus
4 Intestinal surface of uterus
5 Uterine cavity (endometrium)
6 Vesical surface (toward bladder)
7 Rectouterine pouch (cul de sac)
8 Fallopian tube
9 Ovary
10 Round ligament
11 Cervix
12 Supravaginal portion of cervix
13 Vaginal portion of cervix
14 Cervical os (external)
15 Anterior lip
16 Posterior lip
17 Cervical canal
18 Vagina
19 Bladder
20 Rectum

Adapted from MediClip, *Color Anatomy 2.* Williams and Wilkins, 1996.

Figure 3. Parts of the Uterus (C55.9)

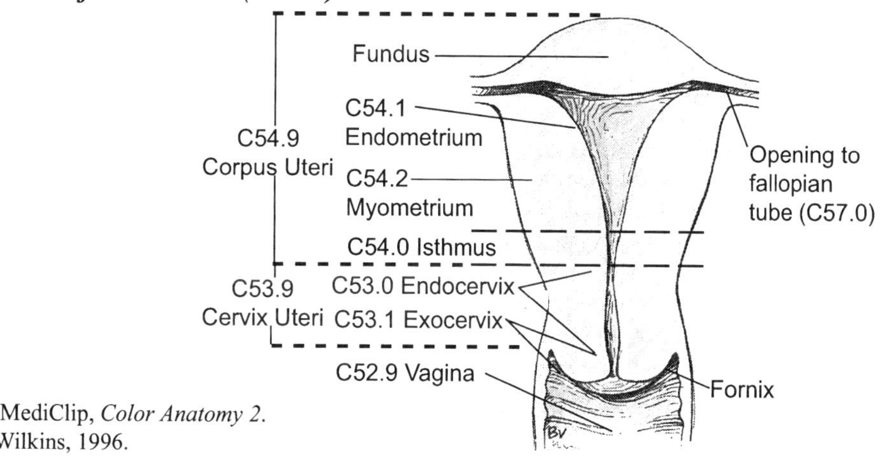

Adapted from MediClip, *Color Anatomy 2.* Williams and Wilkins, 1996.

Anatomy, *continued*

The cervix is the lower opening of the uterus; the fallopian tubes provide two additional openings to the uterus.

The fundus of the uterus is the portion that lies above a line drawn between the entrances of the fallopian tubes into the upper uterus.

The body of the uterus has three layers:

Endometrium—innermost mucosal surface consisting of epithelial and mucous membrane; no muscularis mucosae or submucosa; no blood vessels or lymphatics; most common site of cancer in uterus

Myometrium—middle muscular layer; origin of sarcomas

Serosa or perimetrium—outer serosal surface; connective tissue that surrounds the uterus and separates the cervix from the bladder; part of visceral peritoneum; extends between the serosal layers of the broad ligaments from the uterus to the pelvic walls

The lower third of the uterus is the ***cervix*** (C53.9) or neck of the uterus**,** which is subdivided into the endocervix (endo = inner) and the exocervix (exo = outer). The upper two-thirds of the cervix (endocervix, C53.0) contains mucin-secreting columnar glandular epithelium. The central opening or endocervical canal is normally about 8 mm wide. Adenosquamous carcinoma may arise here. The lower third of the cervix (exocervix or ectocervix, C53.1) is comprised of stratified squamous epithelium extending onto the lip of the cervix. The point at which the columnar epithelium of the endocervix transitions into the squamous epithelium of the exocervix is called the squamocolumnar junction (C53.8), which is visible through a colposcope. The squamo-columnar junction is the most common primary site within the cervix.

The cervix projects into the ***vagina*** about 1 cm, and the circular trough formed at the upper end of the vagina around the cervix is the fornix or vaginal vault. There are four fornices: two lateral, anterior, and posterior. The lip or portio (portio vaginalis) is the portion of the cervix that extends into the vagina. The cervix opens into the vagina through the external cervical ***os***.

Other Structures of the Female Genital System (Figure 1)

The ***broad ligament***, a fold of peritoneum, supports all of the internal female genital organs. The ovaries are suspended between the layers of the broad ligament, and attached by the ***suspensory*** or ***infundibulopelvic ligament*** to the lateral pelvic wall. The ***cardinal ligament*** (also called the lateral cervical or transverse cervical ligament), which is located at the base of the broad ligament and attached to the cervix and upper part of the vagina, contains the uterine artery and vein. Another ligament, the ***round*** or ***ovarian ligament***, attaches the medial edge of the ovary to the uterus just below the entrance of the fallopian tube into the uterus. These ligaments, together with the fallopian tubes and the ovaries, are collectively referred to as the ***adnexa***.

The Pouch of Douglas (rectouterine pouch or cul de sac) is the space between the rectum and the uterus. This is the lowest part of the abdominal cavity.

REGIONAL LYMPH NODES

The regional lymph nodes of the female genital tract are primarily in the shadow of the pelvic bones (pelvic lymph nodes, NOS). Figure 4 shows the regional lymph node chains of the cervix and corpus uteri. Review Table 1 to identify which nodes are regional by site.

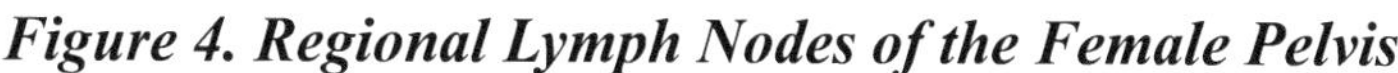

Figure 4. Regional Lymph Nodes of the Female Pelvis

1 External iliac
2 Common iliac
3 Internal iliac
4 Lateral sacral
5 Aortic
6 Inguinal

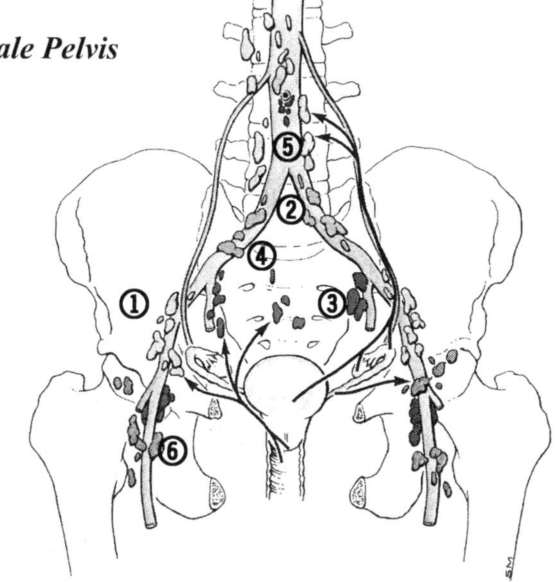

Adapted from MediClip, Grant's Atlas Images 3: Perineum, Pelvis and Lower Limb. Williams and Wilkins, 1998.

Table 1. Regional Lymph Node Chains by Primary Site

Lymph node chain	Cervix	Corpus
Aortic (para-, peri-, lateral)		■
Hypogastric (obturator)	■	■
Iliac, common	■	■
Iliac, external	■	■
Iliac, internal	■	■
Paracervical	■	■
Parametrial	■	■
Pelvic, NOS	■	■
Sacral, NOS	■	■
Sacral, lateral	■	■
Sacral, middle	■	■
Sacral, pre-	■	■
Sacral, utero-	■	■

Note: Para-aortic lymph nodes are distant for cervix, if involved.

DISTANT METASTASES

For corpus cancer, the most common mode of distant spread is direct extension to the vagina. Distant lymph nodes include the inguinal and infraclavicular nodes. Discontinuous metastases to the surfaces of intra-abdominal organs may be seen with certain cell types. Hematogenous metastases may involve the lung, liver, bone and brain.

The most common mode of distant spread for cervical cancer is direct extension to the vagina or other pelvic organs. Distant lymph nodes include the para-aortic, inguinal, mediastinal, and supraclavicular nodes. Cervical cancer can also spread hematogenously to lung, bone, spine and pelvic nerves.

MULTIPLE PRIMARY RULES

Uterine cancers are included in the "Other Sites" multiple primary and histology coding rules. The uterus is not a lateral site. The site-specific rules for multiple primaries provide a detailed priority for determining the primary site.

Features of "Other Sites" Rules

- 18 multiple primaries rules, of which 7 are specific to certain primary sites (prostate, ovary, thyroid, Kaposi sarcoma, retinoblastoma) and will not be discussed here.
- ONE year between diagnoses
- Bilateral tumors are multiple primaries except if described as a metastasis (not applicable to uterine cancers)
- Histology coding rules in five sections (31 rules total)
    - 6 rules (H1 – H6) in Single Tumor: In Situ module
    - 1 rule (H7) in Single Tumor: Invasive and In Situ module
    - 10 rules (H8 – H17) in Single Tumor: Invasive module
    - 14 rules (H18 – H31) in Multiple Tumors Abstracted as a Single Primary module
- Histology coding rules refer to a chart in the site-specific Terms and Definitions providing priorities for most specific histology code

Summary of Multiple Primary Rules

This is only a summary of the multiple primary rules for uterine cancers. Details of the rules are provided in the official published documents available from www.seer.cancer.gov/tools/mphrules. Refer to the General Instructions for information about coding more specific terms, missing pathology or cytology reports, and other aspects of the rules for this and other sets of site-specific rules. **Always** refer to the site-specific rules themselves in your preferred format when determining how many abstracts to prepare or the correct histology code for an individual abstract. The published rules include more discussion, examples, and notes.

The standard three modules of the multiple primaries rules are present: unknown if single or multiple tumors, single tumor, and multiple tumors.

- Count only macroscopic, non-metastatic tumors when deciding which module applies.

The first module, unknown if single or multiple tumors, is the same for all site-specific sets of rules:

M1. Number of tumors (single or multiple) can't be determined = single

Uterine cancer rules are similar to most other multiple primary rules in that there is only one rule for single tumors:

M2. Single tumor = single

The priority of the multiple tumors rules is as follows:

M3 – M9. Site-specific rules not applicable to uterine cancers
M10. Diagnosis dates more than 1 year apart = multiple
M11. Topography code different at 2nd or 3rd character = multiple
M12. Site-specific rule not applicable to uterine cancers.
M13. Frank in situ/invasive adenocarcinoma and in situ/invasive tumor in a polyp = single
M14. Multiple in situ/malignant polyps = single
M15. Invasive carcinoma after in situ more than 60 days = multiple
M16. Non-specific and specific histology codes = single
M17. Histology different at first, second, or third digit = multiple
M18. All other scenarios = single

HISTOLOGIC CELL TYPES OF UTERINE CANCER

CORPUS

The corpus of the uterus is primarily a glandular organ, so most cancers are adenocarcinomas.

- The most common malignancy of the endometrium is adenocarcinoma (814_/3). This cell type represents about 75% of all endometrial carcinoma cases. Adenocarcinoma arises in the glandular tissue of the endometrium.
  Note: Endometrioid carcinoma (8380) is a descriptive term meaning that the (adeno)carcinoma has characteristics of a glandular carcinoma of the endometrium. Endometrioid carcinoma is usually primary in the ovary, but in recent years pathologists have been using the term endometrioid to describe primary adenocarcinoma of the endometrium that is hormonally sensitive. Endometrioid carcinoma in other sites should not be coded as metastatic from the endometrium nor should the endometrium be coded as a metastatic site unless histologically proven. Review the case carefully for a description of the primary site. If the final diagnosis is endometrioid adenocarcinoma of the endometrium, use code 8380.
- Clear cell carcinoma (8310/3; 1% of all cases)
- Papillary serous carcinoma (8460/3; 6% of all cases)
- Adenoacanthoma (8570/3; adenocarcinoma with a benign-looking squamous component)
- Adenosquamous carcinoma (8560/3; 18% of all cases)—mixed adenocarcinoma and squamous carcinoma; arises at the squamocolumnar junction
- Endometrial stromal sarcoma (8930/3, 8931/3)—a sarcoma that arises in the glandular tissues of the endometrium. This cell type should not be coded or staged as a soft tissue tumor. Endometrial stromal sarcoma is subcategorized as high grade (8930/3) or low grade (8931/3).
- Choriocarcinoma (9100/3)—a high grade malignancy of placental (chorionic) tissue. The primary site should be coded as placenta rather than endometrium.

Atypical adenomatous hyperplasia is a benign condition regarded by some as a precursor to endometrial carcinoma. It should not be reported to a cancer registry.

Sarcomas arise from the smooth muscle of the myometrium and, unless another primary site is specified, should be coded to C54.2 myometrium.

- Carcinosarcoma (8980/3), formerly called malignant mixed Mullerian tumor (8950/3), or malignant mesodermal mixed tumor (8951/3)
- Leiomyosarcoma* (8890/3, 8891/3; 1% of all cases)
- Endometrial stromal sarcoma* (8930/3, 8931/3)—arise in the supporting connective tissue of the endometrium
- Adenosarcoma* (8933/3)—low grade sarcomatous mesenchymal malignancy with a benign epithelial component

* These sarcomas are staged separately from carcinomas of the corpus; see TNM staging and Collaborative Stage Data Collection System (CS) later in this chapter.

FIGO Grade

Grade or differentiation is one of the principal prognostic factors for endometrial cancer. FIGO developed criteria for grading endometrial cancers that correspond to varying survival rates for clinical stage I cancers. Information about the tumor growth pattern, which is part of the definition of the FIGO grades, is recorded in CS Site-Specific Factor 7 (refer to CS SSF7 later in this chapter). The FIGO grades can be recorded as the 6th digit of the ICD-O-3 morphology code as follows:

FIGO Grade, *continued*

	FIGO Grade and definition	ICD-O Grade	5 yr Surv.
I	≤ 5% of a nonsquamous or nonmorular solid growth pattern	1	94%
II	6 – 50% of a nonsquamous or nonmorular solid growth pattern	2	88%
III	> 50% of a nonsquamous or nonmorular solid growth pattern	3	79%

Note: Occasionally, it is not possible to determine whether the primary is in the corpus or cervix. In such cases, after all diagnostic workup is complete, assign adenocarcinomas to a corpus primary and epidermal (squamous) carcinomas to a cervical primary.

CERVIX

The cervix is essentially a tube lined with epithelial cells.

- Ninety percent of all cervical cancers are squamous cell carcinoma (8070/3), which develops mostly in the lower third of the cervix and the lip of the cervix, although it can also extend into the vagina. This cell type is also called epidermoid carcinoma.
  Squamous carcinomas can be subcategorized as
  - Keratinizing (8071/3)
  - Non-keratinizing (8072/3)
    - large cell nonkeratinizing (8072/3)
    - small cell nonkeratinizing (8073/3)
  - Spindle cell type (8074/3)
- Squamous carcinoma in situ (8070/2; showing no stromal invasion)
- Squamous carcinoma in situ with questionable stromal invasion (8076/2)
- Squamous carcinoma in situ with microinvasion (8076/3) This is a pathologic determination where the invasion of the stroma is less than 3 mm.
- Cervical intraepithelial neoplasia, grade III (8077/2; see comments below)
- **Synonyms for in situ carcinoma**: Bowen's disease, Stage 0, CIN grade III, confined to epithelium, intraepithelial, involvement up to but not including the basement membrane, noninfiltrating, noninvasive, no stromal involvement
- Adenocarcinoma (8140/3; 10% of cases)—arises in the upper two-thirds of the cervical canal
- Adenosquamous carcinoma (85603—mixed adenocarcinoma and epidermoid carcinoma)—arises at the squamocolumnar junction
- Small cell carcinoma (8041/3)—rare
- Sarcoma (cell types vary)—rare
- Lymphoma (many cell types)—rare

Cervical Intraepithelial Neoplasia (CIN) and The Bethesda Cytology Reporting System

This pathologic descriptive system consists of two categories, low grade squamous intraepithelial lesions (LGSIL) and high grade squamous intraepithelial lesions (HGSIL). The low grade SIL is the equivalent of CIN I; the high grade is comprised of CIN II (moderate dysplasia) and CIN III (severe dysplasia and carcinoma in situ). When a cervical lesion is described simply as high grade SIL, there is no way to differentiate whether it is CIN II or CIN III. Even within CIN III, there is no way to determine whether the lesion is severe dysplasia or carcinoma in situ. The case is not reportable if the pathology report describes only severe dysplasia. Consequently, as the Bethesda System descriptors have been adopted by pathologists, the descriptions that determine the reportability of carcinoma in situ have blurred. Because the true carcinomas in situ cannot be distinguished from all of the dysplasias, central cancer registries in North America have made the decision not to require accessioning of cervical carcinoma in situ. Adenocarcinoma in situ is still reportable to some central cancer registries.

Pap Smears

The mortality rate for cervical cancer has declined in the past 40 years due to improvements in the early detection of the disease. The 50% decrease in deaths from cervical cancer can be attributed almost entirely to the development of the Pap smear as a screening tool. The Pap smear was originally reported in the terms Class I through Class V (frank malignancy) (Table 2).

Table 2. Papanicolaou's Scale

I	Absence of atypical or abnormal cells; negative
II	Atypical cytology, dysplastic, borderline but not neoplastic
III	Cytology suggestive of but not inclusive of malignancy (suspect is a term that is used)
IV	Cytology strongly suggestive of or strongly suspect malignancy
V	Cytology conclusive of malignancy; cancer cells present
	Note: A Class V Pap smear on this scale is the equivalent of carcinoma in situ.

However, the use of descriptive terms by the pathologist or cytologist conveys more information to the clinician. Suggested descriptive terminology includes:

- Unsatisfactory specimen
- No abnormal cells
- Mild squamous atypia: metaplasia, inflammation, regeneration/repair, radiation or viral effect
- Dysplastic or atypical cells—mild, moderate, severe (Cervical Intraepithelial Neoplasia)
- Carcinoma in situ
- Invasive malignant cells

Note: Microinvasive tumor has invaded the stroma microscopically. This is a localized lesion and is no longer in situ. In situ tumor with microinvasion should not be coded as carcinoma in situ.

HISTOLOGY CODING RULES

Uterine cancers are included in the "Other Sites" multiple primary and histology coding rules. For these sites, there are four modules based on behavior and number of tumors. Make sure you are looking at the rules in the correct section. The first few rules may seem repetitive, but this makes each module self-contained so the reader doesn't have to jump from one place to another in the rules.

The Histology Coding Rules for "Other Sites" include an important new concept.

- A rule has been added that, when a tumor has both an invasive histology and a different in situ histology, the invasive histology should be coded. Pathologists generally agree that it is the invasive part of the tumor that has the potential to do the most harm to the patient; thus the in situ component should be disregarded and the histology of the invasive component should be assigned to the case.
- In the non-specific/specific coding rules (H4, H13 and H29), the following terms indicate a more specific type:
    - Invasive cancers: type, subtype, predominantly, with features of, major, with [something] differentiation
    - In situ cancers: pattern, architecture, type, subtype, predominantly, with features of, major, with [something] differentiation

Single Tumor: In situ Only

H1. If no pathology/cytology report available, code the histology stated by the clinician.

H2. If only one histology is stated, code that.

H3. This rule deals with how to code an adenocarcinoma arising in a polyp. This occurs very rarely in the uterus, so it will not be explained in detail here.

Histology Coding Rules, *continued*

H4. Code the more specific histology when one term is NOS and the other is more specific.
   - NOS terms: cancer, NOS; carcinoma, NOS; adenocarcinoma, NOS; squamous cell carcinoma, NOS; melanoma, NOS; sarcoma, NOS

H5. Use a mixed or combination code from Table 2 (in MP/H manual) for a single tumor with multiple specific histologies or a non-specific histology and multiple specific histologies.

H6. If no other rule applies, use the numerically higher ICD-O-3 code as a last priority.

Single Tumor: Invasive and In Situ

H7. Code invasive histology; ignore in situ terms.

Single Tumor: Invasive Only

H8. If no pathology/cytology report available, code the histology stated by the clinician. This is the same rule as H1 but applies to single, invasive tumors.

H9. Code histology from a metastatic site if there is no tissue or cells from the primary site.

H10. Prostate-specific rule.

H11. If only one histology is stated, code that.

H12. This rule deals with how to code an adenocarcinoma arising in a polyp. This occurs very rarely in the uterus, so it will not be explained in detail here.

H13. Code the more specific histology when one term is NOS and the other is more specific.
   - NOS terms: cancer, NOS; carcinoma, NOS; adenocarcinoma, NOS; squamous cell carcinoma, NOS; melanoma, NOS; sarcoma, NOS

H14. Thyroid-specific rule.

H15. Thyroid-specific rule.

H16. Use a mixed or combination code from Table 2 (in MP/H manual) for a single tumor with multiple specific histologies or a non-specific histology and multiple specific histologies.

H17. If no other rule applies, use the numerically higher ICD-O-3 code as a last priority.

Multiple Tumors Abstracted as a Single Primary

H18. If no pathology/cytology report available, code the histology stated by the clinician. This is the same rule as H8 but applies to multiple tumors abstracted as a single primary.

H19. Code histology from a metastatic site if there is no tissue or cells from the primary site.

H20. Prostate-specific rule.

H21. Code 8077/2 for squamous intraepithelial neoplasias described as in situ or reportable by agreement—vulva (VIN III), vagina (VAIN III), cervix (CIN III) and anus (AIN III).

H22. Code 8148/2 for glandular intraepithelial neoplasias described as in situ or reportable by agreement—prostate (PIN III) and pancreas (PAIN III).

H23. If only one histology is stated, code that.

H24. Extramammary Paget disease rule for anus, perianal region or vulva only.

H25. This rule deals with how to code an adenocarcinoma arising in a polyp. This occurs very rarely in the uterus, so it will not be explained in detail here.

H26. Thyroid-specific rule.

H27. Thyroid-specific rule.

H28. Code single invasive histology for invasive-in situ combinations.

H29. Code the more specific histology when one term is NOS and the other is more specific.
   - NOS terms: cancer, NOS; carcinoma, NOS; adenocarcinoma, NOS; squamous cell carcinoma, NOS; melanoma, NOS; sarcoma, NOS

H30. Use a mixed or combination code from Table 2 (in MP/H manual) for a single tumor with multiple specific histologies or a non-specific histology and multiple specific histologies.

H31. If no other rule applies, use the numerically higher ICD-O-3 code as a last priority.

Histology Coding Rules, *continued*

IMPORTANT NOTE: USING CODE 8323
Rules H5, H16 and H30 refer to Table 2 for combination codes to be used when a tumor contains multiple specific histologies. In that table, there are instructions for using 8323, mixed cell adenocarcinoma, for GYN malignancies, particularly ovary and endometrium. Specifically, if a GYN tumor contains two or more of the following cell types, use code 8323 even though the final diagnosis may not say "mixed cell adenocarcinoma." The cell types included in this rule are combinations of clear cell, endometroid, mucinous, papillary, serous, squamous, and transitional (Brenner).

UTERINE CANCER ABSTRACTING GUIDELINES

Review the medical record for the following diagnostic and staging procedures. Look for information (positive and negative) that describes the tumor location, tumor size, presence of multiple tumors, lymph node involvement, extension beyond the organ of origin, seeding, implants, or metastasis to distant sites/organs.

HISTORY

The most common symptoms of uterine cancer are abnormal bleeding and pain. More than 90% of women diagnosed with endometrial cancer have abnormal vaginal bleeding. Other corpus cancer symptoms include irregular, prolonged, or excessive menstrual bleeding or spotting between menses or more than one year after the completion of menopause.

Cervical cancer is generally asymptomatic in its early stages, which is why regular screening is so important. Symptoms of more advanced cervical cancer include persistent abnormal (yellow, odorous) vaginal discharge, unexplained vaginal spotting or bleeding, pelvic or low back pain, painful urination, and dyspareunia (painful sexual intercourse).

Where to look in the patient's record

- History and physical exam report
- Consultation report(s)
- Physician's progress notes

What information to select and record (record all dates)
Unless your facility requires documentation of presenting symptoms or chief complaint, record only those signs and symptoms that document

- Date of onset and type of symptoms
- Personal history of cancer, in particular breast, colon, or ovarian that may indicate a genetic tendency toward developing uterine cancer

Other information to note (but does not document location, tumor size, or extent of disease)

- History of pregnancies and deliveries (sometimes written as "para [number] gravida [number]")
- History of estrogen use or hormone replacement therapy (for corpus cancer)
- History of human papilloma virus (HPV) infection, HIV infection, or STDs (sexually transmitted diseases (for cervical cancer)
- For cervical cancer, history of receiving Gardasil or Cervarix vaccine
- Family history of cancer (similar to personal history of cancer, above)

PHYSICAL EXAM

A careful pelvic examination should be part of the overall physical examination of the patient. However, because of the location of the uterus deep in the pelvis, it may not be possible to palpate the regional (pelvic) lymph nodes directly.

- **Pelvic examination** — manual or speculum evaluation of the cervix, vagina, rectum, external genitalia. Digital examination of the rectum and vagina is also called a rectovaginal exam.
- "**Sounding**" of the uterus — measuring the depth of the uterus by inserting a probe and measuring the distance from the back of the uterine cavity to the external os. The depth may be measured in inches or centimeters. A D & C may also give this information. The size and depth of the uterus has some prognostic significance, but uterine enlargement may also be caused by fibroids or adenomyosis. A description that the uterus is "the size of *xx* weeks pregnancy" is not adequate to differentiate different kinds of tumors.
- **Examination under Anesthesia (EUA)**—bimanual examination (Figure 5) of the pelvis and external abdomen while patient is anesthetized, using one hand in the pelvis and the other hand to press on the organs externally.

Figure 5. Bimanual Pelvic Exam

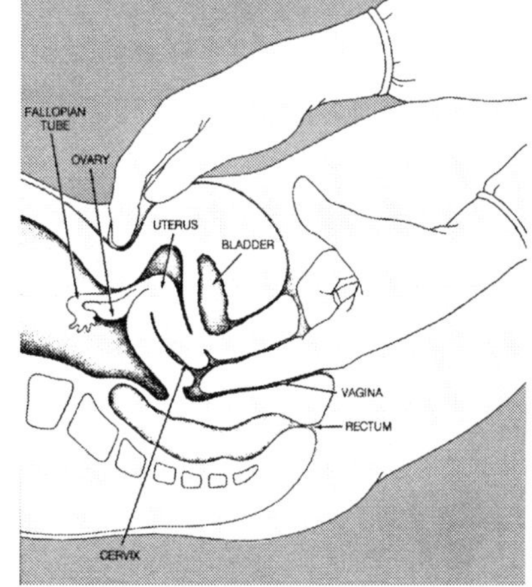

Image source: National Cancer Institute. In the public domain.

Where to look in the patient's record

- History and physical exam report
- Consultation report(s)
- Physician's progress notes
- Operative reports

What information to select and record (record all dates)

Pertinent findings that detail what the physician sees and feels when the patient is examined:

- Pelvic examination: palpable pelvic masses, status of external genitalia
- Size of uterus from sounding or palpation
- Mention of masses or enlarged organs ("-megaly" such as hepatomegaly—enlargement of the liver)
- Size of tumor if visualized by physician
- Palpation of accessible lymph nodes: supraclavicular, other distant lymph nodes
- General survey of rest of the body (overall physical condition)

IMAGING *(see also Diagnoatic Tests and Tumor Markers chapter)*

Tests may be performed on an outpatient basis both pre-and post-admission. The most common sites of distant metastases from uterine cancers are lung and liver.

- **Pelvic Ultrasound—**assessing the structures in the pelvis on images created by sound waves. A probe or transducer is inserted into the vagina (transvaginal) or passed back and forth across the external pelvis. The sound waves can delineate the uterus, ovaries, cervix, fallopian tubes, and bladder.

Imaging, ***continued***

X-rays and Scans —The following imaging procedures may be used to look for distant metastases. See definitions in the Diagnostic Tests and Tumor Markers chapter of this CASEbook.

- **Chest X-ray**
- **Intravenous pyelography (IVP)**—evaluation for involvement of ureters or bladder
- **CT Scans** of chest, abdomen, pelvis or head
- **MRI** of abdomen, pelvis chest or head
- **PET scans**
- **Bone scans**

What information to select and record (record all dates)
Pertinent findings on radiology report from each study including:

- Name of procedure (chest x-ray, CT abdomen, etc.)
- Area of the body being examined
- Both positive and negative findings
- Location of tumor stated by radiologist, if noted
- Size of tumor stated by radiologist, if noted
- Extent of disease – regional or distant spread
- Status of liver
- Lymph node status

LABORATORY TESTS AND TUMOR MARKERS *(see also Diagnostic Tests and Tumor Markers chapter)*

In general, laboratory tests and tumor markers are infrequently used as diagnostic procedures for uterine cancers. However, they may be ordered as follow-up to monitor for recurrence.

CORPUS

- **CA-125**—nonspecific for corpus cancer, but may be a marker for ovarian cancer that has spread to the corpus, or as a follow-up marker for endometrial cancer
- **Estrogen Receptor Assay (ERA)**—a laboratory test to determine the responsiveness of the tumor to endocrine therapy or to removal of the ovaries. Tumors that are negative for estrogen receptors rarely respond to hormone manipulation; about 55% of ER positive tumors will respond to endocrine therapy. The unit of measurement is femtomoles (fmoles) per milligram of tumor.
  Types of ERA: Quantified (measured in femtomoles or fmoles)
  Immunohistochemical—a qualitative measurement of the observed number of hormone responsive cells, reported as positive or negative
  Test results—negative: 3 fmoles or less. ERA may not be performed if tumor is less than 1.0 cm in size or if tumor is completely in situ.
- **Progesterone Receptor Assay (PRA)**—A laboratory test to determine the responsiveness of the tumor to endocrine therapy or to removal of the ovaries. Progesterone receptor assay increases the reliability of estrogen receptor assay results: a positive progesterone receptor assay indicates greater likelihood that the patient will respond to hormone therapy. The unit of measurement is femtomoles (fmoles) per milligram of tumor.
  Types of PRA: Quantified (measured in femtomoles or fmoles)
  Immunohistochemical—a qualitative measurement of the observed number of hormone responsive cells, reported as positive or negative
  Test results—negative: 5 fmoles or less. Test may not be performed if tumor is less than 1.0 cm in size or if tumor is completely in situ.

Laboratory Tests and Tumor Markers, *continued*

CERVIX

- **SCC (Squamous Cell Carcinoma) Antigen**—monitors tumor burden after treatment for squamous cell carcinoma; used in advanced cases; non-specific to cervical carcinoma but specific to squamous cell carcinoma

ENDOSCOPY (Scopes)

Endoscopy, specifically colposcopy, is the best way to locate and inspect a lesion on the exocervix. Figure 6 shows how different type of exocervical lesions look through a colposcope. Other types of endoscopies are used to evaluate the extent of tumor spread from the primary site. All of these procedures use a fiberoptic instrument to examine the organ.

- **Colposcopy**—examination of the vagina and cervix through a colposcope, an instrument containing a magnifying lens that is inserted into the vagina
- **Hysteroscopy**—examination of the uterus
- **Laparoscopy—**examination of the external surfaces of pelvic organs with a scope inserted into the abdomen through a small incision below the navel
- **Cystoscopy—**examination of the bladder
- **Proctosigmoidoscopy**—examination of the rectum and sigmoid

Figure 6. Exocervical Lesions

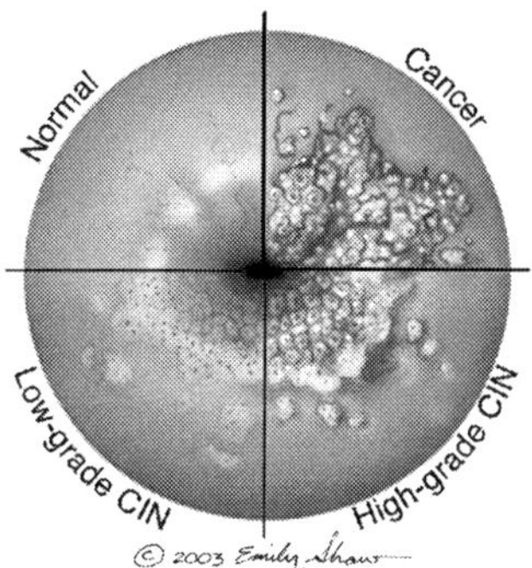

Image source: © Emily Shaw. Used with permission.

What to select and record (record all dates)

- Name of procedure (colposcopy, laparoscopy, hysteroscopy)
- Pertinent findings as described by the physician
    - Location of the tumor
    - Size of the tumor
    - Mention of organ involvement by direct extension or metastases

OPERATIVE FINDINGS

Operative reports from diagnostic, exploratory procedures and/or cancer directed definitive treatment may provide supplementary information on the status of the primary tumor, lymph nodes, or tumor extension and distant metastases. Record the pertinent findings of what the surgeon observed during any of the procedures listed in the Endoscopy section of this chapter, the diagnostic procedures, or the cancer-directed surgeries of the primary site, regional lymph nodes, or distant metastases.

What information to select and record (record all dates)

Pertinent findings as described by the surgeon:

- Size of tumor, if noted
- Status of pelvic lymph nodes
- Gross involvement of surgical margin(s)
- Gross (visual) extent of tumor within cervix or corpus
- Seeding, studding, talcum powder appearance of any other organs
- If surgery is performed to a regional and/or distant site only, indicate this
- Presence and location of any gross tumor not resected by the surgeon
- If no findings are documented, record "findings not recorded"
- Reason, if no cancer-directed surgery to the cervix or corpus was performed

DIAGNOSTIC PROCEDURES

CYTOLOGY REPORTS

- **Pap Smear** or **Pap test**—aspiration, scraping or brushing of the cervix for cytologic evaluation. A Pap smear will diagnose in situ or invasive cervical cancer but is not a reliable method for ruling out endometrial cancer when used by itself. The Pap smear was named after Dr. George Papanicolaou, a Greek-American cytologist and pathologist who developed the cytodiagnostic test for the detection of early cervical cancer in the 1920s.
- **Dilatation and Curettage (D & C)**—also called D and C. Dilation of the cervix with a speculum and scraping or aspirating the contents of the uterus for cytologic examination
- **Endometrial or pelvic washings**—instillation of saline solution into the endometrium or pelvic cavity that is then suctioned out and analyzed for malignant cells

HISTOLOGY

- **Fractional Curettage**—separate scraping of material from the endocervix and walls of uterus in a set order to determine which site may be the source of the malignancy. This is the preferred diagnostic procedure for endometrial cancer but can also identify cervical cancer that has spread to the corpus.
- **Cervical biopsy**—removal of tissue from the cervix by conization, LEEP, or other procedure (see Cervix Treatment below)
- **Endometrial biopsy**—removal of a small piece of the lining of the uterus (endometrium) for microscopic analysis
- **Omentectomy**—removal of the fatty "apron" that covers the abdomen to look for metastases from endometrial cancer. This procedure is separate from the hysterectomy and is not usually done for cervical cancer. Omentectomy for corpus cancer is coded in CS Site-Specific Factor 8.
- **Cytoreduction or debulking**—if the endometrial or cervical cancer is widespread in the pelvis or abdomen, the surgeon may try to reduce the amount of tumor tissue so that chemotherapy or radiation will be more effective
- **Staging Procedures**—procedures that will yield tissue specimens that can document spread beyond the uterus
    - **Peritoneal biopsies**—tissue samples from the lining of the pelvis and abdomen
    - **Lymph node dissection, lymph node sampling, or lymph node biopsies**—pelvic and para-aortic nodes are regional for corpus; pelvic nodes are regional for cervix.
    - **Bilateral salpingo-oophorectomy**—corpus cancers can spread to the adnexa

PATHOLOGY REPORTS

Pathologic evaluation of any resected tissue not only establishes a diagnosis, but also provides important staging (and therefore prognostic) information. All parts of the pathology report—the gross examination of the specimen, the microscopic examination, the final diagnosis and comments—should be reviewed for staging, grade, and histology information, but only the final diagnosis should be used to code the histology.

If a CAP checklist (outline format provided by the College of American Pathologists) is provided, the information may be easier to find in that section of the pathology report than in the gross and microscopic narrative sections. The CAP checklist is also called a synoptic report or CAP protocol. An example of a CAP protocol is shown in Table 3.

Pathology Reports, ***continued***

When reviewing pathology reports for cytologies, biopsies and/or surgical resections, note the following:

What information to select and record (record date tissue was collected)

Final Diagnosis

- Histology (cell type)—Follow the histology coding rules for using this information. Remember, for corpus and cervix, the ICD-O morphology code is based only from the final diagnosis.
- Behavior and grade
  - FIGO grade
  - Standard terminology: well-, moderately-, poorly-differentiated
- Mixed histology information, especially for corpus carcinoma

Gross

- Specimen source (resection, biopsy, cytology)
- Site (cervix, corpus, lymph node, metastatic site, other)
- Tumor size (if complete resection)

Microscopic pathology

- Biopsy: FNA of cells or tissue
  - Site(s) of positive biopsies

Table 3. Example of College of American Pathologists (CAP) Corpus (Endometrium) Cancer Protocol

TUMOR SUMMARY

Specimen Type	Hysterectomy
Tumor Site	Corpus
Tumor Size	2 x 2 x 1.5 cm
Closest Margin to Tumor	Cervical/vaginal (distance from tumor 2 cm) Right parametrial (distance from tumor 1cm) Left parametrial (distance from tumor (1 cm)
Other Organs Involved	None
Histologic Type	Serous adenocarcinoma
Histologic grade	G1: 5% or less non-squamous solid growth
Myometrial invasion	Early superficial noted
Depth of invasion	2-3 mm
Myometrial thickness	1.7 cm
Extent of Invasion	T1a (IA): Tumor invades up to or less than 1/2 of myometrium.
Margins	Uninvolved by tumor Distance of tumor from closest margin 1 cm
Blood/lymphatic Vessel Invasion	Absent
Regional lymph Nodes	NO: No regional lymph node metastasis # examined 20
Distant Metastasis	Not assessed
Additional Pathologic Findings	Hyperplasia Complex (adenomatous)

DIAGNOSIS

1) Nine benign right external iliac lymph nodes
2) Three benign right internal iliac lymph nodes
3) Three benign right obturator lymph nodes
4) One benign left external lymph node
5) Two benign left internal lymph nodes
6) Two benign left obturator lymph nodes
7) Panhysterectomy specimen showing grade 1 serous carcinoma of the endometrium

Pathology Reports, *continued*

- Resection:
  - Presence of tumor on serosal surface
  - Involvement of adjacent structures (ovaries, fallopian tubes, vagina)
  - Status of margins
- Names and number of examined lymph nodes
- Number of lymph nodes positive/number examined
- Findings from any other organ biopsies/resections
- Stage as reported by the pathologist
  - FIGO stage
  - TNM stage

UTERINE CANCER DISEASE MANAGEMENT

Most women who develop endometrial cancer are past child-bearing age. The standard treatment is total abdominal hysterectomy and bilateral salpingo-oophorectomy if the tumor is well or moderately differentiated, involves the upper two-thirds of the corpus, has negative peritoneal cytology, has no involvement of vascular spaces, and/or has less than 50% myometrial invasion.

Either radiation therapy or radical hysterectomy and bilateral lymph node dissection results in cure rates of 85% to 90% for patients with low stage invasive cervical cancer. The choice depends on patient factors and available local expertise. Advantages of surgical treatment include preservation of ovarian function, less of the patient's time taken for treatment, maintenance of vaginal function, decreased possibility of local recurrence, more accurate staging due to assessment of pelvic and para-aortic lymph nodes, and elimination of radiation-induced injury to other pelvic organs. Carcinoma in situ of the cervix is best treated surgically (see below).

SURGERY

Surgical Options for Early Cervical Cancer

Cervical cancer is a disease of younger women in whom preservation of reproductive capability is a consideration. Cervical cancer can be diagnosed while the patient is pregnant. If a carcinoma in situ is diagnosed during pregnancy, no therapy is warranted, although expert colposcopy is recommended to exclude invasive cancer.

If invasive cancer is diagnosed during pregnancy, the treatment depends on the stage of the cancer and the gestational age at diagnosis. Traditionally, immediate therapy appropriate for the disease stage has been recommended when the cancer is diagnosed before fetal maturity, and to delay therapy only if the cancer is detected in the final trimester. More recent studies have recommended deliberate delay for early stage I cancers to allow improved fetal outcome.

For Stage 0, carcinoma in situ cases (80% of all cervical cancers), treatment options include cryo-therapy, laser therapy, thermal ablation, D&C or conization, or hysterectomy. These procedures can be coded as curative treatment for in situ cancers if the procedure is not followed by a hysterectomy. If a hysterectomy is performed, the hysterectomy becomes the cancer-directed surgery.

What information to record (record all dates)

- Definitive (cancer-directed) treatment (name of procedure)
- Reason if no resection is attempted

Surgery, ***continued***

Surgery of Primary Site

The following codes are listed in Appendix B of the American College of Surgeons' *Facility Oncology Registry Data Standards* (FORDS) manual and in Appendix C of the *SEER Program Coding and Staging Manual*. Note that this is not a complete list of codes available. Certain codes differ for corpus (Cor) and cervix (Cer) as indicated below, but the definitions are the same. Many of these procedures can be performed either laparoscopically or through an incision in the pelvis (open). Some types of hysterectomy can be performed vaginally (through the vagina rather than a pelvic incision. Robotic-assisted laparoscopic surgeries are also being performed at some centers.

Cor Cer

10 10 **Local tumor destruction**, NOS (no specimen sent to pathology for codes 10-17)

11 11 **Photodynamic therapy (PDT)**—treatment that uses a drug, called a photosensitizer or photosensitizing agent, and a particular type of light. When the photosensitizer is exposed to a specific wavelength of light, it produces a form of oxygen that kills nearby cells; under clinical evaluation for cervical cancer

12 12 **Electrocautery or fulguration**—destruction of tumor tissue by applying an electrical current directly to the lesion; not a common procedure for cervical cancer

13 13 **Cryosurgery**—freezing the lesion to kill cancer cells (Figure 7)

14 14 **Laser therapy**—destruction of abnormal cells by applying a high-intensity beam of light (laser); see note below

15 15 **Loop Electrocautery Excision Procedure (LEEP)**—see description at cervix code 28

    16 **Laser ablation**—total destruction of the lesion using a laser; see note below

16 17 **Thermal ablation**—heating the tumor to kill cancer cells

Figure 7. Cryosurgery

- **Note:** according to the Inquiry and Response System of the Commission on Cancer, if the surgical notes use the term "ablation" when a laser was used and there was no specimen obtained for pathologic analysis, use code 16 for laser ablation. If the surgical notes simply show that laser was used but do not specify "ablation," assume "destruction" and code 14. If laser ablation was identified and a pathologic specimen was obtained, use code 23.

Image source for Figures 7–9: © Emily Shaw. Used with permission.

20 20 **Local tumor excision, NOS; simple excision, NOS** (specimen sent to pathology for codes 20-29)

24 26 **Excisional biopsy, NOS**

25 **Polypectomy** — removal of an endometrial polyp (specimen sent to pathology)

26 **Myomectomy** — removal of a tumor (myoma or fibroid) from the uterine muscular wall

    27 **Cone biopsy**—also called conization, cold knife cone; surgery to remove a cone-shaped piece of tissue from the cervix and cervical canal for biopsy (Figure 8). This procedure is performed in the operating room with a scalpel (cold knife).

    24 **Cone biopsy with gross excision of lesion**

    29 **Trachelectomy; removal of cervical stump; cervicectomy**—surgical removal of the cervix without removal of the rest of the uterus; used for Stage IA2 and IB cervical cancers

Figure 8. Conization

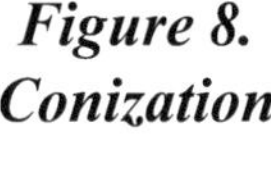

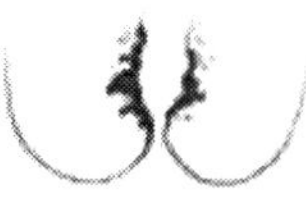

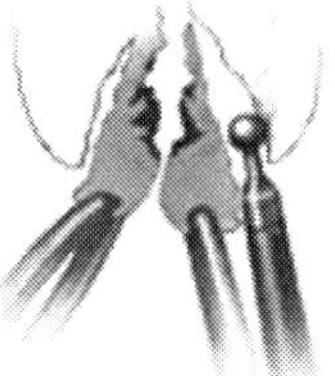

- **Note:** A procedure coded 20/20, 24/26, Cer24, Cor25, Cor26, Cer27, or Cer29 with one of the following techniques is coded to the technique (specimen sent to pathology for these procedures).

21 21 **Electrocautery**

22 22 **Cryosurgery**

23 23 **Laser ablation or excision**

Surgery of Primary Site, *continued*

Cor Cer

25 **Dilatation and curettage (D&C); endocervical curettage**—dilation of the cervix with a speculum and scraping or aspirating the contents for cytologic examination; specimen sent to pathology. This procedure is defined as a cancer-directed treatment for carcinoma in situ of the cervix *only*. For invasive cancer, D&C is coded as an incisional biopsy (code 02) in the Surgical Diagnostic and Staging Procedures field.

28 **Loop Electrocautery Excision Procedure (LEEP)**—best procedure for treating lesions of the exocervix and can be performed in the clinician's office; specimen sent to pathology for this procedure

Figure 9. LEEP

- **LEEP** (Loop Electrocautery Excision Procedure)—an excisional procedure (Figure 9) that uses an electrical energy generator attached to a fine wire loop that when energized functions as a precise and rapid surgical tool to diagnose and/or treat cervical lesions in women with abnormal Pap tests. Other names for this procedure are LLEC (Large Loop Excision of the Cervix), LEETZ (Large Loop Excision of Transformation Zone), Loop Cone Biopsy.

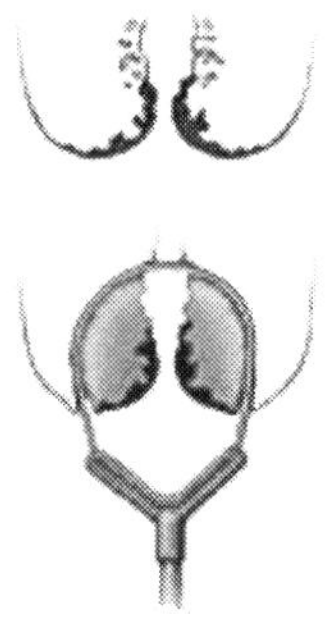

30 **Subtotal hysterectomy**/supracervical hysterectomy/fundectomy with or without removal of tubes and ovaries — partial hysterectomy removing corpus or fundus of uterus leaving cervix in place; use this code if it is not known whether tubes and ovaries are also removed

31 **Subtotal hysterectomy without tubes and ovaries** — hysterectomy as above without salpingo-oophorectomy

32 **Subtotal hysterectomy with tubes and ovaries** — hysterectomy as above with salpingo-oophorectomy; see note under code 50/40.

40 30 **Total hysterectomy**—also called simple hysterectomy or panhysterectomy; removal of cervix and corpus plus a margin of vagina but not the fallopian tubes, ovaries, parametrium, or uterusacral ligaments; resection through an incision in the abdomen. No lymph nodes removed with this procedure.

50 40 **Total (abdominal) hysterectomy with removal of tubes and ovaries**—also called TAH-BSO; the standard procedure for invasive cervical cancer, removing the cervix and corpus and a margin of vagina as well as the fallopian tubes and ovaries

Note: If the patient had a previous unilateral salpingo-oophorectomy for another medical issue, this cancer-directed procedure is coded as a bilateral salpingo-oophorectomy to indicate that both tubes and ovaries had been surgically removed.

60 50 **Modified radical hysterectomy or extended hysterectomy; radical hysterectomy; extended radical hysterectomy**—total abdominal hysterectomy that also includes a 2–3 cm portion of the vagina (more than vaginal cuff) and removal of some lymph nodes; use this code if more tissue is removed than with a standard TAH and BSO but the specific procedure is not described; code lymph node removal in Scope of Regional Lymph Node Surgery

61 51 **Modified radical hysterectomy**—total abdominal hysterectomy and partial vaginectomy with partial removal of parametrium (uterosacral ligament, cardinal ligament and uterine artery) halfway to pelvic wall; usually with lymph node dissection (code the lymph node dissection in Scope of Regional Lymph Node Surgery)

62 52 **Extended hysterectomy**—traditional hysterectomy and lymphadenectomy with a wider margin of tissue (code the lymphadenectomy in Scope of Regional Lymph Node Surgery)

63 53 **Radical hysterectomy; Wertheim procedure**—also called Meigs procedure and Wertheim-Meigs procedure; traditional hysterectomy, partial (upper 1/3) vaginectomy; lymphadenectomy and complete removal of parametrium to pelvic wall (code the lymphadenectomy in Scope of Regional Lymph Node Surgery)

Surgery of Primary Site, *continued*

Cor Cer

64 54 **Extended radical hysterectomy**—Wertheim/Meigs procedure with full mobilization of the ureters past the bladder to allow removal of more paracervical tissue

65 60 **Hysterectomy, NOS** with or without removal of tubes and ovaries—use this code when the specific type of hysterectomy is not named or described

66 61 **Hysterectomy, NOS without removal of tubes and ovaries**—use this code when the specific type of hysterectomy is not named or described but it is known that the tubes and ovaries were *not* removed

67 62 **Hysterectomy, NOS with removal of tubes and ovaries**—use this code when the specific type of hysterectomy is not named or described but it is known that the tubes and ovaries were removed; see note at code 50/40.

75 70 **Pelvic exenteration**—removal of female genital tract and other organs of pelvis; see below. If the bladder and/or part of the colon are removed, the functionality of these organs must be surgically reconstructed.

- **Note:** For codes 76/71 to 79/74, code removal of lymph nodes in Scope of Regional Lymph Node Surgery. The definitions below list specific organs that are removed as part of the procedure. Do not code these organs again in Surgical Procedure of Other Site because they are removed in continuity with the uterus as part of the procedure. For example, removal of the bladder is part of an anterior exenteration. Do not code bladder removal in Surgical Procedure of Other Site.

76 71 **Anterior exenteration**—removal of uterus, tubes, ovaries, vagina, distal ureters and bladder plus pelvic lymph nodes and ligamentous attachments

77 72 **Posterior exenteration**—removal of uterus, tubes, ovaries, rectum and rectosigmoid plus pelvic lymph nodes and ligamentous attachments

78 73 **Total exenteration**—combination of anterior and posterior exenteration procedures; removes all pelvic organs

79 74 **Extended exenteration**—total exenteration plus removal of pelvic blood vessels or portion of bony pelvis

RADIATION THERAPY

What information to select and record (record all dates)

- Treatment start and stop dates
- Method of delivery (beam, brachytherapy, radioisotopes)
- Radiation treatment modality (regional or boost)
- Radiation source (photons, electrons, etc.)
- Total radiation dose (cGy)
- Target site(s) (also called volume)

CORPUS

Most patients whose tumors have extended more than half-way through the myometrium or beyond the corpus itself should have postoperative radiation therapy and either intracavitary or external beam.

- **Intracavitary (brachytherapy)**—also called vault radiation; code intracavitary brachytherapy as 51 in the Regional Treatment Modality and Boost Treatment Modality fields. Low dose rate brachytherapy treatment takes one to four days to complete. The patient is immobile while the radiation source is inserted into the vagina.

Radiation Therapy—Corpus, *continued*

- **High-dose-rate brachytherapy**—uses higher doses of radiation for a shorter amount of time; can be given in daily or weekly doses, usually three or more. Code as 52 in Regional and Boost Treatment Modality fields.
- **External beam radiation (XRT)**—also called whole pelvic irradiation. External beam radiation is given 5 days per week for 4–6 weeks. Code external beam radiation in the range 20-29 (depending on the type of energy) in the Regional and Boost Treatment Modality fields.
- **Intensity Modulated Radiation Therapy (IMRT)** is an advanced form of three-dimensional external beam radiation therapy. In addition to aiming beams from several directions, the intensity (or strength) of the beams can be adjusted to minimize the dose of radiation reaching the most sensitive normal tissues while delivering a uniformly high dose to the cancer. Code IMRT as 31 in the Regional and Boost Treatment Modality fields.

CERVIX

Radiation therapy is the preferred treatment for higher stage cervical cancers, with or without adjuvant chemotherapy. Radiation in the range of 5,000 cGy over 6–7 weeks plus chemotherapy with cisplatin with or without fluorouracil (5-FU) should be considered in patients with positive pelvic nodes, positive surgical margins, and residual parametrial disease.

- Pre-operative **intracavitary (brachytherapy)** or postoperative **external beam radiation** (XRT) is frequently used for treating extensive cervical cancer. Code intracavitary brachytherapy as 51 in the Regional Treatment Modality and Boost Treatment Modality fields. Code external beam radiation in the range 20-29 (depending on the type of energy) in the Regional Treatment Modality and Boost Treatment Modality fields.
- **High-dose-rate and low-dose-rate brachytherapy**—see above
- **Chemoradiation**—radiation therapy plus chemotherapy with cisplatin or cisplatin/5-FU for bulky tumors; code the radiation fields and chemotherapy fields appropriately
- **Radioactive phosphorus (P^{32})** may be used for intraperitoneal treatment of metastases. Code radioactive phosphorus as 60 in the Regional Treatment Modality and Boost Treatment Modality fields

Corpus-Cervix

SYSTEMIC TREATMENT

Chemotherapy/Hormone Therapy/Immunotherapy/Other Therapy
What information to record

- Treatment start date and ending date
- Name of regimen(s)
- Names of agents administered
- Number of cycles

CORPUS

Chemotherapy

There has been limited success with chemotherapy for endometrial cancer. Chemotherapy is primarily used for palliation of advanced stage endometrial cancer. Only a few drugs and regimens have shown cytotoxic activity, including:

- Carboplatin (Paraplatin)
- Cisplatin (Platinol)
- Doxorubicin (Adriamycin, Doxil)
- Paclitaxel (Taxol, Paxene)

Systemic Treatment—Corpus, *continued*

Regimens

- Doxorubicin and cisplatin
- Paclitaxel and doxorubicin
- Doxorubicin, cisplatin and paclitaxel with granulocyte colony stimulating factor (G-CSF)
- For carcinosarcoma, ifosfamide with or without carboplatin, cisplatin or paclitaxel

Hormones

The uterus, as an organ of reproduction, is highly sensitive to hormone levels, and therefore the growth of endometrial cancer is also sensitive to the presence of hormones. Hormone therapy, primarily progestins, has been used to treat metastatic or recurrent endometrial cancer. The progestins counteract the estrogens that cause endometrial cancer to grow. Hormone therapy is also an option for patients who are unable to undergo surgery or radiation. Common progestational agents include:

- Medroxyprogesterone acetate (Depo-Provera)
- Hydroxyprogesterone (Delalutin)
- Megestrol acetate (Megace)

Tamoxifen is an anti-estrogen that has shown some efficacy when used in combination with a progestational agent to treat recurrent or advanced endometrial cancer. Aromatase inhibitors can block estrogens from being formed in body fat. Aromatase inhibitors under investigation for endometrial cancer include letrozole (Femara), anastrozole (Arimidex), and exemestane (Aromasin).

If the woman's ovaries are left in place following hysterectomy, one more class of hormones may be effective against endometrial cancer. These are the gonadotropin-releasing hormone agonists (GNRH) that shut down the production of estrogen by the ovaries, including gosrelin (Zoladex) and leuprolide (Lupron).

Biological Response Modifiers

Treatment with biological response modifiers is under clinical evaluation. There are currently no BRMs effective for corpus cancer.

CERVIX

Chemotherapy

A few drugs and combinations have shown response rates for cervical cancer. These include:

- Cisplatin
- Ifosfamide (Ifos)
- Paclitaxel (Taxol)
- Topotecan (Hycamptin)
- Fluorouracil (5-FU)
- Irinotecan (for patients previously treated with chemotherapy)

Chemotherapy regimens for cervical cancer include:

- Ifosfamide–cisplatin
- Paclitaxel–cisplatin
- Cisplatin–gemcitabine
- Cisplatin–topotecan
- Cisplatin–vinorelbine (for recurrence)
- 5-FU with or without mitomycin C (an older combination used with radiation for recurrence)

Systemic Treatment—Cervix, *continued*

Hormones
Hormone treatment is not effective for cervical cancer.

Biological Response Modifiers
Treatment with biological response modifiers is under clinical evaluation. There are currently no BRMs effective for cervical cancer.

- **Gardasil vaccine**—***Do not code*** Gardasil or Cervarix vaccine as immunotherapy for cervical cancer. Gardasil was approved by the Food and Drug Administration in 2006 to prevent cervical cancer by immunizing the patient against several types of human papilloma virus (HPV) that are associated with cervical cancer development. Cervarix was FDA-approved in 2009.

'USUAL' TREATMENT BY PRIMARY SITE AND STAGE GROUP (from NCI PDQ)

CORPUS CARCINOMA

Stage I and Stage IIA (endocervical glandular involvement only)

- Total abdominal hysterectomy and bilateral salpingo-oophorectomy, with or without removal of selected pelvic lymph nodes. If lymph nodes are negative, no postoperative treatment is indicated.
- Postoperative brachytherapy with a vaginal cylinder for selected patients
- If the patient is not a surgical candidate, external beam or intracavitary radiation is an option.

Stage IIB

- Hysterectomy, bilateral salpingo-oophorectomy, and node sampling followed by post-operative irradiation
- Preoperative intracavitary and external-beam radiation therapy followed by hysterectomy and bilateral salpingo-oophorectomy, with biopsy of para-aortic nodes at time of surgery
- Radical hysterectomy and pelvic lymphadenectomy in selected cases

Stage III

- Hysterectomy, bilateral salpingo-oophorectomy, and node sampling followed by post-operative irradiation
- For unresectable tumor, combination intracavitary and external-beam radiation therapy
- If lymph nodes are positive, postoperative total pelvic irradiation including common iliac nodes
- Progestational agents for patients who are not surgical or radiation candidates
- Chemotherapy with doxorubicin and cisplatin with or without paclitaxel
- Clinical trials for patients who are found to have more extensive disease at operation than estimated clinically prior to surgery

Stage IV
Treatment is determined by the metastatic site and related symptoms:

- Bulky pelvic disease: intracavitary and external beam radiation therapy
- Pulmonary metastases: hormonal therapy (progestational agents)
- Chemotherapy with doxorubicin and cisplatin with or without paclitaxel
- Clinical trials with single-agent or combination chemotherapy, including doxorubicin, paclitaxel, and cisplatin

Usual Treatment by Stage, *continued*

CORPUS SARCOMA

Stage I and Stage II

- Total abdominal hysterectomy, bilateral salpingo-oophorectomy, pelvic and peri-aortic selective lymphadenectomy
- Surgery as above plus pelvic external beam radiation therapy
- Surgery as above plus adjuvant chemotherapy
- Surgery as above plus adjuvant chemotherapy in a clinical trial

Stage III

- Total abdominal hysterectomy, bilateral salpingo-oophorectomy, pelvic and peri-aortic selective lymphadenectomy, and resection of all gross tumor
- Clinical trials of surgery as above plus pelvic radiation therapy or adjuvant chemotherapy

Stage IV

- No standard therapy; patients should be entered into a clinical trial

CERVIX

Stage 0

Exocervical lesions in patients of childbearing age

- Loop electrosurgical excision procedure (LEEP)
- Laser therapy
- Conization
- Cryotherapy

Endocervical canal lesions in patients of childbearing age

- Laser or cold-knife conization for selected patients

Patients past childbearing age

- Total abdominal or vaginal hysterectomy, particularly when tumor extends to the inner cone margin

Patients who are not surgical candidates

- Intracavitary insertion with tandem and ovoids (brachytherapy)

Stage IA

- Total hysterectomy without lymph node dissection with or without oophorectomy for T1a1 lesions
- Conization in patients wishing to preserve fertility for T1a1 lesions
- Modified radical hysterectomy with pelvic node dissection for T1a2 lesions
- Intracavitary radiation alone for T1a1 lesions in patients who are not surgical candidates

Stage IB

- External beam pelvic irradiation combined with 2 or more intracavitary (low dose rate or high dose rate) applications with or without radiosensitizing chemotherapy
- Radical hysterectomy and bilateral pelvic lymphadenectomy
- Postoperative total pelvic irradiation plus chemotherapy following radical hysterectomy and bilateral pelvic lymphadenectomy
- Radiation therapy plus chemotherapy with cisplatin or cisplatin/5-FU for bulky tumors

Stage IIA

- Intracavitary (low dose rate or high dose rate) radiation combined with external beam pelvic irradiation with or without radiation to para-aortic nodes
- Radical hysterectomy and pelvic lymphadenectomy

Usual Treatment by Stage—Cervix, *continued*

- Postoperative total pelvic irradiation plus chemotherapy following radical hysterectomy and bilateral pelvic lymphadenectomy

Stage IIB – III – IVA

- Intracavitary (low dose rate or high dose rate) radiation and external beam pelvic irradiation combined with cisplatin or cisplatin/fluorouracil

Stage IVB

- Radiation therapy to palliate central disease or distant metastases
- Chemotherapy, single agent or combination (see Chemotherapy for cervix above)
- Clinical trials

COLLABORATIVE STAGE DATA COLLECTION SYSTEM (CS) CORPUS UTERI

Review the medical record for the diagnostic and staging procedures listed previously in this chapter under Cancer Abstracting Guidelines for corpus and cervix. Look for information (positive and negative) that describes the tumor location (cervix versus corpus), depth of invasion into or through the myometrium (corpus), tumor size, histologic grade, lymph node involvement, extension to adjacent organs and structures, or metastasis to distant sites or organs. All of this information can be coded in CS.

Make sure that your CS manual is complete by downloading any replacement pages from www.cancerstaging.org/cstage/manuals/index.html. Review carefully the notes preceding each table of the corpus or cervix schema in the Collaborative Stage Data Collection System Coding Instructions version 02.03.02. Use the notes and comments in this section to supplement the information in the CS documentation. Remember that all of the general rules in Part I of the CS documentation apply to the site schema.

- In the seventh edition of TNM and therefore in CS version 2, there are three separate schemas for corpus cancers based on histology. TNM had adopted a decision made by FIGO in 2009 to stage carcinomas differently from sarcomas and adenosarcomas. In CS, the site specific factors for the three schemas are the same but the extension codes and the mapping to T, N, and M values are different. The three schemas are:
  - CorpusCarcinoma (ICD-O morphology codes 8000-8790–carcinomas, 8950–Mullerian mixed tumor (MMMT), 8951–mesodermal mixed tumor, 8980-8981–carcinosarcomas, 9700-9701–mycosis fungoides and Sezary syndrome). 8950 and 8951 are older terms for carcinosarcoma.
  - CorpusAdenosarcoma (8933–adenosarcoma)
  - CorpusSarcoma (8800-8932, 8934-8941, 8959–8974–soft tissue sarcomas), 8982-9136–additional soft tissue malignancies, 9141-9582–more non-carcinoma malignancies
- CS for corpus uteri and corpus, NOS uses the following common (standard) tables, which will not be discussed in detail here.

  CS Tumor Size
  CS TS/Ext Eval
  CS Reg Nodes Eval
  Reg LN Pos
  Reg LN Exam
  CS Mets Eval

Collaborative Staging–Corpus Carcinoma, ***continued***

- Collaborative Staging uses the same eight Site-Specific Factors for the three corpus schemas.
- The corpus schemas exclude placental tumors, which have their own schema.

CS Extension

- Be sure that you are using the correct schema when you code a corpus uteri malignancy.
- The corpus CS Extension codes reference FIGO stages. FIGO is the "Federation Internationale de Gynecologie et d'Obstetrique." The definition of each code corresponds to the FIGO stages. The American Joint Committee on Cancer developed the tumor (T) component of the TNM staging system to correspond to FIGO staging, and these were carried forward into the CS Extension codes.
- Examples of CS Extension codes are shown in Figures 10–13.
- Involvement of the muscular layer of the uterus (myometrium) has prognostic significance (Figure 10). If invasion of the myometrium is described as superficial, less than 50%, or less than half-way, use code 120. If invasion of the myometrium is described as deep, 50% or more, or half-way through, use code 130. If depth of invasion into the myometrium is not stated, use code 140.
- The corpus schema is one of the few CS schemas in which discontinuous metastases are recorded in the Extension field. In the code tables, direct extension to or discontinuous metastases to organs in the pelvis are coded the same way.
- Codes are available to use when the clinician states a specific FIGO stage. However, codes that provide precise information about extension to other organs take priority over codes for FIGO stage.

Figure 10. CS Extension Codes and TNM T1 Category Mappings

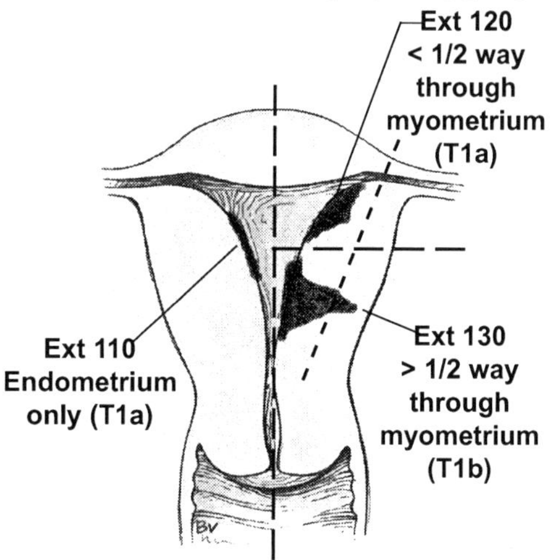

- Other codes are available when the information in the medical record is not specific enough to assign a FIGO, TNM or specific CS code, for example, codes 140, 400, and 500.
- Code 500 is extension to the cervix, NOS. Involvement of the corpus and cervix is Stage II, sometimes referred to as "corpus et collum."
- Extension from the corpus into the endocervical glands (epithelial lining of the cervical canal) is no longer a factor in CS version 2, but was T2a in the sixth edition of TNM (Figure 11). In CSv2, endocervical gland involvement is coded according to the depth of myometrial invasion.
- Code 520 is extension from the corpus into the stroma or muscular tissue of the cervix (Figure 11).
- Tumor confined to other female genital organs is coded in the range 550–640 (Figure 12).
- Tumor confined to the true pelvis is coded in the range 635-663 (Figure 12). Use the highest applicable code if multiple organs are involved.
- Extension to the mucosa of the bowel or bladder must be biopsy-proven. There must be evidence of actual tumor on the interior (mucosal) surface of the bladder or rectum in order for the tumor to be coded as 715 in CS Extension (Figure 13).

Figure 11. CS Extension Codes and TNM T2 Category Mappings

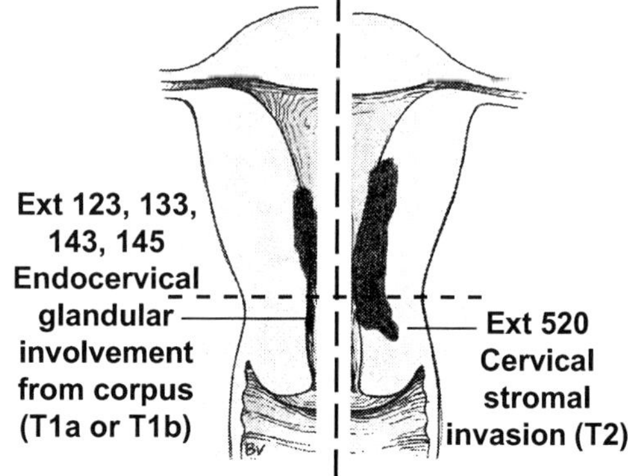

Figure 12. CS Extension Codes and TNM T3 Category Mappings

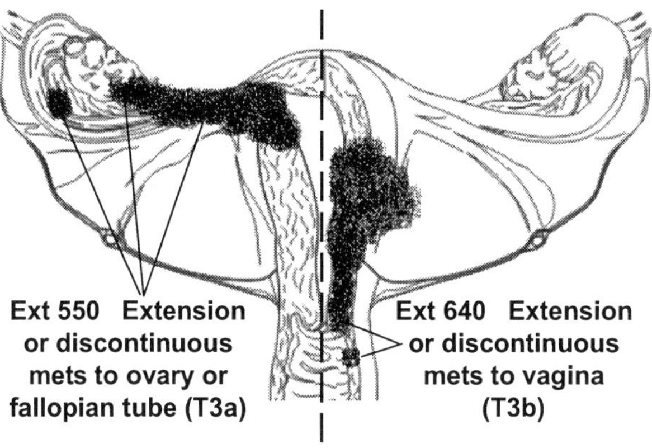

Figure 13. CS Extension Codes and TNM T4 Category Mappings

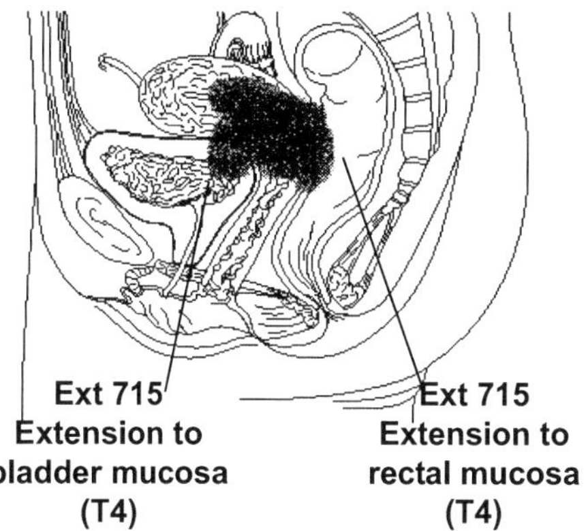

Collaborative Staging–Corpus Carcinoma, *continued*

Bullous edema (a blister-like appearance of the mucosa of the bowel or bladder) is not sufficient to code as 715.

- Positive peritoneal cytology is no longer a factor in TNM seventh edition, but is a staging element for TNM sixth edition and Summary Stage 2000. Information about peritoneal cytology is coded in site-specific factor 2.

CS Lymph Nodes

- This field records involved regional lymph nodes only (Note 1).
- Regional lymph nodes can be coded as negative if
  - the clinician says "adnexa palpated" and does not mention lymph nodes (Note 2)
  - the surgeon does not mention lymph nodes in the operative report of an exploratory laparotomy or hysterectomy (Note 3)
- Bilaterality or involvement of contralateral lymph nodes does not affect the coding of regional lymph nodes.
- Specific regional lymph node chains are listed in codes 100 and 200.
- Any involved regional node makes the case TNM Stage Group IIIC. Occasionally the clinician will call the case IIIC without referencing lymph nodes. When this happens, use code 50.
- FIGO and TNM seventh edition distinguish specific lymph node chains as N1 (FIGO IIIC1) and N2 (FIGO IIIC2). There are extra codes available of the physician indicates lymph node involvement but does not name the specific lymph node chain(s).

CS Mets at Dx

- Distant lymph nodes include superficial inguinal (code 11) and deep inguinal (code 12). All other distant lymph nodes are code 12.
- Abdominal lymph nodes, except para-aortic lymph nodes, are distant (code 12).
- Code 40 includes any specific distant visceral metastases.
- Seeding, implants, and tumor nodules in the omentum, abdominal mesentery, kidney(s), large intestine (except rectum and sigmoid colon), pancreas, pericolic gutter, spleen, stomach or retroperitoneal portion of the ureter(s), or on the surface of the diaphragm or liver are abdominal metastases. By definition, these organs are distant disease and coded as 40 in CS Mets at Dx.

Corpus-Cervix

Collaborative Staging—Corpus Carcinoma, *continued*

- Code 40 ***does not include*** seeding, implants, or tumor nodule metastases to the pelvic serosa, adnexa or vagina. These pelvic sites are coded in CS Extension.
- Both pleural effusion and abdominal ascites must be cytologically proven to be coded as 40 in CS Mets at Dx.
- Code 60 can be used when distant metastases are mentioned by specific sites are not named (distant metastases, NOS) or when the tumor is described as M1 with no further information.

CORPUS SITE-SPECIFIC FACTORS 1 – 8

Note: Part I Section 2 of the CS Coding Manual Version 02.03 includes extensive discussion of the site-specific factors for every schema. Rather than rewrite those coding instructions for inclusion in this CASEbook chapter, refer to Part I Section 2 if questions arise. The discussion that follows provides more rationale for why those site-specific factors were included in the corpus schemas.

- All three histology-specific corpus uteri schemas use the same eight site-specific factors.

SSF1—FIGO Stage

- As previously noted, FIGO is the French acronym for the International Federation of Gynecology and Obstetrics (see also Other Staging Systems later in this chapter). FIGO staging is similar to the TNM stage group but does not have separate elements for T, N, and M. FIGO stage uses Roman numerals from I to IV with Arabic letter subcategories A, B and C. Each female genital organ has a FIGO staging system, and they differ slightly.
- The code structure for this site-specific factor parallels the structure of the FIGO stage. The first digit is the Roman numeral expressed as a number, for example Stage II is 2. The middle digit is the Arabic letter subcategory expressed as a number, such as C is 3. The third digit is the numeric sub-subcategory, if used. For example, corpus stage IIIC2 is code 332.
- Code the FIGO stage from a statement by the physician. Do not convert T, N, and M or TNM Stage Group into FIGO stage to code this field. If FIGO Stage is not stated, use code 999.

SSF2—Peritoneal Cytology

- Peritoneal cytology looks for malignant cells in the fluids present in the abdomen and pelvis (ascites) or in peritoneal washings (saline solution added to the body cavity, then suctioned out and sent for cytology).
- Peritoneal cytology is a factor for Summary Stage 2000 in Regional Direct Extension. It is not a factor in either sixth or seventh edition TNM or FIGO stage. In CS version 2, information about peritoneal cytology was removed from CS Extension (code made obsolete) and is now coded in Site-Specific Factor 2.
- Information to code this field may be found in a pathology report or cytology report. Codes are available for positive cytology, negative cytology, and suspicious or undetermined cytology. Also review the operative report to see if the surgeon took samples of peritoneal fluid. If no peritoneal fluid sample was sent to the laboratory for analysis, use code 998. If there is no mention of peritoneal cytology, use code 999.

SSF3—Number of Positive Pelvic Nodes
SSF4—Number of Examined Pelvic Nodes

- Refer to Figure 4 and Table 1 to identify pelvic lymph nodes.
- This pair of site-specific factors documents the number of pelvic lymph nodes removed and examined by the pathologist (SSF4) and the number of pelvic lymph nodes found to be positive (SSF3).
- The code structures and definitions for these two fields are the same as for Regional Nodes Positive (SSF3) and Regional Nodes Examined (SSF4), but the counts are only for pelvic lymph nodes. Refer to the CS Coding Instructions Part I Section 1 for coding instructions.

Collaborative Staging—Corpus Carcinoma, *continued*

SSF5—Number of Positive Para-aortic Nodes
SSF6—Number of Examined Para-aortic Nodes

- This pair of site-specific factors documents the number of para-aortic lymph nodes removed and examined by the pathologist (SSF6) and the number of para-aortic lymph nodes found to be positive (SSF5). Refer to Figure 4 and Table 1 to identify para-aortic lymph nodes.
- The code structures and definitions for these two fields are the same as for Regional Nodes Positive (SSF5) and Regional Nodes Examined (SSF6), but the counts are only for pelvic lymph nodes. Refer to the CS Coding Instructions Part I Section 1 for coding instructions.

SSF7—Percentage of Non-Endometrioid Cell Type in Mixed Histology Tumors

- This site-specific factor describes the content of adenocarcinomas with mixed histology. A higher percentage of non-squamous or non-morular (non-glandular) growth pattern is an indication of a more aggressive tumor.
- The proportions in codes 001–003 are based on one version of the FIGO grade called the architectural grade or growth pattern (the other version is called nuclear grade). The pathologist looks for and grades the differentiation of the glandular portion of the tumor.
- Assign the code based on the pathologist's description of the growth pattern. If the architectural grade or growth pattern is not stated, use code 999.
- Use code 987 when a case is coded using either the CorpusSarcoma or CorpusAdenosarcoma schema.

SSF8—Omentectomy

- Omentectomy (removal of the fatty "apron" in front of the abdomen) is not usually performed for corpus carcinoma, but some studies have shown that omentectomy can detect microscopic metastases to the omentum that upstage the case. Codes for omentectomy are not part of the Surgery of Primary Site codes for corpus.
- The codes are straightforward: use 000 if the first course of treatment did not include omentectomy; use 010 if the first course surgery included omentectomy, and use 998 if there was no surgery during first course of treatment. Read the operative report and pathology report to determine whether the omentum was removed.

Collaborative Stage Data Collection System (CS) Corpus Adenosarcoma and Sarcomas (Leiomysarcoma and Endometrial Stromal Sarcoma)

- Be sure that you are using the correct schema when you code a corpus uteri malignancy.
- Because the schemas for CorpusAdenosarcoma and Corpus Sarcoma were adapted from the CorpusCarcinoma schema, the code structure for CS Extension is very similar. However, the mapping into the TNM T category is different for the adenosarcomas and the uterine sarcomas. For leiomyosarcoma and endometrial stromal sarcoma, the size of the primary tumor differentiates T1a and T1b.
- The tables for CS Lymph Nodes and CS Mets at Dx are the same for all three corpus schemas.
- The site-specific factors are the same for all three corpus schemas, but SSF7 should always be coded as 987 for CorpusAdenosarcoma and CorpusSarcoma.

COLLABORATIVE STAGE DATA COLLECTION SYSTEM (CS) CERVIX UTERI

Review the medical record for the diagnostic and staging procedures listed previously in this chapter under Cancer Abstracting Guidelines for corpus and cervix. Look for information (positive and negative) that describes the tumor location (cervix versus corpus), tumor size, histologic grade, lymph node involvement, extension to adjacent organs and structures, or metastasis to distant sites or organs. All of this information can be coded in CS.

Make sure that your CS manual is complete by downloading any replacement pages from www.cancerstaging.org/cstage/manuals/index.html. Review carefully the notes preceding each table of the corpus or cervix schema in the Collaborative Stage Data Collection System Coding Instructions version 02.03.02. Use the notes and comments in this section to supplement the information in the CS documentation. Remember that all of the general rules in Part I of the CS documentation apply to the site schema.

- CS for cervix uteri uses the following common (standard) tables, which will not be discussed in detail here.
  - CS Reg Nodes Eval
  - Reg LN Pos
  - Reg LN Exam
  - CS Mets Eval
- CS uses nine Site-Specific Factors for cervix.

CS Tumor Size

- Cervix uses the common table for CS Tumor Size. The only difference from other schemas is a note that the horizontal spread or surface diameter of the cervical lesion is to be coded in CS Tumor Size.

CS Extension

- The cervix CS Extension codes reference FIGO stages. The definition of each extension code corresponds to the FIGO stages. The American Joint Committee on Cancer developed the tumor (T) component of the TNM staging system to correspond to FIGO staging, and these were carried forward into the CS Extension codes.
- Codes are available to use when the clinician states a specific FIGO stage. However, codes that provide precise information about extension to other organs take priority over codes for FIGO stage (Note 1).
  - If the physician refers to FIGO Stage IIIB, determine whether that is on the basis of tumor extension or lymph node involvement. If on the basis of tumor extension, code in CS Extension. If on the basis of lymph node involvement or if the basis is not specified, use code 200 or 300 in CS Lymph Nodes (Note 2).
  - If the physician refers to FIGO Stage IV, determine whether that is on the basis of tumor extension or distant metastases. If on the basis of tumor extension, code in CS Extension. If on the basis of distant metastases or if the basis is not specified, use code 80 in CS CS Mets at Dx (Note 2).
- Carcinoma in situ of the cervix (CIS) (Extension code 000) and cervical intraepithelial neoplasia grade III (Extension code 010) are not reportable to most central cancer registries in the U.S., but can be coded with the cervix schema.
  - FIGO no longer recognizes Stage 0 (Tis) for cervix (Note 3), but AJCC/TNM does.

Collaborative Staging–Cervix, ***continued***

- Codes 110, 120, 200, 360, 370, 380 and 390 are based on the depth of invasion, not the horizontal diameter of the lesion.
- For codes 110 and 120, tumor not visible to the clinician's eye may be seen via colposcopy. Very minimal invasive carcinoma must be measured by the pathologist in order to differentiate between code 110 and 120.
- Tumor that is larger or deeper than the dimensions in code 120 should be assigned to code 200 if the dimensions are stated.
- Any tumor visible to the naked eye should be coded to 250 if no tumor size is stated (Figure 14) (Note 4).
- Supplementary codes are available when the information in the medical record is not specific enough to assign a FIGO, TNM, or specific Collaborative Stage code, for example, codes 250 and 300.
- In the TNM system involvement of the corpus uteri (Figure 15) does not affect the T classification. However, in the Summary Staging system, direct tumor extension from the cervix to the corpus is staged as regional direct extension. Codes 360 through 390 should be assigned when there is tumor extension from the cervix to the corpus.
- Codes 400 and 500 (Figure 15) define further spread of cervical cancer into other adjacent female genital organs (vagina, parametrium, ligaments) and map to T2.
- Involvement of the vaginal wall (code 400) includes extension to the anterior septum (connective tissue between the vagina and bladder) and the posterior septum (connective tissue between the vagina and rectum (Note 5).
- Codes 605 (Figure 16) to 685 define further extension to other structures in the true pelvis, including ovary, fallopian tube, vulva, urethra and ureter. Extension to any of these sites maps to T3. Use the highest applicable code if multiple organs are involved.
- In code 700 (Figure 16), extension to the mucosa of the bowel or bladder must be biopsy-proven. There must be evidence of actual tumor on the interior (mucosal) surface of the bladder or rectum in order for the tumor to be coded as 700 in CS Extension. Bullous

Figure 14. CS Extension Codes 250 and 350 with T Category Mappings

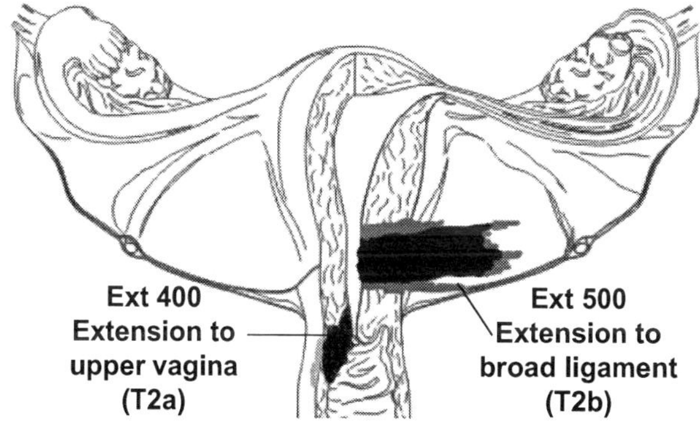

Figure 15. CS Extension Codes 400 and 500 with T Category Mappings

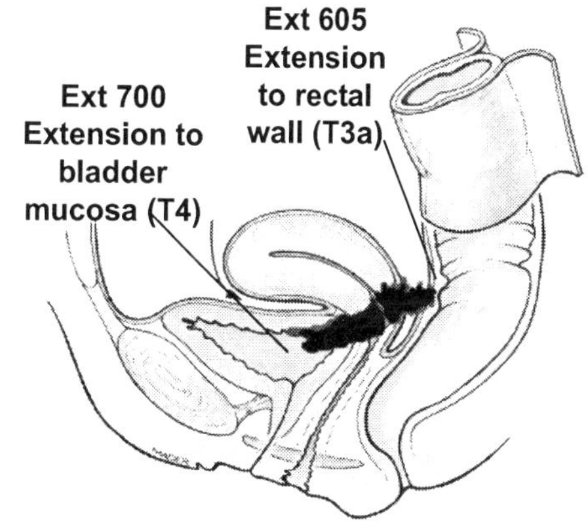

Figure 16. CS Extension Codes 605 and 700 with T Category Mappings

Collaborative Staging–Cervix, *continued*

edema (a blister-like appearance of the mucosa of the bowel or bladder) is not sufficient to code as 700.

- Hydronephrosis and non-functioning kidney in code 635 may be due to blockage of the ureter by cervical cancer or other causes. Hydronephrosis is an accumulation of urine in the kidney because of an obstruction in the ureter (a kidney stone, blood clot, or tumor blockage of the ureter). Radiology or ultrasound of the kidney may reveal swelling or dilation of the kidney. If the hydronephrosis is prolonged, permanent damage to the filtering units of the kidney may occur, resulting in a non-functioning kidney, which is visible on radiology.
- Contiguous tumor extension beyond the true pelvis is coded in 800.

CS TS/Ext Eval

- Cervix uses the common table for the Tumor Size/Extension Eval field. For carcinoma in situ of the cervix, if a conization procedure removed all tumor (clear margins), TS/Ext Eval should be coded as 3 (pathologic). If there are positive margins or residual tumor, code the conization information as Eval code 1.

CS Lymph Nodes

- This field records involved regional lymph nodes only (Note 1).
- Regional lymph nodes can be coded as clinically negative if
  - the clinician says "adnexa palpated" and does not mention lymph nodes (Note 4)
  - the surgeon does not mention lymph nodes in the operative report of an exploratory laparotomy or hysterectomy (Note 3)
- Bilaterality or involvement of contralateral lymph nodes does not affect the coding of regional lymph nodes.
- If the physician refers to FIGO Stage IIIB, determine whether that is on the basis of tumor extension or lymph node involvement. If on the basis of tumor extension, code in CS Extension. If on the basis of lymph node involvement or if the basis is not specified, use code 200 in CS Lymph Nodes (Note 2)
- Specific regional lymph node chains are listed in code 100.
- Code 800 should only be used when it is not possible to identify involved nodes as regional or distant. Any regional node involvement should be coded in 100.

CS Mets at Dx

- Distant lymph nodes include aortic, inguinal, and mediastinal. All distant lymph nodes are code 10.
- Code 40 includes any named distant visceral metastases. Code 60 can be used when distant metastases are described but the location(s) is not specified.
- Seeding, implants, and tumor nodules in the omentum, abdominal mesentery, kidney(s), large intestine (except rectum and sigmoid colon), pancreas, pericolic gutter, spleen, stomach or retroperitoneal portion of the ureter(s), or on the surface of the diaphragm or liver are abdominal metastases. By definition, these organs are distant disease and coded as 40 in CS Mets at Dx.
- Both pleural effusion and abdominal ascites must be cytologically proven to be coded as 40 in CS Mets at Dx.
- Any combination of distant lymph nodes and visceral metastases should be coded to 50.
- If the physician refers to FIGO Stage IV, determine whether that is on the basis of tumor extension or distant metastases. If on the basis of tumor extension, code in CS Extension. If on the basis of distant metastases or if the basis is not specified, use code 80 in CS CS Mets at Dx (Note 2).

Collaborative Staging–Cervix, *continued*

CERVIX SITE-SPECIFIC FACTORS 1 – 9

Note: Part I Section 2 of the CS Coding Manual Version 02.03 includes extensive discussion of the site-specific factors for every schema. Rather than rewrite those coding instructions for inclusion in this CASEbook chapter, refer to Part I Section 2 if questions arise. The discussion which follows provides more rationale for why those site-specific factors were included in the corpus schemas.

Note for SSFs 3, 5, 7, and 9: Part I Section 2 page 100 incorrectly states that the assessment method is coded for positive nodes only. There is a CAnswer Forum question and response discussing this issue and instructing registrars to disregard the word 'positive' in the first sentence of the third full paragraph on that page. Assessment method is for both positive and negative nodes.

SSF1 — FIGO Stage

- Refer to SSF1, FIGO Stage, under CS for Corpus and the discussion of FIGO at the end of this chapter.

SSF2 — Pelvic Nodal Status
SSF3 — Assessment Method of Pelvic Nodal Status

- This pair of site-specific factors records whether the pelvic lymph nodes (only) are involved (Status, SSF2) and what diagnostic method(s) were used to make that determination (Assessment Method, SSF3).
- Refer to Figure 4 and Table 1 to identify pelvic lymph nodes.
- In SSF2, code whether the pelvic lymph nodes are negative (010) or positive (020). In SSF3 code how the lymph nodes were evaluated. Higher codes in the 010–040 range take priority.
- If lymph nodes were not assessed, code both fields as 998.

SSF4 — Para-aortic Nodal Status
SSF5 — Assessment Method of Para-aortic Nodal Status

- This pair of site-specific factors records whether the para-aortic lymph nodes (only) are involved (Status, SSF4) and what diagnostic method(s) were used to make that determination (Assessment Method, SSF5).
- Refer to Figure 4 and Table 1 to identify para-aortic lymph nodes. Para-aortic lymph nodes are distant lymph nodes and coded in CS Mets at Dx.
- In SSF4, code whether the para-aortic lymph nodes are negative (010) or positive (020). In SSF5 code how the lymph nodes were evaluated. Higher codes in the 010–040 range take priority.
- If lymph nodes were not assessed, code both fields as 998.

SSF6 — Mediastinal Nodal Status
SSF7 — Assessment Method of Mediastinal Nodal Status

- This pair of site-specific factors records whether the mediastinal lymph nodes (only) are involved (Status, SSF6) and what diagnostic method(s) were used to make that determination (Assessment Method, SSF7).
- Mediastinal lymph nodes (in the thoracic cavity) are distant lymph nodes and coded in CS Mets at Dx.
- In SSF6, code whether the mediastinal lymph nodes are negative (010) or positive (020). In SSF7 code how the lymph nodes were evaluated. Higher codes in the 010–040 range take priority.
- If lymph nodes were not assessed, code both fields as 998.

Collaborative Staging–Cervix, *continued*

SSF8 — Scalene Nodal Status
SSF9 — Assessment Method of Scalene Nodal Status

- This pair of site-specific factors records whether the scalene lymph nodes (only) are involved (Status, SSF8) and what diagnostic method(s) were used to make that determination (Assessment Method, SSF9).
- Scalene lymph nodes are above the clavicles toward the side of the neck. When para-aortic lymph nodes are involved from cervical cancer, there is about a one in six chance that scalene lymph nodes are also positive. Scalene lymph nodes are distant lymph nodes and coded in CS Mets at Dx.
- In SSF8, code whether the scalene lymph nodes are negative (010) or positive (020). In SSF9, code how the lymph nodes were evaluated. Higher codes in the 010–040 range take priority.
- If lymph nodes were not assessed, code both fields as 998.

OTHER STAGING SYSTEMS

AJCC (TNM)—CORPUS

Much of the structure of the Collaborative Staging schema for corpus cancer is based on information contained in the *AJCC Cancer Staging Manual, seventh edition.*

- As previously noted, there are two separate staging systems for malignancies of the corpus uteri in the seventh edition of TNM based on histology. TNM had adopted a decision made by FIGO in 2009 to stage carcinomas differently from sarcomas and adenosarcomas. The two systems are:
    - Uterine carcinoma
    - Uterine sarcoma, which includes adenosarcoma, leiomyosarcoma, and endometrial stromal sarcoma. Within this staging system, the T classification for leiomyosarcoma and endometrial stromal sarcoma is different from that for adenosarcoma.

Criteria for TNM Clinical Staging for corpus malignancies is uncommon, but may be obtained from:

- Physical examination and history
- Histologic confirmation of malignancy
- Palpation of abdomen
- Abdominal imaging
- Endoscopy
- Colposcopy
- Endocervical curettage
- Fractional curettage
- Sounding of uterine cavity
- Intravenous urography
- Imaging for distant metastases

Criteria for TNM Pathologic Staging

FIGO and TNM staging of endometrial malignancies is primarily pathologic. Information may be obtained from:

- Surgical observation (laparotomy)
- Hysterectomy
- Pathologic assessment of pelvic lymph nodes (strongly advocated)

AJCC (TNM) ABSTRACTING GUIDELINES—CORPUS CARCINOMA

- FIGO no longer includes Tis/Stage 0, but it is included in TNM.
- Stage I is tumor confined to the endometrium and/or myometrium.
- Involvement of the cervix is at least Stage II.

AJCC (TNM)—Corpus, *continued*

- Extension to the uterine serosa, ovary(ies), fallopian tube(s), parametrium, or vagina is at least Stage III.
- Stage III *includes* discontinuous metastases to organs in the true pelvis, ascites, or peritoneal washings.
- Seeding, implants, and tumor nodules outside the true pelvis in the omentum, peritoneum or on the diaphragm are classified as distant disease (M1, Stage IVB).
- Bullous edema is a blister-like appearance of the interior surface of the bladder or rectum, which is not to be considered evidence of a T4 lesion.
- There must be evidence of actual tumor on the interior (mucosal) surface of the bladder or rectum in order for the tumor to be assigned to the T4 (Stage IVA) category.
- Regional lymph nodes have been sub-categorized into N1 (pelvic) and N2 (peri-aortic) to correspond to FIGO stages IIIC1 and IIIC2, respectively.

AJCC (TNM) ABSTRACTING GUIDELINES—CORPUS SARCOMA

- For leiomyosarcoma and endometrial stromal sarcoma confined to the uterus, the size of the tumor differentiates T1a (5 cm or less) and T1b (more than 5 cm).
- Involvement of abdominal tissues—not just protrusion of the tumor mass into the abdominal cavity—is subcategorized T3a (one site) and T3b (more than one site).
- Regional lymph nodes for corpus sarcomas are simply N0 and N1. The M category is simply M0 and M1.
- Stage grouping is the same for all corpus sarcomas.

AJCC (TNM)—CERVIX

As previously noted, the AJCC TNM staging system for cervical cancer is based FIGO staging. It is primarily a clinical staging system. There were no changes in the T, N, and M definitions between the sixth and seventh editions.

Criteria for TNM Clinical Staging of the cervix may be obtained from:

- Physical examination and history
- Histologic confirmation of malignancy
- Inspection and palpation of genitalia and abdomen
- Colposcopy
- Endocervical curettage
- Endoscopies of uterus, rectum and bladder
- Intravenous urography
- Imaging for lung and bone metastases
- If indicated, biopsies of bladder or rectal mucosa

Information from the following diagnostic procedures may help determine treatment but should not be part of clinical staging:

- CT scans
- Magnetic resonance imaging (MRI)
- PET scans
- Invasive contrast imaging of lymph nodes, veins or arteries

- Information obtained from CT, MRI, PET, or lymphangiography may be used to plan treatment but should not be used to determine stage. Cervical cancer staging is used internationally, and these imaging methods are not available in all parts of the world.

Criteria for TNM Pathologic Staging

- Findings from surgical observation and the resected specimen should be recorded but should not be used to alter the clinically established stage at diagnosis.

AJCC (TNM)—Cervix, *continued*

AJCC (TNM) ABSTRACTING GUIDELINES—CERVIX

- FIGO no longer includes Tis/Stage 0, but it is included in TNM.
- Ignore extension into the corpus when determining stage.
- Any cervix lesion that is visible to the naked eye is at least T1b/FIGO IB.
- Extension to the vagina is at least Stage II; extension to ovary is at least Stage III.
- Bullous edema is a blister-like appearance of the interior surface of the bladder or rectum, which is not to be considered evidence of a T4 lesion.
- Nephrosis or non-functioning kidney due to stenosis of the ureter from tumor extension assigns the case to stage III.
- Involvement of the anterior or posterior septum (fornix) is coded as involvement of the vaginal wall.
- Seeding, implants, and tumor nodules in the omentum, peritoneum or on the diaphragm are distant disease (Stage IV).
- There must be evidence of actual tumor on the interior (mucosal) surface of the bladder or rectum in order for the tumor to be assigned to the T4 (Stage IVA) category.
- Both pleural effusion and ascites must be cytologically proven to affect TNM staging.

FIGO STAGING

FIGO is the French acronym for Federation Internationale de Gynecologie et d'Obstetrique, which in English is the International Federation of Gynecology and Obstetrics. The first staging system ever developed was for cervical cancer. Originally published as the League of Nations staging system in the 1929, responsibility for cervical and other gynecologic staging was assumed by FIGO in 1954. The cervical cancer staging has been revised several times, most recently in 2008.

The principles of FIGO staging have been adapted to the TNM format and incorporated into both AJCC/UICC staging and Collaborative Staging. In contrast to TNM, FIGO staging uses Roman numerals and subscripts for its stages—no T, N, or M. The following stages are divided into substages based on certain prognostic criteria within the stage, such as size of lesion or specific organs involved.

Stage 0	In situ carcinoma
Stage I	Similar to localized: confined to organ of origin
Stage II	Extension locally beyond site of origin to involve adjacent organs or structures in the pelvis
Stage III	More extensive involvement, including regional lymph nodes
Stage IV	Metastatic (discontinuous or hematogenous) disease

FIGO STAGING—CORPUS

- FIGO staging for endometrial has been surgical since 1988.
- FIGO subcategorizes Stage IB Endometrial cancer by the grade of tumor, AJCC does not.
- Endocervical extension can only be established by fractional curettage or scraping of the cervix submitted as a separate specimen at D and C.

Table 4 is a comparison of the structure of FIGO definitions, the T category of TNM, and the CS Extension field for corpus carcinoma.

FIGO Staging, ***continued***

FIGO STAGING—CERVIX

- To maintain international compatibility, especially in low resource countries where cervical cancer remains a major health problem, FIGO is a clinical staging system, based on careful clinical examination before any definitive therapy has begun. Information from specialized procedures, such as CT and MRI scanning, is limited, as these procedures may not be available in all countries.

Table 5 is a comparison of the structure of FIGO definitions, the T category of TNM, and the CS Extension field for cervical cancer.

Table 4. Comparison of FIGO, TNM and CS Extension for Corpus Carcinoma Staging

AJCC	FIGO	Definition		CS Extension code(s)
Tis	0	In situ		000
T1	I	Confined to corpus		100, 143, 145, 180
T1a	IA	Limited to endometrium or inner half of myometrium		110, 120, 123, 125
T1b	IB	≥ half of myometrium		130, 133, 135
T2	II	Invades cervix		500, 525
T3/N1	III	Local and/or regional as specified below		680
T3a	IIIA	Serosa/adnexa/positive peritoneal cytology		540, 545, 550, 630
T3b	IIIB	Vaginal involvement		635, 640, 645, 655, 660, 662, 665
T4	IVA	Mucosa of bladder or bowel		715, 800, 810, 820
N1	IIIB	Regional lymph node metastasis	**CS Lymph Nodes**	100, 140, 160, 200, 210, 250, 500, 800
M1	IVB	Distant metastasis	**CS Mets at Dx**	11, 12, 40, 50, 55, 60, 70

Table 5. Comparison of FIGO, TNM and CS Extension for Cervix Cancer Staging

AJCC	FIGO	Definition		CS Extension code(s)
Tis	0	In situ		000
Tis		CIN III		010
T1	I	Confined to uterus		310, 350
T1a	IA	Microscopic finding only		135, 140
T1a1	IA1	≤ 3 mm deep and ≤7 mm horizontal spread		110, 360
T1a2	IA2	> 3–5 mm deep and ≤7 mm horizontal spread		120, 370, 380, 390
T1b	IB	Clinically visible, or microscopic lesion more than T1a in size		200, 250
T1b1	IB1	Clinically visible, ≤ 4.0 cm in size		210
T1b2	IB2	Clinically visible, > 4.0 cm in size		220
T2	II	Beyond uterus but not to pelvic wall or lower 1/3 of vagina		410, 550
T2a	IIA	No parametrial invasion		450
T2a1	IIA1	Clinically visible, ≤ 4.0 cm in size		420
T2a2	IIA2	Clinically visible, > 4.0 cm in size		440
T2b	IIB	Parametrial invasion		500
T3/N1	III	Pelvic wall and/or lower 1/3 of vagina and/or with hydronephrosis or non-functioning kidney		685, 690
T3a	IIIA	Lower 1/3 of vagina, but not to pelvic wall		605, 622, 625
T3b	IIIB	Pelvic wall and/or hydronephrosis or non-functioning kidney		635, 655, 660
T4	IVA	Mucosa of bladder or bowel or extension beyond true pelvis		700, 800, 850, 860
N1	IIIB	Regional lymph node metastasis	**CS Lymph Nodes**	100, 200, 300, 800
M1	IVB	Distant metastasis	**CS Mets at Dx**	10, 40, 50, 60, 70, 80

SUMMARY STAGE

There isn't much new to be said about summary staging for uterine cancers. Be sure to read the summary staging guidelines at the end of each section. The *SEER Summary Staging Manual 2000* (SSSM2000) includes the definitions for the various FIGO/TNM stages where they fit in the summary stage categories.

Note: There are two typographical errors in the cervical cancer staging section, one in the original printing of SSSM2000, and one in the second printing.

- In the first printing of SSSM2000 (red and white cover), the definition of FIGO stage IA2 should read "> 3 mm and ≤ 5 mm in depth".
- In the second printing of SSSM2000 (red, white, and blue cover), that typo was fixed, but another one showed up in the definition of FIGO Stage IB, which should read "tumor > 5 mm in depth and/or > 7 mm in horizontal spread".

EPIDEMIOLOGY AND ETIOLOGY

CORPUS

- Endometrial cancer is the fourth most common cancer among women in the U.S. and the most common female reproductive cancer.
- Uterine (corpus and uterus, NOS) cancer is the fifth most common cancer among women worldwide.
- Incidence worldwide is highest in developed countries, and the highest rates in the world are in North America.
- Corpus cancer is primarily a disease of postmenopausal women; the average age at diagnosis is 63.
- In the U.S., endometrial cancer is more common among whites than other races.
- Fortunately, the mortality rate for endometrial cancer is declining.

Risk Factors

- Estrogens without progesterones
- Obesity
- High consumption of dietary fats
- History of breast or rectal cancer
- Tamoxifen use
- Late menopause
- Age (95% of patients are age 50 – 70)
- Hemorrhagic menses
- Diabetes
- Nulliparity

Prognostic Factors

- Histologic grade (FIGO grade criteria)
- Cell type (histology)
- Stage at diagnosis (FIGO or TNM)
- Depth of myometrial invasion
- Adnexal involvement
- Positive peritoneal cytology
- Lymph node involvement

Epidemiology and Etiology, *continued*

CERVIX

- Cervical cancer is the second most common cancer in women worldwide.
- Cervical cancer is the seventh most common cancer worldwide in men and women combined.
- 83% of new invasive cases occur in the less developed world.
- The highest rates of cervical cancer are in India, eastern and southern Africa, Melanesia, central and south America, the Caribbean, southeast and southcentral Asia.

Risk Factors

- Women of childbearing age
- Human papilloma virus (HPV) infection
- Intercourse at early age; multiple sexual partners
- History of STD (sexually transmitted disease)
- Smoking
- Immunosuppression (HIV)

Prognostic Factors

- Localized disease
    - Lymphovascular involvement
    - Tumor size
    - Depth of invasion
    - Lymph node metastasis
- Regional and distant disease
    - Stage
    - Lymph node metastasis
    - Tumor volume
    - Age
    - Performance status

Page left blank.

Abstracting, Staging, and Coding Exercises

CORPUS

This section includes twelve brief corpus cancer cases to be coded in ICD-O-3, Summary Stage 2000, TNM seventh edition (clinical and pathologic), and CS version 0203.

NOTE: For the purposes of these brief cases, assume that all other tests not mentioned in the case are negative for malignancy.

- Identify the primary site and schema.
- Assign the codes for primary site, histology, behavior, and grade.
- Assign codes to all applicable CS fields.
- Assume that your facility does offer a test and that the standards setters for your facility require the data field. In other words, avoid using code 988 (not applicable).
- 20XX is the diagnosis year, and where applicable, 20YY is the following year.

CERVIX

This section includes twelve brief cervical cancer cases to be coded in ICD-O-3, Summary Stage 2000, TNM seventh edition (clinical and pathologic), and CS version 0203.

NOTE: For the purposes of these brief cases, assume that all other tests not mentioned in the case are negative for malignancy.

- Identify the primary site and schema.
- Assign the codes for primary site, histology, behavior, and grade.
- Assign codes to all applicable CS fields.
- Assume that your facility does offer a test and that the standards setters for your facility require the data field. In other words, avoid using code 988 (not applicable).
- 20XX is the diagnosis year, and where applicable, 20YY is the following year.

CORPUS CASE 1

HISTORY AND PHYSICAL EXAM
Irregular bleeding, no pain. Normal vulva, vagina, cervix. Somewhat enlarged uterus. No adnexal masses.

X-RAYS AND SCANS
5-6-20XX Pelvic Ultrasound: Shows uterus to be 7 x 7 x 7 cm (slightly larger than normal) with no endometrial thickening.
5-6-20XX Chest x-ray: Negative for metastatic disease.

LABORATORY None.

ENDOSCOPIC PROCEDURES None.

OPERATIVE REPORT
5-18-20XX TAH-BSO: Liver, spleen, gallbladder, stomach and other organs normal. No palpable retroperitoneal, aortic or pelvic nodes. Uterus has multiple large myofibromata on its surface and intramurally. No other visible abnormalities.

PATHOLOGY REPORTS
5-18-20XX TAH-BSO: Adenosquamous carcinoma of endometrium, deeply invasive with involvement of anterior serosal surface, lymphatics and lumen of R fallopian tube. Cervix: No evidence of tumor.

TREATMENT
5-18-20XX Total abdominal hysterectomy and bilateral salpingo-oophorectomy

Site Code ___ ___ ___.___
Histology/Behavior/Grade ___ ___ ___ ___/___ ___
Grade Path Value ___
Grade Path System ___
Lymph Vascular Invasion ___
Ambiguous Terminol ___
Date Conclusive Terminol ___ ___ ___ ___ ___ ___ ___ ___
Date Conclus Dx Flag ___ ___
Multiplicity Counter ___ ___
Date Mult Tumors ___ ___ ___ ___ ___ ___ ___ ___
Date Mult Tumors Flag ___ ___
Mult Tum Reported as One Prim ___ ___
Summary Stage 2000 ___

cT ___ cN ___ cM ___
Clin Stage Group _____
pT ___ pN ___ M ___
Path Stage Group _____
CS Tumor Size ___ ___ ___
CS Extension ___ ___ ___
CS TS/Ext Eval ___
CS LN ___ ___ ___
CS Reg Nodes Eval ___
Reg LN Pos ___ ___
Reg LN Exam ___ ___
CS Mets at Dx ___ ___
CS Mets at Dx - Bone ___ Brain ___ Liver ___ Lung ___
CS Mets Eval ___

SSF1 FIGO Stage ___ ___ ___
SSF2 Periton Cytol ___ ___ ___
SSF3 # Pos Pelvic LN ___ ___ ___
SSF4 # Exam Pelvic LN ___ ___ ___
SSF5 # Pos Para-Aortic LN ___ ___ ___
SSF6 # Exam Para-Aortic LN ___ ___ ___
SSF7 % Non-Endomet Cell Type ___ ___ ___
SSF8 Omentectomy ___ ___

CORPUS CASE 2

HISTORY AND PHYSICAL EXAM
Crampy abdominal pain with vaginal bleeding.
8-8-20XX Physical exam: No lymphadenopathy, no abdominal masses. No abnormal findings.
8-8-20XX Pelvic exam: Uterus normal size and anteverted. Cervix normal.

X-RAYS AND SCANS
8-14-20XX MRI Pelvis: Decreased signal in right fundal endometrium consistent with endometrial carcinoma. No evidence of deep invasion.
8-14-20XX Chest x-ray: Negative.
8-31-20XX CT abdomen/pelvis: No evidence of urinary tract obstruction. No adenopathy.

LABORATORY None.

ENDOSCOPIC PROCEDURES None.

OPERATIVE REPORT
8-24-20XX TAH-BSO: Uterus slightly increased in size with normal external contour. Small lesion noted in the fundus without gross evidence of invasion. Ovaries and tubes bilat. WNL. Liver, kidneys within normal limits. No pelvic or periaortic adenopathy noted.

PATHOLOGY REPORTS
D&C (prior to admission): Moderately well-differentiated adenocarcinoma, endometrium.
Endocervical curettage (prior to admission): Negative
8-24-20XX TAH-BSO: Adenocarcinoma, grade ii of endometrium. No myometrial invasion. Tumor size 2 x 1.2 x 1 cm. Tubes and ovaries: No malignancy.

TREATMENT
8-24-20XX Total abdominal hysterectomy and bilateral salpingo-oophorectomy

Corpus-Cervix

Site Code ___ ___ ___.___	cT ___ cN ___ cM ___	SSF1 FIGO Stage ___ ___ ___
Histology/Behavior/Grade ___ ___ ___ ___/___ ___	Clin Stage Group _____	SSF2 Periton Cytol ___ ___ ___
Grade Path Value ___	pT ___ pN ___ M ___	SSF3 # Pos Pelvic LN ___ ___ ___
Grade Path System ___	Path Stage Group _____	SSF4 # Exam Pelvic LN ___ ___ ___
Lymph Vascular Invasion ___	CS Tumor Size ___ ___ ___	SSF5 # Pos Para-Aortic LN ___ ___ ___
Ambiguous Terminol ___	CS Extension ___ ___ ___	SSF6 # Exam Para-Aortic LN ___ ___ ___
Date Conclusive Terminol ___ ___ ___ ___ ___ ___ ___ ___	CS TS/Ext Eval ___	SSF7 % Non-Endomet Cell Type ___ ___ ___
Date Conclus Dx Flag ___ ___	CS LN ___ ___ ___	SSF8 Omentectomy ___ ___ ___
Multiplicity Counter ___ ___	CS Reg Nodes Eval ___	
Date Mult Tumors ___ ___ ___ ___ ___ ___ ___ ___	Reg LN Pos ___ ___	
Date Mult Tumors Flag ___ ___	Reg LN Exam ___ ___	
Mult Tum Reported as One Prim ___ ___	CS Mets at Dx ___ ___	
Summary Stage 2000 ___	CS Mets at Dx - Bone ___ Brain ___ Liver ___ Lung ___	
	CS Mets Eval ___	

CORPUS CASE 3

HISTORY AND PHYSICAL EXAM

61 year old female presented with abdominal distention and pain. History of right tube and ovary removed many years ago for ectopic pregnancy.

7-21-20XX Physical exam: Large mass palpable in pelvis on bimanual examination. No lymph-adenopathy or organomegaly.

X-RAYS AND SCANS

7-24-20XX Chest x-ray: No evidence of disease.
7-24-20XX CT abdomen/pelvis: Mass of unknown identity present in pelvis.

LABORATORY

7-21-20XX CEA within normal limits. CA-125 elevated.
7-27-20XX ER positive, PR positive

ENDOSCOPIC PROCEDURES None.

OPERATIVE REPORT

7-27-20XX TAH-LSO: Large uterine mass noted, not resectable en bloc. Mass transected during surgery to remove bulk of mass, then remainder removed. Gross tumor spillage onto parametrium during resection.

PATHOLOGY REPORTS

7-27-20XX TAH-LSO: Adenocarcinoma, grade II with 50% myometrial invasion. Cervix: Secondary endometrial adenocarcinoma invading endocervical canal stroma. Left tube negative; left ovary: polycystic ovarian disease. Pelvic lavage: Positive for tumor cells.

TREATMENT

7-27-20XX Total abdominal hysterectomy and left salpingo-oophorectomy
8-21-20XX to 9-15-20XX External beam radiation to pelvis in 25 fractions
10-2-20XX Single cesium insertion using ovoids

Site Code ___ ___ ___.___	Summary Stage 2000 _____	CS Mets at Dx - Bone ___ Brain ___ Liver ___ Lung ___
Histology/Behavior/Grade ___ ___ ___ ___/___ ___	cT ___ cN ___ cM ___	CS Mets Eval ___
Grade Path Value ___	Clin Stage Group _____	SSF1 FIGO Stage ___ ___ ___
Grade Path System ___	pT ___ pN ___ M ___	SSF2 Periton Cytol ___ ___ ___
Lymph Vascular Invasion ___	Path Stage Group _____	SSF3 # Pos Pelvic LN ___ ___ ___
Ambiguous Terminol ___	CS Tumor Size ___ ___ ___	SSF4 # Exam Pelvic LN ___ ___ ___
Date Conclusive Terminol ___ ___ ___ ___ ___ ___ ___ ___	CS Extension ___ ___ ___	SSF5 # Pos Para-Aortic LN ___ ___ ___
Date Conclus Dx Flag ___ ___	CS TS/Ext Eval ___	SSF6 # Exam Para-Aortic LN ___ ___ ___
Multiplicity Counter ___ ___	CS LN ___ ___ ___	SSF7 % Non-Endomet Cell Type ___ ___ ___
Date Mult Tumors ___ ___ ___ ___ ___ ___ ___ ___	CS Reg Nodes Eval ___	SSF8 Omentectomy ___ ___ ___
Date Mult Tumors Flag ___ ___	Reg LN Pos ___ ___	
Mult Tum Reported as One Prim ___ ___	Reg LN Exam ___ ___	
	CS Mets at Dx ___ ___	

CORPUS CASE 4

HISTORY AND PHYSICAL EXAM
Post-menopausal bleeding. Entire physical exam within normal limits.

X-RAYS AND SCANS
2-19-20XX Intravenous pyelogram: Negative.
2-19-20XX Chest x-ray: Negative.

LABORATORY
2-19-20XX CBC: Slightly anemic.

ENDOSCOPIC PROCEDURES
None.

OPERATIVE REPORT
3-1-20XX TAH-BSO: Superficial invasion involving entire endometrial cavity. Ovaries and tubes: No evidence of involvement.

PATHOLOGY REPORTS
2-22-20XX Endometrial biopsy: Moderately differentiated adenocarcinoma, grade II. Non-squamous growth pattern 10%. Fragments of highly dysplastic squamous epithelium (at least CIN III).
2-24-20XX Endometrial curettage: Moderately well-differentiated adenocarcinoma.
3-1-20XX TAH/BSO, pelvic lymph node dissection: Well differentiated adenocarcinoma with papillary features invading upper third of myometrium. Tumor size 0.7 x 0.2 cm. None of six pelvic lymph nodes involved with tumor.

TREATMENT
3-1-20XX Total abdominal hysterectomy with bilateral salpingo-oophorectomy and pelvic lymph node dissection

Site Code ___ ___ ___.___
Histology/Behavior/Grade ___ ___ ___ ___/___ ___
Grade Path Value ___
Grade Path System ___
Lymph Vascular Invasion ___
Ambiguous Terminol ___
Date Conclusive Terminol ___ ___ ___ ___ ___ ___ ___ ___
Date Conclus Dx Flag ___ ___
Multiplicity Counter ___ ___
Date Mult Tumors ___ ___ ___ ___ ___ ___ ___ ___
Date Mult Tumors Flag ___ ___
Mult Tum Reported as One Prim ___ ___
Summary Stage 2000 ___

cT ___ cN ___ cM ___
Clin Stage Group ___
pT ___ pN ___ M ___
Path Stage Group ___
CS Tumor Size ___ ___ ___
CS Extension ___ ___ ___
CS TS/Ext Eval ___
CS LN ___ ___ ___
CS Reg Nodes Eval ___
Reg LN Pos ___ ___
Reg LN Exam ___ ___
CS Mets at Dx ___ ___
CS Mets at Dx - Bone ___ Brain ___ Liver ___ Lung ___
CS Mets Eval ___

SSF1 FIGO Stage ___ ___
SSF2 Periton Cytol ___ ___ ___
SSF3 # Pos Pelvic LN ___ ___ ___
SSF4 # Exam Pelvic LN ___ ___ ___
SSF5 # Pos Para-Aortic LN ___ ___ ___
SSF6 # Exam Para-Aortic LN ___ ___ ___
SSF7 % Non-Endomet Cell Type ___ ___ ___
SSF8 Omentectomy ___ ___ ___

CORPUS CASE 5

HISTORY AND PHYSICAL EXAM
Post menopausal bleeding.
5-16-20XX Cervix: Necrotic ulcer extending to vaginal fornix. No abdominal masses. Uterus normal; confirmed by rectovaginal examination. Parametria free of masses. No lymphadenopathy.

X-RAYS AND SCANS
5-16-20XX MRI of pelvis: Endometrial carcinoma with deep myometrial invasion. Tumor extends to lower uterine segment. Invasion of proximal cervix cannot beruled out. No tumor extension through the serosal surface or into adnexal areas. No pelvic adenopathy.
5-31-20XX Chest x-ray: Negative.

LABORATORY None significant.

ENDOSCOPIC PROCEDURES
5-24-20XX Colposcopy: 2 cm tumor on posterior lip of cervix with some extension down to vaginal apex.
5-27-20XX Sigmoidoscopy and cystoscopy: Negative for tumor.

OPERATIVE REPORT
6-8-20XX Endocervical curettage: Ulcerated cervix seen. Uterus enlarged. No adnexal masses or parametrial invasion.

PATHOLOGY REPORTS
6-1-20XX Endocervical curettage: Adenocarcinoma, grade III with clear cell and secretory features.
6-20-20XX TAH-BSO: Adenocarcinoma, grade 3 with focal secretory and squamous differentiation. 75% myometrial invasion. Severe inflammatory reaction, but no tumor involvement of cervix. No other spread of tumor. Peritoneal washings benign.

TREATMENT
6-8-20XX Intracavitary cesium implant
6-20-20XX Total abdominal hysterectomy-bilateral salpingo-oophorectomy
7-12-20XX to 8-3-20XX External beam radiation to pelvis. 45Gy Conformal technique

Site Code ___ ___ ___.___
Histology/Behavior/Grade ___ ___ ___ ___ / ___ ___
Grade Path Value ___
Grade Path System ___
Lymph Vascular Invasion ___
Ambiguous Terminol ___
Date Conclusive Terminol ___ ___ ___ ___ ___ ___ ___ ___
Date Conclus Dx Flag ___ ___
Multiplicity Counter ___ ___
Date Mult Tumors ___ ___ ___ ___ ___ ___ ___ ___

Date Mult Tumors Flag ___ ___
Mult Tum Reported as One Prim ___ ___
Summary Stage 2000 ___
cT ___ cN ___ cM ___
Clin Stage Group ___
pT ___ pN ___ M ___
Path Stage Group ___
CS Tumor Size ___ ___ ___
CS Extension ___ ___ ___
CS TS/Ext Eval ___
CS LN ___ ___ ___

CS Reg Nodes Eval ___
Reg LN Pos ___ ___
Reg LN Exam ___ ___
CS Mets at Dx ___ ___
CS Mets at Dx - Bone ___ Brain ___ Liver ___ Lung ___
CS Mets Eval ___
SSF1 FIGO Stage ___ ___ ___
SSF2 Periton Cytol ___ ___ ___
SSF3 # Pos Pelvic LN ___ ___ ___

Corpus Case 5, continued

SSF4 # Exam Pelvic LN ___ ___ ___	**SSF6 # Exam Para-Aortic LN** ___ ___ ___	**SSF8 Omentectomy** ___ ___ ___
SSF5 # Pos Para-Aortic LN ___ ___ ___	**SSF7 % Non-Endomet Cell Type** ___ ___ ___	

CORPUS CASE 6

HISTORY AND PHYSICAL EXAM

Small bladder capacity with some incontinence.
Pelvic: enlarged uterus. No other significant findings.

X-RAYS AND SCANS

1-21-20XX IVP:Normal kidneys and ureters. Compression of bladder by large pelvic mass.
1-24-20XX MRI of pelvis: Bilateral iliac lymphadenopathy. Bladder and rectum: no evidence of disease. Impression: Possible uterine sarcoma of mixed mullerian type.
1-24-20XX Chest x-ray: No evidence of disease.

LABORATORY

1-21-20XX CEA: 10 (patient is smoker).

ENDOSCOPIC PROCEDURES None.

OPERATIVE REPORTS

1-26-20XX Endometrial biopsy in MD office: No information from procedure.
2-7-20XX Radical hysterectomy: Enlarged uterus, no abnormal findings of parametrium or other pelvic structures.

PATHOLOGY REPORTS

1-26-20XX Biopsy, endometrial: High grade stromal sarcoma vs. carcinosarcoma
2-7-20XX Uterus, tubes, ovaries, lymph nodes: High grade carcinosarcoma, involving 10% of myometrium. No tumor on serosal surface of corpus. Cervix, ovaries, fallopian tubes all negative. 5 of 24 pelvic lymph nodes involved with metastases. FIGO IIIC.

TREATMENT

2-7-20XX Radical hysterectomy and bilateral salpingo-oophorectomy, pelvic node dissection
2-24-20XX Started combination chemotherapy in MD office

Site Code ___ ___ ___.___	**Multiplicity Counter** ___ ___	**Path Stage Group** _____
Histology/Behavior/Grade ___ ___ ___ ___/___ ___	**Date Mult Tumors** ___ ___ ___ ___ ___ ___ ___ ___	**CS Tumor Size** ___ ___ ___
Grade Path Value ___	**Date Mult Tumors Flag** ___ ___	**CS Extension** ___ ___ ___
Grade Path System ___	**Mult Tum Reported as One Prim** ___ ___	**CS TS/Ext Eval** ___
Lymph Vascular Invasion ___	**Summary Stage 2000** ___	**CS LN** ___ ___ ___
Ambiguous Terminol ___	**cT** ___ **cN** ___ **cM** ___	**CS Reg Nodes Eval** ___
Date Conclusive Terminol ___ ___ ___ ___ ___ ___ ___ ___	**Clin Stage Group** _____	**Reg LN Pos** ___ ___
Date Conclus Dx Flag ___ ___	**pT** ___ **pN** ___ **M** ___	**Reg LN Exam** ___ ___
		CS Mets at Dx ___ ___

Corpus Case 6, continued

CS Mets at Dx - Bone ___ Brain ___ Liver ___ Lung ___	SSF2 Periton Cytol ___ ___ ___	SSF6 # Exam Para-Aortic LN ___ ___ ___
CS Mets Eval ___	SSF3 # Pos Pelvic LN ___ ___ ___	SSF7 % Non-Endomet Cell Type ___ ___ ___
SSF1 FIGO Stage ___ ___ ___	SSF4 # Exam Pelvic LN ___ ___ ___	SSF8 Omentectomy ___ ___ ___
	SSF5 # Pos Para-Aortic LN ___ ___ ___	

CORPUS CASE 7

HISTORY AND PHYSICAL EXAMINATION

47 year old female complaining of discomfort and fullness in low abdomen and intermittent low back pain.
Physical exam: Obese patient with no palpable lymphadenopathy in neck, axilla or groin. No palpable hepatosplenomegaly. Pelvic exam essentially normal except for possibly enlarged uterus.

X-RAYS AND SCANS

11-8-20XX CT abdomen and pelvis: Enlarged uterus with ill-defined mass in left adnexa
11-20-20XX PET scan post surgery: Subtle areas of increased activity in distal esophagus and possibly in sigmoid colon.
12-24-20XX CT abdomen and pelvis: Uterus and adnexa removed. New mass in low abdomen with mesenteric and peritoneal implants. Stricture in proximal rectum with impending obstruction.

LABORATORY

11-8-20XX CA-125 slightly elevated. CEA slightly elevated. All other lab work normal.

ENDOSCOPIC PROCEDURES

11-28-20XX Esophagogastroduodenoscopy and colonoscopy: Circumferential submucosal bulging in rectum of uncertain significance.

OPERATIVE REPORT

11-12-20XX TAH-BSO: Locally advanced disease with extension through the uterus and the cul-de-sac involving the left broad ligament, as well as rectovaginal space. FIGO Stage IIIA.

PATHOLOGY REPORTS

11-12-20XX TAH-BSO: High grade leiomyosarcoma.

TREATMENT

11-12-20XX TAH-BSO
12-20-20XX to 12-27-20XX 10.8 Gy 3D conformal radiation therapy to whole pelvis (discontinued)
12-30-20XX Diverting colostomy
01-10-20YY Tumor embolization of pelvic mass. Started on Tamoxifen

CLINICAL COURSE

Soon after starting her radiation therapy, the patient noted increasing symptoms similar to her initial presentation.

continued on next page

Corpus Case 7, continued

Abdominal examination revealed findings of recurrent pelvic disease. The patient was discharged and offered the options of hospice versus consideration of palliative chemotherapy.

Site Code ___ ___ ___.___	**Summary Stage 2000** _____	**CS Mets at Dx -** **Bone** ___ **Brain** ___
Histology/Behavior/Grade ___ ___ ___ ___ / ___ ___	**cT** ___ **cN** ___ **cM** ___	**Liver** ___ **Lung** ___
	Clin Stage Group _____	
Grade Path Value ___		**CS Mets Eval** ___
Grade Path System ___	**pT** ___ **pN** ___ **M** ___	**SSF1 FIGO Stage** ___ ___ ___
Lymph Vascular Invasion ___	**Path Stage Group** _____	**SSF2 Periton Cytol** ___ ___ ___
Ambiguous Terminol ___	**CS Tumor Size** ___ ___ ___	**SSF3 # Pos Pelvic LN** ___ ___ ___
Date Conclusive Terminol ___ ___ ___ ___ ___ ___ ___ ___	**CS Extension** ___ ___ ___	
	CS TS/Ext Eval ___	**SSF4 # Exam Pelvic LN** ___ ___ ___
Date Conclus Dx Flag ___ ___	**CS LN** ___ ___ ___	
Multiplicity Counter ___ ___	**CS Reg Nodes Eval** ___	**SSF5 # Pos Para-Aortic LN** ___ ___ ___
Date Mult Tumors ___ ___ ___ ___ ___ ___ ___ ___	**Reg LN Pos** ___ ___	**SSF6 # Exam Para-Aortic LN** ___ ___ ___
	Reg LN Exam ___ ___	
Date Mult Tumors Flag ___ ___	**CS Mets at Dx** ___ ___	**SSF7 % Non-Endomet Cell Type** ___ ___ ___
Mult Tum Reported as One Prim ___ ___		**SSF8 Omentectomy** ___ ___ ___

CORPUS CASE 8

HISTORY AND PHYSICAL EXAMINATION

Recent history of abdominal bloating.
Physical exam: Abdominal pelvic mass that fills the cul-de-sac. Mass is firm, compatible with ovary or uterine malignancy, likely adenocarcinoma of ovary vs. uterine vs. uterine carcinoma/sarcoma.

X-RAYS AND SCANS

9-21-20XX CXR: No evidence of metastases.
Bilateral mammogram: Within normal limits.

LABORATORY None.

ENDOSCOPIC PROCEDURES None.

OPERATIVE REPORT

9-24-20XX Laparotomy, TAH and BSO. Observations at surgery: Abdomen—no evidence of seeding; pelvis—huge cystic mass replacing left ovary.
Right ovary and remaining adnexa appear normal.

PATHOLOGY REPORTS

9-24-20XX Left ovary: Invasive w-d mucinous cystadenocarcinoma. 27 mm area of tumor within large cystic mass. Right ovary, bilateral tubes, cervix: Negative for tumor. All other biopsies and removed tissues negative for tumor. Lymph nodes removed (number not stated): all negative. Tumor confined to left ovary; no tumor on ovarian surface.
Endometrium: P-d endometrial adenocarcinoma.

continued on next page

Corpus Case 8, continued

TREATMENT

9-24-20XX Exploratory laparotomy, TAH and BSO, bilateral pelvic-periaortic lymphadenectomy, omentectomy, cul-de-sac biopsy, liver biopsies, diaphragm biopsies, bladder peritoneum biopsy and ascitic fluid for cell block

Site Code ___ ___ ___.___	Summary Stage 2000 _____	CS Mets at Dx - Bone ___ Brain ___ Liver ___ Lung ___
Histology/Behavior/Grade ___ ___ ___ ___/___ ___	cT ___ cN ___ cM ___	CS Mets Eval ___
Grade Path Value ___	Clin Stage Group _____	SSF1 FIGO Stage ___ ___ ___
Grade Path System ___	pT ___ pN ___ M ___	SSF2 Periton Cytol ___ ___ ___
Lymph Vascular Invasion ___	Path Stage Group _____	SSF3 # Pos Pelvic LN ___ ___ ___
Ambiguous Terminol ___	CS Tumor Size ___ ___ ___	SSF4 # Exam Pelvic LN ___ ___ ___
Date Conclusive Terminol ___ ___ ___ ___ ___ ___ ___ ___	CS Extension ___ ___ ___	SSF5 # Pos Para-Aortic LN ___ ___ ___
Date Conclus Dx Flag ___ ___	CS TS/Ext Eval ___	SSF6 # Exam Para-Aortic LN ___ ___ ___
Multiplicity Counter ___ ___	CS LN ___ ___ ___	SSF7 % Non-Endomet Cell Type ___ ___ ___
Date Mult Tumors ___ ___ ___ ___ ___ ___ ___ ___	CS Reg Nodes Eval ___	SSF8 Omentectomy ___ ___ ___
Date Mult Tumors Flag ___ ___	Reg LN Pos ___ ___	
Mult Tum Reported as One Prim ___ ___	Reg LN Exam ___ ___	
	CS Mets at Dx ___ ___	

CORPUS CASE 9

HISTORY AND PHYSICAL EXAMINATION

One year history of blood-tinged vaginal discharge; irregular periods.

3-2-20YY Physical exam: Essentially normal pelvic exam.
No adenopathy or organomegaly.

X-RAYS AND SCANS

12-17-20XX Ultrasound: Essentially normal pelvis.

LABORATORY

12-17-20XX CA-125: 54 (normal 0 - 35 U/mL)

1-29-20YY CA-125: 94 (normal 0 – 35 U/mL)

ENDOSCOPIC PROCEDURES None.

OPERATIVE REPORT

3-17-20YY Radical hysterectomy: Upper abdomen grossly unremarkable. Tumor extends from corpus into right parametria. Right ureter stuck down to tumor but dissected free. No gross residual tumor at end of procedure.

PATHOLOGY REPORTS

3-2-20YY Endometrial biopsy: Endometrial carcinoma.

3-17-20YY Uterus, adenexa, right parametrium and omentum: FIGO grade I adenosquamous carcinoma with lymphovascular invasion involving uterus with extension to

continued on next page

Corpus Case 9, continued

endocervical stroma, left and right adnexa, and right parametrial tissue. Final margins contained no tumor. Right pelvic lymph nodes (8): No metastatic tumor. Obturator lymph node (1): No metastatic tumor. Common iliac node (1): No metastatic tumor. Omentum: No metastatic tumor. Pelvic washings: Atypical cells present worrisome for adenocarcinoma. ER: Neg. PR: Weakly positive.

TREATMENT

3-17-20YY Modified radical hysterectomy and right pelvic lymphadenectomy with upper vaginectomy, bilateral salpingo-oophorectomy and omentectomy

4-25-20YY to 5-31-20YY 3D Conformal external beam radiation therapy to whole pelvis, 45 Gy in 25 fractions

6-18-20YY to 6-19-20YY High dose rate brachytherapy boost to vaginal cuff

7-14-20YY Started chemotherapy with Cisplatin, Adriamycin and Taxol

Site Code ___ ___ ___.___	Summary Stage 2000 _____	CS Mets at Dx - Bone ___ Brain ___
Histology/Behavior/Grade ___ ___ ___ ___/___ ___	cT ___ cN ___ cM ___	Liver ___ Lung ___
	Clin Stage Group _____	
Grade Path Value ___		CS Mets Eval ___
Grade Path System ___	pT ___ pN ___ M ___	SSF1 FIGO Stage ___ ___ ___
Lymph Vascular Invasion ___	Path Stage Group _____	SSF2 Periton Cytol ___ ___ ___
Ambiguous Terminol ___	CS Tumor Size ___ ___ ___	SSF3 # Pos Pelvic LN ___ ___ ___
Date Conclusive Terminol ___ ___ ___ ___ ___ ___ ___ ___	CS Extension ___ ___ ___	
	CS TS/Ext Eval ___	SSF4 # Exam Pelvic LN ___ ___ ___
Date Conclus Dx Flag ___ ___	CS LN ___ ___ ___	
Multiplicity Counter ___ ___	CS Reg Nodes Eval ___	SSF5 # Pos Para-Aortic LN ___ ___ ___
Date Mult Tumors ___ ___ ___ ___ ___ ___ ___ ___	Reg LN Pos ___ ___	SSF6 # Exam Para-Aortic LN ___ ___ ___
	Reg LN Exam ___ ___	
Date Mult Tumors Flag ___ ___	CS Mets at Dx ___ ___	SSF7 % Non-Endomet Cell Type ___ ___ ___
Mult Tum Reported as One Prim ___ ___		SSF8 Omentectomy ___ ___ ___

CORPUS CASE 10

HISTORY AND PHYSICAL EXAMINATION

Postmenopausal female with history of intermittent vaginal bleeding for six months. Physical exam: Essentially normal exam. No evidence of lesions in vagina or exocervix on speculum exam. No adenopathy or organomegaly.

X-RAYS AND SCANS

5-25-20XX Chest x-ray: Within normal limits.

6-05-20XX CT abdomen and pelvis: No metastatic lesions noted. Uterus normal size.

LABORATORY None.

ENDOSCOPIC PROCEDURES

4-12-20XX Hysteroscopy and fractional D&C.

continued on next page

Corpus Case 10, continued

OPERATIVE REPORT

6-13-20XX TAH-BSO: No seeding in pelvis or abdomen. Uterus thickened but no apparent tumor on surfaces of pelvic organs.

PATHOLOGY REPORTS

4-12-20XX PATH: 1) ENDOCERVIX, BIOPSY: High grade adenocarcinoma, papillary serous type.
2) ENDOMETRIAL CURETTINGS: High grade adenocarcinoma, papillary serous type.
PATH ADDENDUM: On re-examination of the endocervix biopsy (Specimen #1), and endometrial curettings (Specimen #2), it is concluded that this tumor is best characterized as "High-grade, endometrioid adenocarcinoma with papillary features", rather than "High-grade adenocarcinoma, papillary serous type." Approximately 35% is non-morular.

6-13-20XX TAH-BSO: Histology similar to previous tissue; invasion through 3/4 of myometrium (FIGO Stage IB), 00 of 23 lymph nodes showing malignancy.

TREATMENT

4-12-20XX Hysteroscopy and fractional dilatation and curettage
6-13-20XX TAH-BSO and pelvic lymph node dissection
12-11-20XX Excisional biopsy of left vaginal wall recurrence
12-17-20XX to 1-23-20YY 4500 cGy to pelvis
2-21-20YY to 2-22-20YY 3 treatments high dose rate Iridium 192 vaginal implants

Site Code ___ ___ ___.___	Summary Stage 2000 _____	CS Mets at Dx - Bone ___ Brain ___ Liver ___ Lung ___
Histology/Behavior/Grade ___ ___ ___ ___ / ___ ___	cT ___ cN ___ cM ___	CS Mets Eval ___
Grade Path Value ___	Clin Stage Group _____	SSF1 FIGO Stage ___ ___ ___
Grade Path System ___	pT ___ pN ___ M ___	SSF2 Periton Cytol ___ ___ ___
Lymph Vascular Invasion ___	Path Stage Group _____	SSF3 # Pos Pelvic LN ___ ___ ___
Ambiguous Terminol ___	CS Tumor Size ___ ___ ___	SSF4 # Exam Pelvic LN ___ ___ ___
Date Conclusive Terminol ___ ___ ___ ___ ___ ___ ___ ___	CS Extension ___ ___ ___	SSF5 # Pos Para-Aortic LN ___ ___ ___
Date Conclus Dx Flag ___ ___	CS TS/Ext Eval ___	SSF6 # Exam Para-Aortic LN ___ ___ ___
Multiplicity Counter ___ ___	CS LN ___ ___ ___	SSF7 % Non-Endomet Cell Type ___ ___ ___
Date Mult Tumors ___ ___ ___ ___ ___ ___ ___ ___	CS Reg Nodes Eval ___	SSF8 Omentectomy ___ ___ ___
Date Mult Tumors Flag ___ ___	Reg LN Pos ___ ___	
Mult Tum Reported as One Prim ___ ___	Reg LN Exam ___ ___	
	CS Mets at Dx ___ ___	

CORPUS CASE 11

HISTORY AND PHYSICAL EXAMINATION

52-year-old female approximately 10 years postmenopausal with recent light pink spotting. No abdominal or pelvic pain, but some urinary incontinence with coughing and sneezing. No dysuria or urinary frequency.
Pelvic exam: Normal external genitalia. Normal vagina and cervix without lesions on speculum exam. Bimanual exam limited secondary to patient's obesity. Uterus mobile and non-tender; size difficult to determine. No obvious masses. Rectovaginal exam: grade 2-3 rectocele, no rectal masses.

X-RAYS AND SCANS

11-15-20XX Pelvic ultrasound: Uterus 10 x 3.7 x 5.4 cm, arcuate uterus with a thickened endometrial stripe of 0.8 cm.
11-27-20XX Chest x-ray: No lymphadenopathy or masses in lungs or mediastinum
11-27-20XX CT abdomen and pelvis: No masses, adenopathy or any other abnormalities.

LABORATORY None.

ENDOSCOPIC PROCEDURES None.

OPERATIVE REPORT

11-30-20XX TAH-BSO: No significant findings.

PATHOLOGY REPORTS

11-6-20XX Pap smear: Parabasal cells consistent with post-menopause.
11-15-20XX Endometrial biopsy: FIGO Grade 1 adenocarcinoma
11-30-20XX TAH-BSO: 1) Adipose tissue (omentum), left and right fallopian tubes, left and right ovaries: No diagnostic abnormality.
2) Uterus: Uterine cervix: Chronic cervicitis. Endomyometrium: Endometrioid adenocarcinoma, FIGO grade 2, with superficial myometrial invasion. Myometrial leiomyoma.
Tumor Site: Not specified
Tumor Size: Cannot be determined (present multifocally throughout endometrium)
Histologic Type: Endometrioid adenocarcinoma
Histologic Grade: Grade 2
Myometrial Invasion: Invasion present.
Depth of Invasion: 1 to 2 mm, total thickness of myometrium 2.2 cm
Regional Lymph Nodes: None in specimen–cannot be assessed
Margins: Uninvolved by invasive carcinoma
Distance of Invasive Carcinoma from Closest Margin: 2 cm (serosal margin).
Venous/Lymphatic Invasion: Absent

TREATMENT

11-30-20XX Total abdominal hysterectomy and bilateral salpingo-oophorectomy with pelvic lymph node dissection

Corpus Case 11, continued

Site Code	___ ___ ___.___	Summary Stage 2000	_____	CS Mets at Dx - Bone ___ Brain ___ Liver ___ Lung ___	
Histology/Behavior/Grade	___ ___ ___ ___/___ ___	cT ___ cN ___ cM ___		CS Mets Eval	___
		Clin Stage Group _____			
Grade Path Value	___	pT ___ pN ___ M ___		SSF1 FIGO Stage	___ ___ ___
Grade Path System	___	Path Stage Group _____		SSF2 Periton Cytol	___ ___ ___
Lymph Vascular Invasion	___	CS Tumor Size	___ ___ ___	SSF3 # Pos Pelvic LN	___ ___ ___
Ambiguous Terminol	___	CS Extension	___ ___ ___	SSF4 # Exam Pelvic LN	___ ___ ___
Date Conclusive Terminol	___ ___ ___ ___ ___ ___ ___ ___	CS TS/Ext Eval	___	SSF5 # Pos Para-Aortic LN	___ ___ ___
Date Conclus Dx Flag	___ ___	CS LN	___ ___ ___	SSF6 # Exam Para-Aortic LN	___ ___ ___
Multiplicity Counter	___ ___	CS Reg Nodes Eval	___	SSF7 % Non-Endomet Cell Type	___ ___ ___
Date Mult Tumors	___ ___ ___ ___ ___ ___ ___ ___	Reg LN Pos	___ ___	SSF8 Omentectomy	___ ___ ___
Date Mult Tumors Flag	___ ___	Reg LN Exam	___ ___		
Mult Tum Reported as One Prim	___ ___	CS Mets at Dx	___ ___		

CORPUS CASE 12

PHYSICAL EXAMINATION

3-2-20XX Dysfunctional vaginal bleeding. Physical exam unremarkable. Exam under anesthesia showed 16-18 week size uterus, irregular in shape but mobile.

X-RAYS AND SCANS

3-7-20XX CXR: No acute process.

LABORATORY None.

ENDOSCOPIC PROCEDURES None.

OPERATIVE REPORTS

3-7-20XX D&C: Enlarged mobile uterus; no adnexal masses

3-16-20XX TAH and BSO: No remarkable findings

PATHOLOGY REPORTS

3-7-20XX Endometrium curettage: Well-differentiated adenocarcinoma.

3-16-20XX TAH and BSO: Adenoacanthoma, myometrial invasion more than half-way through. 16 pelvic and iliac nodes negative. 1 para-aortic node positive. Adnexa benign.

TREATMENT

3-16-20XX TAH and BSO with regional lymph node dissection

Site Code	___ ___ ___.___	Lymph Vascular Invasion	___	Multiplicity Counter	___ ___
Histology/Behavior/Grade	___ ___ ___ ___/___ ___	*Ambiguous Terminol*	___	Date Mult Tumors	___ ___ ___ ___ ___ ___ ___ ___
Grade Path Value	___	Date Conclusive Terminol	___ ___ ___ ___ ___ ___ ___ ___	Date Mult Tumors Flag	___ ___
Grade Path System	___	Date Conclus Dx Flag	___ ___		

Corpus Case 12, continued

Mult Tum Reported as One Prim __ __

Summary Stage 2000 ____

cT __ cN __ cM __

Clin Stage Group ____

pT __ pN __ M __

Path Stage Group ____

CS Tumor Size __ __ __

CS Extension __ __ __

CS TS/Ext Eval __

CS LN __ __ __

CS Reg Nodes Eval __

Reg LN Pos __ __

Reg LN Exam __ __

CS Mets at Dx __ __

CS Mets at Dx -
Bone __ Brain __
Liver __ Lung __

CS Mets Eval __

SSF1 FIGO Stage __ __ __

SSF2 Periton Cytol __ __ __

SSF3 # Pos Pelvic LN __ __ __

SSF4 # Exam Pelvic LN __ __ __

SSF5 # Pos Para-Aortic LN __ __ __

SSF6 # Exam Para-Aortic LN __ __ __

SSF7 % Non-Endomet Cell Type __ __ __

SSF8 Omentectomy __ __ __

ANSWERS TO CORPUS UTERI STAGING EXERCISES

—— CORPUS CASE 1 ——

Site Code	C54.1	Endometrium			
Histology	8560/39	Adenosquamous carcinoma, grade not stated			
Grade Path Value	Blank	Does not apply			
Grade Path System	Blank	Does not apply			
Lymph Vascular Invasion	9	Lymph-vascular invasion not mentioned in path report			
Ambiguous Terminology	0	Conclusive terminology			
Date Conclusive Terminol	Blank	Diagnosis made by conclusive terminology			
Date Conclus Dx Flag	11	Not applicable			
Multiplicity Counter	01	One tumor only			
Date Multiple Tumors	Blank	Not applicable			
Date Mult Tumors Flag	15	Single tumor only (multiplicity counter is coded 01)			
Type Mult Tum as 1 Prim	00	Single tumor			
Summary Stage	2	Regional direct extension			
CLINICAL	T X	N X	M 0	Stage Group	Unstageable
PATHOLOGIC	T 3a	N X	cM 0	Stage Group	III
CS Tumor Size	999	Size of uterus is not size of tumor			
CS Extension	550	Involvement of fallopian tube			
CS TS/Ext Eval	3	Based on pathology report			
CS Lymph Nodes	000	No palpable nodes at surgery observation			
CS Reg Nodes Eval	1	Based on surgery observation without biopsy			
Reg Nodes Pos	98	No nodes examined			
Reg Nodes Exam	00	No nodes removed			
CS Mets at Dx	00	CXR negative			
CS Mets at Dx–Bone	0	No bone metastases			
CS Mets at Dx–Brain	0	No brain metastases			
CS Mets at Dx–Liver	0	No liver metastases			
CS Mets at Dx–Lung	0	No lung metastases			
CS Mets Eval	0	Based on imaging			
SSF1 FIGO Stage	999	FIGO stage not documented			
SSF2 Peritoneal Cytol	998	Test not done			
SSF3 # Pos Pelvic LN	098	No pelvic nodes examined			
SSF4 # Exam Pelvic LN	000	No pelvic nodes examined			
SSF5 # Pos Para-aortic LN	098	No para-aortic nodes examined			
SSF6 # Exam Para-aort LN	000	No para-aortic nodes examined			
SSF7 % Non-Endomet Cell	999	Not documented in patient record			
SSF8 Omentectomy	000	Omentectomy not performed			

This case will map to pT3a cN0 cM0 Stage Group IIIA.

Technically, this case cannot be TNM stage-grouped because no lymph nodes were mentioned clinically or removed for examination. However, the T3a puts the case into at least Stage III whether or not regional lymph nodes are involved. Another principle of TNM is that if the substage cannot be determined, it is OK to assign the whole stage (general rules 12).

—— CORPUS CASE 2 ——

Site Code	C54.1	Endometrium		
Histology	8140/32	Moderately differentiated adenocarcinoma		
Grade Path Value	Blank	Does not apply		
Grade Path System	Blank	Does not apply		
Lymph Vascular Invasion	9	Lymph-vascular invasion not mentioned in path report		
Ambiguous Terminology	0	Conclusive terminology		
Date Conclusive Terminol	Blank	Diagnosis made by conclusive terminology		
Date Conclus Dx Flag	11	Not applicable		
Multiplicity Counter	01	One tumor only		
Date Multiple Tumors	Blank	Not applicable		
Date Mult Tumors Flag	15	Single tumor only (multiplicity counter is coded 01)		
Type Mult Tum as 1 Prim	00	Single tumor		
Summary Stage	1	Localized		
CLINICAL	T X	N 0	M 0	Stage Group Unstageable
PATHOLOGIC	T 1a	N X	cM 0	Stage Group Unstaged
CS Tumor Size	020	Size of uterus is not size of tumor		
CS Extension	110	Confined to endometrium		
CS TS/Ext Eval	3	Based on pathology report		
CS Lymph Nodes	000	Note 3: no mention of nodes during exploration, assumed to be negative		
CS Reg Nodes Eval	1	Based on surgery observation without biopsy		
Reg Nodes Pos	98	No nodes examined		
Reg Nodes Exam	00	No nodes removed		
CS Mets at Dx	00	CXR negative		
CS Mets at Dx–Bone	0	No bone metastases		
CS Mets at Dx–Brain	0	No brain metastases		
CS Mets at Dx–Liver	0	No liver metastases		
CS Mets at Dx–Lung	0	No lung metastases		
CS Mets Eval	0	Based on imaging		
SSF1 FIGO Stage	999	FIGO stage not documented		
SSF2 Peritoneal Cytol	998	Test not done		
SSF3 # Pos Pelvic LN	098	No pelvic nodes examined		
SSF4 # Exam Pelvic LN	000	No pelvic nodes examined		
SSF5 # Pos Para-aortic LN	098	No para-aortic nodes examined		
SSF6 # Exam Para-aort LN	000	No para-aortic nodes examined		
SSF7 % Non-Endomet Cell	999	Growth pattern not documented		
SSF8 Omentectomy	000	Omentectomy not performed		

This case will map to pT1a cN0 cM0 Stage Group IA.

For TNM, no lymph nodes were removed for pathologic examination, so case cannot be staged grouped. FIGO stage is IA. The stated Grade II is a histologic grade; SSF2 needs a statement of percentage.

—— CORPUS CASE 3 ——

Site Code	C54.1	Endometrium		
Histology	8140/32	Moderately differentiated adenocarcinoma		
Grade Path Value	Blank	Does not apply		
Grade Path System	Blank	Does not apply		
Lymph Vascular Invasion	9	Lymph-vascular invasion not mentioned in path report		
Ambiguous Terminology	0	Conclusive terminology		
Date Conclusive Terminol	Blank	Diagnosis made by conclusive terminology		
Date Conclus Dx Flag	11	Not applicable		
Multiplicity Counter	01	One tumor only		
Date Multiple Tumors	Blank	Not applicable		
Date Mult Tumors Flag	15	Single tumor only (multiplicity counter is coded 01)		
Type Mult Tum as 1 Prim	00	Single tumor		
Summary Stage	2	Regional direct extension		
CLINICAL	T X	N 0	M 0	Stage Group Unstageable
PATHOLOGIC	T 1b	N X	cM 0	Stage Group Unstaged
CS Tumor Size	999	No size stated		
CS Extension	130	Tumor invades > 50% of myometrium		
CS TS/Ext Eval	3	Evidence acquired during surgery, surgical resection		
CS Lymph Nodes	000	Note 3: no mention of nodes during exploration, assumed to be negative		
CS Reg Nodes Eval	1	Based on surgery observation without biopsy		
Reg Nodes Pos	98	No nodes examined		
Reg Nodes Exam	00	No nodes removed		
CS Mets at Dx	00	CXR negative		
CS Mets at Dx–Bone	0	No bone metastases		
CS Mets at Dx–Brain	0	No brain metastases		
CS Mets at Dx–Liver	0	No liver metastases		
CS Mets at Dx–Lung	0	No lung metastases		
CS Mets Eval	0	Based on imaging		
SSF1 FIGO Stage	999	FIGO stage not documented		
SSF2 Peritoneal Cytol	010	Pelvic lavage positive		
SSF3 # Pos Pelvic LN	098	No pelvic nodes examined		
SSF4 # Exam Pelvic LN	098	No pelvic nodes examined		
SSF5 # Pos Para-aortic LN	098	No para-aortic nodes examined		
SSF6 # Exam Para-aort LN	000	No para-aortic nodes examined		
SSF7 % Non-Endomet Cell	999	Growth pattern not stated		
SSF8 Omentectomy	000	Omentectomy not performed		

This case will map to pT1b cN0 cM0 Stage Group IB.

This case cannot be TNM stage-grouped without pathologic information about the lymph nodes. However, because FIGO does not take into consideration the status of the lymph nodes, the case is at least FIGO Stage IB due to the 50% myometrial invasion. The gross tumor spillage and resulting positive pelvic washings are coded in SSF2 and do not affect the seventh edition stage. GYN surgeons will upstage the case because of the gross tumor spillage during the procedure and will recommend additional postoperative treatment. The stated Grade II is a histologic grade; SSF2 needs a statement of percentage.

—— CORPUS CASE 4 ——

Site Code	C54.1	Endometrium
Histology	8260/32	Adenocarcinoma with papillary features = papillary adenocarcinoma; code to higher grade in biopsy
Grade Path Value	Blank	Does not apply
Grade Path System	Blank	Does not apply
Lymph Vascular Invasion	9	Lymph-vascular invasion not mentioned in path report
Ambiguous Terminology	0	Conclusive terminology
Date Conclusive Terminol	Blank	Diagnosis made by conclusive terminology
Date Conclus Dx Flag	11	Not applicable
Multiplicity Counter	01	One tumor only
Date Multiple Tumors	Blank	Not applicable
Date Mult Tumors Flag	15	Single tumor only (multiplicity counter is coded 01)
Type Mult Tum as 1 Prim	00	Single tumor
Summary Stage	1	Localized

CLINICAL	T X	N 0	M 0	Stage Group Unstageable
PATHOLOGIC	T 1b	N 0	cM 0	Stage Group IB

CS Tumor Size	007	Tumor size on path report
CS Extension	120	Upper third is less than half of myometrium
CS TS/Ext Eval	3	Based on pathology report
CS Lymph Nodes	000	No involved nodes on pathology report
CS Reg Nodes Eval	3	Based on pathology report
Reg Nodes Pos	00	No nodes involved
Reg Nodes Exam	06	Six nodes examined
CS Mets at Dx	00	CXR negative
CS Mets at Dx–Bone	0	No bone metastases
CS Mets at Dx–Brain	0	No brain metastases
CS Mets at Dx–Liver	0	No liver metastases
CS Mets at Dx–Lung	0	No lung metastases
CS Mets Eval	0	Based on imaging
SSF1 FIGO Stage	999	FIGO stage not documented
SSF2 Peritoneal Cytol	998	Test not done
SSF3 # Pos Pelvic LN	000	No positive pelvic nodes
SSF4 # Exam Pelvic LN	006	Six pelvic nodes examined
SSF5 # Pos Para-aortic LN	098	No para-aortic nodes examined
SSF6 # Exam Para-aort LN	000	No para-aortic nodes examined
SSF7 % Non-Endomet Cell	002	Stated as 10% non-squamous growth pattern
SSF8 Omentectomy	000	Omentectomy not performed

This case will map to pT1b pN0 cM0 Stage Group IB.

—— CORPUS CASE 5 ——

Site Code	C54.1	Endometrium
Histology	8140/33	Poorly differentiated adenocarcinoma; disregard "focal" descriptors
Grade Path Value	Blank	Does not apply
Grade Path System	Blank	Does not apply
Lymph Vascular Invasion	9	Lymph-vascular invasion not mentioned in path report
Ambiguous Terminology	0	Conclusive terminology
Date Conclusive Terminol	Blank	Diagnosis made by conclusive terminology
Date Conclus Dx Flag	11	Not applicable
Multiplicity Counter	01	One tumor only
Date Multiple Tumors	Blank	Not applicable
Date Mult Tumors Flag	15	Single tumor only (multiplicity counter is coded 01)
Type Mult Tum as 1 Prim	00	Single tumor
Summary Stage	2	Regional direct extension
CLINICAL	T 3b	N 0 M 0 Stage Group I
PATHOLOGIC	yT 1b	N X cM 0 Stage Group Unstaged
CS Tumor Size	999	Tumor on cervix is not the primary site (and turns out to be just an ulcer)
CS Extension	640	Extends to vaginal apex per colposcopy
CS TS/Ext Eval	5	Clinical information prior to cesium implant (pre-operative treatment). Reading the dates of treatment is important!
CS Lymph Nodes	00	No pelvic adenopathy on MRI
CS Reg Nodes Eval	0	Per MRI scan prior to treatment
Reg Nodes Pos	98	No nodes examined
Reg Nodes Exam	00	No nodes removed
CS Mets at Dx	00	CXR negative
CS Mets at Dx–Bone	0	No bone metastases
CS Mets at Dx–Brain	0	No brain metastases
CS Mets at Dx–Liver	0	No liver metastases
CS Mets at Dx–Lung	0	No lung metastases
CS Mets Eval	0	Based on imaging
SSF1 FIGO Stage	999	FIGO stage not documented
SSF2 Peritoneal Cytol	000	Peritoneal washings benign
SSF3 # Pos Pelvic LN	098	No pelvic nodes examined
SSF4 # Exam Pelvic LN	098	No pelvic nodes examined
SSF5 # Pos Para-aortic LN	098	No para-aortic nodes examined
SSF6 # Exam Para-aort LN	000	No para-aortic nodes examined
SSF7 % Non-Endomet Cell	999	Growth pattern not stated
SSF8 Omentectomy	000	Omentectomy not performed

This case will map to cT3b cN0 cM0 Stage Group IIIB.

For TNM, clinical T3b (extends to vaginal apex) is based on colposcopy involvement of the vagina, although this turns out to be a benign ulcer after cesium treatment. The "lower uterine segment" is part of the corpus. Although unstaged in TNM, this case is FIGO Stage IIIB. The stated Grade 3 is a histologic grade; SSF2 needs a statement of percentage.

—— CORPUS CASE 6 ——

Site Code	C54.1	Endometrium
Histology	8980/34	Carcinosarcoma; stated as high grade on resection
Grade Path Value	Blank	Does not apply
Grade Path System	Blank	Does not apply
Lymph Vascular Invasion	9	Lymph-vascular invasion not mentioned in path report
Ambiguous Terminology	0	Conclusive terminology
Date Conclusive Terminol	Blank	Diagnosis made by conclusive terminology
Date Conclus Dx Flag	11	Not applicable
Multiplicity Counter	01	One tumor only
Date Multiple Tumors	Blank	Not applicable
Date Mult Tumors Flag	15	Single tumor only (multiplicity counter is coded 01)
Type Mult Tum as 1 Prim	00	Single tumor
Summary Stage	3	Regional to lymph nodes

CLINICAL	T X	N 1	M 0	Stage Group Unstageable
PATHOLOGIC	T 1b	N 1	cM 0	Stage Group IIIC

CS Tumor Size	999	No size stated
CS Extension	120	10% involvement of myometrium is less than half
CS TS/Ext Eval	3	Based on pathology report
CS Lymph Nodes	100	Pelvic lymph nodes involved
CS Reg Nodes Eval	3	Based on pathology report
Reg Nodes Pos	05	Five nodes involved
Reg Nodes Exam	24	24 pelvic lymph nodes examined
CS Mets at Dx	00	CXR negative
CS Mets at Dx–Bone	0	No bone metastases
CS Mets at Dx–Brain	0	No brain metastases
CS Mets at Dx–Liver	0	No liver metastases
CS Mets at Dx–Lung	0	No lung metastases
CS Mets Eval	0	Based on imaging
SSF1 FIGO Stage	330	Stated as FIGO IIIC
SSF2 Peritoneal Cytol	998	Test not done
SSF3 # Pos Pelvic LN	005	Five pelvic nodes positive
SSF4 # Exam Pelvic LN	024	24 pelvic nodes examined
SSF5 # Pos Para-aortic LN	098	No para-aortic nodes examined
SSF6 # Exam Para-aort LN	000	No para-aortic nodes examined
SSF7 % Non-Endomet Cell	987	Not applicable, not an adenocarcinoma morphology
SSF8 Omentectomy	000	Omentectomy not performed.

This case will map to pT1a pN1 cM0 Stage Group IIIC.

Use Corpus Carcinoma schema that includes carcinosarcoma. Grade is stated as high grade on the resection. This terminology translates to grade 4 according to the grade coding guidelines in FORDS. The positive lymph nodes upstage the case to IIIC.

—— CORPUS CASE 7 ——

Site Code	C54.2	Myometrium		
Histology	8890/34	Leiomyosarcoma, NOS, high grade		
Grade Path Value	Blank	Does not apply		
Grade Path System	Blank	Does not apply		
Lymph Vascular Invasion	9	Lymph-vascular invasion not mentioned in path report		
Ambiguous Terminology	0	Conclusive terminology		
Date Conclusive Terminol	Blank	Diagnosis made by conclusive terminology		
Date Conclus Dx Flag	11	Not applicable		
Multiplicity Counter	01	One tumor only		
Date Multiple Tumors	Blank	Not applicable		
Date Mult Tumors Flag	15	Single tumor only (multiplicity counter is coded 01)		
Type Mult Tum as 1 Prim	00	Single tumor		
Summary Stage	7	Distant (cul-de-sac)		
CLINICAL	T 3a	N 0	M 0	Stage Group IIIA
PATHOLOGIC	T X	N X	cM 0	Stage Group Unstageable
CS Tumor Size	999	Tumor size not stated		
CS Extension	665	Extension to cul-de-sac on operative report		
CS TS/Ext Eval	1	Based on surgical observation		
CS Lymph Nodes	000	No mention of lymph nodes at surgery (note 3)		
CS Reg Nodes Eval	0	Clinical assessment		
Reg Nodes Pos	98	No nodes examined		
Reg Nodes Exam	00	No nodes removed		
CS Mets at Dx	00	No distant metastases		
CS Mets at Dx–Bone	0	No bone metastases		
CS Mets at Dx–Brain	0	No brain metastases		
CS Mets at Dx–Liver	0	No liver metastases		
CS Mets at Dx–Lung	0	No lung metastases		
CS Mets Eval	0	Based on imaging		
SSF1 FIGO Stage	310	FIGO Stage IIIA per operative report		
SSF2 Peritoneal Cytol	998	Test not done		
SSF3 # Pos Pelvic LN	098	No pelvic nodes examined		
SSF4 # Exam Pelvic LN	000	No pelvic nodes examined		
SSF5 # Pos Para-aortic LN	098	No para-aortic nodes examined		
SSF6 # Exam Para-aort LN	000	No para-aortic nodes examined		
SSF7 % Non-Endomet Cell	987	Not applicable, not an adenocarcinoma morphology		
SSF8 Omentectomy	000	Omentectomy not performed		

This case will map to cT3a cN0 cM0 Stage Group IIIA.

Use the Corpus Sarcoma schema that includes the code for leiomyosarcoma. Leiomyosarcoma is a soft tissue sarcoma of the uterine muscle. The case maps to Distant summary stage because of the observed involvement of the cul-de-sac at the time of surgery. Even though the mesenteric and peritoneal implants were found within 5 weeks of surgery, they are progression of disease and are not included in the initial staging of the case.

—— CORPUS CASE 8 ——

Site Code	C54.1	Endometrium		
Histology	8140/33	Poorly differentiated adenocarcinoma		
Grade Path Value	Blank	Does not apply		
Grade Path System	Blank	Does not apply		
Lymph Vascular Invasion	9	Lymph-vascular invasion not mentioned in path report		
Ambiguous Terminology	0	Conclusive terminology		
Date Conclusive Terminol	Blank	Diagnosis made by conclusive terminology		
Date Conclus Dx Flag	11	Not applicable		
Multiplicity Counter	01	One tumor only		
Date Multiple Tumors	Blank	Not applicable		
Date Mult Tumors Flag	15	Single tumor only (multiplicity counter is coded 01)		
Type Mult Tum as 1 Prim	00	Single tumor		
Summary Stage	1	Localized		
CLINICAL	T X	N X	M X	Stage Group Unstageable
PATHOLOGIC	T 1a	N 0	cM 0	Stage Group IA
CS Tumor Size	999	Tumor size of endometrial carcinoma not stated		
CS Extension	110	Tumor confined to endometrium		
CS TS/Ext Eval	3	Based on resected specimen (incidental finding)		
CS Lymph Nodes	000	No regional lymph nodes involved		
CS Reg Nodes Eval	3	Based on resected specimen		
Reg Nodes Pos	00	No nodes involved		
Reg Nodes Exam	97	Lymphadenectomy = dissection; number examined unknown		
Mets at Dx	00	CXR negative		
CS Mets at Dx–Bone	0	No bone metastases		
CS Mets at Dx–Brain	0	No brain metastases		
CS Mets at Dx–Liver	0	No liver metastases		
CS Mets at Dx–Lung	0	No lung metastases		
CS Mets Eval	0	Based on imaging		
SSF1 FIGO Stage	999	FIGO stage not documented		
SSF2 Peritoneal Cytol	000	Ascitic fluid negative		
SSF3 # Pos Pelvic LN	000	No pelvic nodes positive		
SSF4 # Exam Pelvic LN	097	Pelvic lymph node removal documented as a dissection, but number of nodes not stated		
SSF5 # Pos Para-aortic LN	098	No para-aortic nodes examined		
SSF6 # Exam Para-aort LN	000	No para-aortic nodes examined		
SSF7 % Non-Endomet Cell	999	Not documented		
SSF8 Omentectomy	010	Omentectomy performed		

This case will map to pT1a pN0 cM0 Stage Group IA.

This patient has two primaries of different histologies—cystadenocarcinoma of the ovaries and adenocarcinoma of the endometrium. There is no clinical information available about the endometrial carcinoma because the tumor was an incidental finding at the time of surgery for bilateral ovarian carcinomas. Incidental findings of additional primaries at surgery are reportable malignancies. Answers for the ovarian primary in the Ovary chapter, case 6.

—— CORPUS CASE 9 ——

Site Code	C54.1	Endometrium		
Histology	8560/31	Adenosquamous carcinoma, grade I		
Grade Path Value	Blank	Does not apply		
Grade Path System	Blank	Does not apply		
Lymph Vascular Invasion	1	Lymph-vascular invasion present		
Ambiguous Terminology	0	Conclusive terminology		
Date Conclusive Terminol	Blank	Diagnosis made by conclusive terminology		
Date Conclus Dx Flag	11	Not applicable		
Multiplicity Counter	01	One tumor only		
Date Multiple Tumors	Blank	Not applicable		
Date Mult Tumors Flag	15	Single tumor only (multiplicity counter is coded 01)		
Type Mult Tum as 1 Prim	00	Single tumor		
Summary Stage	2	Regional direct extension		
CLINICAL	T X	N 0	M 0	Stage Group Unstageable
PATHOLOGIC	T 3a	N 0	cM 0	Stage Group IIIA
CS Tumor Size	999	Tumor size not stated		
CS Extension	635	Extension to right and left adnexa and right parametrium		
CS TS/Ext Eval	3	Based on resected specimen		
CS Lymph Nodes	000	No regional lymph nodes involved		
CS Reg Nodes Eval	3	Based on resected specimen		
Reg Nodes Pos	00	No nodes involved		
Reg Nodes Exam	10	Ten lymph nodes removed and examined		
CS Mets at Dx	00	No distant metastases		
CS Mets at Dx–Bone	0	No bone metastases		
CS Mets at Dx–Brain	0	No brain metastases		
CS Mets at Dx–Liver	0	No liver metastases		
CS Mets at Dx–Lung	0	No lung metastases		
CS Mets Eval	0	Based on physical exam		
SSF1 FIGO Stage	999	FIGO stage not documented		
SSF2 Peritoneal Cytol	000	Atypical cells worrisome for adenocarcinoma; atypical and worrisome are not terms indicating involvement		
SSF3 # Pos Pelvic LN	000	No pelvic nodes positive		
SSF4 # Exam Pelvic LN	010	Right pelvic lymphadenectomy		
SSF5 # Pos Para-aortic LN	098	No para-aortic nodes examined		
SSF6 # Exam Para-aort LN	000	No para-aortic nodes examined		
SSF7 % Non-Endomet Cell	999	Growth pattern not stated		
SSF8 Omentectomy	010	Omentectomy performed		

This case will map to pT3a pN0 cM0 Stage Group IIIA.

The pelvic washings are "worrisome"–not a word considered as involved. If the pelvic washings were definitely involved, it would not change the stage. The stated Grade I is a histologic grade; SSF2 needs a statement of percentage.

—— CORPUS CASE 10 ——

Site Code	C54.1	Endometrium		
Histology	8323/34	Mixed cell adenocarcinoma, high grade; see note		
Grade Path Value	Blank	Does not apply		
Grade Path System	Blank	Does not apply		
Lymph Vascular Invasion	9	Lymph-vascular invasion not mentioned in path report		
Ambiguous Terminology	0	Conclusive terminology		
Date Conclusive Terminol	Blank	Diagnosis made by conclusive terminology		
Date Conclus Dx Flag	11	Not applicable		
Multiplicity Counter	01	One tumor only		
Date Multiple Tumors	Blank	Not applicable		
Date Mult Tumors Flag	15	Single tumor only (multiplicity counter is coded 01)		
Type Mult Tum as 1 Prim	00	Single tumor		
Summary Stage	1	Localized		
CLINICAL	T X	N 0	M 0	Stage Group Unstageable
PATHOLOGIC	T 1b	N 0	cM 0	Stage Group IB
CS Tumor Size	999	Tumor size not stated		
CS Extension	130	Invasion through 3/4 of the myometrium is more than half way		
CS TS/Ext Eval	3	Based on resected specimen		
CS Lymph Nodes	000	No regional lymph nodes involved		
CS Reg Nodes Eval	3	Based on resected specimen		
Reg Nodes Pos	00	No regional nodes involved		
Reg Nodes Exam	23	Twenty-three lymph nodes removed and examined		
CS Mets at Dx	00	CXR and CT Abdomen negative for metastases		
CS Mets at Dx–Bone	0	No bone metastases		
CS Mets at Dx–Brain	0	No brain metastases		
CS Mets at Dx–Liver	0	No liver metastases		
CS Mets at Dx–Lung	0	No lung metastases		
CS Mets Eval	0	Based on imaging		
SSF1 FIGO Stage	120	Stated as FIGO Stage IB		
SSF2 Peritoneal Cytol	998	Test not done		
SSF3 # Pos Pelvic LN	000	No pelvic nodes positive		
SSF4 # Exam Pelvic LN	023	23 nodes in pelvic lymph node dissection		
SSF5 # Pos Para-aortic LN	098	No para-aortic nodes examined		
SSF6 # Exam Para-aort LN	000	No para-aortic nodes examined		
SSF7 % Non-Endomet Cell	002	Stated as 35% non-morular		
SSF8 Omentectomy	000	Omentectomy not performed		

This case will map to pT1b pN0 cM0 Stage Group IB.

In the addendum, the pathologist changes the final diagnosis from papillary serous to endometrioid adenocarcinoma with papillary features. In Table 2 of the “Other Sites” rules, endometrioid and papillary should be coded to 8323, mixed cell adenocarcinoma.

Corpus-Cervix

—— CORPUS CASE 11 ——

Site Code	C54.1	Endometrium		
Histology	8380/32	Endometrioid adenocarcinoma, FIGO Grade 2		
Grade Path Value	Blank	Does not apply		
Grade Path System	Blank	Does not apply		
Lymph Vascular Invasion	0	No lymph-vascular invasion per path report		
Ambiguous Terminology	0	Conclusive terminology		
Date Conclusive Terminol	Blank	Diagnosis made by conclusive terminology		
Date Conclus Dx Flag	11	Not applicable		
Multiplicity Counter	99	Described as multifocal		
Date Multiple Tumors	20XX1130	Earliest date multiple tumors were diagnosed		
Date Mult Tumors Flag	Blank	Valid date provided		
Type Mult Tum as 1 Prim	40	Multiple invasive tumors		
Summary Stage	1	Localized		
CLINICAL	T X	N 0	M 0	Stage Group Unstageable
PATHOLOGIC	T 1a(m)	N X	cM 0	Stage Group Unstageable
CS Tumor Size	999	Tumor size not stated		
CS Extension	120	Superficial myometrial invasion is considerably less than halfway through. The pathologist states depth is 1-2 mm out of 22 mm thickness.		
CS TS/Ext Eval	3	Based on resected specimen		
CS Lymph Nodes	000	No pelvic adenopathy on CT scan		
CS Reg Nodes Eval	0	Based on imaging. No information from operative report.		
Reg Nodes Pos	98	No nodes examined		
Reg Nodes Exam	00	No nodes removed		
CS Mets at Dx	00	CXR and CT abdomen negative		
CS Mets at Dx–Bone	0	No bone metastases		
CS Mets at Dx–Brain	0	No brain metastases		
CS Mets at Dx–Liver	0	No liver metastases		
CS Mets at Dx–Lung	0	No lung metastases		
CS Mets Eval	0	Based on imaging		
SSF1 FIGO Stage	999	FIGO stage not documented		
SSF2 Peritoneal Cytol	998	Test not done		
SSF3 # Pos Pelvic LN	098	No pelvic nodes examined		
SSF4 # Exam Pelvic LN	000	No pelvic nodes examined		
SSF5 # Pos Para-aortic LN	098	No para-aortic nodes examined		
SSF6 # Exam Para-aort LN	000	No para-aortic nodes examined		
SSF7 % Non-Endomet Cell	999	Growth pattern not stated		
SSF8 Omentectomy	010	Omentectomy performed (Adipose tissue stated to be omentum)		

This case will map to pT1a cN0 cM0 Stage Group IA.

Without pathologic information from lymph nodes, the case cannot be pathologically stage-grouped. However, based on the superficial myometrial invasion, the case would be at least FIGO IA. Even though the procedure was listed as a pelvic lymph node dissection, there were no nodes in the specimen, so the case is pNX and Reg Nodes Pos/Reg Nodes Exam are 98 and 00 for no nodes examined. The stated Grade 2 is a histologic grade; SSF2 needs a statement of percentage non-squamous tumor, and this is purely endometrioid..

—— CORPUS CASE 12 ——

Site Code	C54.1	Endometrium
Histology	8570/39	Adenoacanthoma, grade not stated. Do not take grade from biopsy because the cell type is not the same.
Grade Path Value	Blank	Does not apply
Grade Path System	Blank	Does not apply
Lymph Vascular Invasion	9	Lymph-vascular invasion not mentioned in path report
Ambiguous Terminology	0	Conclusive terminology
Date Conclusive Terminol	Blank	Diagnosis made by conclusive terminology
Date Conclus Dx Flag	11	Not applicable
Multiplicity Counter	01	One tumor only
Date Multiple Tumors	Blank	Not applicable
Date Mult Tumors Flag	15	Single tumor only (multiplicity counter is coded 01)
Type Mult Tum as 1 Prim	00	Single tumor

Summary Stage	3	Regional to nodes

CLINICAL	T X	N X	M 0	Stage Group Unstageable
PATHOLOGIC	T 1c	N 1	cM 0	Stage Group IIIC1

CS Tumor Size	999	Tumor size not stated
CS Extension	130	Myometrial invasion more than half way through
CS TS/Ext Eval	3	Based on resected specimen
CS Lymph Nodes	200	Para-aortic lymph node involved
CS Reg Nodes Eval	3	Based on resected specimen
Reg Nodes Pos	01	One lymph node involved
Reg Nodes Exam	17	Seventeen lymph nodes (16 + 1) removed and examined
CS Mets at Dx	00	CXR negative
CS Mets at Dx–Bone	0	No bone metastases
CS Mets at Dx–Brain	0	No brain metastases
CS Mets at Dx–Liver	0	No liver metastases
CS Mets at Dx–Lung	0	No lung metastases
CS Mets Eval	0	Based on imaging
SSF1 FIGO Stage	999	FIGO stage not documented
SSF2 Peritoneal Cytol	998	Test not done
SSF3 # Pos Pelvic LN	000	No pelvic lymph nodes positive
SSF4 # Exam Pelvic LN	016	16 pelvic nodes examined
SSF5 # Pos Para-aortic LN	001	One para-aortic node positive
SSF6 # Exam Para-aort LN	098	Para-aortic nodes surgically removed, but number of lymph nodes not stated and not documented as a sampling or dissection
SSF7 % Non-Endomet Cell	999	Not documented
SSF8 Omentectomy	000	Omentectomy not performed

This case will map to pT1b pN1 cM0 Stage Group IIIC1.

Corpus-Cervix

CERVIX CASE 1

PHYSICAL EXAM

11-12-20XX Endocervical lesion with no parametrial or vaginal extension. No inguinal adenopathy.

X-RAYS AND SCANS

11-13-20XX CT scan abdomen and pelvis: No evidence of lymphadenopathy or local extension.
11-15-20XX Chest x-ray: No evidence of disease.

SCOPES

None

LABORATORY

None

PATHOLOGY REPORTS

11-12-20XX Endocervical biopsy: Infiltrating poorly differentiated squamous cell carcinoma.
11-15-20XX Hysterectomy: Moderately differentiated squamous cell carcinoma of cervix with invasion half-way through cervical wall.

TREATMENT

11-15-20XX Modified radical hysterectomy
12-30-20XX 5-FU and CisPlatinum
1-10-20YY to 1-31-20YY 4500 cGy to pelvis
2-11-20YY High dose radiation (intracavitary)

Site Code ___ ___ ___.___	cT ___ cN ___ cM ___	SSF1 FIGO Stage ___ ___ ___
Histology/Behavior/Grade ___ ___ ___ ___/___ ___	Clin Stage Group _____	SSF2 Pelvic Node Status ___ ___ ___
Grade Path Value ___	pT ___ pN ___ M ___	SSF3 Assess Meth Pelvic Node Status ___ ___ ___
Grade Path System ___	Path Stage Group _____	SSF4 Para-Aortic Node Status ___ ___ ___
Lymph Vascular Invasion ___	CS Tumor Size ___ ___ ___	SSF5 Assess Meth Para-Aortic Note Status ___ ___ ___
Ambiguous Terminol ___	CS Extension ___ ___ ___	SSF6 Mediastinal Node Status ___ ___ ___
Date Conclusive Terminol ___ ___ ___ ___ ___ ___ ___ ___	CS TS/Ext Eval ___	SSF7 Assess Meth Mediastinal Node Status ___ ___ ___
Date Conclus Dx Flag ___ ___	CS LN ___ ___ ___	SSF8 Scalene Node Status ___ ___ ___
Multiplicity Counter ___ ___	CS Reg Nodes Eval ___	SSF9 Assess Meth Scalene Node Status ___ ___ ___
Date Mult Tumors ___ ___ ___ ___ ___ ___ ___ ___	Reg LN Pos ___ ___	
Date Mult Tumors Flag ___ ___	Reg LN Exam ___ ___	
Mult Tum Reported as One Prim ___ ___	CS Mets at Dx ___ ___	
Summary Stage 2000 _____	CS Mets at Dx - Bone ___ Brain ___ Liver ___ Lung ___	
	CS Mets Eval ___	

CERVIX CASE 2

PHYSICAL EXAM
1-24-20XX Normal sized uterus with no palpable adnexal masses

X-RAYS AND SCANS
1-16-20XX Chest X-ray: Normal
1-16-20XX Pelvic Ultrasound: Within normal limits

SCOPES
1-24-20XX Colposcopy with cervical biopsy: Obvious lesion in transformation zone seen easily with Lugol's dye.

LABORATORY
1-22-20XX CBC: Normal ranges .

PATHOLOGY REPORTS
1-4-20XX Cervical biopsy: CIN III.
1-24-20XX Cervical conization: CIN III in endocervical glands, foci of early microinvasion.
3-3-20XX Vaginal hysterectomy: No evidence of residual carcinoma.

TREATMENT
1-24-20XX Cervical conization
3-3-20XX Total vaginal hysterectomy

Site Code ___ ___ ___.___
Histology/Behavior/Grade ___ ___ ___ ___/___ ___
Grade Path Value ___
Grade Path System ___
Lymph Vascular Invasion ___
Ambiguous Terminol ___
Date Conclusive Terminol ___ ___ ___ ___ ___ ___ ___ ___
Date Conclus Dx Flag ___ ___
Multiplicity Counter ___ ___
Date Mult Tumors ___ ___ ___ ___ ___ ___ ___ ___
Date Mult Tumors Flag ___ ___
Mult Tum Reported as One Prim ___ ___
Summary Stage 2000 ___

cT ___ cN ___ cM ___
Clin Stage Group ___
pT ___ pN ___ M ___
Path Stage Group ___
CS Tumor Size ___ ___ ___
CS Extension ___ ___ ___
CS TS/Ext Eval ___
CS LN ___ ___ ___
CS Reg Nodes Eval ___
Reg LN Pos ___ ___
Reg LN Exam ___ ___
CS Mets at Dx ___ ___
CS Mets at Dx - Bone ___ Brain ___ Liver ___ Lung ___
CS Mets Eval ___

SSF1 FIGO Stage ___ ___ ___
SSF2 Pelvic Node Status ___ ___ ___
SSF3 Assess Meth Pelvic Node Status ___ ___ ___
SSF4 Para-Aortic Node Status ___ ___ ___
SSF5 Assess Meth Para-Aortic Note Status ___ ___ ___
SSF6 Mediastinal Node Status ___ ___ ___
SSF7 Assess Meth Mediastinal Node Status ___ ___ ___
SSF8 Scalene Node Status ___ ___ ___
SSF9 Assess Meth Scalene Node Status ___ ___ ___

Corpus-Cervix

CERVIX CASE 3

PHYSICAL EXAM

1-23-20YY Exam under anesthesia: Vagina was somewhat shortened considering radical hysterectomy. Well healed. Minimal induration above the cuff. No evidence of rectovaginal disease.

X-RAYS AND SCANS

1-21-20YY Chest x-ray: Normal.

1-23-20YY CT scan of pelvis: Two applicators, overlying the lower pelvis with residual contrast in the rectum.

LABORATORY

1-21-20YY CA-125: <6.3 (nl 0-35)

PATHOLOGY REPORTS

10-10-20XX (Prior to admission) Radical hysterectomy and BSO with pelvic node dissection: poorly differentiated squamous cell carcinoma of the cervix. Tumor size 3.5 x 4.0 cm. Pelvic nodes positive for metastatic disease; number of lymph nodes not recorded.

TREATMENT

10-10-20XX (Prior to admission) Radical hysterectomy and bilateral salpingo-oophorectomy with pelvic lymph node dissection

11-1-20XX to 11-30-20XX 4500 rads to pelvis

1-23-20YY Intracavitary cesium 127 implant to cervix

Site Code ___ ___ ___.___	cT ___ cN ___ cM ___	SSF1 FIGO Stage ___ ___ ___
Histology/Behavior/Grade ___ ___ ___ ___/___ ___	Clin Stage Group _____	SSF2 Pelvic Node Status ___ ___ ___
Grade Path Value ___	pT ___ pN ___ M ___	SSF3 Assess Meth Pelvic Node Status ___ ___ ___
Grade Path System ___	Path Stage Group _____	SSF4 Para-Aortic Node Status ___ ___ ___
Lymph Vascular Invasion ___	CS Tumor Size ___ ___ ___	SSF5 Assess Meth Para-Aortic Note Status ___ ___ ___
Ambiguous Terminol ___	CS Extension ___ ___ ___	SSF6 Mediastinal Node Status ___ ___ ___
Date Conclusive Terminol ___ ___ ___ ___ ___ ___ ___ ___	CS TS/Ext Eval ___	SSF7 Assess Meth Mediastinal Node Status ___ ___ ___
Date Conclus Dx Flag ___ ___	CS LN ___ ___ ___	SSF8 Scalene Node Status ___ ___ ___
Multiplicity Counter ___ ___	CS Reg Nodes Eval ___	SSF9 Assess Meth Scalene Node Status ___ ___ ___
Date Mult Tumors ___ ___ ___ ___ ___ ___ ___	Reg LN Pos ___ ___	
Date Mult Tumors Flag ___ ___	Reg LN Exam ___ ___	
Mult Tum Reported as One Prim ___ ___	CS Mets at Dx ___ ___	
Summary Stage 2000 ____	CS Mets at Dx - Bone ___ Brain ___ Liver ___ Lung ___	
	CS Mets Eval ___	

CERVIX CASE 4

PHYSICAL EXAM

2-25-20XX Blood in cervical os. Vaginal fornices and cervical mucosa normal. Cervix approx. 5 cm. Tumor extending into right parametrium and uterosacral region. Left parametrium negative.

X-RAYS AND SCANS

2-26-20XX Chest x-ray: Negative.
Abdominal CT scan: Negative.
Pelvic CT scan: Prominent cervix and uterus with two small foci of lucency in the cervical region. Shotty periaortic retroperitoneal adenopathy just above the level of the bifurcation.

LABORATORY

3-5-20XX Alkaline phosphatase: 47 (nl 50-136)

PATHOLOGY REPORTS

2-8-20XX D&C: Poorly differentiated squamous cell carcinoma.
5-13-20XX Cervix: No residual tumor. Uterus and bilateral adnexa: No tumor. Periaortic lymph nodes: Metastatic squamous cell carcinoma.

TREATMENT

2-8-20XX D&C
2-26-20XX to 4-2-20XX 4400 rads to pelvis with cesium implant. Anterior pelvis 7000 rads; posterior pelvis 5240 rads
3-1-20XX CisPlatinum and 5-FU
4-26-20XX Cesium implant 2520 rads
5-13-20XX Modified radical hysterectomy, bilateral salpingo-oophorectomy and periaortic lymph node dissection

Site Code ___ ___ ___.___
Histology/Behavior/Grade ___ ___ ___ ___/___ ___
Grade Path Value ___
Grade Path System ___
Lymph Vascular Invasion ___
Ambiguous Terminol ___
Date Conclusive Terminol ___ ___ ___ ___ ___ ___ ___ ___
Date Conclus Dx Flag ___ ___
Multiplicity Counter ___ ___
Date Mult Tumors ___ ___ ___ ___ ___ ___ ___ ___
Date Mult Tumors Flag ___ ___
Mult Tum Reported as One Prim ___ ___
Summary Stage 2000 ___

cT ___ **cN** ___ **cM** ___
Clin Stage Group ___
pT ___ **pN** ___ **M** ___
Path Stage Group ___
CS Tumor Size ___ ___ ___
CS Extension ___ ___ ___
CS TS/Ext Eval ___
CS LN ___ ___ ___
CS Reg Nodes Eval ___
Reg LN Pos ___ ___
Reg LN Exam ___ ___
CS Mets at Dx ___ ___
CS Mets at Dx - Bone ___ **Brain** ___ **Liver** ___ **Lung** ___
CS Mets Eval ___

SSF1 FIGO Stage ___ ___ ___
SSF2 Pelvic Node Status ___ ___ ___
SSF3 Assess Meth Pelvic Node Status ___ ___ ___
SSF4 Para-Aortic Node Status ___ ___ ___
SSF5 Assess Meth Para-Aortic Note Status ___ ___ ___
SSF6 Mediastinal Node Status ___ ___ ___
SSF7 Assess Meth Mediastinal Node Status ___ ___ ___
SSF8 Scalene Node Status ___ ___ ___
SSF9 Assess Meth Scalene Node Status ___ ___ ___

CERVIX CASE 5

PHYSICAL EXAM
10-31-20XX Pelvic exam normal

X-RAYS AND SCANS
10-31-20XX Chest x-ray: No evidence of disease.

SCOPES
10-31-20XX Colposcopy with biopsy: No unusual findings.

PATHOLOGY REPORTS
10-31-20XX Colposcopic biopsy: CIN III.
11-5-20XX Cervical cone and D&C: Severe dysplasia and carcinoma in situ with one microfocus of invasion.
1-23-20YY Surgery: No residual tumor; 32 regional lymph nodes free of tumor.

TREATMENT
11-5-20XX Cervical conization
1-23-20YY Radical abdominal hysterectomy with bilateral salpingo-oophorectomy and lymph node dissection

Site Code ___ ___ ___.___	cT ___ cN ___ cM ___	SSF1 FIGO Stage ___ ___ ___
Histology/Behavior/Grade ___ ___ ___ ___/___ ___	Clin Stage Group _____	SSF2 Pelvic Node Status ___ ___ ___
Grade Path Value ___	pT ___ pN ___ M ___	SSF3 Assess Meth Pelvic Node Status ___ ___ ___
Grade Path System ___	Path Stage Group _____	SSF4 Para-Aortic Node Status ___ ___ ___
Lymph Vascular Invasion ___	CS Tumor Size ___ ___ ___	SSF5 Assess Meth Para-Aortic Note Status ___ ___ ___
Ambiguous Terminol ___	CS Extension ___ ___ ___	SSF6 Mediastinal Node Status ___ ___ ___
Date Conclusive Terminol ___ ___ ___ ___ ___ ___ ___ ___	CS TS/Ext Eval ___	SSF7 Assess Meth Mediastinal Node Status ___ ___ ___
Date Conclus Dx Flag ___ ___	CS LN ___ ___ ___	SSF8 Scalene Node Status ___ ___ ___
Multiplicity Counter ___ ___	CS Reg Nodes Eval ___	SSF9 Assess Meth Scalene Node Status ___ ___ ___
Date Mult Tumors ___ ___ ___ ___ ___ ___ ___ ___	Reg LN Pos ___ ___	
Date Mult Tumors Flag ___ ___	Reg LN Exam ___ ___	
Mult Tum Reported as One Prim ___ ___	CS Mets at Dx ___ ___	
Summary Stage 2000 ____	CS Mets at Dx - Bone ___ Brain ___ Liver ___ Lung ___	
	CS Mets Eval ___	

CERVIX CASE 6

PHYSICAL EXAM
Patient presented with dizziness, shortness of breath and vaginal discharge. Examination showed tumor involving the right side of the bladder wall and bilateral ureteral obstruction.

X-RAYS AND SCANS
All performed prior to admission.
Summary: Large cervical mass involving the right side of the bladder, extending into the upper third of the vagina with right parametrial area involvement. Tumor extends to pelvic wall and causes hydronephrosis. Metastatic workup negative.

SCOPES
Prior to admission: Cystoscopy: Bullous edema of bladder wall.

PATHOLOGY REPORTS
Prior to admission: Cervical biopsy: Moderately differentiated squamous cell carcinoma.
Prior to admission: Cystoscopic bladder biopsy: Squamous cell carcinoma.

TREATMENT
3600 rads to A/P pelvis

Site Code ___ ___ ___.___
Histology/Behavior/Grade ___ ___ ___ ___/___ ___
Grade Path Value ___
Grade Path System ___
Lymph Vascular Invasion ___
Ambiguous Terminol ___
Date Conclusive Terminol ___ ___ ___ ___ ___ ___ ___ ___
Date Conclus Dx Flag ___ ___
Multiplicity Counter ___ ___
Date Mult Tumors ___ ___ ___ ___ ___ ___ ___ ___
Date Mult Tumors Flag ___ ___
Mult Tum Reported as One Prim ___ ___
Summary Stage 2000 ___

cT ___ cN ___ cM ___
Clin Stage Group ___
pT ___ pN ___ M ___
Path Stage Group ___
CS Tumor Size ___ ___ ___
CS Extension ___ ___ ___
CS TS/Ext Eval ___
CS LN ___ ___ ___
CS Reg Nodes Eval ___
Reg LN Pos ___ ___
Reg LN Exam ___ ___
CS Mets at Dx ___ ___
CS Mets at Dx - Bone ___ Brain ___ Liver ___ Lung ___
CS Mets Eval ___

SSF1 FIGO Stage ___ ___ ___
SSF2 Pelvic Node Status ___ ___ ___
SSF3 Assess Meth Pelvic Node Status ___ ___ ___
SSF4 Para-Aortic Node Status ___ ___ ___
SSF5 Assess Meth Para-Aortic Note Status ___ ___ ___
SSF6 Mediastinal Node Status ___ ___ ___
SSF7 Assess Meth Mediastinal Node Status ___ ___ ___
SSF8 Scalene Node Status ___ ___ ___
SSF9 Assess Meth Scalene Node Status ___ ___ ___

Corpus-Cervix

CERVIX CASE 7

HISTORY

A 31-year-old, gravida 5, para 4 had an abnormal screening Pap smear performed that showed high grade SIL and positive HPV. The patient reports a history of cone biopsy performed three years previously.

PHYSICAL EXAM

11-15-20XX Pelvic exam: Uterus is small, mobile, not likely greater than 6 weeks size. Acetowhite lesion with typical vessels along right aspect of cervix along margins of previous cone biopsy scar with extension within the scar region for approximately 4 to 6 o'clock. Lesion is approximately 2-3 cm wide. Ovaries: no masses. Remainder of exam within normal limits.

X-RAYS AND SCANS

11-18-20XX Chest x-ray normal.

LABORATORY

None significant.

SCOPES

11-15-20XX Colposcopy: A large, thickened acetowhite lesion with atypical vessels extending from 12 o'clock along the patient's left aspect of the cervix to 6 o'clock, approximately 2-3 cm. Transformation zone was noted. Biopsies were taken then at 3 o'clock and 5 o'clock and an ECC was performed.

OPERATIVE FINDINGS

11-30-20XX Hysterectomy: Enlarged 8-week size uterus. Ureters patent bilaterally.

PATHOLOGY REPORTS

11-15-20XX Biopsies and endocervical curettage: CIN 2-3 at both biopsy sites. Endocervical curettage was negative for dysplasia.

11-30-20XX Uterus, hysterectomy: Severe dysplasia (CIN III) and in situ adenocarcinoma, 2 mm focus. All margins are free. Secretory endometrium. Myometrium with no histopathologic abnormalities.

TREATMENT

11-15-20XX Biopsies and endocervical curettage

11-30-20XX Total vaginal hysterectomy

Site Code ___ ___ ___.___

Histology/Behavior/Grade ___ ___ ___ ___/___ ___

Grade Path Value ___

Grade Path System ___

Lymph Vascular Invasion ___

Ambiguous Terminol ___

Date Conclusive Terminol ___ ___ ___ ___ ___ ___ ___ ___

Date Conclus Dx Flag ___ ___

Multiplicity Counter ___ ___

Date Mult Tumors ___ ___ ___ ___ ___ ___ ___ ___

Date Mult Tumors Flag ___ ___

Mult Tum Reported as One Prim ___ ___

Summary Stage 2000 ___

cT ___ **cN** ___ **cM** ___

Clin Stage Group ___

pT ___ **pN** ___ **M** ___

Path Stage Group ___

CS Tumor Size ___ ___ ___

CS Extension ___ ___ ___

CS TS/Ext Eval ___

CS LN ___ ___ ___

CS Reg Nodes Eval ___

Cervix Case 7, continued

Reg LN Pos ___ ___	**SSF2 Pelvic Node Status** ___ ___ ___	**SSF6 Mediastinal Node Status** ___ ___ ___
Reg LN Exam ___ ___	**SSF3 Assess Meth Pelvic Node Status** ___ ___ ___	**SSF7 Assess Meth Mediastinal Node Status** ___ ___ ___
CS Mets at Dx ___ ___	**SSF4 Para-Aortic Node Status** ___ ___ ___	**SSF8 Scalene Node Status** ___ ___ ___
CS Mets at Dx - **Bone** ___ **Brain** ___ **Liver** ___ **Lung** ___	**SSF5 Assess Meth Para-Aortic Note Status** ___ ___ ___	**SSF9 Assess Meth Scalene Node Status** ___ ___ ___
CS Mets Eval ___		
SSF1 FIGO Stage ___ ___ ___		

CERVIX CASE 8

HISTORY
66-year-old diabetic female evaluated for renal failure and found to have cervical carcinoma with distal ureteral obstruction, which was stented at another facility.

PHYSICAL EXAM
6-18-20XX Abdomen distended and bloated; no abdominal pain. Rectal examination negative. Gyn examination limited by immobility of vagina. Pap smear performed.

X-RAYS AND SCANS
6-21-20XX CT of abdomen and pelvis: left hydronephrosis and ascites. Ill-defined mass extending from distal uterus towards left pelvic wall. Small pelvic lymph nodes noted.
6-24-20XX Chest x-ray: pleural effusions and mediastinal adenopathy consistent with metastatic carcinoma
7-3-20XX PET Scan: periaortic, pericaval, mediastinal and bilateral groin lymphadenopathy

LABORATORY
Prior to admission: Kidney panel: borderline renal function.
Prior to admission: SMA-20: Fasting glucose 245 (elevated).

SCOPES
None

OPERATIVE FINDINGS
None

PATHOLOGY REPORTS
6-24-20XX PAP smear: poorly differentiated adenosquamous carcinoma
6-26-20XX Thoracentesis: malignant cells present
6-26-20XX Needle biopsies of lung and liver: metastatic adenosquamous cell carcinoma

TREATMENT
Prior to admission: Placement of ureteral stent.
7-10-20XX Began four courses of Cisplatin and Taxotere

Cervix Case 8, continued

Site Code ___ ___ ___.___
Histology/Behavior/Grade ___ ___ ___ ___/___ ___
Grade Path Value ___
Grade Path System ___
Lymph Vascular Invasion ___
Ambiguous Terminol ___
Date Conclusive Terminol ___ ___ ___ ___ ___ ___ ___ ___
Date Conclus Dx Flag ___ ___
Multiplicity Counter ___ ___
Date Mult Tumors ___ ___ ___ ___ ___ ___ ___ ___
Date Mult Tumors Flag ___ ___
Mult Tum Reported as One Prim ___ ___
Summary Stage 2000 ___

cT ___ cN ___ cM ___
Clin Stage Group _____
pT ___ pN ___ M ___
Path Stage Group _____
CS Tumor Size ___ ___ ___
CS Extension ___ ___ ___
CS TS/Ext Eval ___
CS LN ___ ___ ___
CS Reg Nodes Eval ___
Reg LN Pos ___ ___
Reg LN Exam ___ ___
CS Mets at Dx ___ ___
CS Mets at Dx - Bone ___ Brain ___ Liver ___ Lung ___
CS Mets Eval ___

SSF1 FIGO Stage ___ ___ ___
SSF2 Pelvic Node Status ___ ___ ___
SSF3 Assess Meth Pelvic Node Status ___ ___ ___
SSF4 Para-Aortic Node Status ___ ___ ___
SSF5 Assess Meth Para-Aortic Note Status ___ ___ ___
SSF6 Mediastinal Node Status ___ ___ ___
SSF7 Assess Meth Mediastinal Node Status ___ ___ ___
SSF8 Scalene Node Status ___ ___ ___
SSF9 Assess Meth Scalene Node Status ___ ___ ___

CERVIX CASE 9

INDICATIONS

The patient is a 38-year-old with a clinically staged adeno-carcinoma of the cervix, biopsied in the office in October 200X, who presents for surgical treatment. She was offered surgery versus radiation and elected to proceed with surgery. She understands that both are equally curative. Physical examination, gynecologic evaluation and CT scans of the chest, abdomen and pelvis show no evidence of malignancy outside the cervix.

OPERATIVE FINDINGS

11-29-20XX Laparotomy and radical hysterectomy: No findings to suggest extracervical disease

PATHOLOGY REPORT

11-29-20XX Radical hysterectomy: 1) UTERUS, AND UPPER PORTION OF VAGINA: Moderately differentiated adenocarcinoma, endometrioid type, 2 cm in radial dimension invading underlying stroma to a depth of 0.6 cm. Margins free (deep margin 0.8 cm from tumor and ectocervical margin 0.7 cm from tumor)

2) VAGINAL CUFF: Squamous mucosa; no tumor.
3) LYMPH NODES, LEFT INTERNAL AND EXTERNAL ILIAC, BIOPSY: Three lymph nodes with no evidence of metastatic tumor.
4) LYMPH NODES, LEFT OBTURATOR, BIOPSY: Two lymph nodes with no evidence of metastatic tumor.
5) LYMPH NODE, LEFT COMMON ILIAC, BIOPSY: One lymph node with no evidence of metastatic tumor.
6) LYMPH NODE, LEFT PERIAORTIC, BIOPSY: One lymph node with no evidence of metastatic tumor.
7) LYMPH NODES, RIGHT INTERNAL AND EXTERNAL ILIAC, BIOPSIES: Four lymph nodes with no evidence of metastatic tumor.

continued on next page

Cervix Case 9, continued

8) LYMPH NODES, RIGHT OBTURATOR, BIOPSY: Five lymph nodes with no evidence of metastatic tumor.
9) LYMPH NODES, RIGHT COMMON ILIAC, BIOPSY: One lymph node with no evidence of metastatic tumor.
10) LYMPH NODE, PRECAVAL, BIOPSY: One lymph node with no evidence of metastatic tumor.

TREATMENT

11-29-20XX Exploratory laparotomy and radical hysterectomy with bilateral pelvic and periaortic lymph node dissection with bilateral ovarian transposition. Pelvic washings

Site Code ___ ___ ___.___	cT ___ cN ___ cM ___	SSF1 FIGO Stage ___ ___ ___
Histology/Behavior/Grade ___ ___ ___ ___/___ ___	Clin Stage Group _____	SSF2 Pelvic Node Status ___ ___ ___
Grade Path Value ___	pT ___ pN ___ M ___	SSF3 Assess Meth Pelvic Node Status ___ ___ ___
Grade Path System ___	Path Stage Group _____	SSF4 Para-Aortic Node Status ___ ___ ___
Lymph Vascular Invasion ___	CS Tumor Size ___ ___ ___	SSF5 Assess Meth Para-Aortic Note Status ___ ___ ___
Ambiguous Terminol ___	CS Extension ___ ___ ___	SSF6 Mediastinal Node Status ___ ___ ___
Date Conclusive Terminol ___ ___ ___ ___ ___ ___ ___ ___	CS TS/Ext Eval ___	SSF7 Assess Meth Mediastinal Node Status ___ ___ ___
Date Conclus Dx Flag ___ ___	CS LN ___ ___ ___	SSF8 Scalene Node Status ___ ___ ___
Multiplicity Counter ___ ___	CS Reg Nodes Eval ___	SSF9 Assess Meth Scalene Node Status ___ ___ ___
Date Mult Tumors ___ ___ ___ ___ ___ ___ ___ ___	Reg LN Pos ___ ___	
Date Mult Tumors Flag ___ ___	Reg LN Exam ___ ___	
Mult Tum Reported as One Prim ___ ___	CS Mets at Dx ___ ___	
Summary Stage 2000 ___	CS Mets at Dx - Bone ___ Brain ___ Liver ___ Lung ___	
	CS Mets Eval ___	

CERVIX CASE 10

HISTORY

64-year-old white female with vaginal spotting. History of COPD.

PHYSICAL EXAM

10-10-20XX GYN exam: Endocervical lesion visible on right side.

X-RAYS AND SCANS

10-16-20XX CT Scan Abdomen and Pelvis: Cystic left adnexal mass. No evidence of pelvic or abdominal lymphadenopathy or distant metastases.

10-18-20XX Pelvic ultrasound: Confirms two cystic masses in left adnexal/ovarian area.

SCOPES

None

continued on next page

Cervix Case 10, continued

LABORATORY

10-18-20XX CA-125: Within normal range.

OPERATIVE FINDINGS

10-10-20XX D&C: Friable lesion on endocervix.

10-23-20XX Conization and exam under anesthesia: Lesion appears to be confined to endocervix. On bimanual exam, no apparent extension to paracervical or parametrial tissues.

PATHOLOGY REPORTS

10-23-20XX Cervix conization: High grade squamous intraepithelial lesion (severe dysplasia/ carcinoma in situ, CIN III).

Endocervix biopsy: High grade squamous intraepithelial lesion (severe dysplasia/ carcinoma in situ, CIN III).

Endocervix curettings: Squamous cell carcinoma with focal features consistent with stromal invasion arising in association with high grade squamous intraepithelial lesion (severe dysplasia/carcinoma in situ/CIN III).

TREATMENT

12-3-20XX to 1-16-20YY 45 Gy to pelvis

12-18-20XX Cesium 137 brachytherapy (Fletcher Suit applicator), 31 Gy to cervix

Site Code ___ ___ ___.___	cT ___ cN ___ cM ___	SSF1 FIGO Stage ___ ___ ___
Histology/Behavior/Grade ___ ___ ___ ___ / ___ ___	Clin Stage Group _____	SSF2 Pelvic Node Status ___ ___ ___
Grade Path Value ___	pT ___ pN ___ M ___	SSF3 Assess Meth Pelvic Node Status ___ ___ ___
Grade Path System ___	Path Stage Group _____	SSF4 Para-Aortic Node Status ___ ___ ___
Lymph Vascular Invasion ___	CS Tumor Size ___ ___ ___	SSF5 Assess Meth Para-Aortic Note Status ___ ___ ___
Ambiguous Terminol ___	CS Extension ___ ___ ___	SSF6 Mediastinal Node Status ___ ___ ___
Date Conclusive Terminol ___ ___ ___ ___ ___ ___ ___ ___	CS TS/Ext Eval ___	SSF7 Assess Meth Mediastinal Node Status ___ ___ ___
Date Conclus Dx Flag ___ ___	CS LN ___ ___ ___	SSF8 Scalene Node Status ___ ___ ___
Multiplicity Counter ___ ___	CS Reg Nodes Eval ___	SSF9 Assess Meth Scalene Node Status ___ ___ ___
Date Mult Tumors ___ ___ ___ ___ ___ ___ ___ ___	Reg LN Pos ___ ___	
Date Mult Tumors Flag ___ ___	Reg LN Exam ___ ___	
Mult Tum Reported as One Prim ___ ___	CS Mets at Dx ___ ___	
Summary Stage 2000 ___	CS Mets at Dx - Bone ___ Brain ___ Liver ___ Lung ___	
	CS Mets Eval ___	

CERVIX CASE 11

HISTORY
54 year old white female presented to emergency department complaining of vaginal bleeding, passing large clots, abdominal pain and dyspareunia. History of abnormal Pap smear six years previously that she did not follow up.

PHYSICAL EXAM
8-19-20XX PE in hospital: Large mass in cervix. Remainder of exam essentially normal except for diffuse tenderness in suprapubic abdomen.

X-RAYS AND SCANS
8-26-20XX CT scan: 8.6 x 6.0 cm cervical mass involving upper vaginal wall. No evidence of hydronephrosis or lymphadenopathy.

SCOPES
9-6-20XX Cystoscopy: no abnormalities in bladder or urethra.
9-6-20XX Proctoscopy: no abnormalities to 18 cm.

LABORATORY
8-19-20XX Hct 23 (severely anemic).

OPERATIVE FINDINGS
None

PATHOLOGY REPORTS
8-20-20XX Cervical biopsy: well-differentiated invasive squamous cell carcinoma.

TREATMENT
9-9-20XX to 10-18-20XX Concurrent daily pelvic radiation 50 Gy and weekly Cisplatin

Site Code ___ ___.___	cT ___ cN ___ cM ___	SSF1 FIGO Stage ___ ___ ___
Histology/Behavior/Grade ___ ___ ___ ___/___ ___	Clin Stage Group _____	SSF2 Pelvic Node Status ___ ___ ___
Grade Path Value ___	pT ___ pN ___ M ___	SSF3 Assess Meth Pelvic Node Status ___ ___ ___
Grade Path System ___	Path Stage Group _____	SSF4 Para-Aortic Node Status ___ ___ ___
Lymph Vascular Invasion ___	CS Tumor Size ___ ___ ___	SSF5 Assess Meth Para-Aortic Note Status ___ ___ ___
Ambiguous Terminol ___	CS Extension ___ ___ ___	SSF6 Mediastinal Node Status ___ ___ ___
Date Conclusive Terminol ___ ___ ___ ___ ___ ___ ___ ___	CS TS/Ext Eval ___	SSF7 Assess Meth Mediastinal Node Status ___ ___ ___
Date Conclus Dx Flag ___ ___	CS LN ___ ___ ___	SSF8 Scalene Node Status ___ ___ ___
Multiplicity Counter ___ ___	CS Reg Nodes Eval ___	SSF9 Assess Meth Scalene Node Status ___ ___ ___
Date Mult Tumors ___ ___ ___ ___ ___ ___ ___ ___	Reg LN Pos ___ ___	
Date Mult Tumors Flag ___ ___	Reg LN Exam ___ ___	
Mult Tum Reported as One Prim ___ ___	CS Mets at Dx ___ ___	
Summary Stage 2000 _____	CS Mets at Dx - Bone ___ Brain ___ Liver ___ Lung ___	
	CS Mets Eval ___	

CERVIX CASE 12

HISTORY

30 year old woman with 12 month history of unprovoked vaginal bleeding, dragging sensation in the vagina and protrusion of a mass from the vagina on urination. Occasional vaginal discharge when no bleeding was present. There was associated lower abdominal pain, lower abdominal mass and low back ache. Long history of drug abuse and had been sexually active since the age of 14.

PHYSICAL EXAM

4-2-20XX PE: Abdominal examination showed a suprapubic mass. No abnormalities detected on examination of other systems.

X-RAYS AND SCANS

4-6-20XX Ultrasound: Hour glass appearance of the uterus due to bulky cervix.

LABORATORY

4-4-20XX ELISA (enzyme-linked immunosorbent assay): seroreactivity to HIV-1 antibodies.

OPERATIVE FINDINGS

4-2-20XX Examination under anesthesia with biopsies: Bulky hemorrhagic friable mass in the vagina down to the vestibule continuous with the uterus, which was bulky and the margins flush with vaginal walls. There was extension to the pelvic side walls.

PATHOLOGY REPORTS

4-2-20XX Incisional biopsy of cervix: Squamous cell carcinoma (large cell keratinizing), poorly differentiated.

TREATMENT

4-10-20XX to 4-26-20XX External beam radiation therapy to cervix and pelvis, 2100 rads

OUTCOME

She was placed on antiretroviral drugs but developed full blown AIDS and died after few weeks.

Site Code ___ ___ ___.___

Histology/Behavior/Grade ___ ___ ___ ___/___ ___

Grade Path Value ___

Grade Path System ___

Lymph Vascular Invasion ___

Ambiguous Terminol ___

Date Conclusive Terminol ___ ___ ___ ___ ___ ___ ___ ___

Date Conclus Dx Flag ___ ___

Multiplicity Counter ___ ___

Date Mult Tumors ___ ___ ___ ___ ___ ___ ___ ___

Date Mult Tumors Flag ___ ___

Mult Tum Reported as One Prim ___ ___

Summary Stage 2000 ___

cT ___ **cN** ___ **cM** ___

Clin Stage Group ___

pT ___ **pN** ___ **M** ___

Path Stage Group ___

CS Tumor Size ___ ___ ___

CS Extension ___ ___ ___

CS TS/Ext Eval ___

CS LN ___ ___ ___

CS Reg Nodes Eval ___

Reg LN Pos ___ ___

Reg LN Exam ___ ___

CS Mets at Dx ___ ___

CS Mets at Dx - **Bone** ___ **Brain** ___ **Liver** ___ **Lung** ___

CS Mets Eval ___

SSF1 FIGO Stage ___ ___ ___

SSF2 Pelvic Node Status ___ ___ ___

SSF3 Assess Meth Pelvic Node Status ___ ___ ___

SSF4 Para-Aortic Node Status ___ ___ ___

SSF5 Assess Meth Para-Aortic Note Status ___ ___ ___

SSF6 Mediastinal Node Status ___ ___ ___

SSF7 Assess Meth Mediastinal Node Status ___ ___ ___

SSF8 Scalene Node Status ___ ___ ___

SSF9 Assess Meth Scalene Node Status ___ ___ ___

ANSWERS TO CERVICAL CANCER CASE EXERCISES

—— CERVIX CASE 1 ——

Site Code	C53.0	Endocervix
Histology	8070/33	Poorly differentiated squamous cell carcinoma
Grade Path Value	Blank	Does not apply
Grade Path System	Blank	Does not apply
Lymph Vascular Invasion	9	Lymph-vascular invasion not mentioned in path report
Ambiguous Terminology	0	Conclusive terminology
Date Conclusive Terminol	Blank	Diagnosis made by conclusive terminology
Date Conclus Dx Flag	11	Not applicable
Multiplicity Counter	01	One tumor only
Date Multiple Tumors	Blank	Not applicable
Date Mult Tumors Flag	15	Single tumor only (multiplicity counter is coded 01)
Type Mult Tum as 1 Prim	00	Single tumor
Summary Stage	1	Localized
CLINICAL	T 1b	N 0 M 0 Stage Group IB
PATHOLOGIC	T 1	N X cM 0 Stage Group Unstageable
CS Tumor Size	999	Tumor size not stated
CS Extension	250	Lesion visible on physical exam, confined to cervix
CS TS/Ext-Eval	3	Based on resected specimen
CS Lymph Nodes	000	No inguinal adenopathy
CS Reg Nodes Eval	0	Based on physical exam
Reg LN Pos	98	No lymph nodes removed for examination
Reg LN Exam	00	No lymph nodes examined
CS Mets at DX	00	No distant metastases
CS Mets at Dx–Bone	0	No bone metastases
CS Mets at Dx–Brain	0	No brain metastases
CS Mets at Dx–Liver	0	No liver metastases
CS Mets at Dx–Lung	0	No lung metastases
CS Mets Eval	0	Based on imaging
SSF1 FIGO Stage	999	FIGO stage not documented
SSF2 Pelvic Nodal Status	000	CT abdomen and pelvis negative
SSF3 Assess Meth Pelv Nodes	020	Radiology
SSF4 Para-Aortic Nodal Status	000	CT abdomen and pelvis negative
SSF5 Assess Meth Para-Aortic	020	Radiology
SSF6 Mediastinal Nodal Status	000	CXR states no evidence of disease
SSF7 Assess Meth Mediastin	020	Radiology
SSF8 Scalene Nodal Status	999	Physical exam performed but no statement of lymph node status
SSF9 Assess Meth Scalene Nodes	999	No information

This case will map to pT1bNOS cN0 cM0 Stage Group IB.

Because the size of the lesion is not known, the case cannot be stage grouped. However, because the lesion is clinically visible, the stage is *at least* IB.

—— CERVIX CASE 2 ——

Site Code	C53.9	Cervix uteri, NOS
Histology	8077/39	Cervical intraepithelial neoplasia grade III (8077) with microinvasion (change /2 to /3)
Grade Path Value	Blank	Does not apply
Grade Path System	Blank	Does not apply
Lymph Vascular Invasion	9	Lymph-vascular invasion not mentioned in path report
Ambiguous Terminology	0	Conclusive terminology
Date Conclusive Terminol	Blank	Diagnosis made by conclusive terminology
Date Conclus Dx Flag	11	Not applicable
Multiplicity Counter	01	One tumor only
Date Multiple Tumors	Blank	Not applicable
Date Mult Tumors Flag	15	Single tumor only (multiplicity counter is coded 01)
Type Mult Tum as 1 Prim	00	Single tumor
Summary Stage	1	Localized
CLINICAL	T 1b	N 0 M 0 Stage Group IB
PATHOLOGIC	T 1b	N X cM 0 Stage Group Unstageable
CS Tumor Size	990	Microscopic focus of invasion
CS Extension	250	Clinically visible microinvasive tumor on colposcopy
CS TS/Ext-Eval	3	Based on resected specimen
CS Lymph Nodes	000	Assume lymph nodes negative if not mentioned
CS Reg Nodes Eval	0	Based on physical exam
Reg LN Pos	98	No lymph nodes removed for examination
Reg LN Exam	00	No lymph nodes examined
CS Mets at DX	00	No distant metastases
CS Mets at Dx–Bone	0	No bone metastases
CS Mets at Dx–Brain	0	No brain metastases
CS Mets at Dx–Liver	0	No liver metastases
CS Mets at Dx–Lung	0	No lung metastases
CS Mets Eval	0	Based on imaging
SSF1 FIGO Stage	999	FIGO stage not documented
SSF2 Pelvic Nodal Status	000	Pelvic ultrasound within normal limits
SSF3 Assess Meth Pelv Nodes	020	Ultrasound
SSF4 Para-Aortic Nodal Status	999	Unknown para-aortic nodal status
SSF5 Assess Meth Para-Aortic	999	No information
SSF6 Mediastinal Nodal Status	000	Chest x-ray normal
SSF7 Assess Meth Mediastin	020	Chest x-ray
SSF8 Scalene Nodal Status	999	Physical exam performed but no statement of lymph node status
SSF9 Assess Meth Scalene Nodes	999	No information

This case will map to pT1bNOS cN0 cM0 Stage Group IB.

The size of the lesion is microscopic only, but the computer algorithm can calculate a stage group.

—— CERVIX CASE 3 ——

Site Code	C53.9	Cervix uteri, NOS
Histology	8070/33	Poorly differentiated squamous cell carcinoma
Grade Path Value	Blank	Does not apply
Grade Path System	Blank	Does not apply
Lymph Vascular Invasion	9	Lymph-vascular invasion not mentioned in path report
Ambiguous Terminology	0	Conclusive terminology
Date Conclusive Terminol	Blank	Diagnosis made by conclusive terminology
Date Conclus Dx Flag	11	Not applicable
Multiplicity Counter	01	One tumor only
Date Multiple Tumors	Blank	Not applicable
Date Mult Tumors Flag	15	Single tumor only (multiplicity counter is coded 01)
Type Mult Tum as 1 Prim	00	Single tumor
Summary Stage	3	Regional to nodes
CLINICAL	T X	N X M 0 Stage Group Unstageable
PATHOLOGIC	T 1	N 1 cM 0 Stage Group IIIB
CS Tumor Size	040	Tumor size stated as 4.0 cm
CS Extension	300	Confined to cervix, NOS (unknown if clinically visible)
CS TS/Ext-Eval	3	Based on resected specimen
CS Lymph Nodes	100	Pelvic lymph nodes involved
CS Reg Nodes Eval	3	Based on resected specimen
Reg LN Pos	97	Lymph nodes positive, unknown how many
Reg LN Exam	97	Lymph nodes examined, procedure stated as dissection; unknown how many lymph nodes
CS Mets at DX	00	No distant metastases
CS Mets at Dx–Bone	0	No bone metastases
CS Mets at Dx–Brain	0	No brain metastases
CS Mets at Dx–Liver	0	No liver metastases
CS Mets at Dx–Lung	0	No lung metastases
CS Mets Eval	0	Based on imaging
SSF1 FIGO Stage	999	FIGO stage not documented
SSF2 Pelvic Nodal Status	010	Positive pelvic nodes
SSF3 Assess Meth Pelv Nodes	040	Lymphadenectomy (lymph node dissection)
SSF4 Para-Aortic Nodal Status	999	Unknown para-aortic nodal status
SSF5 Assess Meth Para-Aortic	999	No information
SSF6 Mediastinal Nodal Status	999	Unknown mediastinal nodal status
SSF7 Assess Meth Mediastin	999	No information
SSF8 Scalene Nodal Status	999	Unknown scalene nodal status
SSF9 Assess Meth Scalene Nodes	999	No information

This case will map to pT1NOS pN1 cM0 Stage Group IIIB.

—— CERVIX CASE 4 ——

Site Code	C53.9	Cervix uteri, NOS
Histology	8070/33	Poorly differentiated squamous cell carcinoma
Grade Path Value	Blank	Does not apply
Grade Path System	Blank	Does not apply
Lymph Vascular Invasion	9	Lymph-vascular invasion not mentioned in path report
Ambiguous Terminology	0	Conclusive terminology
Date Conclusive Terminol	Blank	Diagnosis made by conclusive terminology
Date Conclus Dx Flag	11	Not applicable
Multiplicity Counter	01	One tumor only
Date Multiple Tumors	Blank	Not applicable
Date Mult Tumors Flag	15	Single tumor only (multiplicity counter is coded 01)
Type Mult Tum as 1 Prim	00	Single tumor
Summary Stage	7	Distant (periaortic lymph nodes)
CLINICAL	T 2b	N X M 0 Stage Group Unstageable
PATHOLOGIC	yT 0	yN X ypM 1 Stage Group yIVB
CS Tumor Size	999	Tumor size not stated
CS Extension	500	Parametrial extension
CS TS/Ext-Eval	5	Chemo and radiation administered prior to surg, pre-operative clinical information coded
CS Lymph Nodes	000	Lymph nodes not mentioned on imaging or surgery
CS Reg Nodes Eval	0	Based on clinical assessment
Reg LN Pos	98	No regional lymph nodes removed for examination
Reg LN Exam	00	No regional lymph nodes examined
CS Mets at DX	10	Periaortic (distant) lymph nodes involved
CS Mets at Dx–Bone	0	No bone metastases
CS Mets at Dx–Brain	0	No brain metastases
CS Mets at Dx–Liver	0	No liver metastases
CS Mets at Dx–Lung	0	No lung metastases
CS Mets Eval	6	Distant lymph node identified after pre-operative treatment
SSF1 FIGO Stage	999	FIGO stage not documented
SSF2 Pelvic Nodal Status	000	CT scan only mentions periaortic nodes (assume pelvic nodes are negative)
SSF3 Assess Meth Pelv Nodes	020	Imaging
SSF4 Para-Aortic Nodal Status	010	Positive para-aortic node
SSF5 Assess Meth Para-Aortic	040	Lymphadenectomy
SSF6 Mediastinal Nodal Status	000	Chest x-ray negative
SSF7 Assess Meth Mediastin	020	Imaging
SSF8 Scalene Nodal Status	999	Physical exam performed but no statement of lymph node status
SSF9 Assess Meth Scalene Nodes	999	No information

This case will map to ypT2b cN0 ypM1 Stage Group IV.

For TNM, the regional lymph nodes are not described clinically or pathologically (NX). Periaortic lymph nodes are distant for cervical cancer. For CS, we can assume that regional lymph nodes are negative (code 00) if they are not mentioned.

—— CERVIX CASE 5 ——

Site Code	C53.9	Cervix uteri, NOS
Histology	8010/39	Microinvasive carcinoma in situ
Grade Path Value	Blank	Does not apply
Grade Path System	Blank	Does not apply
Lymph Vascular Invasion	9	Lymph-vascular invasion not mentioned in path report
Ambiguous Terminology	0	Conclusive terminology
Date Conclusive Terminol	Blank	Diagnosis made by conclusive terminology
Date Conclus Dx Flag	11	Not applicable
Multiplicity Counter	01	One tumor only
Date Multiple Tumors	Blank	Not applicable
Date Mult Tumors Flag	15	Single tumor only (multiplicity counter is coded 01)
Type Mult Tum as 1 Prim	00	Single tumor
Summary Stage	1	Localized
CLINICAL	T 1A	N X M 0 Stage Group Unstageable
PATHOLOGIC	T 1A	N 0 cM 0 Stage Group IA
CS Tumor Size	990	Microscopic focus of invasion
CS Extension	135	Minimal microscopic stromal invasion
CS TS/Ext-Eval	3	Based on resected specimen
CS Lymph Nodes	000	No involved lymph nodes
CS Reg Nodes Eval	3	Based on path report
Reg LN Pos	00	No lymph nodes involved
Reg LN Exam	32	32 lymph nodes examined
CS Mets at DX	00	No distant metastases
CS Mets at Dx–Bone	0	No bone metastases
CS Mets at Dx–Brain	0	No brain metastases
CS Mets at Dx–Liver	0	No liver metastases
CS Mets at Dx–Lung	0	No lung metastases
CS Mets Eval	0	Based on imaging
SSF1 FIGO Stage	999	FIGO stage not documented
SSF2 Pelvic Nodal Status	000	Negative pelvic lymph nodes
SSF3 Assess Meth Pelv Nodes	040	Lymph node dissection
SSF4 Para-Aortic Nodal Status	999	Unknown para-aortic nodal status
SSF5 Assess Meth Para-Aortic	999	No information
SSF6 Mediastinal Nodal Status	000	Chest x-ray states no evidence of disease
SSF7 Assess Meth Mediastin	020	Imaging
SSF8 Scalene Nodal Status	999	Physical exam performed but no statement of lymph node status
SSF9 Assess Meth Scalene Nodes	999	No information

This case will map to pT1a pN0 cM0 Stage Group IA.

The morphology from the larger specimen (the conization) is stated as carcinoma in situ (8010/2), not squamous carcinoma in situ (8076/2) or CIN III (8077/2). To account for the microinvasion, change the /2 to /3. For staging, the size of the microinvasion is not stated, so code the NOS category.

Corpus-Cervix

—— CERVIX CASE 6 ——

Site Code	C53.9	Cervix uteri, NOS
Histology	8070/32	Moderately differentiated squamous cell carcinoma
Grade Path Value	Blank	Does not apply
Grade Path System	Blank	Does not apply
Lymph Vascular Invasion	9	Lymph-vascular invasion not mentioned in path report
Ambiguous Terminology	0	Conclusive terminology
Date Conclusive Terminol	Blank	Diagnosis made by conclusive terminology
Date Conclus Dx Flag	11	Not applicable
Multiplicity Counter	01	One tumor only
Date Multiple Tumors	Blank	Not applicable
Date Mult Tumors Flag	15	Single tumor only (multiplicity counter is coded 01)
Type Mult Tum as 1 Prim	00	Single tumor
Summary Stage	7	Distant (extension to bladder mucosa)
CLINICAL	T 4	N X M 0 Stage Group IVA
PATHOLOGIC	T 4	N X cM 0 Stage Group IVA
CS Tumor Size	999	Tumor size not stated
CS Extension	700	Bladder mucosa involved
CS TS/Ext-Eval	3	Based on path report prior to admission
CS Lymph Nodes	999	Status of regional lymph nodes not mentioned, high stage primary, no surgery performed
CS Reg Nodes Eval	0	Based on clinical assessment
Reg LN Pos	98	No regional lymph nodes removed for examination
Reg LN Exam	00	No regional lymph nodes examined
CS Mets at DX	00	Imaging studies performed prior to admission do not mention distant metastases
CS Mets at Dx–Bone	0	No bone metastases
CS Mets at Dx–Brain	0	No brain metastases
CS Mets at Dx–Liver	0	No liver metastases
CS Mets at Dx–Lung	0	No lung metastases
CS Mets Eval	0	Based on imaging
SSF1 FIGO Stage	999	FIGO stage not documented
SSF2 Pelvic Nodal Status	999	Pelvic nodal status unknown
SSF3 Assess Meth Pelv Nodes	999	No information
SSF4 Para-Aortic Nodal Status	000	Metastatic workup negative
SSF5 Assess Meth Para-Aortic	010	Clinical assessment
SSF6 Mediastinal Nodal Status	000	Metastatic workup negative
SSF7 Assess Meth Mediastin	010	Clinical assessment
SSF8 Scalene Nodal Status	000	Metastatic workup negative
SSF9 Assess Meth Scalene Nodes	010	Clinical assessment

This case will map to pT4 cNX cM0 Stage Group IVA.

Lymph nodes cannot be assumed to be negative due to the extensive nature of the primary tumor. The case maps to pathologic Stage Group IVA because of the biopsy-proven bladder mucosa involvement. "Any N" includes NX.

—— CERVIX CASE 7 ——

Site Code	C53.9	Cervix uteri, NOS
Histology	8140/29	Adenocarcinoma in situ, grade not stated
Grade Path Value	Blank	Does not apply
Grade Path System	Blank	Does not apply
Lymph Vascular Invasion	0	No lymph-vascular invasion (carcinoma in situ tumor cannot invade lymphatic or vascular channels)
Ambiguous Terminology	0	Conclusive terminology
Date Conclusive Terminol	Blank	Diagnosis made by conclusive terminology
Date Conclus Dx Flag	11	Not applicable
Multiplicity Counter	01	One tumor only
Date Multiple Tumors	Blank	Not applicable
Date Mult Tumors Flag	15	Single tumor only (multiplicity counter is coded 01)
Type Mult Tum as 1 Prim	00	Single tumor
Summary Stage	0	In situ
CLINICAL	T 1b1	N 0 M 0 Stage Group IB1
PATHOLOGIC	T is	cN 0 cM 0 Stage Group 0
CS Tumor Size	002	TS stated as 2 mm on pathology report
CS Extension	000	In situ per hysterectomy path report
CS TS/Ext-Eval	3	Based on resected specimen
CS Lymph Nodes	000	No nodes identified on physical exam
CS Reg Nodes Eval	0	Based on physical exam
Reg LN Pos	98	No lymph nodes removed for examination
Reg LN Exam	00	No lymph nodes examined
CS Mets at DX	00	No distant metastases on chest x-ray
CS Mets at Dx–Bone	0	No bone metastases
CS Mets at Dx–Brain	0	No brain metastases
CS Mets at Dx–Liver	0	No liver metastases
CS Mets at Dx–Lung	0	No lung metastases
CS Mets Eval	0	Based on imaging
SSF1 FIGO Stage	987	Carcinoma in situ (FIGO no longer recognizes Stage 0 for in situ
SSF2 Pelvic Nodal Status	000	In situ tumor
SSF3 Assess Meth Pelv Nodes	999	Not documented
SSF4 Para-Aortic Nodal Status	000	In situ tumor
SSF5 Assess Meth Para-Aortic	999	Not documented
SSF6 Mediastinal Nodal Status	000	Chest x-ray normal; in situ tumor
SSF7 Assess Meth Mediastin	020	Imaging
SSF8 Scalene Nodal Status	000	Physical exam within normal limits; in situ tumor
SSF9 Assess Meth Scalene Nodes	999	Not documented

This case will map to pTis cN0 cM0 Stage Group 0.

The lesion seen clinically turned out to be severe dysplasia with a tiny focus of adenocarcinoma in situ. According to AJCC, pTis cN0 cM0 is *clinical* Stage Group 0.

—— CERVIX CASE 8 ——

Site Code	C53.9	Cervix uteri, NOS
Histology	8560/33	Poorly differentiated adenosquamous carcinoma
Grade Path Value	Blank	Does not apply
Grade Path System	Blank	Does not apply
Lymph Vascular Invasion	9	Lymph-vascular invasion not mentioned in path report
Ambiguous Terminology	0	Conclusive terminology
Date Conclusive Terminol	Blank	Diagnosis made by conclusive terminology
Date Conclus Dx Flag	11	Not applicable
Multiplicity Counter	01	One tumor only
Date Multiple Tumors	Blank	Not applicable
Date Mult Tumors Flag	15	Single tumor only (multiplicity counter is coded 01)
Type Mult Tum as 1 Prim	00	Single tumor
Summary Stage	7	Distant
CLINICAL	T 3b	N X M 1 Stage Group IVB
PATHOLOGIC	T X	N X pM 1 Stage Group IVB
CS Tumor Size	999	Tumor size not stated
CS Extension	635	Hydronephrosis seen on CT scan
CS TS/Ext-Eval	0	Based on imaging
CS Lymph Nodes	000	"Small" pelvic nodes on CT not considered involved
CS Reg Nodes Eval	0	Based on imaging
Reg LN Pos	98	No lymph nodes removed for examination
Reg LN Exam	00	No lymph nodes examined
CS Mets at DX	50	Distant lymph nodes and lung and liver metastases
CS Mets at Dx–Bone	0	No bone metastases
CS Mets at Dx–Brain	0	No brain metastases
CS Mets at Dx–Liver	1	Liver metastases
CS Mets at Dx–Lung	1	Lung metastases
CS Mets Eval	3	Based on pathology from biopsies of distant sites
SSF1 FIGO Stage	999	FIGO stage not documented
SSF2 Pelvic Nodal Status	000	CT abdomen and pelvis negative
SSF3 Assess Meth Pelv Nodes	020	Imaging
SSF4 Para-Aortic Nodal Status	000	CT abdomen and pelvis negative
SSF5 Assess Meth Para-Aortic	020	Imaging
SSF6 Mediastinal Nodal Status	010	Positive mediastinal lymph nodes
SSF7 Assess Meth Mediastin	020	Radiology imaging (biopsy was of lung, not nodes)
SSF8 Scalene Nodal Status	999	Physical exam performed but no statement of lymph node status
SSF9 Assess Meth Scalene Nodes	999	No information about scalene nodes

This case will map to cT3b cN0 pM1 Stage Group IVB.

All of the lymph nodes seen on the PET scan are distant for cervix, although the term "lymphadenopathy" cannot be used to code involvement in CS. The case is stage IVB regardless of the lymph node status. Biopsies of the distant metastatic sites allow the case to be pathologically staged.

—— CERVIX CASE 9 ——

Site Code	C53.9	Cervix uteri, NOS
Histology	8380/32	Moderately differentiated endometrioid adenocarcinoma
Grade Path Value	Blank	Does not apply
Grade Path System	Blank	Does not apply
Lymph Vascular Invasion	9	Lymph-vascular invasion not mentioned in path report
Ambiguous Terminology	0	Conclusive terminology
Date Conclusive Terminol	Blank	Diagnosis made by conclusive terminology
Date Conclus Dx Flag	11	Not applicable
Multiplicity Counter	01	One tumor only
Date Multiple Tumors	Blank	Not applicable
Date Mult Tumors Flag	15	Single tumor only (multiplicity counter is coded 01)
Type Mult Tum as 1 Prim	00	Single tumor
Summary Stage	1	Localized
CLINICAL	T X	N 0 M 0 Stage Group I
PATHOLOGIC	T 1a2	N 0 cM 0 Stage Group IA2
CS Tumor Size	020	Tumor size 2 cm per path report (code the radial or horizontal dimension not the depth)
CS Extension	200	Lesion larger than dimensions in code 120
CS TS/Ext-Eval	3	Based on resected specimen
CS Lymph Nodes	000	No regional lymph nodes involved
CS Reg Nodes Eval	3	Based on resected specimen
Reg LN Pos	00	No lymph nodes involved
Reg LN Exam	16	16 regional lymph nodes; periaortic and precaval nodes are distant for cervix
CS Mets at DX	00	Preadmission CT scans negative for metastases
CS Mets at Dx–Bone	0	No bone metastases
CS Mets at Dx–Brain	0	No brain metastases
CS Mets at Dx–Liver	0	No liver metastases
CS Mets at Dx–Lung	0	No lung metastases
CS Mets Eval	0	Based on imaging
SSF1 FIGO Stage	999	FIGO stage not documented
SSF2 Pelvic Nodal Status	000	No pelvic lymph nodes positive per path report
SSF3 Assess Meth Pelv Nodes	040	Lymphadenectomy
SSF4 Para-Aortic Nodal Status	000	No para-aortic lymph nodes positve per path report
SSF5 Assess Meth Para-Aortic	040	Lymphadenectomy
SSF6 Mediastinal Nodal Status	000	CT chest negative
SSF7 Assess Meth Mediastin	020	Imaging
SSF8 Scalene Nodal Status	000	Physical exam negative
SSF9 Assess Meth Scalene Nodes	010	Clinical assessment

This case will map to pT1b1 cN0 cM0 Stage Group IB1.

Lesions larger than those defined in T1a map to T1b. Endometrioid cancer is not a cancer metastatic from the endometrium; it is an unusual but correct histology in the cervix.

—— CERVIX CASE 10 ——

Site Code	C53.0	Endocervix
Histology	8070/39	Squamous cell carcinoma, grade not stated
Grade Path Value	Blank	Does not apply
Grade Path System	Blank	Does not apply
Lymph Vascular Invasion	9	Lymph-vascular invasion not mentioned in path report
Ambiguous Terminology	0	Conclusive terminology
Date Conclusive Terminol	Blank	Diagnosis made by conclusive terminology
Date Conclus Dx Flag	11	Not applicable
Multiplicity Counter	01	One tumor only
Date Multiple Tumors	Blank	Not applicable
Date Mult Tumors Flag	15	Single tumor only (multiplicity counter is coded 01)
Type Mult Tum as 1 Prim	00	Single tumor
Summary Stage	1	Localized
CLINICAL	T 1b	N 0 M 0 Stage Group IB
PATHOLOGIC	T 1b	N X cM 0 Stage Group Unstageable
CS Tumor Size	999	Tumor size not stated
CS Extension	250	Lesion visible on physical exam, confined to cervix
CS TS/Ext-Eval	1	Based on exam under anesthesia and biopsies
CS Lymph Nodes	000	No abdominal lymphadenopathy
CS Reg Nodes Eval	0	Based on imaging
Reg LN Pos	98	No lymph nodes removed for examination
Reg LN Exam	00	No lymph nodes examined
CS Mets at DX	00	No distant metastases
CS Mets at Dx–Bone	0	No bone metastases
CS Mets at Dx–Brain	0	No brain metastases
CS Mets at Dx–Liver	0	No liver metastases
CS Mets at Dx–Lung	0	No lung metastases
CS Mets Eval	0	Based on imaging
SSF1 FIGO Stage	999	FIGO stage not documented
SSF2 Pelvic Nodal Status	000	CT abdomen and pelvis negative
SSF3 Assess Meth Pelv Nodes	020	Imaging
SSF4 Para-Aortic Nodal Status	000	CT abdomen and pelvis negative
SSF5 Assess Meth Para-Aortic	020	Imaging
SSF6 Mediastinal Nodal Status	999	Mediastinal nodal status unknown
SSF7 Assess Meth Mediastin	999	No information
SSF8 Scalene Nodal Status	999	Physical exam limited to GYN exam
SSF9 Assess Meth Scalene Nodes	999	No information

This case will map to pT1bNOS cN0 cM0 Stage Group IB

Because the lesion is clinically visible, the stage is *at least* IB.

—— CERVIX CASE 11 ——

Site Code	C53.9	Cervix uteri, NOS
Histology	8070/31	Well differentiated squamous cell carcinoma
Grade Path Value	Blank	Does not apply
Grade Path System	Blank	Does not apply
Lymph Vascular Invasion	9	Lymph-vascular invasion not mentioned in path report
Ambiguous Terminology	0	Conclusive terminology
Date Conclusive Terminol	Blank	Diagnosis made by conclusive terminology
Date Conclus Dx Flag	11	Not applicable
Multiplicity Counter	01	One tumor only
Date Multiple Tumors	Blank	Not applicable
Date Mult Tumors Flag	15	Single tumor only (multiplicity counter is coded 01)
Type Mult Tum as 1 Prim	00	Single tumor
Summary Stage	2	Regional direct extension only
CLINICAL	T 2a	N 0 M 0 Stage Group IIA
PATHOLOGIC	T X	N X cM 0 Stage Group Unstageable
CS Tumor Size	999	Tumor size not stated; do not code clinical size of "mass" as that could mean anything
CS Extension	400	Extension to upper vaginal wall on CT scan
CS TS/Ext-Eval	0	Based on imaging
CS Lymph Nodes	000	No lymphadenopathy on CT scan
CS Reg Nodes Eval	0	Based on imaging
Reg LN Pos	98	No lymph nodes removed for examination
Reg LN Exam	00	No lymph nodes examined
CS Mets at DX	00	No distant metastases
CS Mets at Dx–Bone	0	No bone metastases
CS Mets at Dx–Brain	0	No brain metastases
CS Mets at Dx–Liver	0	No liver metastases
CS Mets at Dx–Lung	0	No lung metastases
CS Mets Eval	0	Based on imaging
SSF1 FIGO Stage	999	FIGO stage not documented
SSF2 Pelvic Nodal Status	000	CT scan negative
SSF3 Assess Meth Pelv Nodes	020	Imaging
SSF4 Para-Aortic Nodal Status	999	Para-aortic nodal status unknown
SSF5 Assess Meth Para-Aortic	999	No information
SSF6 Mediastinal Nodal Status	999	Mediastinal nodal status unknown
SSF7 Assess Meth Mediastin	999	No information
SSF8 Scalene Nodal Status	000	Physical exam negative
SSF9 Assess Meth Scalene Nodes	010	Clinical assessment

This case will map to cT2a cN0 cM0 Stage Group IIA.

Corpus-Cervix

—— CERVIX CASE 12 ——

Site Code	C53.9	Cervix uteri, NOS
Histology	8071/33	Poorly differentiated large cell nonkeratinizing squamous cell carcinoma
Grade Path Value	Blank	Does not apply
Grade Path System	Blank	Does not apply
Lymph Vascular Invasion	9	Lymph-vascular invasion not mentioned in path report
Ambiguous Terminology	0	Conclusive terminology
Date Conclusive Terminol	Blank	Diagnosis made by conclusive terminology
Date Conclus Dx Flag	11	Not applicable
Multiplicity Counter	01	One tumor only
Date Multiple Tumors	Blank	Not applicable
Date Mult Tumors Flag	15	Single tumor only (multiplicity counter is coded 01)
Type Mult Tum as 1 Prim	00	Single tumor
Summary Stage	2	Regional direct extension only
CLINICAL	T 3b	N 0 M 0 Stage Group IIIB
PATHOLOGIC	T X	N X cM 0 Stage Group Unstageable
CS Tumor Size	999	Tumor size not stated
CS Extension	655	Extension to pelvic sidewalls on exam under anesthesia
CS TS/Ext-Eval	1	Exam under anesthesia is surgery observation without biopsy
CS Lymph Nodes	999	Cannot assume nodes are not involved when extension is high
CS Reg Nodes Eval	0	Based on physical exam
Reg LN Pos	98	No lymph nodes removed for examination
Reg LN Exam	00	No lymph nodes examined
CS Mets at DX	00	No distant metastases
CS Mets at Dx–Bone	0	No bone metastases
CS Mets at Dx–Brain	0	No brain metastases
CS Mets at Dx–Liver	0	No liver metastases
CS Mets at Dx–Lung	0	No lung metastases
CS Mets Eval	0	Based on imaging
SSF1 FIGO Stage	999	FIGO stage unknown
SSF2 Pelvic Nodal Status	000	Pelvic nodes not mentioned on ultrasound (assume negative)
SSF3 Assess Meth Pelv Nodes	020	Ultrasound
SSF4 Para-Aortic Nodal Status	999	Para-aortic nodal status not documented
SSF5 Assess Meth Para-Aortic	999	No information
SSF6 Mediastinal Nodal Status	999	Mediastinal nodal status not documented
SSF7 Assess Meth Mediastin	999	No information
SSF8 Scalene Nodal Status	000	Physical exam negative
SSF9 Assess Meth Scalene Nodes	010	Clinical assessment

This case will map to cT3b cNX cM0 Stage Group IIIB.

CANCER OF THE OVARY, FALLOPIAN TUBE, AND PLACENTA

Cancers of the female reproductive tract include primaries in the cervix uteri, corpus uteri (endometrium) and ovary. Together these sites represent about 12% of all women's cancers diagnosed in the past ten years. Although ovarian cancer is less common than uterine cancer, it is very deadly because it is usually found at a late stage. Over 21,880 new ovarian cancer cases were estimated to be diagnosed in the United States in 2010. This chapter focuses on ovary, fallopian tube and placenta primaries.

ETIOLOGY AND NATURAL HISTORY

Each of the cancers of the female genital system has its own set of risk factors and symptoms. Ovarian cancer is a disease of older women (postmenopausal). Although the causes of ovarian cancer are unknown, some of the risk factors are similar to those of corpus cancer. For example, when early menarche and late menopause are combined to produce a long period of fertility, the risk of ovarian cancer increases. Similarly, infertility treatments and nulliparity (no children), estrogen replacement therapy after menopause, obesity, and a family history of ovarian cancer or a personal history of breast or endometrial cancer are also risk factors for ovarian cancer. A unique risk factor is the use of talcum powder containing asbestos fibers on the genital area, although commercial talcum powders have been asbestos free for at least two decades.

When a woman comes to her doctor, her presenting symptoms can help identify the site of the possible cancer. Unfortunately, ovarian cancer symptoms do not appear until later stages of the disease, and then the symptoms are rather non-specific. Abdominal bloating, edema, abdominal pain, increased tightness of clothes with or without weight gain, weight loss, constipation and flatulence (caused by extrinsic obstruction of the colon or rectum), nausea, and ascites (excess fluid in the abdominal cavity) are all possible symptoms of ovarian cancer as well as other conditions. By the time the differential diagnoses are narrowed down to ovarian cancer, it is usually in an advanced stage.

ANATOMY OF THE FEMALE GENITAL SYSTEM AND REGIONAL LYMPH NODES AS THEY RELATE TO STAGING

The female genital system consists of the vulva, vagina, cervix uteri, corpus uteri, two fallopian tubes, two ovaries, placenta, supporting ligaments, and miscellaneous small glands (Figures 1 and 2). These organs are situated in the true pelvis along with the bladder, lower ureters, urethra and rectum. In this chapter, the focus is on the ovaries, with some discussion of placenta and fallopian tubes. Cancers of the uterus—cervix and corpus—are covered in a separate chapter.

The organs of the female genital system have a variety of names and descriptors.

- Word roots that may refer to the uterus as a whole are utero-, metra-, and hyster-. These may also be specific to the corpus uteri.
- The cervix is also called the uterine cervix, cervix uteri, and cervical canal. The common adjective is cervico-.
- The corpus is also called the corpus uteri, uterus, and uterine body. Word roots referring to the corpus include utero-, endometrio-, and uterine.
- The ovaries are also called the female gonads. Adjectives referring to the ovary are ovarian and the word roots oophor- and ovar-.
- The fallopian tubes are also called the oviducts, uterine tubes, or just tubes. Word roots referring to the fallopian tubes are salpingo- and tubo-.
- The fallopian tubes, ovaries and the supporting ligaments of the internal genitalia are referred to collectively as the adnexa.
- The ovary and fallopian tube are referred to collectively as salpingo-oophor- or tubo-ovarian.
- The placenta may be called products of conception or fetal membranes; placental cancer is also referred to as gestational trophoblastic tumor (GTT).

Ovaries

The ovaries are paired organs that lie on the posterior wall of the pelvis lateral to each side of the uterus. Each ovary is almond shaped, approximately 2.5 to 5 cm in transverse length and 0.5 to 1 cm in thickness.

There are three functional elements in each ovary:

- germ cells that produce the eggs (ova)
- stromal cells that hold the ovary together and make the female hormones
- epithelial cells that cover the outer surface of the ovary and are surrounded by a layer of connective tissue called the capsule

Unlike most other primary cancers of solid organs, the majority of ovarian cancers begin in the epithelium. Because they arise so near the surface, if the tumor invades through the capsule, tumor cells can circulate throughout the pelvis and peritoneum via the ascitic fluid and establish secondary tumors called implantation metastases. If these discontinuous metastases are diagnosed within the pelvis or peritoneal cavity, they are staged as regional disease. Ovarian cancer is one of the few primary sites where discontinuous metastases (seeding or studding) on the surface of organs within the pelvis or peritoneum are classified in the same way as direct extension to these pelvic or abdominal organs.

Figure 1. Anatomy of Internal Female Genital Organs *(partial cutaway anterior view)*

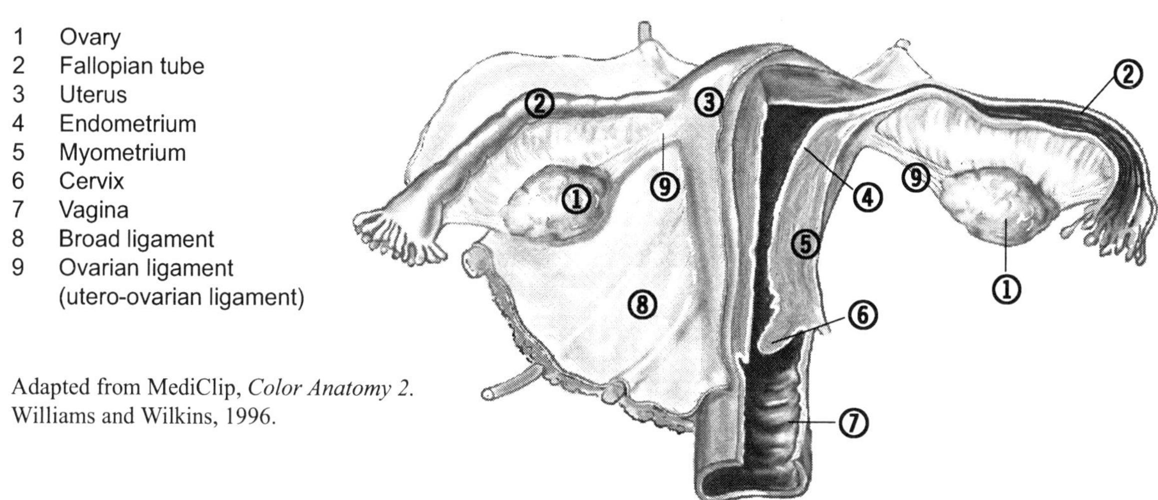

Adapted from MediClip, *Color Anatomy 2.* Williams and Wilkins, 1996.

Figure 2. Anatomy of Female Genital and Pelvic Organs *(sagittal view)*

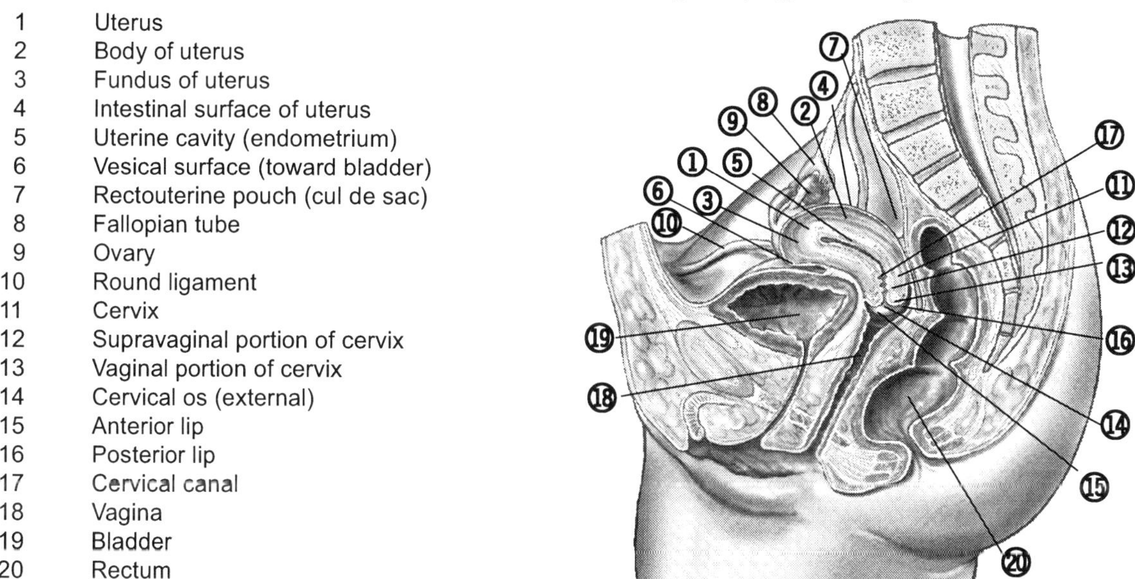

Adapted from MediClip, *Color Anatomy 2.* Williams and Wilkins, 1996.

Other Structures of the Female Genital System (Figure 1)
The ***fallopian tubes*** are detached ducts that "catch" the ovum as it is expelled from the ovary and channel it to the uterus. The paired fallopian tubes are hollow organs and staged independently from the ovaries.

The ***broad ligament***, a fold of peritoneum, supports all of the internal female genital organs. The ovaries are suspended between the layers of the broad ligament, and attached by the ***suspensory*** or ***infundibulopelvic ligament*** to the lateral pelvic wall. A third ligament, the ***round*** or ***ovarian ligament***, attaches the medial edge of the ovary to the uterus just below the entrance of the fallopian tube into the uterus. These ligaments, together with the fallopian tubes and the ovaries, are collectively referred to as the ***adnexa***.

The ***placenta*** is formed from the endometrial lining of the corpus when the ovum has been fertilized by sperm. Malignancies of the placenta may develop during pregnancy or after an abortion. The

Other Structures of the Female Genital System, *continued*

patient exhibits symptoms of pregnancy although only placental-like tissue develops (called a molar pregnancy or hydatidiform mole). Tumors of the placenta are rare but highly curable.

The ***Pouch of Douglas*** (rectouterine pouch or cul de sac) is the space between the rectum and the uterus. This is the lowest part of the abdominal cavity and a common site of seeding from ovarian cancer.

REGIONAL LYMPH NODES

The regional lymph nodes of the female genital tract are primarily in the shadow of the pelvic bones, although the para-aortic lymph nodes are above the iliac crest. The regional lymph nodes of the ovary also include lymph nodes in the retroperitoneum and at the inguinal ligament. Figure 3 shows the regional lymph node chains for ovary.

The hypogastric lymph nodes lie along the hypogastric vessels, which branch from the internal iliac artery. The obturator lymph nodes are also part of the interal iliac nodes and lie along the obturator artery. The sacral lymph nodes may also be called pre-sacral or lateral sacral.

Figure 3. Regional Lymph Nodes of Female Pelvis

1 External iliac
2 Common iliac
3 Internal iliac (hypogastric)
4 Sacral
5 Aortic
6 Inguinal

Not shown: Retroperitoneal, NOS nodes
Pelvic, NOS
Utero-ovarian nodes
Round ligament nodes

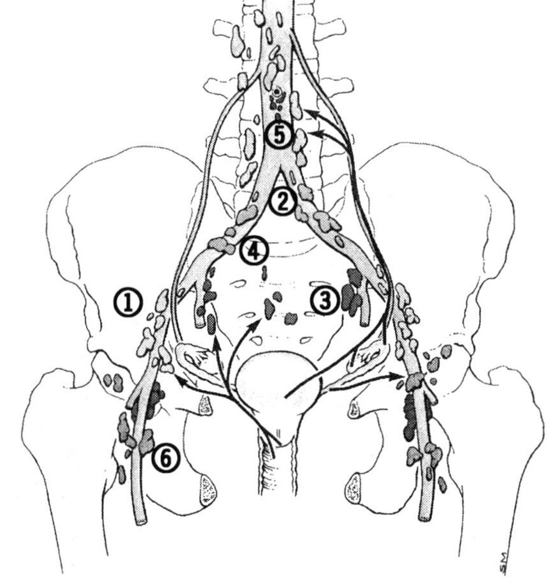

Adapted from MediClip, Grant's Atlas
Images 3: Perineum, Pelvis and Lower Limb.
Williams and Wilkins, 1998.

Other lymph nodes in the pelvis, such as paracervical, parametrial, middle sacral, and uterosacral nodes that are regional for corpus and cervix, are distant lymph nodes for the ovaries.

DISTANT METASTASES

Ovarian cancer tends to spread via implantation metastases (shedding malignant cells across the serosal surfaces of the pelvis and abdomen rather than directly invading other organs). The omentum, under surface of the diaphragm, appendix, bowel, and surface of the liver become involved this way. Ovary is unusual in TNM and the Collaborative Stage Data Collection System (CS) in that these discontinuous implantation metastases are classified in the T category and CS Extension fields, not as distant metastases. Lymphatic spread is infrequent. Distant hematogenous metastases are unusual but may include lung, pleura, and the parenchyma of the liver. Patients succumb from extensive abdominal disease.

MULTIPLE PRIMARY RULES

The ovaries are included in the "Other Sites" multiple primary and histology coding rules. Ovaries are a paired organ.

Features of "Other Sites" Rules

- 18 multiple primaries rules, of which 6 are specific to certain primary sites (prostate, thyroid, Kaposi sarcoma, retinoblastoma) and will not be discussed here
- ONE year between diagnoses
- Bilateral tumors are multiple primaries except if described as a metastasis (bilateral epithelial carcinoma of the ovaries diagnosed within 60 days is an exception to this rule)
- Histology coding rules in four sections (31 rules total)
    - 6 rules (H1 – H6) in Single Tumor: In Situ module
    - 1 rule (H7) in Single Tumor: Invasive and In Situ module
    - 10 rules (H8 – H17) in Single Tumor: Invasive module
    - 14 rules (H18 – H31) in Multiple Tumors Abstracted as a Single Primary module
- Histology coding rules refer to a chart in the site-specific Terms and Definitions providing priorities for most specific histology code

Summary of Multiple Primary Rules

This is only a summary of the multiple primary rules for the ovarian primaries. Details of the rules are provided in the official published documents available from www.seer.cancer.gov/tools/mphrules. Refer to the General Instructions for information about coding more specific terms, missing pathology or cytology reports, and other aspects of the rules for this and other sets of site-specific rules. **Always** refer to the site-specific rules themselves in your preferred format when determining how many abstracts to prepare or the correct histology code for an individual abstract. The published rules include more discussion, examples, and notes.

The standard three modules of the multiple primaries rules are present: unknown if single or multiple tumors, single tumor, and multiple tumors.

- Count only macroscopic, non-metastatic tumors when deciding which module applies.

The first module, unknown if single or multiple tumors, is the same as for all other site-specific sets of rules:

M1. Number of tumors (single or multiple) can't be determined = single

Ovary rules are similar to the other multiple primary rules: there is only one rule for single tumors:

M2. Single tumor = single

The priority of the multiple tumors rules is as follows:

M3 – M6. Site-specific rules not applicable to ovary
M7. Bilateral epithelial tumors of the ovary diagnosed within 60 days of each other = single
M8 – M9. Site-specific rules not applicable to ovary
M10. Diagnosis dates more than 1 year apart = multiple
M11. Topography code different at 2nd or 3rd character = multiple
M12. Site-specific rule not applicable to ovary
M13. Frank in situ/invasive adenocarcinoma and in situ/invasive tumor in a polyp = single
M14. Multiple in situ/malignant polyps = single
M15. Invasive carcinoma after in situ more than 60 days = multiple
M16. Non-specific and specific histology codes = single
M17. Histology different at first, second, or third digit = multiple
M18. All other scenarios = single

HISTOLOGIC CELL TYPES OF OVARIAN, FALLOPIAN TUBE, AND PLACENTAL CANCER

All types of cancer should be coded in CS. In contrast, certain cell types may be staged in the TNM system but the instructions in the AJCC Cancer Staging Manual are to analyze them separately. These exceptions are noted below.

Three types of cancers can develop in the different functional areas of the ovaries:

I. **Epithelial tumors** (about 85% of all ovarian cancers) in the ICD-O-3 code range 8000 to 8799 develop from the cells that cover the outer surface of the ovary. The major epithelial histologic types, according to the World Health Organization publication on ovarian tumors, are (ICD-O-3 morphology code is in parenthesis):
   A. Serous cystadenocarcinomas (8441/3), including papillary cystadenocarcinoma (8450/3)—40% of all ovarian cancers
   B. Mucinous cystadenocarcinomas (8470/3)—12% of ovarian cancers
   C. Endometrioid adenocarcinomas (8380/3)—15%, similar in appearance to endometrial adenocarcinoma
   Note: Endometrioid carcinoma may be primary in the ovary. This diagnosis should not be coded as metastatic from the endometrium, nor should the endometrium be coded as a metastatic site unless histologically proven.
   D. Clear cell adenocarcinomas (8310/3)—6%; also called mesonephroma
   E. Brenner tumor, malignant (9000/3)—also called transitional cell carcinoma
   F. Undifferentiated carcinoma (8020/3)—5%; too poorly differentiated to be classified to groups A through E
   G. Mixed epithelial tumors (mixed cell adenocarcinoma, 8323/3)—tumors comprised of two or more of groups A through E

Ovarian epithelial tumors of borderline malignancy (about 10-15% of the epithelial tumors) may be staged according to the TNM system, but must be reported separately. Epithelial tumors of low malignant potential (borderline malignancy) were changed from /3 to /1 in ICD-O-3 (2001). Borderline ovarian tumors may be collected as reportable-by-agreement cases if there is interest in them by the facility's medical staff. Some central cancer registries still collect these tumors as well.

- Serous cystadenoma (8442/_)
- Papillary cystadenoma (8451/_)
- Serous papillary cystadenoma (8562/_)
- Mucinous cystadenoma (8472/_)
- Papillary mucinous cystadenoma (8473/_)

II. **Germ cell tumors** (about 15%) develop in the cells that produce the ova. These include:
   - Dysgerminoma (9060/3)—counterpart to male seminoma; most common in children; most radiosensitive
   - Endodermal sinus tumor (9071/3)—also called yolk sac tumor; aggressive tumor; sensitive to chemotherapy
   - Embryonal carcinoma (9070/3)—rare
   - Choriocarcinoma (9100/3)—very rare
   - Teratoma (9082/3)—rare
   - Polyembryoma (9072/3)—rare
   - Mixed germ cell type (codes vary; rare)

Histologic Cell Types—Ovary, *continued*

III. **Sex cord-stromal tumors** (NOS, 8590/1) (about 1%) develop from the connective tissue cells that support the other cells of the ovary and produce female hormones. These include:
- Granulosa-stromal cell tumor (8620/3)—produces estrogens
- Androblastoma (8630/3)
- Others—usually benign or borderline
  - Sertoli-Leydig cell tumor (8631/0)—also called arrhenoblastoma; usually benign; causes masculinization
  - Gynandroblastoma (8632/1)—mixed granulosa-Sertoli cell tumors
  - Other unclassified sex cord stromal tumors (many cell types)

Both germ cell tumors and sex cord stromal tumors occur in younger women. They are staged according to the TNM system, but must be analyzed separately from the epithelial malignancies.

Other Ovarian Tumors (excluded from AJCC staging for ovarian cancer)—lymphomas and sarcomas of the ovary account for less than 1% of all ovarian malignancies.
- Lipid cell tumors (8670/0)
- Gonadoblastoma (9073/1)
- Nonspecific soft tissue tumors (sarcomas—many cell types)
- Lymphomas (many cell types)

Simultaneous Bilateral Ovarian Involvement
Both ovaries are commonly found to be involved simultaneously. In some cases, the pathology report will state whether these are concurrent primaries or if tumor in one ovary has metastasized to the other. If this information is not apparent from the pathology report, it needs to be clarified, because it does affect staging, counting of multiple primaries, and coding of laterality.

Other Terms
The following terms may be found in medical records. They are excluded from AJCC staging for ovarian cancer.
- **Krukenberg tumor** (8490/6; also called metastatic signet ring cell carcinoma)—metastatic tumor ***to*** the ovary ***from*** a primary in the gastrointestinal tract; should not be coded or staged as an ovarian primary. Coding of Krukenberg tumors is explained in more detail in the second errata to ICD-O-3, available at http://seer.cancer.gov/icd-o-3/errata.d05062003.pdf.
- **Pseudomyxoma peritonei** (8480/6)—widespread metastases in the peritoneum from mucinous cystadenocarcinoma. The peritoneum becomes filled with a jellylike material that causes abdominal distention and compresses the bowel, requiring periodic surgical debulking.

FALLOPIAN TUBE
Fallopian tube is another bilateral organ. The malignancies of the oviducts are the same as the epithelial adenocarcinomas of the ovaries:

A. Serous cystadenocarcinomas (8441/3)
B. Mucinous cystadenocarcinomas (8470/3)
C. Endometrioid adenocarcinomas (8380/3)
D. Clear cell adenocarcinomas (8310/3)
E. Transitional cell carcinoma (8120/3, non-Brenner; 9000/3, Brenner)
F. Undifferentiated carcinoma (8020/3)

Fallopian tube is also covered in the "Other Sites" Multiple Primary and Histology Coding Rules.

Histologic Cell Types, ***continued***

PLACENTA

- Hydatidiform mole (9100/0)—products of conception that lack an intact fetus with gross cyst-like swelling of chorionic villi
- Choriocarcinoma (9100/3)—highly malignant gestational trophoblastic neoplasms occurring in a hydatidiform mole; occurs in about 1 in 20,000 pregnancies
- Chorioadenoma destruens (9100/1)—locally invasive; rarely metastatic
- Placental-site trophoblastic tumor (9104/1)—rare tumor arising from placental implantation site with infiltration of myometrium

Placenta is also covered in the "Other Sites" Multiple Primary and Histology Coding Rules.

PRIMARY PERITONEAL CARCINOMA

Extra-ovarian primaries may arise from the coelomic epithelium in the peritoneum. These malignancies are histologically identical to epithelial ovarian cancer but the ovaries are not involved. They are diagnosed as primary papillary peritoneal adenocarcinoma (8461/3) with a primary site of C48._. They may be staged with the ovary TNM classification but must be reported separately. In CS, these tumors are coded with their own schema, PeritoneumFemale Gen.

HISTOLOGY CODING RULES

Ovary is included in the "Other Sites" multiple primary and histology coding rules. For these sites, there are four modules based on behavior and number of tumors. Make sure you are looking at the rules in the correct section. The first few rules may seem repetitive, but this was done so that each module is self-contained and avoids having the reader jump from one place to another in the rules.

The 2007 Histology Coding Rules for "Other Sites" include an important new concept.

- A rule has been added that, when a tumor has both an invasive histology and a different in situ histology, the invasive histology should be coded. Pathologists generally agree that it is the invasive part of the tumor that has the potential to do the most harm to the patient; thus the in situ component should be disregarded and the histology of the invasive component should be assigned to the case.
- In the non-specific/specific coding rules (H4, H13 and H29), the following terms indicate a more specific type:
  - Invasive cancers: type, subtype, predominantly, with features of, major, with [something] differentiation
  - In situ cancers: pattern, architecture, type, subtype, predominantly, with features of, major, with [something] differentiation

Single Tumor: In situ Only

H1. If no pathology/cytology report available, code the histology stated by the clinician.
H2. If only one histology is stated, code that.
H3. This rule deals with how to code an adenocarcinoma arising in a polyp. This occurs very rarely in the ovary, so it will not be explained in detail here.
H4. Code the more specific histology when one term is NOS and the other is more specific.
- NOS terms: cancer, NOS; carcinoma, NOS; adenocarcinoma, NOS; squamous cell carcinoma, NOS; melanoma, NOS; sarcoma, NOS

H5. Use a mixed or combination code from Table 2 (in MP/H manual) for a single tumor with multiple specific histologies or a non-specific histology and multiple specific histologies
H6. If no other rule applies, use the numerically higher ICD-O-3 code as a last priority.

Histology Coding Rules – Single Tumor, *continued*

Single Tumor: Invasive and In Situ

H7. Code invasive histology; ignore in situ terms.

Single Tumor: Invasive Only

H8. If no pathology/cytology report available, code the histology stated by the clinician. This is the same rule as H1 but applies to single, invasive tumors.
H9. Code histology from a metastatic site if there is no tissue or cells from the primary site.
H10. Prostate-specific rule.
H11. If only one histology is stated, code that.
H12. This rule deals with how to code an adenocarcinoma arising in a polyp. This occurs very rarely in the ovary, so it will not be explained in detail here.
H13. Code the more specific histology when one term is NOS and the other is more specific.
- NOS terms: cancer, NOS; carcinoma, NOS; adenocarcinoma, NOS; squamous cell carcinoma, NOS; melanoma, NOS; sarcoma, NOS

H14. Thyroid-specific rule.
H15. Thyroid-specific rule.
H16. Use a mixed or combination code from Table 2 (in MP/H manual) for a single tumor with multiple specific histologies or a non-specific histology and multiple specific histologies.
H17. If no other rule applies, use the numerically higher ICD-O-3 code as a last priority.

Multiple Tumors Abstracted as a Single Primary

H18. If no pathology/cytology report available, code the histology stated by the clinician. This is the same rule as H8 but applies to multiple tumors abstracted as a single primary.
H19. Code histology from a metastatic site if there is no tissue or cells from the primary site.
H20. Prostate-specific rule.
H21. Squamous intraepithelial neoplasia rule for vulva, vagina, and anus only.
H22. Code 8148/2 for PAIN III (pancreatic glandular intraepithelial neoplasia).
H23. If only one histology is stated, code that.
H24. Extramammary Paget disease rule for anus, perianal region or vulva only.
H25. This rule deals with how to code an adenocarcinoma arising in a polyp. This occurs very rarely in the ovary, so it will not be explained in detail here.
H26. Thyroid-specific rule.
H27. Thyroid-specific rule.
H28. Code single invasive histology for invasive-in situ combinations.
H29. Code the more specific histology when one term is NOS and the other is more specific.
- NOS terms: cancer, NOS; carcinoma, NOS; adenocarcinoma, NOS; squamous cell carcinoma, NOS; melanoma, NOS; sarcoma, NOS

H30. Use a mixed or combination code from Table 2 (in MP/H manual) for a single tumor with multiple specific histologies or a non-specific histology and multiple specific histologies.
H31. If no other rule applies, use the numerically higher ICD-O-3 code as a last priority.

IMPORTANT NOTE: USING CODE 8323

Rules H5, H16 and H30 refer to Table 2 for combination codes to be used when a tumor contains multiple specific histologies. In that table, there are instructions for using 8323, mixed cell adenocarcinoma, for GYN malignancies, particularly ovary and endometrium. Specifically, if a GYN tumor contains two or more of the following cell types, use code 8323 even though the final diagnosis may not say "mixed cell adenocarcinoma." The ovarian cell types included in this rule are combinations of clear cell, endometroid, mucinous, papillary, serous, squamous, and transitional (Brenner).

Ovary

OVARIAN CANCER ABSTRACTING GUIDELINES

Review the medical record for the following diagnostic and staging procedures. Look for information (positive and negative) that describes the tumor size, presence of multiple tumors, lymph node involvement, extension beyond the organ of origin, seeding or implants in the pelvis or abdomen, or metastasis to distant sites/organs.

HISTORY

The most common symptoms of ovarian cancer are, unfortunately, quite non-specific to cancer. They include bloating, ascites (abnormal buildup of fluid in the abdomen), and generalized fatigue. A woman may notice that her skirt or pants are becoming tight without any significant weight gain. Symptoms may persist for many months before the woman sees her doctor.

Where to look in the patient's record

- History and physical exam report
- Consultation report(s)
- Physician's progress notes

What information to select and record (record all dates)

Unless your facility requires documentation of presenting symptoms/chief complaint, record only those signs and symptoms that document

- Date of onset and type of symptoms
- Personal history of cancer, in particular breast, colorectal, or endometrial, that may indicate a genetic tendency toward developing ovarian cancer

Other information to note (but does not document location, tumor size, or extent of disease)

- Family history of cancer (similar to personal history of cancer, above)

PHYSICAL EXAM

Physical findings are uncommon in patients with early disease. Findings on physical exam for more advanced disease include ovarian or pelvic mass(es), ascites, pleural effusion, abdominal mass, or bowel obstruction. A careful pelvic examination should be part of the overall physical examination of the patient. However, because of the location of the ovaries deep in the pelvis, it may not be possible to palpate the regional (pelvic) lymph nodes directly.

- **Pelvic examination**—manual or speculum evaluation of the cervix, vagina, rectum, external genitalia. Digital examination of the rectum and vagina is also called a rectovaginal exam.
- **Examination under Anesthesia (EUA)**—bimanual examination of the pelvis and external abdomen while patient is anesthetized, using one hand in the pelvis and the other hand to press on the organs externally.

Where to look in the patient's record

- History and physical exam report
- Consultation report(s)
- Physician's progress notes
- Operative report

Physical Exam, *continued*

What information to select and record (record all dates)

Pertinent findings that detail what the physician sees and feels when the patient is examined:

- Pelvic examination: palpable pelvic masses, status of external genitalia
- Size of ovarian mass(es) from palpation
- Mention of masses or enlarged organs ("-megaly" such as hepatomegaly—enlargement of the liver)
- Palpation of accessible lymph nodes: supraclavicular, other distant lymph nodes
- General survey of rest of the body (overall physical condition)

IMAGING *(See also Diagnostic Tests and Tumor Markers chapter)*

Tests may be performed on an outpatient basis both pre-and post-admission. The most common sites of discontinuous metastases from ovarian cancer are the pelvic and abdominal cavities. These metastases are coded the same as direct tumor extension into regional organs. Occasionally, however, the patient may have lung or parenchymal liver metastases.

- **Abdominal or Pelvic Ultrasound**—assessing the structures in the abdomen and pelvis on images created by sound waves. A probe or transducer is passed back and forth across the external pelvis or may be inserted into the vagina (transvaginal). The sound waves can delineate the uterus, ovaries, cervix, fallopian tubes, and bladder. Ultrasonography can find a mass in the ovary but cannot distinguish whether it is benign or malignant.

X-rays and Scans—the following imaging procedures may be used to look for spread of tumor beyond the ovaries or distant metastases (see the Diagnostic Tests and Tumor Markers chapter of this book for definitions):

- **Chest X-ray**—looks for lung metastases or pleural effusion
- **Intravenous pyelography (IVP)**—to evaluate for involvement of ureters or bladder
- **Barium enema or Upper GI series**—if the patient has gastrointestinal symptoms
- **CT Scans** of pelvis and abdomen—can estimate the size of the tumor and identify involvement of other pelvic or abdominal organs and lymph nodes. CT scans of the head and chest are not commonly performed to diagnose distant metastases.
- **MRI** of abdomen, pelvis chest or head—not commonly performed unless patient is symptomatic for distant metastases
- **Positron emission tomography (PET) scan**—useful for identifying small masses of tumor cells away from the primary site, such as seeding or studding of tumor in the upper part of the abdomen

What information to select and record (record all dates)

Pertinent findings on radiology report from each study including:

- Name of procedure (chest x-ray, CT abdomen, etc.)
- Area of the body being examined
- Both positive and negative findings
- Location of tumor stated by radiologist, if noted
- Size of tumor stated by radiologist, if noted
- Extent of disease – regional or distant spread
- Status of liver
- Lymph node status

LABORATORY TESTS AND TUMOR MARKERS *(see also Diagnostic Tests and Tumor Markers chapter)*

In addition to routine blood work (CBC and chemistry screening panel), a patient suspected of ovarian cancer may have any or all of the following laboratory tests and tumor markers:

- **CA-125 (Cancer Antigen-125)**—a tumor marker useful for monitoring for ovarian cancer by measuring an antigen to epithelial neoplasms circulating in blood serum. An elevated CA-125 is not diagnostic of ovarian cancer but is used as a marker for recurrence. Normal range: 0 - 35 U/mL. Normal range may vary somewhat according to institutional experience. Levels above 35 suggest the presence of ovarian tumor, but other conditions can cause elevated CA-125 levels. When the CA-125 level is elevated, it must be investigated to determine whether the cause is an ovarian malignancy. Consequently, CA-125 is not and should not be used as a routine screening test for ovarian cancer.
- **CEA (Carcinoembryonic Antigen)**—a blood test measuring the presence of an antigen in malignancies arising in endodermal (embryonic) or gastrointestinal tissue. CEA assay is nonspecific for identifying a primary site, but it does indicate the presence of malignancy. Smokers may have an elevated CEA without malignant disease. Normal range: < 2.5 ng/ml. Normal range may vary somewhat according to institutional experience. Levels > 10 ng/ml suggest extensive disease and levels > 20 ng/ml suggest metastatic disease.
- **Liver Function Tests (LFT)**—a series of blood chemistry tests measuring enzymes excreted by the liver during abnormal functioning due to metastases, obstruction or other conditions. Also called liver panel. A liver panel may contain several of the following tests: alkaline phosphatase, lactic dehydrogenase (LDH), transaminase, SGOT, SGPT, leucine amino-peptidase, bilirubin. If any one of these tests is outside the normal range of values, the test should be reported as abnormal.
- *Other tumor markers* may help differentiate the cell type of an ovarian tumor, such as keratin, vimentin, glial fibrillary acidic protein, S-100, epithelial membrane antigen, human placental alkaline phosphatase, alpha fetoprotein, LeuM1, muscle-specific actin, SMA.

For Germ Cell Tumors

- **Alpha-fetoprotein**—a blood serum test used as a tumor marker for teratoma or embryonal carcinoma of the ovary. Elevated alpha-fetoprotein levels are not found in other histologies of ovarian cancer, although they may be found in patients with hepatocellular cancer.
  Note: Observe the date of an alpha-fetoprotein study carefully. Record a pre-operative study only. Alpha-fetoprotein is also used as a marker postoperatively to monitor residual tumor. Also called: αFP, AFP, alpha-fetoglobulin. Normal range: Adults: < 15 ng/ml.
- **Beta Subunit HCG (Human Chorionic Gonadotropin)**—A serum test used as a tumor marker for germ cell ovarian carcinoma. When the presence of B-HCG is detected in serum it always indicates a malignancy. Also called: β-HCG, beta-HCG, beta chain HCG.
  Note: Observe the date of the beta-HCG study carefully. Record a pre-operative study only. Beta-HCG is also used as a marker postoperatively to monitor residual tumor and the effectiveness of therapy. In patients with germ cell ovarian cancer who have had an oophorectomy, the presence of beta-HCG will confirm the patient has residual cancer that requires further treatment. However, when beta-HCG does not exist in the serum, the presence of active cancer cannot be excluded, especially in patients who have been previously treated. Normal range: 0 ng/ml.

For Placental Tumors

- **Beta Subunit HCG** (human chorionic gonadotropin)—See description and discussion above.
- *Other markers:* human placental lactogen, human placental alkaline phosphatase, keratin

ENDOSCOPY (Scopes)

Endoscopy, specifically laparoscopy, may provide visual information about the extent of ovarian cancer if the patient is not a surgical candidate. Other types of endoscopies are used to evaluate the extent of tumor spread from ovarian cancer.

- **Laparoscopy**—examination of the external surfaces of pelvic organs through a fiberoptic instrument inserted into the abdomen through a small incision below the navel
- **Cystoscopy**—examination of the bladder for metastases using a fiberoptic instrument
- **Hysteroscopy**—examination of the inside of the uterus using a fiberoptic instrument
- **Proctosigmoidoscopy**—examination of the rectum for metastases using a fiberoptic instrument

What to select and record (record all dates)

- Name of procedure (laparoscopy, hysteroscopy)
- Pertinent findings as described by the physician
  - Location of the tumor
  - Size of the tumor
  - Mention of organ involvement by direct extension or metastases

OPERATIVE FINDINGS

The surgeon's opinion of the volume of tumor present in the pelvis or abdomen is critical information for determining ovarian cancer staging. The operative report should note the appearance of both ovaries, extent of involvement of other abdominal organs (adnexae, pelvic wall, pelvic tissues, omentum), encasement, nodularity on or of viscera, frozen pelvis, any tumor on or in the liver that is not biopsied, nodules or evidence of tumor on the diaphragm that is not biopsied, which organs were biopsied or removed, amount of tumor not resected (to estimate residual tumor bulk), and any other areas where tumor was not removed.

- The terms *seeding, talcum powder appearance*, *salting, implants*, *tumor nodules* and *studding* are terms that indicate involvement of the pelvis or abdomen, depending on which organs are involved. *Omental caking* is term that indicates a large amount of tumor in the omentum.
- The operative report should also note whether rupture of one or both ovarian capsules occurred prior to laparotomy, spontaneously during the procedure, or was caused by the surgeon (iatrogenic rupture). Rupture of the ovarian capsule affects the stage at diagnosis.
- Implantation metastases (tumors on the serosal surface of other organs) are part of the T2 and T3 categories in the TNM system. Metastases on the capsule (surface) of the liver are classified as T3. Surface metastases are visible by surgical observation during laparotomy or laparoscopy and (less likely) by imaging.
- The size of the largest tumor nodule or deposit described in the operative report when the surgeon enters the abdominal cavity before tumor debulking (cytoreduction) determines the subcategory of T3/FIGO Stage III: T3a/IIIA (microscopic), T3b/IIIB (largest tumor nodule less than 2 cm) or T3c/IIIC (largest tumor nodule more than 2 cm).
- Adequate staging procedures during laparotomy should include evaluation of the undersurface of the diaphragm, pelvic and abdominal peritoneum biopsies, pelvic and para-aortic lymph node biopsies, peritoneal washings, and biopsies of any suspicious nodules or masses. The surgeon should report the results of these procedures.
- The surgeon should also include in the operative report an estimate of how much tumor was left behind at the end of the debulking procedure.

Operative Findings, *continued*

- **Intraoperative Evaluation of Diaphragm**—visual and manual inspection of the diaphragm, particularly the right leaf, during laparotomy for treatment of ovarian cancer. Optimally, the intraoperative evaluation of the diaphragm should occur prior to any dissection of pelvic organs. Evaluation of the diaphragm is an important part of good staging of ovarian cancer.
- **Peritoneal washings**—see Washings (pelvic or abdominal) in Cytology below.

What information to select and record (record all dates)
Pertinent findings as described by the surgeon:

- Size of tumor, if noted
- Implants on the serosal surface on other organs in the pelvis and abdomen
- Seeding, studding, tumor nodules, talcum powder appearance of any other organs
- Gross (visual) extent of tumor within pelvis and/or abdomen
- Status of pelvic and periaortic lymph nodes
- If surgery is performed to a regional and/or distant site only, indicate this
- Location and amount of any gross tumor not resected by the surgeon (usually described as the size of the largest residual tumor in centimeters)
- If no findings are documented, record "findings not recorded"
- Reason, if no cancer-directed surgery to the ovary(ies) was performed

DIAGNOSTIC PROCEDURES

If ovarian cancer is suspected clinically, the patient should undergo a diagnostic surgical procedure. Fine-needle aspiration or percutaneous biopsy of an adnexal mass in lieu of laparotomy will only delay appropriate diagnosis and treatment. However, in patients with widespread metastases or ascites without an obvious ovarian mass, a fine-needle aspiration or diagnostic paracentesis is appropriate.

CYTOLOGY REPORTS

- **Paracentesis**—drainage of excess fluid or ascites by inserting a needle into the abdomen. If ovarian cancer is suspected, the fluid is sent to the laboratory to be microscopically examined for malignant cells.
- **Washings (pelvic or abdominal)**—instillation of approximately 200 ml. of saline solution into the abdomen or pelvis during laparotomy; also called peritoneal lavage. After the solution is allowed to contact surfaces in the area for about five minutes, it is aspirated and sent for cytologic examination. This procedure is used to determine whether tumor is present in the abdomen in the absence of ascites. If malignant cells are present, the stage of the case increases.
  Note: The presence of non-malignant ascites does not affect staging in any of the three systems.
- **Thoracentesis**—removal of fluid from the chest (pleural space) for relief of symptoms or to look for malignant cells

HISTOLOGY

- **Staging laparotomy**—an adequate staging procedure during a laparotomy should include removal of the ovaries, fallopian tubes, and uterus; removal of the pelvic and para-aortic lymph nodes; evaluation of the undersurface of the diaphragm, surface of the liver, and parenchymal liver nodules if apparent; biopsies of the pelvic and abdominal peritoneum; removal of the omentum; other regional lymph node biopsies; peritoneal washings; and biopsies of any other suspicious nodules or masses. Each of these biopsies may be listed

Diagnostic Procedures—Histology, *continued*

separately in the pathology report. Read the pathology report carefully to note any abdominal organ involvement, as this increases the stage of the tumor.

PATHOLOGY REPORTS

Pathologic evaluation of any resected tissue not only establishes a diagnosis, but also provides important staging (and therefore prognostic) information. All parts of the pathology report—the gross examination of the specimen, the microscopic examination, the final diagnosis and comments—should be reviewed for staging, grade, and histology information, but only the final diagnosis should be used to code the histology. If a CAP checklist (outline format provided by the College of American Pathologists) is provided, the information may be easier to find in that section of the pathology report than in the gross and microscopic narrative sections. The CAP checklist is also called a synoptic report or CAP protocol. An example of a CAP protocol is shown in Table 1. When reviewing pathology reports for cytologies, biopsies and/or surgical resections, note the following:

What information to select and record (record date tissue was collected)

Final Diagnosis

- Histology (cell type)—Follow the histology coding rules for using this information. Remember, for ovary, the ICD-O-3 morphology code is based only on the final diagnosis.
- Behavior and grade
- Mixed histology information

Gross

- Specimen source (resection, biopsy, cytology)
- Site of specimen—particularly important for an ovarian staging procedure (ovary, corpus, liver, other pelvic and abdominal structures, lymph nodes, metastatic site)
- Tumor size (if complete resection)

Microscopic pathology

- Biopsy: FNA of cells or tissue
  - Site(s) of positive biopsies
- Resection
  - Presence of tumor on serosal surface
  - Involvement of adjacent structures (fallopian tubes, ligaments, corpus, intestine, abdominal structures, diaphragm, etc.)
- Results of multiple staging biopsies including:
  - Omentum
  - Mesentery
  - Pelvic and para-aortic lymph nodes
  - Diaphragm
  - Liver
  - Any other suspected metastatic sites
- Ascites (excess fluid in the abdominal cavity)—if present, check cytology report for malignant cells
- Pelvic or abdominal washings sent for cytologic examination
- Pleural effusion (excess fluid in the pleural space in the chest) – if present, check cytology for presence of malignant cells
- Status of margins, if applicable
- Evidence of tumor rupture

Diagnostic Procedures—Pathology Reports, *continued*

- Names and number of lymph nodes positive/number examined
- Findings from any other organ biopsies/resections
- Stage as reported by the pathologist
  - FIGO Stage
  - TNM Stage

Table 1. Example of College of American Pathologists (CAP) Ovarian Cancer Protocol

SUMMARY REPORT

MACROSCOPIC

Specimen type: Right salpingo-oophorectomy (part of specimen 3).
Left salpingo-oophorectomy (specimen 2).
Total hysterectomy (part of specimen 3).
Omentectomy (Specimen 1).

Primary tumor site: LEFT OVARY: Parenchymal growth. Growth on surface cannot be assessed (ruptured).
RIGHT OVARY: Uninvolved.

Specimen integrity: RIGHT OVARY: Intact.
LEFT OVARY: Ruptured.

Tumor size: LEFT OVARY: Involves almost the entire left adnexa, 7.2 x 5.9 x 4.3, plus additional fragments aggregating to 7 x 7 x 1.5 cm.

MICROSCOPIC

Histologic type: Serous carcinoma.

Histologic grade: G3: Poorly differentiated.

Pathologic staging (pTNM [FIGO]):

Primary tumor (pT): pT3c and/or N1 [IIIC]: Peritoneal metastases beyond pelvis more than 2 cm in greatest dimension.

Regional lymph nodes (pN): pNX: Cannot be assessed.

Distant metastasis (pM): pMX: Cannot be assessed.

Summary of organ/tissues microscopically involved by tumor:

One ovary (left)
Omentum
Uterus (left cornual nodules, left anterior and left posterior parametrium)

Venous/lymphatic (Large/small vessel) invasion (V/L): Present, numerous foci.

Additional Pathologic Findings

A. Cervix: Cervical transformation excised, atrophy of exocervical squamous epithelium, negative for intraepithelial lesion or malignancy.
B. Endometrium: Benign endometrial polyp in a background of benign cystic atrophy, negative for hyperplasia, negative for malignancy.
C. Myometrium: Single small leiomyoma.
D. Cul-de-sac: Histologically normal, negative for metastatic malignancy.
E. Right fallopian tube: Post tubal ligation status, benign paratubal cyst, otherwise histologically normal, negative for metastatic carcinoma.
F. Right ovary: Benign, atrophic, negative for neoplasia.

DIAGNOSIS

1. OMENTUM, PARTIAL OMENTECTOMY:
   METASTATIC SEROUS CARCINOMA.
2. LEFT FALLOPIAN TUBE AND OVARY:
   SEROUS CARCINOMA, INVOLVING ALMOST ENTIRE ADNEXA, RUPTURED, INVOLVING PAINTED MARGINS.
3. TOTAL HYSTERECTOMY AND SEPARATE RIGHT SALPINGO-OOPHORECTOMY:
   METASTATIC SEROUS CARCINOMA, INVOLVING LEFT CORNUAL NODULE, LEFT ANTERIOR PARAMETRIUM AND LEFT POSTERIOR PARAMETRIUM WITH INVOLVEMENT OF PAINTED MARGINS.

REMAINDER OF FINDINGS NOTED IN SYNOPTIC REPORT ABOVE.

OVARIAN CANCER DISEASE MANAGEMENT

Total abdominal hysterectomy and bilateral salpingo-oophorectomy (TAH-BSO) are not only part of the treatment for all stages of ovarian cancer, but are also crucial for adequate staging of the disease to determine whether further treatment is warranted. Following a thorough staging laparotomy, no further treatment is usually needed for well- and moderately well-differentiated Stage IA and IB epithelial carcinomas. Higher stage cancers, poorly differentiated tumors confined to the ovary(ies), densely adherent tumors, or tumors with positive peritoneal washings warrant adjuvant chemotherapy, either intraperitoneally for Stage III disease with minimal residual, or systemic chemotherapy for more extensive tumor.

SURGERY

Surgery of Primary Site

What information to record (record all dates)

- Planned definitive cancer treatment (name of procedure)
- Reason if no resection is attempted

The treatment of choice is total abdominal hysterectomy and bilateral salpingo-oophorectomy with omentectomy. The code structure of Surgery of Primary Site is based on salpingo-oophorectomy with or without hysterectomy and with or without omentectomy. The following procedures should be performed by a specially trained gynecologic oncologist, rather than a gyn surgeon.

- **Staging Laparotomy**—Opening the abdomen and pelvis of the patient for careful inspection. The procedure should include review of the undersurface of the diaphragm, biopsies of the pelvic and abdominal peritoneum, regional lymph node biopsies, peritoneal washings and biopsies of any suspicious nodules or masses. Be sure to look for documentation about the size of the largest metastasis, as this can affect stage. Staging laparotomy is a separate exploratory procedure that is usually included in the following cancer-directed operations.
- **Oophorectomy**—surgical removal of an ovary. If the fallopian tube is removed with the ovary as is usually the case, the procedure is called a salpingo-oophorectomy.
    - **Wedge resection of ovary** or **partial/subtotal oophorectomy**—surgical removal of entire tumor but less than an entire ovary; the fallopian tube is not removed in this procedure (Surgery of Primary Site code 25–28 depending on whether hysterectomy was performed).
    - **Unilateral (salpingo-)oophorectomy**—removal of one ovary (Surgery of primary site code 35–37 depending on whether hysterectomy was performed).
    - **Bilateral (salpingo-)oophorectomy**—removal of both ovaries (Surgery of primary site code 50–52 depending on whether hysterectomy was performed).

  Note: If a resection of one ovary is performed for diagnosis and a more complete procedure, such as resection of the other ovary, is done as cancer directed surgery, code the more complete surgical procedure. For example, if a left oophorectomy was done in the past for a previous primary or other problem and a right oophorectomy is now being performed for a new primary, code the current procedure as bilateral oophorectomy. The surgical code should indicate the status of the primary(s) organ at the completion of the procedure.
- **Omentectomy**—surgical removal of the omentum, the fatty "apron" covering in the anterior abdomen attached to the transverse colon and stomach and a common site of metastases from the ovary. The omentum can then be examined for nonpalpable metastases. This may be

Surgery, ***continued***

either a partial (infracolic) or complete omentectomy. Oophorectomy with omentectomy is coded in the 55–57 range in Surgery of Primary Site depending on whether a hysterectomy was performed.

- **Debulking** (cytoreductive surgery, tumor reduction surgery)—the surgical removal of as much macroscopic ovarian tumor as possible in the pelvis and abdomen. The purpose of the procedure is to reduce the size of the largest residual tumor so that the effect of postoperative chemotherapy or radiation is maximized. Residual disease after debulking refers to the size of the largest tumor mass left in the pelvis and abdomen. Optimal debulking is defined as reducing the size of the largest individual residual tumor nodule to less than 1.0 cm in greatest dimension (also called minimal residual) so that the patient's total tumor mass is minimal. So-called suboptimal debulking results in individual residual tumor nodule(s) more than 1.0 cm in size (also called macroscopic residual). The effectiveness of postoperative adjuvant radiation and chemotherapy is increased when the tumor burden is smallest. Omentectomy alone and multiple lymph node samplings and/or biopsies of suspicious areas for staging purposes are separate procedures not included in debulking.
  Debulking is coded in the range 60–63 in Surgery of Primary Site, depending on other organs removed as part of the procedure.
- **Pelvic exenteration**—removal of female genital tract and other organs of the pelvis; see below. Pelvic exenteration is coded as 70 in Surgery of Primary Site.
- **Anterior exenteration**—removal of uterus, tubes, ovaries, vagina, distal ureters and bladder plus pelvic lymph nodes and ligamentous attachments. Anterior exenteration is coded as 71 in Surgery of Primary Site.
- **Posterior exenteration**—removal of uterus, tubes, ovaries, rectum and rectosigmoid plus pelvic lymph nodes and ligamentous attachments. Posterior exenteration is coded as 72 in Surgery of Primary Site.
- **Total exenteration**—combination of anterior and posterior exenteration procedures; removes all pelvic organs. Total exenteration is coded as 73 in Surgery of Primary Site.
- **Extended exenteration**—total exenteration plus removal of pelvic blood vessels or portion of bony pelvis. Extended exenteration is coded as 74 in Surgery of Primary Site.
- If the operative report states that the adnexa were palpated but does not mention nodes, assume that the lymph nodes are negative.
- If exploratory or definitive surgery is performed and lymph nodes are not mentioned in the operative report, assume that the lymph nodes are negative.
- Fallopian tube carcinoma may be determined to be primary only if tumor is confined to the tube and any ovarian involvement is on the surface.
- **"Second-look" operation**—After completion of chemotherapy (usually about 12 months after diagnosis) patients may undergo a second-look laparotomy to evaluate response to therapy. In the past, a second look operation was commonly performed; more recently the efficacy of the procedure has been controversial in that it does not improve survival and has its own morbidity. A second-look procedure is not coded as first-course treatment or subsequent treatment because it is an exploratory procedure.

RADIATION THERAPY

Radiation therapy for epithelial ovarian cancers is usually reserved for treatment of metastases or as adjuvant treatment for high grade, low stage cancers. For germ cell tumors, prophylactic irradiation to the mediastinal and supraclavicular lymph nodes may be considered.

Radiation Therapy, *continued*

Radioactive phosphorus (P-32 or P^{32}) instilled into the peritoneum can control ascites but causes adhesions and bowel complications. P-32 is no longer commonly used to treat ovarian cancer.

External beam radiation my be used as treatment for ovarian cancer, but brachytherapy is rarely used.

What information to select and record

- Treatment start and stop dates
- Method of delivery (beam, brachytherapy, radioisotopes)
- Radiation treatment modality (regional or boost)
- Radiation source (photons, electrons, etc.)
- Total radiation dose (cGy)
- Target site(s) (also called volume)

SYSTEMIC TREATMENT

Chemotherapy/Hormone Therapy/Immunotherapy/Other Therapy
What information to record

- Treatment start date and ending date
- Name of regimen(s)
- Names of agents administered
- Number of cycles

CHEMOTHERAPY

After surgical debulking of tumor and a thorough evaluation of residual tumor, chemotherapy is the treatment of choice for maintaining a long disease-free interval.

Paclitaxel (Taxol) and platinum drugs (Cisplatin, Carboplatin) have revolutionized the treatment and prognosis of ovarian cancer. Other drugs effective in the treatment of ovarian cancer include Alkeran, Cytoxan (cyclophosphamide), Adriamycin (doxorubicin), Hycamptin (topotecan), Navelbine (vinorelbine), Ifos (ifosfamide), VP-16 (etoposide), and Gemzar (gemcitabine).

Intraperitoneal chemotherapy with Taxol and Cisplatin may be administered for microscopic tumor or small residual tumor bulk, or the patient may undergo whole-abdomen radiation.

The most effective of the newer targeted therapy drugs is bevacizumab (Avastin), an anti-angiogenesis agent that blocks the growth of new blood vessels that feed the tumor. Other targeted therapy drugs under clinical investigation are poly(ADP-ribose) polymerase inhibitors (PARPs) that make cancers without BRCA mutations more sensitive to certain kinds of chemotherapy and radiation.

Consolidation therapy, also called maintenance therapy, is continuation of one or more drugs after the completion of the initial chemotherapy regimen for the purpose of reducing recurrences. Clinical trials have shown that consolidation therapy can prolong the disease-free interval but does not improve survival. Investigation is ongoing.

Chemotherapy for epithelial tumors

- Platinum-based chemotherapy (Cisplatin or carboplatin) alone
- Platinum-based chemotherapy in combination with Paclitaxel (Taxol)

Systemic Therapy—Chemotherapy, *continued*

Other combinations

- CP (cisplatin and cyclophosphamide)
- CC (cyclophosphamide and carboplatin)
- CAP (cytoxan, adriamycin, cisplatin)

Intraperitoneal radioimmunoconjugates and targeted drugs are under clinical evaluation.

Chemotherapy for germ cell tumors

- PEB (or BEP) (cisplatin, etoposide, bleomycin) (also effective for ovarian stromal tumors)
- TIP (Taxol, ifosfamide, cisplatin)
- VelP (vinblastine, ifosfamide, cisplatin)
- VIP (VP-16, ifosfamide, cisplatin

HORMONE THERAPY

Hormone therapy is not usually used for ovarian epithelial cancers, but Tamoxifen (an anti-estrogen) can be used for ovarian stromal tumors.

Gonadotropin-releasing hormone agonists such as Zoladex (gosrelin) or Lupron (leuprolide) may be given to premenopausal women to shut down estrogen production by the ovaries.

IMMUNOTHERAPY

Vaccines (oregovomab) are under clinical evaluation. Monoclonal antibodies being investigated, such as farletuzumab and catumaxomab, may help the patient's immune system fight the cancer.

'USUAL' TREATMENT BY HISTOLOGY AND/OR STAGE GROUP (from NCI PDQ)

Ovarian Epithelial Tumors

Ovary Stage I and II

- If well- or moderately well-differentiated, TAH and BSO with omentectomy for Stage IA and IB. A careful staging laparotomy with multiple biopsies is critical.
- Unilateral salpingo-oophorectomy in selected patients with grade I tumor who want to maintain childbearing capacity.
- Adjuvant treatment if the tumor is grade III, densely adherent, or stage IC, such as: intraperitoneal P-32 or radiation therapy, platinum-based systemic chemotherapy with or without alkylating agents, or combination platinum-paclitaxel chemotherapy.

Ovary Stage III and IV

- Adequate staging laparotomy, TAH-BSO with omentectomy, and as much surgical debulking of tumor as can be safely performed.
- Intraperitoneal regimens following surgery, such as cisplatin or paclitaxel following optimal cytoreduction
- Standard intravenous cisplatin, paclitaxel or combinations following suboptimal cytoreduction
- Consolidation or maintenance therapy following combination chemotherapy has not been shown to improve survival.

'Usual' Treatment by Stage, *continued*

Ovarian Germ Cell Tumors

Stage I patients except those with stage I, grade I immature teratoma and stage IA dysgerminoma require postoperative chemotherapy. With platinum-based combination chemotherapy, the prognosis for patients with endodermal sinus tumors, immature teratomas, embryonal carcinomas, choriocarcinomas, and mixed tumors containing one or more of these elements has improved dramatically.

Stage I Dysgerminomas

- Unilateral salpingo-oophorectomy conserving the uterus and opposite ovary for younger patients desiring to preserve fertility or to preserve a pregnancy, assuming a careful intraoperative staging evaluation.
- Adjuvant treatment for incompletely staged patients or those with higher stage tumors, such as radiation therapy or chemotherapy.

Stage I Other Germ Cell Tumors

- Unilateral salpingo-oophorectomy when fertility is to be preserved. Chemotherapy is usually given postoperatively, for example VAC (vincristine, dactinomycin, and cyclophosphamide); BEP (cisplatin, etoposide, and bleomycin).
- Unilateral salpingo-oophorectomy followed by close observation

Stage II Dysgerminomas

- TAH-BSO with adjuvant radiation or chemotherapy
- Unilateral salpingo-oophorectomy when fertility is to be preserved; adjuvant chemotherapy should be given. Adjuvant BEP (cisplatin, etoposide, and bleomycin) is preferred to radiation therapy.

Stage II Other Germ Cell Tumors

- Unilateral salpingo-oophorectomy when fertility is to be preserved. Adjuvant chemotherapy with VAC (vincristine/dactinomycin/cyclophosphamide), or combinations containing bleomycin, etoposide, and cisplatin (BEP).
- Second look laparotomy in selected patients
- Clinical trials

Stage III Germinomas

- TAH-BSO with tumor debulking
- Unilateral salpingo-oophorectomy with chemotherapy if fertility is to be preserved
- Chemotherapy with bleomycin/etoposide/cisplatin (BEP) or PVB (cisplatin/vincristine/bleomycin)
- Clinical trials

Stage III Other Germ Cell Tumors

- TAH-BSO with tumor debulking followed by a cisplatinum-based regimen
- Neoadjuvant chemotherapy prior to TAH-BSO
- Unilateral salpingo-oophorectomy if fertility is to be preserved, with adjuvant chemotherapy, with or without neoadjuvant chemotherapy
- Second look laparotomy in selected patients
- Clinical trials

Stage IV Germinomas

- TAH-BSO with tumor debulking and adjuvant chemotherapy
- Unilateral salpingo-oophorectomy followed by chemotherapy such as BEP if fertility is to be preserved

'Usual' Treatment by Stage, *continued*

Stage IV Other Germ Cell Tumors

- TAH-BSO with tumor debulking with adjuvant chemotherapy, with/without neoadjuvant chemotherapy
- Unilateral salpingo-oophorectomy if fertility is to be preserved, with adjuvant chemotherapy, with/without neoadjuvant chemotherapy
- Clinical trials

Fallopian Tube Cancer

Treatment for these rare cancers is similar to that of ovarian cancer (see above).

Placental Tumors

Hydatidiform Mole (molar pregnancy)

- Removal of the hydatidiform mole (dilation, suction evacuation, and curettage)
- Hysterectomy. Only in rare situations do the ovaries require removal.
- Chemotherapy for recurrence or a diagnosis of choriocarcinoma

Placental-Site Gestational Trophoblastic Tumors

- Hysterectomy; relatively resistant to chemotherapy

Nonmetastatic Gestational Trophoblastic Tumors

- Single agent cytotoxic therapy (methotrexate or dactinomycin)
- Hysterectomy if fertility is not an issue
- Other drugs: methotrexate, etoposide

Good-Prognosis Metastatic Gestational Trophoblastic Tumors

- Single-agent chemotherapy as described for nonmetastatic disease
- Primary hysterectomy followed by single-agent chemotherapy with methotrexate or dactinomycin (if fertility is not an issue)
- Primary chemotherapy followed by secondary hysterectomy for persistent uterine disease (must verify that metastatic disease has totally regressed)
- For refractory disease:
  MAC: methotrexate + dactinomycin + chlorambucil
  Other regimens appear to produce similar survival outcomes but have been studied less extensively or are in less common use. They are:
  EMA-CO: etoposide + methotrexate + dactinomycin and vincristine + cyclophosphamide.

Poor-Prognosis Metastatic Gestational Trophoblastic Tumors

- Multiple-agent chemotherapy
  EMA-CO: etoposide + methotrexate + dactinomycin and vincristine + cyclophosphamide
  EMA-CE, in which etoposide and cisplatin are substituted for vincristine and cyclophosphamide of the EMA-CO regimen
  APE: dactinomycin + cisplatin + etoposide
  PVB: cisplatin + vinblastine + bleomycin
  PEBA: cisplatin + etoposide + bleomycin + adriamycin
  Ifosfamide + carboplatin + etoposide with autologous bone marrow transplant

Additional therapy (including radiation to central nervous system metastases and adjuvant surgery) is often necessary.

COLLABORATIVE STAGE DATA COLLECTION SYSTEM (CS) OVARY

STAGING WORK-UP

Review the medical record for the diagnostic and staging procedures listed previously in this chapter under Ovarian Cancer Abstracting Guidelines. Look for information (positive and negative) that describes the tumor location, tumor size, presence of multiple tumors, lymph node involvement, or metastasis to distant sites or organs. All of this information can be coded in CS.

Make sure that your CS manual is complete by downloading any replacement pages from www.cancerstaging.org/cstage/manuals/index.html. Review carefully the notes preceding each table of the schema in Collaborative Stage Data Collection System Coding Instructions version 02.03.02. Use the notes and comments in this section to supplement the information in the CS Manual. Remember that all of the general rules in Part I of the CS manual apply to the site-specific schema.

- CS for ovary uses the following standard or common tables, which will not be discussed in detail here:
  - CS Tumor Size—not a factor in TNM staging of ovarian cancer, but should be recorded if available
  - CS TS/Ext Eval
  - CS Reg Nodes Eval
  - Reg LN Pos
  - Reg LN Exam
  - CS Mets Eval
- Collaborative Staging for ovary uses five Site-Specific Factors.

CS Extension

- Note that the CS Extension codes reference FIGO stages. FIGO is the "Federation Internationale de Gynecologie et d'Obstetrique." The definition of the Extension codes corresponds to the FIGO stages.
- Use a code corresponding to a FIGO stage when the stated FIGO stage is the only information available. More detailed codes should be used when specific information is documented in the medical record (Note 2).
  - If the physician refers to FIGO Stage IIIC, determine whether that is on the basis of tumor extension or lymph node involvement. If on the basis of tumor extension, code in CS Extension. If on the basis of lymph node involvement or if the basis is not specified, use code 510 in CS Lymph Nodes.
- Carcinoma in situ of the ovary is considered an impossible diagnosis by FIGO and AJCC. Extension code 000 will map to TX in the seventh edition of the AJCC Cancer Staging Manual (Note 1).
- In the ovary CS schema, discontiguous tumor nodules are coded in CS Extension rather than in CS Mets at Dx.
- If borderline ovarian tumors are included in a registry as reportable-by-agreement, the CS Extension should be coded to 999 (Note 10).
- The presence of malignant ascites or positive peritoneal washings alters the stage of disease (Note 3).
  - Ignore ascites and peritoneal washings found to be negative or not specified as positive or negative (NOS); this does not affect the choice of code.

CS Extension–Ovary, *continued*

- Within code range 100–360, malignant cells in ascites or peritoneal washings changes the code to the 410–440 range, depending on other tumor characteristics.
- Within code range 500–610, the presence of malignant cells in ascites or peritoneal washings changes the code to the 620–640 range, depending on whether other pelvic structures are involved.

- Codes 100-360 define tumor confined to one or both ovaries (Stage I) (Figure 4).
- Notes 4 and 7 are perhaps the most important notes in CS Extension. Note 4 lists the structures in the pelvis that, if involved either directly or by implants, would be coded in the range 500–650, equivalent to TNM/FIGO Stage II (Figure 5). They include:
  Adnexae, NOS (broad and round ligaments, fallopian tubes)
  Bladder, bladder serosa
  Broad ligament (mesovarium)
  Cul-de-sac
  Fallopian tube(s)
  Parametrium
  Pelvic peritoneum (peritoneum below the pelvic brim)
  Pelvic wall
  Rectosigmoid
  Rectum
  Sigmoid colon; sigmoid mesentery
  Ureter (pelvic portion)
  Uterus, including vagina and cervix; uterine serosa

Figure 4. CS Extension 200 T1b/FIGO Stage IB Tumor limited to both ovaries

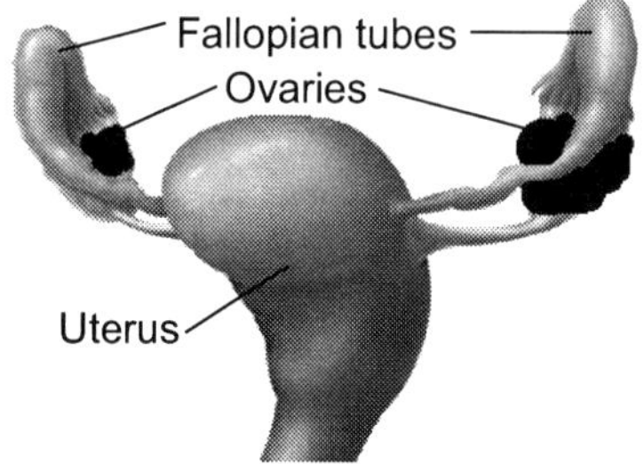

- Note 7 lists the structures in the abdomen that, if involved either directly or by implants, would be coded in the range 700–750, equivalent to TNM/FIGO Stage III (Figure 6). They include:
  Abdominal mesentery
  Diaphragm
  Gallbladder
  Infracolic omentum
  Kidney(s)
  Large intestine (except rectum, rectosigmoid, and sigmoid colon)
  Liver (peritoneal surface)
  Omentum
  Pancreas
  Pericolic gutter
  Peritoneum, NOS
  Small intestine
  Spleen
  Stomach
  Ureter(s) (retroperitoneal portion)

  There must be histologic confirmation of a metastasis outside the pelvis in order to be coded in the 700–750 range and classified as T3/Stage III.
- Note 5 lists synonyms for implants (discontinuous tumor nodules in the pelvis or abdomen).
- If tumor implants are mentioned, review the medical record to determine whether they are in the pelvis

Figure 5. CS Extension 500–520 T2a/FIGO Stage IIA Tumor on adnexa or uterus

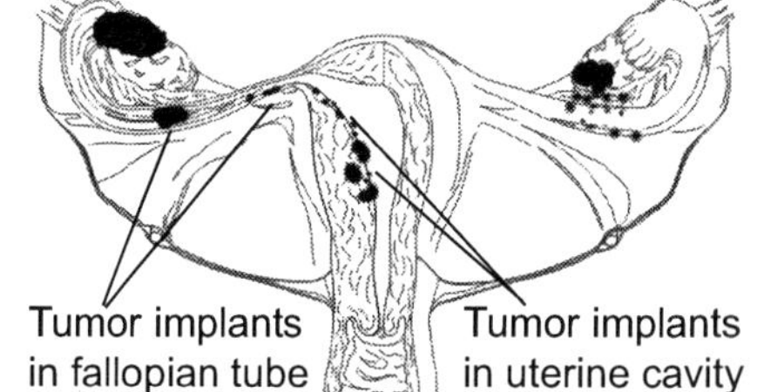

Figure 6. CS Extension 710–730 T3/FIGO Stage III (based on size of implants)

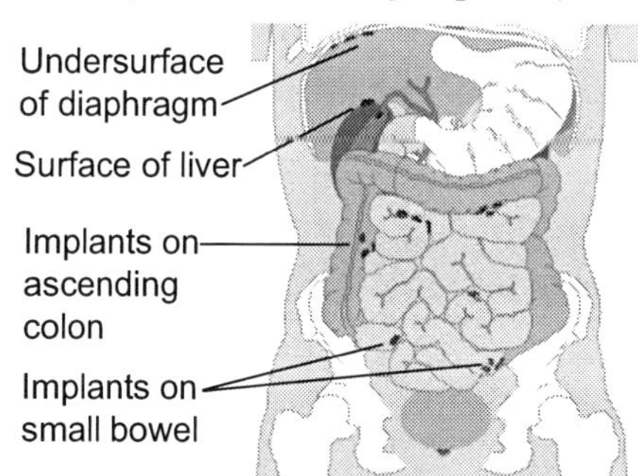

CS Extension–Ovary, *continued*

(codes 600–650) or in the abdomen (codes 700–730). If the location cannot be determined, use code 750. (Note 6)

- The size of the discontinuous tumor nodules in the abdomen (codes 710–730) is based on the surgeon's assessment prior to debulking, not on the size of the largest individual tumor nodule left after the procedure.
- Note 8 differentiates between tumor nodules ON the liver (peritoneal implants, CS Extension codes 700–730 depending on size) and tumor IN the liver (hematogenous metastases, CS Mets at Dx code 40) (Figure 7). If there is liver involvement but no mention of whether the metastases are on the surface (Extension codes) or in the parenchyma (Mets at Dx), assign the lower category and code in CS Extension.

Figure 7. Liver Involvement

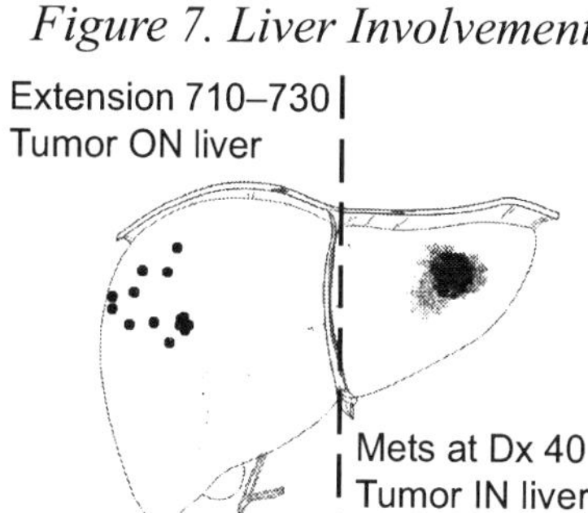

CS Lymph Nodes

- This field records involved regional lymph nodes only (Note 1).
- Bilaterality or involvement of contralateral lymph nodes does not affect the coding of regional lymph nodes (Note 2).
- Regional lymph nodes can be coded as negative if
  - the clinician says "adnexa palpated" and does not mention lymph nodes (Note 4).
  - the surgeon does not mention lymph nodes in the operative report of an exploratory laparotomy or hysterectomy (Note 5).
- Regional lymph nodes lie in the shadow of the pelvic bone and along the aorta. They were discussed in the anatomy section of this chapter.
- If multiple named lymph node chains are involved, use code 400 or 440.
- If the physician refers to FIGO Stage IIIC, determine whether that is on the basis of tumor extension or lymph node involvement. If on the basis of tumor extension, code in CS Extension. If on the basis of lymph node involvement or if the basis is not specified, use code 510 in CS Lymph Nodes.

CS Mets at Dx

- Distant lymph nodes are code 10.
- Code 40 includes any named, distant visceral metastases and specifically mentions positive pleural effusion, metastases within the parenchyma of the liver (see Figure 7), and carcinomatosis. Code 60 is used for unspecified distant metastases or a statement of M1 with no further information.
- Code 40 ***does not include*** discontinuous tumor nodules in the pelvis or abdomen, such as tumor seeding of pelvic serosa, large intestine, adnexa or vagina. These are coded in CS Extension.
- Code 50 is used when both distant visceral metastases and distant lymph nodes are involved.

Site-Specific Factors

Note: Part I Section 2 of the CS Coding Manual Version 02.03 includes extensive discussion of the site-specific factors for every schema. Rather than rewrite those coding instructions for inclusion in this CASEbook chapter, refer to Part I Section 2 if questions arise. The discussion that follows provides more rationale for why those site-specific factors were included in the ovary schema.

- The CS Ovary schema uses five site-specific factors. The default code for SSFs 6–25 is 988.

Site-Specific Factors–Ovary, *continued*

SSF1 — Carbohydrate Antigen 125 (CA-125)

- CA-125 is a tumor marker for recurrent ovarian cancer. This test of blood serum monitors for disease progression. Other names are cancer antigen 125 and carbohydrate antigen 125. Normal range is less than 35 U/ml (SI: < 35 kU/L). A normal value does not rule out cancer.
- Record the clinician's interpretation of the highest value prior to treatment, based on the reference range used by the lab.
  - 010 Positive/elevated
  - 020 Negative/normal
  - 030 Borderline; undetermined whether positive or negative
- **Note:** CA-125 is not a screening test, nor is it specific to ovarian cancer. However, any value over 35 is highly correlated with cancer. Borderline values can be up to 65 u/ml. A value of greater than 200 is unlikely to be due to a benign condition. CA-125 monitors for success of treatment and recurrence.
- After obtaining a baseline value prior to treatment, a lower result on a subsequent test indicates a response to treatment, and an increasing value indicates possible recurrence.

SSF2 — FIGO Stage

- This site-specific factor records the FIGO stage as stated in the medical record. Code the FIGO stage from a statement by the physician. Do not convert T, N, and M or TNM Stage Group into FIGO stage to code this field. If FIGO Stage is not stated, use code 999.
- As previously noted, FIGO is the French acronym for the International Federation of Gynecology and Obstetrics (see also Other Staging Systems later in this chapter). FIGO staging is similar to the TNM stage group but does not have separate elements for T, N, and M. FIGO stage uses Roman numerals from I to IV with Arabic letter subcategories A, B and C. Each female genital organ has a FIGO staging system, and they differ slightly.
- The code structure for this site-specific factor parallels the structure of the FIGO stage. The first digit is the Roman numeral expressed as a number, for example Stage II is 2. The middle digit is the Arabic letter subcategory expressed as a number, such as C is 3. The third digit is the numeric sub-subcategory, if it is used. For example, ovary stage IIIA is code 310.
- See also the discussion of FIGO Stage at the end of this chapter.

SSF3 — Residual Tumor Status and Size After Primary Cytoreduction Surgery

- The purpose of cytoreduction or debulking surgery is to remove as much tumor as is safely possible in order to make combination chemotherapy more effective. The amount of tumor left behind is an important prognostic factor.
- This site-specific factor records two pieces of information: the size of the largest residual tumor and whether the patient had neoadjuvant chemotherapy (chemotherapy before the debulking surgery). Code a statement by the surgeon in the operative report regarding the size of the largest residual tumor. Obtain information about neoadjuvant chemotherapy from the patient's history.
- Gynecologic oncologists use 1 centimeter as the boundary between successful and not-so-successful debulking surgery.
  - If the procedure is described as "optimal debulking" and the size of the residual tumor is not stated, code as 992 without neoadjuvant chemotherapy or 993 if the patient did have neoadjuvant chemotherapy.
  - If the procedure is described as "suboptimal debulking" and the size of the residual tumor is not stated, use code 990 or 992 as appropriate.
- If the surgery is not considered cytoreductive (for example, a basic salpingo-oophorectomy), use code 998.

Site-Specific Factors–Ovary, ***continued***

SSF4 — Tumor Location After Primary Cytoreduction (Debulking) Surgery

- This field is the companion to Site-Specific Factor 3 and identifies the specific location(s) of residual tumor after cytoreduction surgery. The number of sites of residual tumor has prognostic implications for the patient.
- This field is somewhat unusual in its structure. The code definitions are both cumulative and include information about whether the patient had neoadjuvant chemotherapy. For example, code 060 means that there was residual tumor in the pelvis (code 050) and in the ovary (code 010) or in the fallopian tube or uterus (code 020). Code 070 means that there was residual tumor in the pelvis, and ovary or fallopian tube/uterus and the patient had received neoadjuvant treatment. Read the code definitions carefully. Use the code that covers the most amount of residual tumor as described by the surgeon in the operative report.
- In CSv0203, there is not a good code to use when there is no cytoreduction surgery or when there is no residual tumor. According to the responses to questions posted in the CAnswer Forum (http://cancerbulletin.facs.org/forums), use code 999 (not documented) when there is no cytoreduction surgery (code 998 in SSF3) and when there is no residual tumor (code 000 in SSF3).

SSF5 — Malignant Ascites

- Malignant ascites is the abnormal buildup of natural fluids in the abdomen and pelvis that contain cancer cells. Malignant ascites upstages cases in Stage IA and IB to IC, and cases in IIA and IIB to IIC. Non-malignant ascites to not affect the stage. This field records the amount of malignant ascites in milliliters. Do not record amounts of peritoneal washings (saline fluid instilled by the surgeon and suctioned out) in this field.
- Code amounts in the range 001–979 milliliters for malignant ascites only. If the amount reported is greater than 979 milliliters (which happens frequently), use code 980. Quarts and liters (1000 milliliters) are roughly equivalent, so if the surgeon describes a quart or more of malignant ascites, use code 980.
- If ascites are present but non-malignant, use code 991. If no cytology is performed on the ascites, use code 998.
- In CSv0203, there is not a good code to use when there is no ascites. According to the response to a question posted in the CAnswer Forum (http://cancerbulletin.facs.org/forums), use code 999 (not documented) when there is no ascites reported.

COLLABORATIVE STAGE DATA COLLECTION SYSTEM (CS) FALLOPIAN TUBE

- The code structure of CS for fallopian tube is very similar to that of ovary, so it will not be discussed in detail. The fallopian tube schema uses seven site-specific factors, of which six are different from ovary.
- In CS version 01.04.00, the CS Extension field for fallopian tube was extensively revised due to an issue with incorrect identification of pelvic and abdominal organs (the difference between Stage II involvement and Stage III involvement) in previous versions. Notes were added, a few codes were split, and a few codes were made obsolete. More revisions were made in CS versions 02.00 and 02.03 resulting in additional obsolete codes. Be sure to read the CS Extension notes carefully and pay attention to inclusions and exceptions noted in the definitions of the extension codes, as well as new combination codes.

Site-Specific Factors—Fallopian Tube, *continued*

SSF1 — FIGO Stage

- Refer to SSF2, FIGO Stage, under CS for Ovary and the discussion of FIGO at the end of this chapter.

SSF2 — Biopsy of Metastatic Site

- The purpose of this site-specific factor is to document the location of specific metastatic sites that were biopsied.
- Code whether a biopsy of the omentum, small intestine, or liver parenchyma (inside the liver, not just the surface) was performed in the appropriate code, regardless of whether the biopsy result was malignant.
  - If the omentum or small intestine biopsy is positive, code that information in CS extension as well.
  - If the liver parenchyma biopsy is positive, code that information in CS Mets at Dx as well.
- If the source of a metastatic tissue biopsy is not identified, use code 100. If no metastatic tissue is biopsied, use code 998.

SSF3 — Primary Tumor Location

- The location where the fallopian tube tumor started — medial (toward the uterus end) or lateral (toward the open end) — has some prognostic significance, because tumors that arise in the fimbria (open end) can shed cells directly into the peritoneum without extending through the wall of the fallopian tube.
- In order from medial to lateral, the sections are: interstitial, isthmus, ampulla, infundibulum, fimbria. There is a nice drawing of the five sections of the fallopian tube in the CS Coding Instructions Part I Section 2 for this site-specific factor. Code the appropriate anatomic section as identified in the pathology report or elsewhere in the medical record.
- Use code 060 if the tumor is identified as not in the fimbria, but the location is not more specific.
  Use code 999 if the tumor is only identified as arising in the fallopian tube (not otherwise specified).

SSF4 — Number of Positive Pelvic Nodes
SSF5 — Number of Examined Pelvic Nodes

- This pair of site-specific factors documents the number of pelvic lymph nodes removed and examined by the pathologist (SSF4) and the number of pelvic lymph nodes found to be positive (SSF3). Refer to Figure 3 for a diagram of pelvic lymph nodes.
- The code structures and definitions for these two fields are the same as for Regional Nodes Positive (SSF3) and Regional Nodes Examined (SSF4), but the counts are only for pelvic lymph nodes. Refer to the CS Coding Instructions Part I Section 1 for coding instructions.

SSF6 — Number of Positive Para-aortic Nodes
SSF7 — Number of Examined Para-aortic Nodes

- This pair of site-specific factors documents the number of para-aortic lymph nodes removed and examined by the pathologist (SSF7) and the number of para-aortic lymph nodes found to be positive (SSF6). Refer to Figure 3 for a diagram of para-aortic lymph nodes.
- The code structures and definitions for these two fields are the same as for Regional Nodes Positive (SSF6) and Regional Nodes Examined (SSF7), but the counts are only for pelvic lymph nodes. Refer to the CS Coding Instructions Part I Section 1 for coding instructions.

COLLABORATIVE STAGE DATA COLLECTION SYSTEM (CS) PLACENTA

- CS for placenta is somewhat different from other primary sites in a couple of ways: coding of lymph nodes and the prognostic scoring index. There are two site-specific factors.
- This CS schema applies only to trophoblastic tumors that develop after a pregnancy. If a trophoblastic tumor arises in a site other than placenta, such as the ovary, code it with the schema of the appropriate primary site.
- Any extension to genital structures is coded in CS Extension, not CS Mets at Dx.
- In CS Extension, use a code corresponding to a FIGO stage when the stated FIGO stage is the only information available. More detailed extension codes should be used when specific information is documented in the medical record.
- Because there are no lymph nodes to drain placental tumors, all lymph node fields are coded as not applicable.

SSF1 — Prognostic Scoring Index

- Although there is FIGO staging and corresponding TNM chapter for gestational trophoblastic tumors, the stage groups are substaged based largely on a prognostic scoring index which is coded in Site-Specific Factor 1. The registrar may determine the prognostic score if the clinician has not recorded it in the medical record.
- Sum the risk factor "points" and code SSF1 as low risk (score of 6 or less, code 010), high risk (score of 7 or more, code 110), or unknown.
- The notes on SSF1 are hard to read, so the information is laid out as Table 2.

TABLE 2. PLACENTA PROGNOSTIC SCORING INDEX

	SCORE			
RISK FACTOR	**0**	**1**	**2**	**4**
Age	< 40	40+	---	---
Antecedent pregnancy	Hydatidiform mole	Abortion	Term pregnancy	---
Months from index pregnancy	< 4	4 to < 7	7 – 12	> 12
Pretreatment HCG	$< 10^3$ < 1000	$\geq 10^3 - < 10^4$ 1000 – < 10,000	$\geq 10^4 - < 10^5$ 10,000 – < 100,000	$\geq 10^5$ ≥ 100,000
Largest tumor size incl. uterus	< 3	3 to < 5	5 or more	---
Sites of mets	Lung only	Spleen, kidney	GI tract	Liver, brain
Number of mets	0	1 – 4	5 – 8	> 8
Previous failed chemotherapy	---	---	Single drug	2 or more drugs

SSF2 — FIGO Stage

- Refer to SSF2, FIGO Stage, under CS for Ovary and the discussion of FIGO at the end of this chapter.

OTHER STAGING SYSTEMS

AJCC (TNM)

Staging of ovarian cancer in the TNM system requires surgical evaluation; thus according to the AJCC, ovarian cancer staging is pathologic rather than clinical. Complete assessment of stage will include laparoscopy or laparotomy, histopathologic diagnosis, resection of the ovarian mass and hysterectomy, and multiple staging biopsies, including omentum, mesentery, pelvic and retroperitoneal nodes, peritoneal surfaces, diaphragm, and any other suspected metastases such as liver. A sample of ascites or pelvic and abdominal washings should be sent for cytologic examination. Extra-abdominal disease should be documented by cytology or histologic study.

The TNM system for ovarian cancer is based on a system developed by the Federation Internationale de Gynecologie et d'Obstetrique (FIGO). The T categories in TNM correspond to the Roman numeral stage categories in the FIGO system, for example, T1a corresponds to FIGO Stage IA and T2b corresponds to FIGO Stage IIB. N1 is FIGO Stage IIIC and M1 is FIGO Stage IV. There were no changes in ovarian staging between the sixth and seventh editions of the *AJCC Cancer Staging Manual.*

Criteria for TNM Pathologic Staging

- Diagnostic studies to document distant metastases, including radiography of the chest and abdomen; CT scans of the abdomen, pelvis, chest or head; MRI studies of the abdomen, pelvis, chest or head; PET scans; bone scans; liver studies; laboratory tests
- Careful examination of the pelvis and peritoneum during laparotomy
- Resection of ovarian mass(es)
- Hysterectomy
- Removal or biopsy and microscopic examination of any suspicious sites, in particular:
  - omentum
  - mesentery
  - diaphragm
  - pelvic and para-aortic lymph nodes (at least 10)
  - liver
- Cytologic examination of ascites or peritoneal/pelvic washings
- Cytologic examination of pleural effusion, as indicated

Criteria for TNM Clinical Staging

The FIGO staging scheme on which TNM for ovary is based has no provisions for clinical staging. It is used only for patients in poor medical condition who cannot undergo surgical staging.

TNM SITE-SPECIFIC STAGING GUIDELINES—OVARY

- According to the *AJCC Cancer Staging Manual,* seventh edition, TNM staging for ovary can be used for benign and borderline (low malignant potential) epithelial tumors of the ovary, sex-cord stromal tumors, and germ cell tumors. However, these cell types and behaviors must be analyzed separately from the ovarian epithelial malignancies that are the primary focus of the TNM ovarian staging chapter.
- Complete only one abstract when the diagnosis is simultaneous bilateral epithelial ovarian carcinoma. Simultaneous is defined as within sixty days. Bilateral involvement differentiates Stage I cases: Stage IA (one ovary) and T1b/Stage IB (both ovaries involved). Single or bilateral involvement is not a factor in higher stages.
- If both ovaries are involved with the same cell type, it is important to determine whether they are independent primaries (simultaneous bilateral) or tumor from one ovary has metastasized

AJCC (TNM), *continued*

to the other ovary. Bilateral involvement is Stage I, an ovarian primary with metastases to the other ovary is at least Stage II. The pathologist should be able to make this determination.

- T2/Stage II and T3/Stage III disease include both direct extension of the primary ovarian carcinoma to other structures in the pelvis or abdomen, respectively, as well as implantation metastases (seeding)–discontinuous tumor on the surface of pelvic or abdominal organs. Ovary and endometrium are the only sites where tumor seeding is included in the T category.
- FIGO Stage III/TNM Stage Group III is comprised of information from the tumor (T) and lymph node (N) categories. When no lymph nodes are removed or when lymph nodes are not mentioned in the operative report, the case can still be stage grouped IIIA, IIIB or IIIC based on other evidence of involvement in the abdomen.
- The size of tumor seeding or nodules in the abdomen is determined prior to any debulking procedure. Measurement is the horizontal diameter, not the thickness of the nodule. If tumor is identified only microscopically, the classification is T3a/Stage IIIA. Macroscopically identified tumors 2 cm or less in size are T3b/Stage IIIB, and tumors more than 2 cm in size are T3c/Stage IIIC. Macroscopic tumor identified by the surgeon must be confirmed by the pathologist.
- T3a, T3b and T3c and their corresponding stage groups are based on the largest size of any metastatic deposit in the abdominal cavity prior to any debulking or cytoreductive surgery. If the surgeon observes and reports a 3 cm tumor nodule, the case is classified as T3c/Stage IIIC regardless of whether the biopsied tissue was smaller in size.
- For ovarian cancer, a pelvic lymph node dissection usually removes at least 10 regional lymph nodes, but there will be occasions when the number or presence of involved nodes cannot be determined because of extensive pelvic and/or abdominal metastases.
- For correct classification of liver involvement, it is important to determine whether the tumor is on the surface of the liver or in the parenchyma of the liver, as this makes a difference between T-category and M-category involvement. Tumor on the surface or capsule of the liver is classified as T3. Tumor on the inside of the liver is a hematogenous metastasis, having arrived through the blood stream, and is classified as M1 (Stage IV). Parenchymal metastases can be identified during laparotomy by palpating the liver or can be seen on imaging (CT scan).
- Abdominal ascites must be cytologically proven as malignant to increment a stage I, II or III to IC, IIC, or IIIC, respectively. If pleural effusion (excess fluid in the pleural space in the chest) is diagnosed, it too must be cytologically proven, and if so, the case is classified M1/ Stage IV.

FALLOPIAN TUBE

The TNM categories and stage groups for fallopian tube are very similar to those of ovarian cancer and parallel the structure of the FIGO staging system (see below under FIGO).

PLACENTA (Gestational Trophoblastic Tumor)

The TNM categories parallel the FIGO staging system (see below under FIGO).

FIGO STAGING

FIGO is the French acronym for Federation Internationale de Gynecologie et d'Obstetrique, which in English is the International Federation of Gynecology and Obstetrics. The first staging system ever developed for any site was for cervical cancer. Originally published as the League of Nations staging system in the 1929, responsibility for cervical and other gynecologic staging was assumed by FIGO in 1954. FIGO staging of ovarian cancer was most recently modified in 1988.

The principles of FIGO staging have been adapted to the TNM format and incorporated into both AJCC/UICC staging and Collaborative Staging (Tables 3–5). In contrast to TNM, FIGO staging uses Roman numerals and subscripts for its stages—no T, N, or M. The following stages are divided into substages based on certain prognostic criteria within the stage, such as size of lesion or specific organs involved.

Stage 0	In situ carcinoma
Stage I	Similar to localized: confined to organ of origin
Stage II	Extension locally beyond site of origin to involve adjacent organs or structures in the pelvis
Stage III	More extensive involvement, including regional lymph nodes
Stage IV	Metastatic (discontinuous or hematogenous) disease

Table 3. Comparison of FIGO, TNM and CS Extension for Ovarian Cancer Staging

AJCC	FIGO	Definition	CS Extension code(s)
TX		In situ [no longer recognized by TNM or FIGO]	999
T1	I	Confined to one or both ovaries	460
T1a	IA	One ovary, capsule intact, no tumor on ovarian surface	100, 150
T1b	IB	Both ovaries, capsules intact, no tumor on ovarian surfaces	200, 250
T1c	IC	One or both ovaries, capsule ruptured OR tumor on ovarian surface AND/OR malignant ascites or peritoneal washings	350, 360, 410, 430, 440, 450
T2	II	Pelvic extension or implants	660
T2a	IIA	Extension/implants on uterus or tubes	500, 510, 520, 550
T2b	IIB	Extension/implants on other pelvic tissues	600, 605, 610, 615
T2c	IIC	Pelvic extension/implants with malignant ascites or peritoneal washings	620, 625, 650, 640, 645
T3	III	Microscopically confirmed peritoneal mets outside pelvis	730, 750, 780, 800
T3a	IIIA	Microscopic tumor only	700
T3b	IIIB	Macroscopic tumor $\leq$ 2 cm	710
T3c	IIIC	Macroscopic tumor > 2 cm	720
N1	IIIC	Regional lymph node metastasis **CS Lymph Nodes**	100, 120, 200, 300, 400, 440, 500, 510, 800
M1	IV	Distant metastasis **CS Mets at Dx**	10, 40, 50, 65, 70

FIGO Staging, *continued*

Table 4. Comparison of FIGO, TNM and CS Extension for Fallopian Tube Cancer Staging

AJCC	FIGO	Definition	CS Extension code(s)
Tis	0	In situ	000
T1	I	Confined to one or both fallopian tubes	200, 320
T1a	IA	One tube; no penetration of serosal surface	110
T1b	IB	Both tubes; no penetration of serosal surface	120
T1c	IC	One or both tubes with extension onto or through tubal serosa OR malignant ascites or peritoneal washings	130
T2	II	Pelvic extension or implants	655, 670
T2a	IIA	Extension/implants on uterus or ovaries	400, 450, 460
T2b	IIB	Extension/implants on other pelvic tissues	510, 620, 652, 658
T2c	IIC	Pelvic extension/implants with malignant ascites or peritoneal washings	660
T3	III	Microscopically confirmed peritoneal mets outside pelvis	790, 795, 810, 820
T3a	IIIA	Microscopic tumor only	685, 688, 695, 698
T3b	IIIB	Macroscopic tumor ≤ 2 cm	722, 723, 725, 728
T3c	IIIC	Macroscopic tumor > 2 cm	732, 733, 735, 740
N1	IIIC	Regional lymph node metastasis	**CS Lymph Nodes** 100, 120, 200, 220, 300, 500, 550, 800
M1	IV	Distant metastasis	**CS Mets at Dx** 05, 10, 20, 40, 45, 50, 55, 60

PLACENTAL TUMOR STAGING

The US Trophoblastic Disease Centers have developed a clinical staging system based on the following criteria:

- Duration of disease
- Presence of liver or brain metastases
- HCG titer level
- Treatment with chemotherapy
- Occurrence after a full-term pregnancy

Cases are grouped into nonmetastatic and metastatic, which is further subdivided into low risk and high risk.

- Nonmetastatic: tumor confined to the uterus
- Metastatic, good prognosis: last pregnancy less than 4 months prior; HCG titer low; no liver or brain metastases; no prior chemotherapy
- Metastatic, poor prognosis: last pregnancy more than 4 months prior; high HCG titer; liver or brain metastases; prior chemotherapy; occurrence after a full-term pregnancy

A second system proposed by the World Health Organization is a scoring system that determines low-, medium- and high-risk patients, based on such factors as age, previous pregnancy, HCG titer, blood group, size of tumor, metastatic sites, number of metastases, interval between end of previous pregnancy and start of chemotherapy, and history of chemotherapy. The scoring system is similar to that shown in Site-Specific Factor 1 above, with the addition of the HCG titer and blood group as shown below. The scores are grouped into low risk (up to 4), intermediate risk (5–7), and high risk (8 or more).

Placental Tumor Staging, ***continued***

RISK FACTOR	SCORE 0	1	2	4
HCG (IU/L)	≤ 10^3	> 10^3–10^4	> 10^4–10^5	> 10^5
ABO blood groups Female x male		O x A	O x B	

Table 4. Comparison of FIGO, TNM and CS Extension for Placental Tumors (Gestational Trophoblastic Tumors)

AJCC	FIGO	Definition	CS Extension code(s)
T1	I	Confined to uterus	100, 300, 350
	IA	Confined to uterus, low risk	330
	IB	Confined to uterus, high risk	340
T2	II	Extension to or implants on other genital structures	400, 620, 720, 800, 850
	IIA	Genital structures, low risk	810
	IIB	Genital structures, high risk	820
			CS Mets at Dx code(s)
M1		Distant metastasis	84, 85
M1a	III	Lung metastasis	10, 15
M1a	IIIA	Lung metastasis, low risk	12
M1a	IIIA	Lung metastasis, high risk	13
M1b	IV	All other distant metastases	20, 30, 33, 35, 37, 51, 52 55, 60, 70, 80, 81, 83

SUMMARY STAGE

The *SEER Summary Staging Manual 2000* closely parallels the content of the FIGO and TNM staging systems for ovary and fallopian tube.

- Stage I and its substages correspond to localized disease.
- Stage II and its substages correspond to regional direct extension.
- Stage III and IV and their substages correspond to distant metastases.

- Malignant ascites and positive peritoneal washings are defined as distant in Summary Stage 2000. However, since "cancer cells in ascites or in peritoneal washings" was not specifically categorized in the 1977 Summary Staging Guide, it is unclear to which stage previous cases may have been coded.

For placenta, tumor confined to the placenta is localized, tumor involving adjacent structures or other genital structures is regional direct extension, involved regional lymph nodes are coded as regional to lymph nodes, and all other tumor involvement is distant metastases.

EPIDEMIOLOGY AND ETIOLOGY

OVARY

- Ovarian cancer is the sixth most common cancer in women worldwide.
- Ovarian cancer is more common in industrialized countries and less common in underdeveloped countries.
- However, ovarian cancer is the fourth leading cause of cancer deaths in women and the most lethal of the female genital system cancers.
- In the United States, the lifetime risk of developing ovarian cancer is roughly 1 in 58 (1.7%)
- The incidence rate for ovarian cancer is rising.
- The ovarian cancer mortality rate is declining, thanks to more effective chemotherapy agents.
- Approximately 75% of ovarian cancers are diagnosed at advanced stage.
- Caucasian women have the highest incidence of ovarian cancer, followed by African-American, Hawaiian, and Alaska native women.

Risk Factors

- Family history of ovarian cancer (mother, sister or daughter)
- Presence of BRCA1 or BRCA2 gene
- Age > 50
- Nulliparity (no pregnancies)
- Never used birth control pills
- Personal history of breast, endometrial or colon cancer

Prognostic Factors

- Stage at diagnosis (FIGO or TNM)
- Volume of residual tumor after surgery/debulking

FALLOPIAN TUBE

- Fallopian tube cancer is rare—about 1% of all female genital organ cancers.
- Staging, spread of disease, treatment, and prognosis are similar to ovarian cancer.

Risk Factors

- Most commonly diagnosed between ages 50–60
- Presence of BRCA1 gene
- Family history of fallopian tube cancer
- Some association with chronic infection and/or inflammation of the tubes (due to untreated sexually transmitted diseases, for example), but this link has not been definitively proven.

Prognostic Factors—Fallopian Tube

- Similar to those for ovarian cancer

PLACENTA

- Hydatidiform mole (9100/0) occurs in about 1 in 1000 pregnancies. About 2–4% of hydatidiform moles progress to become choriocarcinoma (9100/3). Choriocarcinoma can also develop without a pre-existing hydatidiform mole.

Epidemiology and Etiology, *continued*

Risk Factors

- Age < 20 or > 40 at start of pregnancy
- Previous molar pregnancy
- Low levels of carotene and vitamin A may be associated with higher risk of molar pregnancy.
- Lower socioeconomic status
- Blood type of each parent. For example, risk is increased if the woman has blood type A and the man has blood type O.

Prognostic Factors

- The prognostic factors for gestational trophoblastic tumors are discussed in the Collaborative Staging section on placental tumors in the Prognostic Scoring Index.

Abstracting, Staging, and Coding Exercises

This section includes twelve brief ovarian, fallopian tube, and placenta cancer cases to be coded in ICD-O-3, Summary Stage 2000, TNM seventh Edition (clinical and pathologic), and CS version 0203.

NOTE: For the purposes of these brief cases, assume that all other tests not mentioned in the case are negative for malignancy.

- Identify the primary site and schema.
- Assign the codes for primary site, histology, behavior, and grade.
- Assign codes to all applicable CS fields.
- Assume that your facility does offer a test and that the standards setters for your facility require the data field. In other words, avoid using code 988 (not applicable).
- 20XX is the diagnosis year, and where applicable, 20YY is the following year.

CASE 1

HISTORY AND PHYSICAL EXAMINATION

Patient saw primary care physician for vague symptoms of bloating and gastrointestinal distress.

Pelvic exam: Uterus appears to be contiguous with bilateral masses and some induration is present.

Abd: Palpable mass in midline extending to 2 in. above umbilicus.

X-RAYS AND SCANS

4-27-20XX Ultrasound of abdomen: Involvement of both ovaries with large multicystic masses extending superiorly to umbilicus, at least 2 inches in size. Semicystic and semisolid tumors highly suggestive of ovarian cancer.

4-27-20XX CXR: Negative.

LABORATORY REPORTS

Chemistry screening panel: Within normal limits.

CA-125: 97 (normal 0 - 35 ng/ml)

ENDOSCOPIC PROCEDURES None.

OPERATIVE REPORTS

4-30-20XX TAH-BSO: R and L ovaries multicystic and enlarged. Multiple tumor implants visible in right and left pelvic sidewall. No other evidence of extra-ovarian metastasis. All visible tumor removed.

PATHOLOGY REPORTS

4-30-20XX R and L ovary: Clear cell adenocarcinoma, grade iii, and oviduct. Left and right common iliac lymph nodes and periaortic lymph nodes: metastatic carcinoma. Fibrous and fibrofatty tissue, connective tissue (cul-de-sac and pericolic gutter): Metastatic adenocarcinoma. Left ovary 7 cm; right ovary 7.8 cm.

TREATMENT

4-30-20XX Total abdominal hysterectomy, bilateral salpingo-oophorectomy, bilateral pelvic and periaortic lymphadenectomy; omentectomy; debulking

Site Code ___ ___ ___.___	**Mult Tum Reported as One Prim** ___ ___	**CS Mets at Dx** ___ ___
Histology/Behavior/Grade ___ ___ ___ ___ / ___ ___	**Summary Stage 2000** ____	**CS Mets at Dx - Bone** ___ **Brain** ___ **Liver** ___ **Lung** ___
Grade Path Value ___	**cT** ___ **cN** ___ **cM** ___	**CS Mets Eval** ___
Grade Path System ___	**Clin Stage Group** ____	**SSF1 CA-125** ___ ___ ___
Lymph Vascular Invasion ___	**pT** ___ **pN** ___ **M** ___	**SSF2 FIGO Stage** ___ ___ ___
Ambiguous Terminol ___	**Path Stage Group** ____	**SSF3 Resid Tum Stat/Size after Cytoreduction** ___ ___ ___
Date Conclusive Terminol ___ ___ ___ ___ ___ ___ ___ ___	**CS Tumor Size** ___ ___ ___	**SSF4 Tum Location after Cytoreduction** ___ ___ ___
Date Conclus Dx Flag ___ ___	**CS Extension** ___ ___ ___	**SSF5 Malig Ascites** ___ ___ ___
Multiplicity Counter ___ ___	**CS TS/Ext Eval** ___	
Date Mult Tumors ___ ___ ___ ___ ___ ___ ___ ___	**CS LN** ___ ___ ___	
Date Mult Tumors Flag ___ ___	**CS Reg Nodes Eval** ___	
	Reg LN Pos ___ ___	
	Reg LN Exam ___ ___	

CASE 2

HISTORY AND PHYSICAL EXAMINATION

Patient noticed that jeans no longer fit, but patient had not gained any weight.

Physical exam: Abdomen soft, distended inferiorly by a palpable mass which extended to 2 fingerbreadths below umbilicus. No other masses; no hepatosplenomegaly. Pelvic deferred.

X-RAYS AND SCANS

9-21-20XX US abd/pelvis: Large Rt adnexal mass with cystic and solid components measuring 14 cm. Smaller 4.5 cm left adnexal mass. Uterus with fibroids; no free fluid; no hydronephrosis.

9-21-20XX CT pelvis: Uterus anteriorly displaced by bilateral large cystic and solid masses. Right mass 10 cm; left ovary 4 cm. No ascites or implants in pelvis. No evidence of retroperitoneal lymphadenopathy.

LABORATORY REPORTS None remarkable.

ENDOSCOPIC PROCEDURES None.

OPERATIVE REPORTS

9-27-20XX TAH-BSO: No gross ascites. Small amount of fluid in pelvis removed for cytology. Upper abdomen negative for metastatic disease. Large cystic mass in pelvis stuck behind uterus. Uterus small and normal. Mass appeared to be coming off right ovary. Multiple biopsies taken along with surgical resection.

PATHOLOGY REPORTS

9-27-20XX Cervix, endometrium, myometrium all WNL. Bilateral fallopian tubes: Negative. Bilateral ovaries both containing 40% endometrioid carcinoma, 35% mucinous adenocarcinoma, 15% transitional carcinoma, and 10% serous carcinoma. 8 left pelvic, 7 right pelvic, 3 periaortic lymph nodes: negative. Sigmoid implant: No malignancy. Omentum, bilateral pelvic gutters: No malignancy. Pelvic fluid: Abnormal clusters of epithelial cells with positive cytology similar to concurrent surgical specimen. FNA diaphragm: Benign.

TREATMENT

9-27-20XX TAH-BSO; adhesiolysis, omentectomy, appendectomy, bilateral pelvic and periaortic LN sampling

Site Code ___ ___ ___.___

Histology/Behavior/Grade ___ ___ ___ ___ / ___ ___

Grade Path Value ___

Grade Path System ___

Lymph Vascular Invasion ___

Ambiguous Terminol ___

Date Conclusive Terminol ___ ___ ___ ___ ___ ___ ___ ___

Date Conclus Dx Flag ___ ___

Multiplicity Counter ___ ___

Date Mult Tumors ___ ___ ___ ___ ___ ___ ___ ___

Date Mult Tumors Flag ___ ___

Mult Tum Reported as One Prim ___ ___

Summary Stage 2000 ___

cT ___ cN ___ cM ___

Clin Stage Group ___

pT ___ pN ___ M ___

Path Stage Group ___

CS Tumor Size ___ ___ ___

CS Extension ___ ___ ___

CS TS/Ext Eval ___

CS LN ___ ___ ___

CS Reg Nodes Eval ___

Reg LN Pos ___ ___

Reg LN Exam ___ ___

CS Mets at Dx ___ ___

CS Mets at Dx - Bone ___ Brain ___ Liver ___ Lung ___

CS Mets Eval ___

Ovary

Case 2, continued

SSF1 CA-125 ___ ___ ___	**SSF4 Tum Location after Cytoreduction** ___ ___ ___	
SSF2 FIGO Stage ___ ___ ___	**SSF5 Malig Ascites** ___ ___ ___	
SSF3 Resid Tum Stat/Size after Cytoreduction ___ ___ ___		

CASE 3

HISTORY AND PHYSICAL EXAM

64 year old female G1 P1 complaining of GI symptoms for one year. Recent Pap smear abnormal showing cells suspicious for adenocarcinoma.

10-10-20XX Physical exam: Completely normal. Chest and abdomen: No masses. Pelvis: No organomegaly. Speculum exam: No lesions visualized.

X-RAYS AND SCANS

10-10-20XX CT abdomen and pelvis: Retroperitoneal adenopathy, right iliac adenopathy, tiny low density liver lesions. Small amount of free pelvic fluid.

10-15-20XX PET Scan: Small, equivocally enlarged lymph nodes in the left supraclavicular region. Widespread retroperitoneal, pelvic and periaortic lymphadenopathy measuring 2.8 x 2.1 cm above pelvic brim.

LABORATORY REPORTS None.

ENDOSCOPIC PROCEDURES

12-17-20XX Cystoscopy: No abnormalities within bladder.

12-17-20XX Laparoscopy: White mass on end of R fallopian tube. R ovary, L tube, L ovary, and uterus: WNL. No other significant findings in pelvis or abdomen, but shaggy yellow exudative process seen throughout peritoneal surfaces of abdominal cavity.

OPERATIVE REPORTS

1-9-20YY TAH-BSO: Diaphragm, liver, upper abdominal structures, small and large intestines all within normal limits. Massive adenopathy within right retroperitoneal space and extending along the entire periaortic chain. Procedure terminated at this point due to extensive disease.

PATHOLOGY REPORTS

11-5-20XX CT guided FNA right pelvic lymph node: Metastatic moderately differentiated adenocarcinoma.

12-17-20XX Conization: Metastatic adenocarcinoma of unknown origin. Biopsy, R fallopian tube mass: poorly differentiated serous carcinoma involving fimbriated end.

1-9-20YY Cytology: Four separate washings: pelvic, right gutter, left gutter, diaphragm: No malignant cells

1-9-20YY TAH-BSO: No malignancy found in right pelvic sidewall, cervix, corpus, bilateral fallopian tubes and ovaries, gallbladder, umbilical region, sigmoid colon serosa or omentum. Right side lymph nodes: Metastatic high grade carcinoma in 1 of 2 nodes. Comment: The lymph node metastasis is similar to previous right fallopian tube resection (12/17) and consistent with poorly differentiated serous carcinoma of fallopian tube origin. Tumor extends into perinodal soft tissue where there is vascular/lymphatic invasion.

continued on next page

Case 3, continued

TREATMENT

12-17-20XX D&C, cervical conization, diagnostic cystoscopy, and diagnostic laparoscopy with right salpingectomy
1-11-20YY TAH and completion BSO, total infracolic omentectomy, right-sided pelvic node dissection, washings.

To start chemotherapy as outpatient at GYN oncologist office.

Site Code ___ ___ ___.___	Summary Stage 2000 _____	CS Mets at Dx - Bone ___ Brain ___ Liver ___ Lung ___
Histology/Behavior/Grade ___ ___ ___ ___ / ___ ___	cT ___ cN ___ cM ___	CS Mets Eval ___
Grade Path Value ___	Clin Stage Group _____	SSF1 FIGO Stage ___ ___ ___
Grade Path System ___	pT ___ pN ___ M ___	SSF2 Biopsy Metastatic Site ___ ___ ___
Lymph Vascular Invasion ___	Path Stage Group _____	SSF3 Primary Tumor Location ___ ___ ___
Ambiguous Terminol ___	CS Tumor Size ___ ___ ___	SSF4 # Positive Pelvic Nodes ___ ___ ___
Date Conclusive Terminol ___ ___ ___ ___ ___ ___ ___ ___	CS Extension ___ ___ ___	SSF5 # Examined Pelvic Nodes ___ ___ ___
Date Conclus Dx Flag ___ ___	CS TS/Ext Eval ___	SSF6 # Positive Para-aortic Nodes ___ ___ ___
Multiplicity Counter ___ ___	CS LN ___ ___ ___	SSF7 # Examined Para-aortic Nodes ___ ___ ___
Date Mult Tumors ___ ___ ___ ___ ___ ___ ___ ___	CS Reg Nodes Eval ___	
Date Mult Tumors Flag ___ ___	Reg LN Pos ___ ___	
Mult Tum Reported as One Prim ___ ___	Reg LN Exam ___ ___	
	CS Mets at Dx ___ ___	

CASE 4

HISTORY AND PHYSICAL EXAMINATION

Patient teased by family about being "pregnant".
Large pelvic mass to umbilicus. No other significant findings on PE.

X-RAYS AND SCANS

3-3-20XX CT pelvis: 13.5 x 14 cm solid soft tissue mass contiguous with uterus. Appears benign but cannot rule out malignancy. No lymphadenopathy, liver metastases, peritoneal implants or ascites.
3-3-20XX CXR: WNL.

LABORATORY REPORTS

3-3-20XX CBC and platelets: Normal.
3-3-20XX CA-125: 17 (normal 0-35 ng/ml)

ENDOSCOPIC PROCEDURES None.

OPERATIVE REPORTS

3-15-20XX TAH-BSO: 200 cc. of fluid aspirated from cul-de-sac. Bilateral large adnexal tumors (8-9 cm). Palpation of periaortic nodes revealed a prominent node that was removed. All gross evidence of tumor removed.

continued on next page

Case 4, continued

PATHOLOGY REPORTS

3-15-20XX Bilateral ovaries: Adenocarcinoma, endometrioid type, grade iii, with focal clear cell changes. Tubes: Negative. Uterus and cervix: negative. Omentum: Negative. 25 pelvic lymph nodes negative. Cul de sac cytology: Negative. Periaortic node: Negative.

TREATMENT

3-15-20XX TAH-BSO, omentectomy, LN dissection

FIGO Stage IB. Referred to medical oncologist for multi-agent chemotherapy post-operatively.

Site Code ___ ___ ___.___	Mult Tum Reported as One Prim ___ ___	CS Mets at Dx ___ ___
Histology/Behavior/Grade ___ ___ ___ ___ / ___ ___	Summary Stage 2000 _____	CS Mets at Dx - Bone ___ Brain ___ Liver ___ Lung ___
Grade Path Value ___	cT ___ cN ___ cM ___	CS Mets Eval ___
Grade Path System ___	Clin Stage Group _____	SSF1 CA-125 ___ ___ ___
Lymph Vascular Invasion ___	pT ___ pN ___ M ___	SSF2 FIGO Stage ___ ___ ___
Ambiguous Terminol ___	Path Stage Group _____	SSF3 Resid Tum Stat/Size after Cytoreduction ___ ___ ___
Date Conclusive Terminol ___ ___ ___ ___ ___ ___ ___ ___	CS Tumor Size ___ ___ ___	SSF4 Tum Location after Cytoreduction ___ ___ ___
Date Conclus Dx Flag ___ ___	CS Extension ___ ___ ___	SSF5 Malig Ascites ___ ___ ___
Multiplicity Counter ___ ___	CS TS/Ext Eval ___	
Date Mult Tumors ___ ___ ___ ___ ___ ___ ___ ___	CS LN ___ ___ ___	
Date Mult Tumors Flag ___ ___	CS Reg Nodes Eval ___	
	Reg LN Pos ___ ___	
	Reg LN Exam ___ ___	

CASE 5

HISTORY AND PHYSICAL EXAM

She had two months of nausea, intermittent abdominal pain, and a fifteen to twenty-pound weight loss.

Physical exam: Right ovarian adnexal mass. Review of systems otherwise normal.

X-RAYS AND SCANS

4-13-20XX Sonogram: Right ovarian adnexal mass with surrounding fluid approximately 6 x 3.9 x 1.8 cm with omental caking and ascites.

LABORATORY REPORTS

4-13-20XX CA-125: 3,226 (normal 0-35 ng/ml)

ENDOSCOPIC PROCEDURES None.

OPERATIVE REPORTS

4-22-20XX Staging laparotomy: Extensive intraperitoneal and retroperitoneal carcinoma arising from the tubes and ovaries. Nodular disease on both leaves of the diaphragm. Surface of the liver uninvolved. Greater omentum distorted with a nodular tumor measuring approximately 4 cm by 10 cm with extension into the hilum of the spleen. Both ovaries involved with carcinoma as well as agglutination of the sigmoid in the pelvis.

continued on next page

Case 5, continued

Tumor involved root of mesentery on right side distorting the distal ileum without evidence of obstruction.

PATHOLOGY REPORTS

4-22-20XX Peritoneal cell washings: Metastatic carcinoma, consistent with ovarian primary.

1) Gallbladder and contents, cholecystectomy: Chronic cholecystitis and cholelithiasis.
2) Left tube and ovary: Poorly differentiated mucin-producing adenocarcinoma (3.5 cm). No lymphovascular invasion present. Fallopian tube negative for metastatic carcinoma.
3) Right tube and ovary: Poorly differentiated mucin-producing adenocarcinoma (4 cm). No lymphovascular invasion present. Fallopian tube with focal metastatic mucin-producing tumor.

TREATMENT

4-22-20XX Staging of ovarian malignancy with exploratory laparotomy, bilateral salpingo-oophorectomy, and open cholecystectomy

5-9-20XX Started Taxol and Carboplatin

Site Code ___ ___ ___.___	Mult Tum Reported as One Prim ___ ___	CS Mets at Dx ___ ___
Histology/Behavior/Grade ___ ___ ___ ___/___ ___	Summary Stage 2000 ___	CS Mets at Dx - Bone ___ Brain ___ Liver ___ Lung ___
Grade Path Value ___	cT ___ cN ___ cM ___	CS Mets Eval ___
Grade Path System ___	Clin Stage Group ___	SSF1 CA-125 ___ ___ ___
Lymph Vascular Invasion ___	pT ___ pN ___ M ___	SSF2 FIGO Stage ___ ___ ___
Ambiguous Terminol ___	Path Stage Group ___	SSF3 Resid Tum Stat/Size after Cytoreduction ___ ___ ___
Date Conclusive Terminol ___ ___ ___ ___ ___ ___ ___ ___	CS Tumor Size ___ ___ ___	SSF4 Tum Location after Cytoreduction ___ ___ ___
Date Conclus Dx Flag ___ ___	CS Extension ___ ___ ___	SSF5 Malig Ascites ___ ___ ___
Multiplicity Counter ___ ___	CS TS/Ext Eval ___	
Date Mult Tumors ___ ___ ___ ___ ___ ___ ___ ___	CS LN ___ ___ ___	
Date Mult Tumors Flag ___ ___	CS Reg Nodes Eval ___	
	Reg LN Pos ___ ___	
	Reg LN Exam ___ ___	

CASE 6

HISTORY AND PHYSICAL EXAMINATION

Recent history of abdominal bloating.

Physical exam: Abdominal pelvic mass that fills the cul-de-sac. Mass is firm, compatible with ovary or uterine malignancy, likely adenocarcinoma of ovary vs. uterine vs. uterine carcinoma/sarcoma.

X-RAYS AND SCANS

9-21-20XX CXR: No evidence of metastases .
Bilateral mammogram: Within normal limits.

LABORATORY REPORTS None.

ENDOSCOPIC PROCEDURES None.

OPERATIVE REPORTS

9-24-20XX Exploratory laparotomy: Abdomen—no evidence of seeding; pelvis—huge cystic mass replacing left ovary. Right ovary and remaining adnexa appear normal. Multiple biopsies taken in pelvis and abdomen for staging purposes.

PATHOLOGY REPORTS

9-24-20XX Left ovary: Invasive w-d mucinous cystadenocarcinoma. 27 mm area of tumor within large cystic mass. Right ovary, bilateral tubes, cervix: negative for tumor. All other biopsies and removed tissues and fluids negative for tumor. Lymph nodes removed (number not stated): all negative. Tumor confined to left ovary (FIGO IA); no tumor on ovarian surface. Endometrium: P-d endometrial adenocarcinoma.

TREATMENT

9-24-20XX Exploratory laparotomy, TAH and BSO, bilateral pelvic-periaortic lymphadenectomy, omentectomy, cul-de-sac biopsy, liver biopsies, diaphragm biopsies, bladder peritoneum biopsy and ascitic fluid for cell block

Site Code ___ ___ ___.___

Histology/Behavior/Grade ___ ___ ___ ___ / ___ ___

Grade Path Value ___

Grade Path System ___

Lymph Vascular Invasion ___

Ambiguous Terminol ___

Date Conclusive Terminol ___ ___ ___ ___ ___ ___ ___ ___

Date Conclus Dx Flag ___ ___

Multiplicity Counter ___ ___

Date Mult Tumors ___ ___ ___ ___ ___ ___ ___ ___

Date Mult Tumors Flag ___ ___

Mult Tum Reported as One Prim ___ ___

Summary Stage 2000 ___

cT ___ **cN** ___ **cM** ___

Clin Stage Group ___

pT ___ **pN** ___ **M** ___

Path Stage Group ___

CS Tumor Size ___ ___ ___

CS Extension ___ ___ ___

CS TS/Ext Eval ___

CS LN ___ ___ ___

CS Reg Nodes Eval ___

Reg LN Pos ___ ___

Reg LN Exam ___ ___

CS Mets at Dx ___ ___

CS Mets at Dx - **Bone** ___ **Brain** ___ **Liver** ___ **Lung** ___

CS Mets Eval ___

SSF1 CA-125 ___ ___ ___

SSF2 FIGO Stage ___ ___ ___

SSF3 Resid Tum Stat/Size after Cytoreduction ___ ___ ___

SSF4 Tum Location after Cytoreduction ___ ___ ___

SSF5 Malig Ascites ___ ___ ___

CASE 7

HISTORY AND PHYSICAL EXAM

38 year-old female, nulligravida, with pelvic pain for two months and heavy menstrual period.

7-7-20XX Physical exam: Uterine fibroids and a right adnexal mass extending in midline and over to right lower quadrant. Pelvic exam: Normal external genitalia. Uterus deviated to left due to right adnexal mass and enlarged to about 10 weeks size. Partially mobile right adnexal mass. Tender uterosacral ligaments.

X-RAYS AND SCANS

7-12-20XX Hysterosalpingogram: Large, right sided pelvic mass causing right fallopian tube to be extremely attenuated. Both tubes appeared patent. No intrauterine filling defects, but there appears to be an additional uterine mass consistent with uterine fibroid.

7-12-20XX Pelvic ultrasound: Confirms uterine fibroid 7 cm in greatest dimension. Also separate pelvic mass 7 cm in greatest dimension.

LABORATORY REPORTS

7-20-20XX CA-125: 14 (normal 0-35 ng/ml); consistent with benign process.

ENDOSCOPIC PROCEDURES None.

OPERATIVE REPORTS

8-6-20XX Laparoscopy: Extensive endometriosis and large cystic mass in right adnexa.

8-29-20XX Staging laparotomy: no gross tumor seen; biopsies taken per protocol

PATHOLOGY REPORTS

8-6-20XX Exploratory laparotomy and RSO: Right ovarian cyst: Serous adenocarcinoma, moderately to poorly differentiated (1.5 cm), arising in a borderline serous cystadenoma (6 cm). Tumor is limited to capsule; no tumor on ovarian surface. No lymphovascular invasion identified. Peritoneal washings negative.
Nodule right ovarian cyst: Serous adenocarcinoma, moderately to poorly differerentiated (1.0 cm), arising in a borderline serous cystadenoma.

8-29-20XX TAH and LSO: Anterior pelvic cul-de-sac peritoneum biopsy: Focal intralymphatic metastatic carcinoma. Right uterine serosa: Intralymphatic metastatic carcinoma. Right pelvic peritoneum biopsy: Microscopic foci of metastatic carcinoma. 12 lymph nodes negative. Other tissue negative.

TREATMENT

8-6-20XX Diagnostic operative laparoscopy. CO2 laser vaporization of endometriosis and adhesiolysis. Transuterine tubal lavage. Diagnostic hysteroscopy with D and C. Exploratory laparotomy. Multiple myomectomy. Right salpingo-oophorectomy. Peritoneal washings. Pelvic peritoneal biopsy.

8-29-20XX Staging for ovarian malignancy with total abdominal hysterectomy, left salpingo-oophorectomy, omentectomy, multiple intra-peritoneal biopsies, pelvic peritonectomy, retroperitoneal lymph node sampling, and separate procedure of appendectomy

9-17-20XX Intraperitoneal Porta-Cath placement with instillation of Carboplatin and Taxol

Case 7, continued

Site Code ___ ___ ___.___	Mult Tum Reported as One Prim ___ ___	CS Mets at Dx ___ ___
Histology/Behavior/Grade ___ ___ ___ ___ / ___ ___	Summary Stage 2000 _____	CS Mets at Dx - Bone ___ Brain ___ Liver ___ Lung ___
Grade Path Value ___	cT ___ cN ___ cM ___	
Grade Path System ___	Clin Stage Group _____	CS Mets Eval ___
Lymph Vascular Invasion ___	pT ___ pN ___ M ___	SSF1 CA-125 ___ ___ ___
Ambiguous Terminol ___	Path Stage Group _____	SSF2 FIGO Stage ___ ___ ___
Date Conclusive Terminol ___ ___ ___ ___ ___ ___ ___ ___	CS Tumor Size ___ ___ ___	SSF3 Resid Tum Stat/Size after Cytoreduction ___ ___ ___
	CS Extension ___ ___ ___	
Date Conclus Dx Flag ___ ___	CS TS/Ext Eval ___	SSF4 Tum Location after Cytoreduction ___ ___ ___
Multiplicity Counter ___ ___	CS LN ___ ___ ___	
Date Mult Tumors ___ ___ ___ ___ ___ ___ ___ ___	CS Reg Nodes Eval ___	SSF5 Malig Ascites ___ ___ ___
Date Mult Tumors Flag ___ ___	Reg LN Pos ___ ___	
	Reg LN Exam ___ ___	

CASE 8

HISTORY AND PHYSICAL EXAMINATION
Pelvic exam: enlarged uterus noted. No other abnormal findings.

X-RAYS AND SCANS
12-2-20XX Pelvic ultrasound: 9 cm right adnexal mass and 6 cm left adnexal mass. Normal ovaries could not be delineated from these masses.

LABORATORY REPORTS
Chemistry screening panel: Liver enzymes elevated.
CA-125: 722 (normal 0-35 ng/ml)

ENDOSCOPIC PROCEDURES
None.

OPERATIVE REPORTS
12-7-20XX Laparotomy and TAH-BSO: Widespread metastatic tumor seen in pelvis and abdomen and biopsied.

PATHOLOGY REPORTS
12-7-20XX Bilateral ovaries: Invasive poorly-differentiated papillary serous surface carcinoma with extensive studding of colon, uterine serosa, and myometrial and parametrial soft tissues. Metastases to bladder, appendix, omentum. Metastatic deposits on sigmoid colon. Metastases to 32 of 48 pelvic and periaortic lymph nodes.

ADDITIONAL TREATMENT
12-7-20XX Exploratory laparotomy, TAH-BSO. Rectosigmoid colon resection. Bilateral pelvic and periaortic lymphadenectomy. Total omentectomy.

12-29-20XX Patient started on carboplatin and paclitaxel

Case 8, continued

Site Code ___ ___ ___.___

Histology/Behavior/Grade ___ ___ ___ ___/___ ___

Grade Path Value ___

Grade Path System ___

Lymph Vascular Invasion ___

Ambiguous Terminol ___

Date Conclusive Terminol ___ ___ ___ ___ ___ ___ ___ ___

Date Conclus Dx Flag ___ ___

Multiplicity Counter ___ ___

Date Mult Tumors ___ ___ ___ ___ ___ ___ ___ ___

Date Mult Tumors Flag ___ ___

Mult Tum Reported as One Prim ___ ___

Summary Stage 2000 ___

cT ___ cN ___ cM ___

Clin Stage Group ___

pT ___ pN ___ M ___

Path Stage Group ___

CS Tumor Size ___ ___ ___

CS Extension ___ ___ ___

CS TS/Ext Eval ___

CS LN ___ ___ ___

CS Reg Nodes Eval ___

Reg LN Pos ___ ___

Reg LN Exam ___ ___

CS Mets at Dx ___ ___

CS Mets at Dx - Bone ___ Brain ___ Liver ___ Lung ___

CS Mets Eval ___

SSF1 CA-125 ___ ___ ___

SSF2 FIGO Stage ___ ___ ___

SSF3 Resid Tum Stat/Size after Cytoreduction ___ ___ ___

SSF4 Tum Location after Cytoreduction ___ ___ ___

SSF5 Malig Ascites ___ ___ ___

CASE 9

HISTORY AND PHYSICAL EXAM

Patient is 61-year-old female, G1P1, with abdominal carcinomatosis found during admission for bilateral pulmonary embolisms. Recommendations made at that time for the patient to be treated with chemotherapy.

X-RAYS AND SCANS

2-XX-20XX CT Abdomen and pelvis: Uterus poorly defined and enlarged with abnormal appearance. Mixed cystic and solid masses of bilateral adnexa measuring 7.4 x 5.5 cm on right and 5.3 x 7.1 cm on left. Ascites throughout abdomen with soft tissue masses measuring 2.5 x 4.8 cm, along with nodule in omentum.

LABORATORY REPORTS

2-XX-20XX CA-125: 1522 (normal 0-35 ng/ml)

3-31-20XX CA-125: 237 (normal 0-35 ng/ml)

ENDOSCOPIC PROCEDURES None.

OPERATIVE REPORTS

5-4-20XX TAH-BSO: Carcinomatosis; tumor nodules in cul-de-sac, small and large bowel, omentum, paracolic gutter. Two parenchymal liver nodules on right side. Additional tumor on falciform ligament from peritoneal surfaces intra-abdominally. All visible tumor greater than 2 mm removed except for the two masses within the liver which measured approximately 0.5cm in diameter.

PATHOLOGY REPORTS

2-XX-20XX Paracentesis (2 liters): Consistent with ovarian malignancy.

5-4-20XX TAH-BSO: Right ovary: Papillary serous carcinoma, 1.6 cm papillary tan lesion. No residual ovarian stroma identified. FIGO grade III of III. Left ovary: Surface involvement by papillary serous carcinoma. Uterus: Cervix no diagnostic abnormalities. Endometrium: Endometrial polyps x 3.

continued on next page

Case 9, continued

Myometrium: Leiomyomata. Left fallopian tube negative. Papillary serous carcinoma involving sigmoid colon, lesser omentum, cul-de-sac, nodule of small bowel mesentery, omentum, right utero-sacral ligament, and descending colon.

TREATMENT

2-XX-20XX to 4-2-20XX Carboplatin and Taxol, six cycles

5-4-20XX Exploratory laparotomy, TAH-BSO, total infracolic omentectomy, radical dissection for debulking of ovarian malignancy

Site Code ___ ___ ___.___

Histology/Behavior/Grade ___ ___ ___ ___ / ___ ___

Grade Path Value ___

Grade Path System ___

Lymph Vascular Invasion ___

Ambiguous Terminol ___

Date Conclusive Terminol ___ ___ ___ ___ ___ ___ ___ ___

Date Conclus Dx Flag ___ ___

Multiplicity Counter ___ ___

Date Mult Tumors ___ ___ ___ ___ ___ ___ ___ ___

Date Mult Tumors Flag ___ ___

Mult Tum Reported as One Prim ___ ___

Summary Stage 2000 ___

cT ___ cN ___ cM ___

Clin Stage Group _____

pT ___ pN ___ M ___

Path Stage Group _____

CS Tumor Size ___ ___ ___

CS Extension ___ ___ ___

CS TS/Ext Eval ___

CS LN ___ ___ ___

CS Reg Nodes Eval ___

Reg LN Pos ___ ___

Reg LN Exam ___ ___

CS Mets at Dx ___ ___

CS Mets at Dx - Bone ___ Brain ___ Liver ___ Lung ___

CS Mets Eval ___

SSF1 CA-125 ___ ___ ___

SSF2 FIGO Stage ___ ___ ___

SSF3 Resid Tum Stat/Size after Cytoreduction ___ ___ ___

SSF4 Tum Location after Cytoreduction ___ ___ ___

SSF5 Malig Ascites ___ ___ ___

CASE 10

HISTORY AND PHYSICAL EXAM

44 year old female, G2P2, felt to have had a miscarriage on 10-12-200X with a sonogram showing no fetus. D&C showed chorionic villi of the first trimester with hydropic degeneration and focal trophoblastic proliferation. It was not called a molar pregnancy. However, her beta HCGs have continued to rise. The patient is completely healthy, afebrile, and asymptomatic. Other than fatigue, she has absolutely no complaints.

11-15-200X Physical exam: No supraclavicular or inguinal adenopathy. No palpable masses. EGBUS [external genitalia, Bartholin's glands, urethra and Skene's glands]: Negative. Vagina without lesions. Vaginal apex benign. Bimanual and rectovaginal exam demonstrate no masses or nodularity.

X-RAYS AND SCANS

11-1-20XX CT scan: Abnormal lesions in liver felt to be metastatic from molar pregnancy

11-15-20XX Limited ultrasound of liver: Lesions seen on CT scan are felt to represent hemangiomas.

11-18-20XX Complete radiographic evaluation: No metastatic disease. Question of histoplasmosis in lungs.

LABORATORY REPORTS

HCGs (normal range 0 ng/ml): 10-12-20XX: 160,884; 11-1-20XX: 1774; 11-10-20XX: 6269; 12-19-20XX: 2; 12-28-20XX: < 1; 1-10-20YY: < 1

continued on next page

Case 10, continued

ENDOSCOPIC PROCEDURES None.

OPERATIVE REPORTS

11-15-20XX Suction D&C: Gestational trophoblastic disease, with molar pregnancy, persistent, within the uterus

PATHOLOGY REPORTS

11-15-20XX D&C: 3.5 x 2.5 x 2.0 cm aggregate of tan-red hemorrhagic tissue and blood with changes consistent for hydatidiform mole. Comments: Uterine curettings include several hydropic appearing chorionic villi. Within surrounding blood clot and fibrin there are aggregates of trophoblastic cells.
COMMENT: These findings are consistent with this patient's clinical history of epithelioid trophoblastic tumor.

TREATMENT

10-12-20XX D&C
11-15-20XX Suction dilation and curettage
11-20-20XX Started Methotrexate

Site Code __ __ __.__	**Mult Tum Reported as One Prim** __ __	**CS Mets at Dx** __ __
Histology/Behavior/Grade __ __ __ __/__ __	**Summary Stage 2000** __	**CS Mets at Dx - Bone** __ **Brain** __ **Liver** __ **Lung** __
Grade Path Value __	**cT** __ **cN** __ **cM** __	**CS Mets Eval** __
Grade Path System __	**Clin Stage Group** __	**SSF1 CA-125** __ __ __
Lymph Vascular Invasion __	**pT** __ **pN** __ **M** __	**SSF2 FIGO Stage** __ __ __
Ambiguous Terminol __	**Path Stage Group** __	**SSF3 Resid Tum Stat/Size after Cytoreduction** __ __ __
Date Conclusive Terminol __ __ __ __ __ __ __ __	**CS Tumor Size** __ __ __	**SSF4 Tum Location after Cytoreduction** __ __ __
Date Conclus Dx Flag __ __	**CS Extension** __ __ __	**SSF5 Mallg Ascites** __ __ __
Multiplicity Counter __ __	**CS TS/Ext Eval** __	
Date Mult Tumors __ __ __ __ __ __ __ __	**CS LN** __ __ __	
Date Mult Tumors Flag __ __	**CS Reg Nodes Eval** __	
	Reg LN Pos __ __	
	Reg LN Exam __ __	

CASE 11

HISTORY AND PHYSICAL EXAMINATION

Abdomen: Distended; fullness in LLQ.
Pelvic: Questionable large 10 cm mass on left deviating uterus to right. Rectal: Mass palpable anteriorly and separately from rectosigmoid colon.

X-RAYS AND SCANS

Prior to Admission: CT scan abd/pelvis: 10 cm pelvic mass.
1-4-20XX CXR: negative.

LABORATORY REPORTS

CEA: normal; CA-125 50 (reported as slightly elevated)

continued on next page

Case 11, continued

OPERATIVE REPORTS

1-21-20XX TAH-BSO: 16 cm. left ovarian tumor adjacent to uterine fundus, sigmoid colon, small bowel, and pelvic sidewall peritoneum. Uterus was 12 weeks size. Right ovary and tube adherent deep along right pelvic sidewall but not grossly enlarged. A few enlarged firm right external iliac and right common iliac lymph nodes and one slightly enlarged right periaortic lymph node. These were removed. Omentectomy and optimal debulking performed.

PATHOLOGY REPORTS

1-21-20XX Left pelvic mass (ovary): Papillary carcinoma extending to serosa. Right adnexa: Papillary carcinoma of right ovary. Right tube: Negative. Metastatic carcinoma in small bowel mesenteric fat. Metastasis to 2/4 periaortic lymph nodes. Right pelvic lymph nodes (2) negative. Omentum: Negative. Cervix: Negative. Uterus with papillary carcinoma involving proximal half of endometrial cavity with extensive involvement of myometrium. Abdominal fluid: Suspicious for malignancy. Addendum: final diagnosis is high grade papillary adenocarcinoma; both tumors with ovary and uterus are similar and are high grade papillary adenocarcinoma. Final diagnosis: Primary ovarian cancer with metastases, FIGO IIIC.

TREATMENT

1-21-20XX Total abdominal hysterectomy and bilateral salpingo-oophorectomy; right pelvic and periaortic lymph node dissection; complete omentectomy

Started on carboplatin and paclitaxel postoperatively.

Site Code ___ ___ ___.___

Histology/Behavior/Grade ___ ___ ___ ___ / ___ ___

Grade Path Value ___

Grade Path System ___

Lymph Vascular Invasion ___

Ambiguous Terminol ___

Date Conclusive Terminol

___ ___ ___ ___ ___ ___ ___ ___

Date Conclus Dx Flag ___ ___

Multiplicity Counter ___ ___

Date Mult Tumors

___ ___ ___ ___ ___ ___ ___ ___

Date Mult Tumors Flag ___ ___

Mult Tum Reported as One Prim ___ ___

Summary Stage 2000 ___

cT ___ cN ___ cM ___

Clin Stage Group ___

pT ___ pN ___ M ___

Path Stage Group ___

CS Tumor Size ___ ___ ___

CS Extension ___ ___ ___

CS TS/Ext Eval ___

CS LN ___ ___ ___

CS Reg Nodes Eval ___

Reg LN Pos ___ ___

Reg LN Exam ___ ___

CS Mets at Dx ___ ___

CS Mets at Dx - Bone ___ Brain ___ Liver ___ Lung ___

CS Mets Eval ___

SSF1 CA-125 ___ ___ ___

SSF2 FIGO Stage ___ ___ ___

SSF3 Resid Tum Stat/Size after Cytoreduction ___ ___ ___

SSF4 Tum Location after Cytoreduction ___ ___ ___

SSF5 Malig Ascites ___ ___ ___

CASE 12

HISTORY AND PHYSICAL EXAM

8-8-20XX 70-year-old G3, P3 with acute onset of constipation, suprapubic abdominal pain and cramping, with occasional radiation to the epigastrium. Also increasing distention, particularly of epigastric area and lower belly over the last 2-3 weeks.

continued on next page

Case 12, continued

X-RAYS AND SCANS

8-4-20XX CT abdomen/pelvis: 12.5 x 12.1 cm lobulated complex cystic mass, multiple enhancing septation and wall nodularity. Significant mass effect in the pelvis particularly on the right; hydroureter which is dilated proximally. Previous hysterectomy.

8-4-20XX Pelvic ultrasound: Large predominantly solid mass in the pelvis measuring 15 x 8 x 12 cm with a few areas of cystic component with vascular flow. Appearances would "suggest a sarcoma."

LABORATORY REPORTS

8-4-20XX CA-125: marginally elevated at 35.

OPERATIVE REPORTS

8-8-20XX Laparotomy and BSO: Hemorrhagic, highly vascular mass arising from the right ovary, adherent to peritoneum overlying rectosigmoid mesentery. At completion of surgery, no other evidence of disease. No suspiciously enlarged nodes. No ascites. No other peritoneal disease noted along the bowel.

PATHOLOGY REPORTS

8-8-20XX BSO, debulking, and omentectomy: R fallopian tube and ovary: Malignant mixed mesodermal tumor (MMMT) involving right ovary. No malignancy in R fallopian tube, L fallopian tube and ovary, L posterior cul-de-sac peritoneum, omentum, small bowel adhesion biopsy, R abdominal wall peritoneum, or R pelvic peritoneum. R medial broad ligament: Positive for malignant mixed mesodermal tumor. Lymph node biopsies: L pelvic (1), R pelvic (2), R periaortic (3): no evidence of metastatic tumor.

TREATMENT

8-8-20XX Exploratory laparotomy, tumor debulking with bilateral salpingo-oophorectomy, omentectomy, peritoneal biopsies, and bilateral pelvic and periaortic lymph node dissection.

Patient begun on Cisplatin, Ifosfamide, and Mesna at Hospital B following consultation with medical oncologist.

Site Code ___ ___ ___.___

Histology/Behavior/Grade ___ ___ ___ ___/___ ___

Grade Path Value ___

Grade Path System ___

Lymph Vascular Invasion ___

Ambiguous Terminol ___

Date Conclusive Terminol ___ ___ ___ ___ ___ ___ ___ ___

Date Conclus Dx Flag ___ ___

Multiplicity Counter ___ ___

Date Mult Tumors ___ ___ ___ ___ ___ ___ ___ ___

Date Mult Tumors Flag ___ ___

Mult Tum Reported as One Prim ___ ___

Summary Stage 2000 ___

cT ___ cN ___ cM ___

Clin Stage Group ___

pT ___ pN ___ M ___

Path Stage Group ___

CS Tumor Size ___ ___ ___

CS Extension ___ ___ ___

CS TS/Ext Eval ___

CS LN ___ ___ ___

CS Reg Nodes Eval ___

Reg LN Pos ___ ___

Reg LN Exam ___ ___

CS Mets at Dx ___ ___

CS Mets at Dx - Bone ___ Brain ___ Liver ___ Lung ___

CS Mets Eval ___

SSF1 CA-125 ___ ___ ___

SSF2 FIGO Stage ___ ___ ___

SSF3 Resid Tum Stat/Size after Cytoreduction ___ ___ ___

SSF4 Tum Location after Cytoreduction ___ ___ ___

SSF5 Malig Ascites ___ ___ ___

ANSWERS TO OVARIAN AND OTHER CANCER CASE EXERCISES

—— CASE 1 ——

Site Code	C56.9	Ovary, NOS
Histology	8310	Clear cell adenocarcinoma
Behavior	3	Invasive
Grade/differentiation	3	Stated as grade 3
Grade Path Value	Blank	Does not apply
Grade Path System	Blank	Does not apply
Lymph Vascular Invasion	9	Lymph-vascular invasion not mentioned in path report
Ambiguous Terminology	0	Conclusive terminology
Date Conclusive Terminol	Blank	Diagnosis made by conclusive terminology
Date Conclus Dx Flag	11	Not applicable
Multiplicity Counter	01	One tumor only
Date Multiple Tumors	Blank	Not applicable
Date Mult Tumors Flag	15	Single tumor only (multiplicity counter is coded 01)
Type Mult Tum as 1 Prim	00	Single tumor
Summary Stage	7	Distant (pericolic gutter)
Clinical TNM	cTX	Bilateral ovarian masses cannot be assessed as malignancy
	cNX	No assessment of lymph nodes
	cM0	Chest x-ray negative
Clinical Stage Group	Unstageable	
Pathologic TNM	pT3a	Tumor in pelvis (cul-de-sac) seen by surgeon, tumor in abdomen (pericolic gutter) found microscopically
	pN1	Multiple lymph nodes involved
	M0	Clinical evaluation of mets negative
Pathologic Stage Group	IIIC	
CS Schema used: Ovary		
CS Tumor Size	999	Tumor size not stated; do not code size of ovaries when tumor is multicystic
CS Extension	700	Visible tumor implants in pelvis; however, tumor outside of pelvis (pericolic gutter) identified microscopically
CS TS/Ext Eval	3	Based on pathology
CS Lymph Nodes	400	Both common iliac (10) and periaortic (20) nodes involved
CS Reg Nodes Eval	3	Lymph nodes removed for examination
Reg Nodes Pos	97	Lymph nodes positive, number not stated
Reg Nodes Exam	97	Lymphadenectomy (dissection), number of nodes not stated
CS Mets at Dx	00	Chest x-ray normal
CS Mets at Dx–Bone	0	No bone metastases
CS Mets at Dx–Brain	0	No brain metastases
CS Mets at Dx–Liver	0	No liver metastases
CS Mets at Dx–Lung	0	No lung metastases
CS Mets Eval	0	Based on imaging
SSF1 CA-125	010	Elevated
SSF2 FIGO Stage	999	FIGO Stage not documented
SSF3 Resid Tum Stat/Size after Cytoreduction	000	No visible (gross) tumor remained after surgery

Case 1, continued

SSF4 Tum Location after Cytoreduction	999	Not documented (see comment below)
SSF5 Malig Ascites	999	Ascites not mentioned

Although no gross tumor was noted in the abdomen on the operative report (only implants in pelvis), biopsies of the pericolic gutter were positive for metastatic carcinoma. Pericolic gutter is T3 and listed in CS Extension note 7 as to be coded in the 700-750 range. Because the abdominal metastases were identified only microscopically, the extension code is 700, which maps to pT3a. However, the positive lymph nodes upstage the case to Stage Group IIIC. The surgeon states that all visible (gross) tumor was removed (debulking procedure) so SSF3 is 000. However, there is no corresponding code to indicate no residual tumor in SSF4. According to the response to several questions in the CAnswer Forum, use code 999 (not documented) in CS version 0203 when there is no residual tumor after the cytoreduction sugery.
This case will map to pT3a pN1 cM0 Stage Group IIIC.

—— CASE 2 ——

Site Code	C56.9	Ovary, NOS
Histology	8323	Mixed cell adenocarcinoma
Behavior	3	Invasive
Grade/differentiation	9	Grade not stated
Grade Path Value	Blank	Does not apply
Grade Path System	Blank	Does not apply
Lymph Vascular Invasion	9	Lymph-vascular invasion not mentioned in path report
Ambiguous Terminology	0	Conclusive terminology
Date Conclusive Terminol	Blank	Diagnosis made by conclusive terminology
Date Conclus Dx Flag	11	Not applicable
Multiplicity Counter	02	Two tumors (right and left ovary)
Date Multiple Tumors	20XX0403	Date of diagnosis of multiple tumors
Date Mult Tumors Flag	Blank	Valid date provided
Type Mult Tum as 1 Prim	40	Multiple invasive tumors
Summary Stage	2	Regional direct extension (tumor cells in ascites)
Clinical TNM	cT1b	Bilateral adnexal masses
	cN0	No adenopathy on CT
	cM0	CT pelvis, physical exam stated no organomegaly
Clinical Stage Group	IB	
Pathologic TNM	pT1c	No tumor outside of pelvis, but pelvic fluid positive for malignancy
	pN0	No lymph nodes involved
	M0	Clinical evaluation of mets negative
Pathologic Stage Group	IC	
CS Schema used: Ovary		
CS Tumor Size	999	Tumor size not stated; do not code size of ovaries when tumor is described as adnexal mass.
CS Extension	410	Peritoneal washings positive for malignant cells; all abdominal biopsies negative; tumor confined to pelvis
CS TS/Ext Eval	3	Based on pathology
CS Lymph Nodes	000	Right and left pelvic and periaortic lymph nodes negative
CS Reg Nodes Eval	3	Lymph nodes removed for examination

Ovary

Case 2, continued

Reg Nodes Pos	00	No lymph nodes positive
Reg Nodes Exam	18	8 left pelvic + 7 right pelvic + 3 periaortic nodes = 18 nodes examined
CS Mets at Dx	00	Physical exam normal
CS Mets at Dx–Bone	0	No bone metastases
CS Mets at Dx–Brain	0	No brain metastases
CS Mets at Dx–Liver	0	No liver metastases
CS Mets at Dx–Lung	0	No lung metastases
CS Mets Eval	0	Based on non-invasive clinical evaluation
SSF1 CA-125	999	Not documented
SSF2 FIGO Stage	999	FIGO Stage not documented
SSF3 Resid Tum Stat/Size after Cytoreduction	999	Residual tumor status/size not described by surgeon
SSF4 Tum Location after Cytoreduction	999	Not documented (see comment below)
SSF5 Malig Ascites	990	Pelvic fluid with positive cytology

Ultrasound shows bilateral cystic and solid components of adnexal masses. Sizes reported are not of tumor itself, but sizes of entire masses. Tumor is confined to bilateral ovaries; all other biopsies in pelvis and abdomen are negative. However, pelvic washings show malignant cells, so stage is upgraded to subcategory C within stage I. This case is an example of the use of 8323, mixed cell adenocarcinoma for a tumor that contains multiple histologies. See Table 2 in the "Other Sites" Multiple Primary and Histology Coding rules. There is not a good code in SSF4 to indicate no residual tumor when only the ovaries are involved. According to the response to a question in the CAnswer Forum, use code 999 (not documented) in CS version 0203 when there is no residual tumor because the cancer is confined to the ovary(ies).

This case will map to pT1c pN0 cM0 Stage Group IC.

—— CASE 3 ——

Site Code	C57.0	Fallopian tube
Histology	8441	Serous carcinoma
Behavior	3	Invasive
Grade/differentiation	3	Poorly differentiated (do not code high grade from metastatic site)
Grade Path Value	Blank	Does not apply
Grade Path System	Blank	Does not apply
Lymph Vascular Invasion	1	Lymph-vascular invasion present
Ambiguous Terminology	0	Conclusive terminology
Date Conclusive Terminol	Blank	Diagnosis made by conclusive terminology
Date Conclus Dx Flag	11	Not applicable
Multiplicity Counter	01	One tumor only
Date Multiple Tumors	Blank	Not applicable
Date Mult Tumors Flag	15	Single tumor only (multiplicity counter is coded 01)
Type Mult Tum as 1 Prim	00	Single tumor
Summary Stage	4	Regional direct extension and lymph nodes
Clinical TNM	cTX	No assessment of fallopian tubes
	cN1	Widespread lymphadenopathy on PET scan
	cM0	No distant metastases on PET scan
Clinical Stage Group	IIIC (involved regional nodes)	

Case 3, continued

Pathologic TNM	pT2a	Metastatic carcinoma in cervix
	pN1	Pelvic lymph nodes involved
	M0	PET scan showed only lymph node involvement, no distant metastases
Pathologic Stage Group IIIC		

CS Schema used: Fallopian tube		
CS Tumor Size	999	Tumor size not stated
CS Extension	400	Tumor in fallopian tube and cervix
CS TS/Ext Eval	3	Based on pathology
CS Lymph Nodes	200	Retroperitoneal and periaortic nodes involved
CS Reg Nodes Eval	1	Operative report documents involved lymph nodes in abdomen
Reg Nodes Pos	01	One lymph node positive
Reg Nodes Exam	02	Count only the removed nodes (FNA was from same lymph node chain)
CS Mets at Dx	00	PET scan negative for metastases; disregard equivocal supraclavicular (distant) nodes
CS Mets at Dx–Bone	0	No bone metastases
CS Mets at Dx–Brain	0	No brain metastases
CS Mets at Dx–Liver	0	No liver metastases
CS Mets at Dx–Lung	0	No lung metastases
CS Mets Eval	0	Based on imaging
SSF1 FIGO Stage	999	Not documented
SSF2 Biopsy Mets Site	110	Biopsy of omentum
SSF3 Prim Tum Location	010	Involves fimbria
SSF4 # Pos Pelvic Nodes	001	One positive pelvic node
SSF5 # Exam Pelvic Nodes	002	Two pelvic nodes examined
SSF6 # Pos Para-aortic Nod	098	No para-aortic nodes positive
SSF7 # Exam Para-aor Nod	098	No para-aortic nodes examined

Discontinuous metastases to cervix are reported in T category and CS Extension and would be Stage IIA if lymph nodes were negative. However, there are histologically positive pelvic lymph nodes and visualized "massive adenopathy" in the abdomen that upstage the case to IIIC.
This case will map to pT2a pN1 cM0 Stage Group IIIC.

—— CASE 4 ——

Site Code	C56.9	Ovary, NOS
Histology	8380	Endometrioid adenocarcinoma
Behavior	3	Invasive
Grade/differentiation	3	Stated as grade 3
Grade Path Value	Blank	Does not apply
Grade Path System	Blank	Does not apply
Lymph Vascular Invasion	9	Lymph-vascular invasion not mentioned in path report
Ambiguous Terminology	0	Conclusive terminology
Date Conclusive Terminol	Blank	Diagnosis made by conclusive terminology
Date Conclus Dx Flag	11	Not applicable
Multiplicity Counter	02	One tumor only
Date Multiple Tumors	20XX0315	Date of diagnosis
Date Mult Tumors Flag	Blank	Valid date provided

Ovary

Case 4, continued

Type Mult Tum as 1 Prim	40	Multiple invasive tumors
Summary Stage	1	Localized
Clinical TNM	cTX	No assessment of ovaries
	cN0	No adenopathy on CT pelvis
	cM0	CT pelvis negative, chest x-ray negative
Clinical Stage Group	Unstageable	
Pathologic TNM	pT1b	Bilateral ovarian involvement; all biopsies negative
	pN0	26 pelvic and periaortic lymph nodes negative
	M0	Clinical evaluation of mets negative
Pathologic Stage Group	IB	
CS Schema used: Ovary		
CS Tumor Size	999	Size of malignancy not stated; do not code size of ”tumors” from operative report
CS Extension	200	Bilateral ovary involvement; tubes, uterus, cervix, omentum, cul de sac cytology negative; no other signs of tumor
CS TS/Ext Eval	3	Based on pathology
CS Lymph Nodes	000	All lymph nodes negative; “prominent” periaortic node turns out to be negative
CS Reg Nodes Eval	3	Lymph nodes removed for examination
Reg Nodes Pos	00	All lymph nodes negative
Reg Nodes Exam	26	Twenty-five pelvic + 1 periaortic lymph nodes examined
CS Mets at Dx	00	Chest x-ray and CT scan negative
CS Mets at Dx–Bone	0	No bone metastases
CS Mets at Dx–Brain	0	No brain metastases
CS Mets at Dx–Liver	0	No liver metastases
CS Mets at Dx–Lung	0	No lung metastases
CS Mets Eval	0	Based on imaging
SSF1 CA-125	020	CA-125 normal
SSF2 FIGO Stage	120	Stated as FIGO IB
SSF3 Resid Tum Stat/Size after Cytoreduction	000	All gross tumor removed per operative report
SSF4 Tum Location after Cytoreduction	999	Not documented (see comment below)
SSF5 Malig Ascites	991	200 cc of cul-de-sac fluid was negative

Endometrioid adenocarcinoma is an ovarian malignancy that resembles hormonally sensitive endometrial carcinoma. It is not metastatic to the ovary from the uterus. Focal clear cell changes do not constitute a different histology and are not significant enough to code the case as mixed tumor. There is bilateral ovarian involvement but no additional tumor in the pelvis. The surgeon states that all visible (gross) tumor was removed so SSF3 is 000. However, there is no corresponding code to indicate no residual tumor in SSF4. According to the response to several questions in the CAnswer Forum, use code 999 (not documented) in CS version 0203 when there is no residual tumor after the cytoreduction sugery.
This case will map to pT1b pN0 cM0 Stage Group IB.

—— CASE 5 ——

Site Code	C56.9	Ovary, NOS
Histology	8481	Mucin-producing adenocarcinoma
Behavior	3	Invasive
Grade/differentiation	3	Stated as poorly differentiated
Grade Path Value	Blank	Does not apply
Grade Path System	Blank	Does not apply
Lymph Vascular Invasion	9	Lymph-vascular invasion not mentioned in path report
Ambiguous Terminology	0	Conclusive terminology
Date Conclusive Terminol	Blank	Diagnosis made by conclusive terminology
Date Conclus Dx Flag	11	Not applicable
Multiplicity Counter	02	Two tumors present
Date Multiple Tumors	20XX0422	Date of diagnosis
Date Mult Tumors Flag	Blank	Valid date provided
Type Mult Tum as 1 Prim	40	Multiple invasive tumors
Summary Stage	7	Distant (visible tumor in abdomen)
Clinical TNM	cT3b	Omental caking and ascites seen on sonogram
	cNX	Lymph nodes not assessed clinically
	cM0	Physical exam states no other abnormal findings
Clinical Stage Group	Unstageable (see note below)	
Pathologic TNM	pT2c	Tumor implant on fallopian tube and positive ascites (visible large tumor implants in abdomen greater than 2 cm are not microscopically confirmed)
	pNX	No lymph nodes removed for examination
	M0	Clinical evaluation of mets negative
Pathologic Stage Group	Unstageable (see note below)	
CS Schema used: Ovary		
CS Tumor Size	040	Left ovarian carcinoma stated as 4 cm. Do not add sizes of separate tumors together.
CS Extension	720	Visible tumor implants in abdomen greater than 2 cm on operative report (not confirmed microscopically)
CS TS/Ext Eval	1	Based on operative report
CS Lymph Nodes	999	Lymph node status unknown; cannot use inaccessible sites rule because primary tumor is extensive
CS Reg Nodes Eval	0	Based on clinical assessment
Reg Nodes Pos	98	No lymph nodes removed for examination
Reg Nodes Exam	00	No lymph nodes examined
CS Mets at Dx	00	Physical exam statement "review of systems otherwise normal"
CS Mets at Dx–Bone	0	No bone metastases
CS Mets at Dx–Brain	0	No brain metastases
CS Mets at Dx–Liver	0	No liver metastases
CS Mets at Dx–Lung	0	No lung metastases
CS Mets Eval	0	Based on non-invasive clinical evaluation
SSF1 CA-125	010	Elevated
SSF2 FIGO Stage	999	FIGO stage not documented
SSF3 Resid Tum Stat/Size after Cytoreduction	998	Surgery not cytoreductive

Case 5, continued

SSF4 Tum Location after Cytoreduction	999	No cytoreductive surgery (see comment below)
SSF5 Malig Ascites	990	Peritoneal washings positive

Clinically, this patient has minimal disease in the pelvis, but imaging and surgical observation note a large tumor in the omentum and nodular disease on undersurface of diaphragm. Pathologically, the only tissue resected was both ovaries and an implant on the fallopian tube with positive ascites. However, because there is no mention of lymph nodes clinically and none were removed for microscopic examination, this case is cNX and pNX and therefore is unstageable by TNM rules. However, the case is at least clinical Stage IIIC due to the abdominal involvement. Omentum and diaphragm are T3 and listed in CS Extension note 7 as to be coded in the 700-750 range. The omental tumor measures 4 x 10 cm (greater than 2 cm), so code 720/T3c are appropriate, even though not microscopically confirmed. According to the response to a question in CAnswer Forum, use code 999 for SSF4 when no cytoreductive surgery is performed.
This case will map to cT3c cNX cM0 Stage Group IIIC.

—— CASE 6 ——

Site Code	C56.9	Ovary, NOS
Histology	8470	Mucinous cystadenocarcinoma
Behavior	3	Invasive
Grade/differentiation	1	Stated as well differentiated (wd)
Grade Path Value	Blank	Does not apply
Grade Path System	Blank	Does not apply
Lymph Vascular Invasion	9	Lymph-vascular invasion not mentioned in path report
Ambiguous Terminology	0	Conclusive terminology
Date Conclusive Terminol	Blank	Diagnosis made by conclusive terminology
Date Conclus Dx Flag	11	Not applicable
Multiplicity Counter	01	One tumor only
Date Multiple Tumors	Blank	Not applicable
Date Mult Tumors Flag	15	Single tumor only (multiplicity counter is coded 01)
Type Mult Tum as 1 Prim	00	Single tumor (corpus uteri case is a separate abstract)
Summary Stage	1	Localized
Clinical TNM	cTX	Non-specific description of pelvic mass
	cNX	Lymph nodes not assessed clinically
	cM0	Chest x-ray negative
Clinical Stage Group	Unstageable	
Pathologic TNM	pT1a	Tumor confined to one ovary (small area within large cystic mass)
	pN0	Lymph nodes negative
	M0	Clinical evaluation of mets negative
Pathologic Stage Group	IA	
CS Schema used: Ovary		
CS Tumor Size	027	Tumor area described as 27 millimeters in size (2.7 cm)
CS Extension	100	Tumor limited to one ovary
CS TS/Ext Eval	3	Based on pathology
CS Lymph Nodes	000	No lymph nodes involved
CS Reg Nodes Eval	3	Lymph nodes removed for examination
Reg Nodes Pos	00	No nodes positive

Case 6, continued

Reg Nodes Exam	97	Procedure described as lymphadenectomy; number of nodes examined not stated
CS Mets at Dx	00	Chest x-ray negative
CS Mets at Dx–Bone	0	No bone metastases
CS Mets at Dx–Brain	0	No brain metastases
CS Mets at Dx–Liver	0	No liver metastases
CS Mets at Dx–Lung	0	No lung metastases
CS Mets Eval	0	Based on imaging
SSF1 CA-125	999	CA-125 not documented
SSF2 FIGO Stage	100	Stated as IA
SSF3 Resid Tum Stat/Size after Cytoreduction	998	No cytoreductive surgery
SSF4 Tum Location after Cytoreduction	999	No cytoreductive surgery (see comment below)
SSF5 Malig Ascites	991	Ascites negative

This patient has a very large mass but only a tiny portion of it is malignant. All other biopsies are negative. The biopsies were part of the staging procedure, not cytoreduction. According to the response to a question in CAnswer Forum, use code 999 for SSF4 when no cytoreductive surgery is performed. The endometrial carcinoma is a different cell type and would be abstracted as a separate primary (see Corpus Uteri case 8 for answers).
This case will map to pT1a pN0 cM0 Stage Group IA.

—— CASE 7 ——

Site Code	C56.9	Ovary, NOS
Histology	8441	Serous adenocarcinoma
Behavior	3	Invasive
Grade/differentiation	3	Stated as moderately to poorly differentiated; code the higher grade
Grade Path Value	Blank	Does not apply
Grade Path System	Blank	Does not apply
Lymph Vascular Invasion	0	No lymph-vascular invasion per path report
Ambiguous Terminology	0	Conclusive terminology
Date Conclusive Terminol	Blank	Diagnosis made by conclusive terminology
Date Conclus Dx Flag	11	Not applicable
Multiplicity Counter	02	Two tumors (1.5 cm and 1.0 cm)
Date Multiple Tumors	20XX0806	Date of diagnosis
Date Mult Tumors Flag	Blank	Valid date provided
Type Mult Tum as 1 Prim	40	Multiple invasive tumors
Summary Stage	2	Regional direct extension
Clinical TNM	cTX	No clinical assessment of ovaries, only description of adnexal mass
	cNX	Lymph nodes not assessed clinically
	cM0	Physical exam states no other abnormal findings
Clinical Stage Group	Unstageable	
Pathologic TNM	pT2b	Cul-de-sac and pelvic peritoneum positive for tumor
	pN0	No lymph node involvement
	M0	Clinical evaluation of mets negative
Pathologic Stage Group	IIB	

Case 7, continued

CS Schema used: Ovary		
CS Tumor Size	015	Tumor size 1.5 cm in a larger cystadenoma
CS Extension	610	Tumor on pelvic organs (cul-de-sac and pelvic peritoneum)
CS TS/Ext Eval	3	Based on pathology
CS Lymph Nodes	000	No involved lymph nodes
CS Reg Nodes Eval	3	Lymph nodes removed for examination
Reg Nodes Pos	00	No lymph nodes positive
Reg Nodes Exam	12	Twelve nodes examined
CS Mets at Dx	00	No distant metastases
CS Mets at Dx–Bone	0	No bone metastases
CS Mets at Dx–Brain	0	No brain metastases
CS Mets at Dx–Liver	0	No liver metastases
CS Mets at Dx–Lung	0	No lung metastases
CS Mets Eval	0	Based on non-invasive clinical evaluation
SSF1 CA-125	020	Normal
SSF2 FIGO Stage	999	FIGO stage not documented
SSF3 Resid Tum Stat/Size after Cytoreduction	998	No cytoreductive surgery
SSF4 Tum Location after Cytoreduction	999	No cytoreductive surgery (see comment below)
SSF5 Malig Ascites	999	Ascites not documented

The borderline serous cystadenoma (8442/1) is not reportable to most cancer registries, but the small serous adenocarcinoma is. In addition to the primary in the right ovary, there is a separate nodule of tumor in another ovarian cyst and tumor in the cul-de-sac and the pelvic peritoneum, all of which are confined to pelvic organs (code 610/T2b). The biopsies were part of the staging procedure, not cytoreduction. According to the response to a question in CAnswer Forum, use code 999 for SSF4 when no cytoreductive surgery is performed. Lymph nodes and peritoneal washings are pathologically negative, so this case is TNM/FIGO stage IIB.
This case will map to pT2b pN0 cM0 Stage Group IIB.

—— CASE 8 ——

Site Code	C56.9	Ovary, NOS
Histology	8461	Papillary serous surface adenocarcinoma
Behavior	3	Invasive
Grade/differentiation	3	Stated as poorly differentiated
Grade Path Value	Blank	Does not apply
Grade Path System	Blank	Does not apply
Lymph Vascular Invasion	9	Lymph-vascular invasion not mentioned in path report
Ambiguous Terminology	0	Conclusive terminology
Date Conclusive Terminol	Blank	Diagnosis made by conclusive terminology
Date Conclus Dx Flag	11	Not applicable
Multiplicity Counter	02	Two tumors present
Date Multiple Tumors	20XX1207	Date of diagnosis
Date Mult Tumors Flag	Blank	Valid date supplied
Type Mult Tum as 1 Prim	40	Multiple invasive tumors
Summary Stage	7	Involvement of abdominal organs

Case 8, continued

Clinical TNM	cTX	Description of adnexal "masses" not sufficient to stage clinically
	cNX	Lymph nodes not assessed clinically
	cM0	Physical exam states no other abnormal findings
Clinical Stage Group	Unstageable	
Pathologic TNM	pT3b	Visible tumor implants in pelvis, size not stated (use the downstaging rule to classify as T3b rather than T3c); tumor outside of pelvis (appendix and omentum) confirmed microscopically
	pN1	Extensive lymph node involvement
	M0	Clinical evaluation of mets negative
Pathologic Stage Group	IIIC	

CS Schema used: Ovary		
CS Tumor Size	999	Tumor size not stated; do not code size of mass
CS Extension	730	Visible tumor implants in pelvis, size not stated; tumor outside of pelvis (appendix and omentum) confirmed microscopically
CS TS/Ext Eval	3	Based on pathology
CS Lymph Nodes	400	Both pelvic, NOS (10) and periaortic (20) nodes involved
CS Reg Nodes Eval	3	Lymph nodes removed for examination
Reg Nodes Pos	32	Thirty-two lymph nodes positive
Reg Nodes Exam	48	Forty-eight nodes examined
CS Mets at Dx	00	No distant metastases stated on physical exam
CS Mets at Dx–Bone	0	No bone metastases
CS Mets at Dx–Brain	0	No brain metastases
CS Mets at Dx–Liver	0	No liver metastases
CS Mets at Dx–Lung	0	No lung metastases
CS Mets Eval	0	Based on non-invasive clinical evaluation
SSF1 CA-125	010	Elevated
SSF2 FIGO Stage	999	FIGO stage not stated
SSF3 Resid Tum Stat/Size after Cytoreduction	990	Macroscopic residual tumor, size not stated
SSF4 Tum Location after Cytoreduction	990	Residual tumor, location not stated
SSF5 Malig Ascites	999	Unknown whether ascites present.

This patient has extensive disease in the pelvis and abdomen, which was only biopsied (no attempt at cytoreduction). SSFs 3 and 4 can be coded for macroscopic residual tumor. Microscopic analysis of the omentum and appendix are positive for metastases. Omentum and appendix are T3 and listed in CS Extension note 7 as to be coded in the 700-750 range. Because no size was stated for the abdominal metastases that were visualized and then confirmed microscopically, the extension code is 730, which maps to pT3, NOS. However, the positive lymph nodes upstage the case to Stage Group IIIC.

This case will map to pT3 pN1 cM0 Stage Group IIIC.

—— CASE 9 ——

Site Code	C56.9	Ovary, NOS
Histology	8460	Papillary serous carcinoma
Behavior	3	Invasive
Grade/differentiation	4	Stated as grade III of III (highest grade)
Grade Path Value	3	FIGO Grade III of III
Grade Path System	3	FIGO Grade III of III
Lymph Vascular Invasion	9	Lymph-vascular invasion not mentioned in path report
Ambiguous Terminology	0	Conclusive terminology
Date Conclusive Terminol	Blank	Diagnosis made by conclusive terminology
Date Conclus Dx Flag	11	Not applicable
Multiplicity Counter	02	Two tumors (bilateral ovaries involved)
Date Multiple Tumors	20XX02XX	Date of diagnosis
Date Mult Tumors Flag	Blank	Partial date provided
Type Mult Tum as 1 Prim	40	Multiple invasive tumors
Summary Stage	7	Distant
Clinical TNM	cT3c	Ascites and large (>2 cm) soft tissue masses seen on CT abdomen
	cNX	Lymph nodes not assessed clinically
	cM0	Chest x-ray negative
Clinical Stage Group	Unstageable (see note below)	
Pathologic TNM	ypT3b	Extensive tumor involvement of pelvis and abdomen after neoadjuvant treatment
	ypNX	No pathologic assessment of lymph nodes
	ypM1	Parenchymal liver nodules seen after neoadjuvant treatment
Pathologic Stage Group	yIV	
CS Schema used: Ovary		
CS Tumor Size	016	Tumor area described as 1.6 cm per path report
CS Extension	730	Visible tumor implants in pelvis, size not stated; tumor outside of pelvis (appendix and omentum) confirmed microscopically
CS TS/Ext Eval	6	Based on surgical resection after neoadjuvant therapy
CS Lymph Nodes	999	Lymph node status unknown; cannot use inaccessible sites rule due to carcinomatosis at time of diagnosis
CS Reg Nodes Eval	0	Based on non-invasive clinical assessment
Reg Nodes Pos	98	No lymph nodes removed for examination
Reg Nodes Exam	00	No lymph nodes examined
CS Mets at Dx	40	Parenchymal liver metastases described by surgeon
CS Mets at Dx–Bone	0	No bone metastases
CS Mets at Dx–Brain	0	No brain metastases
CS Mets at Dx–Liver	1	Liver metastases
CS Mets at Dx–Lung	0	No lung metastases
CS Mets Eval	6	Based on surgical observation after neoadjuvant therapy
SSF1 CA-125	010	Elevated
SSF2 FIGO Stage	999	FIGO stage not documented
SSF3 Resid Tum Stat/Size after Cytoreduction	020	All visible tumor greater than 2 mm removed (except liver nodules in parenchyma that are distant metastases)

Case 9, continued

SSF4 Tum Location after Cytoreduction	991	Residual tumor, location not stated, and neoadjuvant chemotherapy given
SSF5 Malig Ascites	980	980 milliliters or more

This patient had known abdominal involvement and had chemotherapy preoperatively. At surgery, metastases inside the liver were noted that had not been noted clinically. The Eval codes for CS Extension and Mets at Dx should identify that this patient had neoadjuvant treatment. In the case of the liver metastases, these were more extensive after the chemotherapy than previously suspected. Visualizing the liver metastases is part of surgical-pathologic staging, even though they were not biopsied or removed. The operative report stated that all tumor was removed down to 2 mm but does not state the location of the residual. Two liters (2000 ml) of ascites were removed by paracentesis, but the largest exact volume that can be coded is 979 ml, so SSF5 must be coded as 980 (980 milliliters or more).
This case will map to ypT3NOS cN0 ypM1 Stage Group IV.

—— CASE 10 ——

Site Code	C58.9	Placenta
Histology	9105	Epithelioid trophoblastic tumor
Behavior	3	Invasive
Grade/differentiation	9	Grade not stated
Grade Path Value	Blank	Does not apply
Grade Path System	Blank	Does not apply
Lymph Vascular Invasion	9	Lymph-vascular invasion not mentioned in path report
Ambiguous Terminology	0	Conclusive terminology
Date Conclusive Terminol	Blank	Diagnosis made by conclusive terminology
Date Conclus Dx Flag	11	Not applicable
Multiplicity Counter	01	One tumor only
Date Multiple Tumors	Blank	Not applicable
Date Mult Tumors Flag	15	Single tumor only (multiplicity counter is coded 01)
Type Mult Tum as 1 Prim	00	Single tumor
Summary Stage	1	Localized
Clinical TNM	cTX	Tumor cannot be assessed clinically
	cNX	Lymph nodes not assessed clinically
	cM0	Liver metastases ruled out. Complete radiographic evaluation negative
Clinical Stage Group	Unstageable	
Pathologic TNM	pT1	Tumor confined to uterus
	pN [blank]	N field not used for this site
	M0	Complete radiographic evaluation of mets negative
Pathologic Stage Group	IA (low risk)	

CS Schema used: Placenta

CS Tumor Size	999	Tumor size not stated
CS Extension	300	Localized, NOS (placenta not mentioned in path report)
CS TS/Ext Eval	3	Based on pathology
CS Lymph Nodes	988	Not applicable
CS Reg Nodes Eval	9	Does not apply
Reg Nodes Pos	99	Not applicable
Reg Nodes Exam	99	Not applicable

Case 10, continued

CS Mets at Dx	00	Complete radiographic evaluation negative
CS Mets at Dx–Bone	0	No bone metastases
CS Mets at Dx–Brain	0	No brain metastases
CS Mets at Dx–Liver	0	No liver metastases
CS Mets at Dx–Lung	0	No lung metastases
CS Mets Eval	0	Based on imaging
SSF1 Prognostic Score	010	Prognostic scoring index 7 or less (low risk)
SSF2 FIGO Stage	999	FIGO stage not documented

The clinician did not give a prognostic scoring index value, but based on the information in the case, it would be counted as age > 40 = 1; antecedent pregnancy—abortion = 1; months from pregnancy < 4 = 0; pretreatment HCG—>100,000 = 4; metastases—none = 0; largest tumor size—3-<5 cm = 1; number of mets—none = 0; previous failed chemotherapy—none = 0. Total score 7.
This case will map to pT1 NA cM0 Stage Group IA.

—— CASE 11 ——

Site Code	C56.9	Ovary, NOS
Histology	8260	Papillary carcinoma (code from addendum)
Behavior	3	Invasive
Grade/differentiation	4	Stated as high grade
Grade Path Value	Blank	Does not apply
Grade Path System	Blank	Does not apply
Lymph Vascular Invasion	9	Lymph-vascular invasion not mentioned in path report
Ambiguous Terminology	0	Conclusive terminology
Date Conclusive Terminol	Blank	Diagnosis made by conclusive terminology
Date Conclus Dx Flag	11	Not applicable
Multiplicity Counter	01	One tumor only
Date Multiple Tumors	Blank	Not applicable
Date Mult Tumors Flag	15	Single tumor only (multiplicity counter is coded 01)
Type Mult Tum as 1 Prim	00	Single tumor
Summary Stage	4	Regional direct extension and lymph nodes
Clinical TNM	cTX	No assessment of ovaries
	cNX	No assessment of lymph nodes
	cM0	Chest x-ray negative
Clinical Stage Group	Unstageable	
Pathologic TNM	pT3	Metastatic carcinoma seen in small bowel (abdominal) mesenteric fat, size of metastasis not stated
	pN1	Periaortic lymph nodes involved
	M0	Clinical evaluation of mets negative
Pathologic Stage Group	IIIC	
CS Schema used: Ovary		
CS Tumor Size	160	Tumor size stated as 16 cm in surgery observation
CS Extension	730	Tumor in small bowel (abdominal) mesenteric fat per path report, size not stated
CS TS/Ext Eval	3	Based on pathology
CS Lymph Nodes	200	Periaortic nodes involved
CS Reg Nodes Eval	3	Lymph nodes removed for examination

Case 11, continued

Reg Nodes Pos	02	Two lymph nodes positive
Reg Nodes Exam	06	4 periaortic + 2 right pelvic = 6 nodes examined
CS Mets at Dx	00	Chest x-ray negative
CS Mets at Dx–Bone	0	No bone metastases
CS Mets at Dx–Brain	0	No brain metastases
CS Mets at Dx–Liver	0	No liver metastases
CS Mets at Dx–Lung	0	No lung metastases
CS Mets Eval	0	Based on imaging
SSF1 CA-125	010	Elevated
SSF2 FIGO Stage	330	Stated as FIGO IIIC
SSF3 Resid Tum Stat/Size after Cytoreduction	992	Procedure described as optimal debulking
SSF4 Tum Location after Cytoreduction	990	Residual tumor, location not stated, without neoadjuvant chemotherapy
SSF5 Malig Ascites	992	Ascites present (abdominal fluid), suspicious (no information whether malignant or non-malignant)

Discontinuous metastases to endometrium and myometrium are reported in T category and CS Extension and would be Stage IIA if small bowel mesenteric fat and lymph nodes were negative. The pathology report also states there is metastasis to the mesenteric fat, but the size of the metastasis is not stated (T3, NOS). The positive lymph nodes upstage the case to Stage Group IIIC. The operative procedure indicates optimal debulking (tumor left behind but no larger than 1 cm) but does not state the location of the residual.
This case will map to pT3, NOS pN1 cM0 Stage Group IIIC.

—— CASE 12 ——

Site Code	C56.9	Ovary, NOS
Histology	8951	Malignant mixed mesodermal tumor
Behavior	3	Invasive
Grade/differentiation	9	Grade not stated
Grade Path Value	Blank	Does not apply
Grade Path System	Blank	Does not apply
Lymph Vascular Invasion	9	Lymph-vascular invasion not mentioned in path report
Ambiguous Terminology	0	Conclusive terminology
Date Conclusive Terminol	Blank	Diagnosis made by conclusive terminology
Date Conclus Dx Flag	11	Not applicable
Multiplicity Counter	01	One tumor only
Date Multiple Tumors	Blank	Not applicable
Date Mult Tumors Flag	15	Single tumor only (multiplicity counter is coded 01)
Type Mult Tum as 1 Prim	00	Single tumor
Summary Stage	2	Regional direct extension
Clinical TNM	cTX	No clinical assessment of ovaries
	cNX	Lymph nodes not assessed clinically
	cM0	Based on clinical assessment
Clinical Stage Group	Unstageable	
Pathologic TNM	pT2b	Tumor in broad ligament (confined to pelvis)
	pN0	No lymph nodes involved
	M0	Based on clinical assessment
Pathologic Stage Group	IIB	

Case 12, continued

CS Schema used: Ovary

CS Tumor Size	999	Tumor size not stated
CS Extension	600	Involvement of broad ligament (other structures in pelvis)
CS TS/Ext Eval	3	Based on surgical resection
CS Lymph Nodes	000	No lymph nodes involved
CS Reg Nodes Eval	3	Based on resected specimen
Reg Nodes Pos	00	No lymph nodes involved
Reg Nodes Exam	06	Six lymph nodes examined
CS Mets at Dx	00	No distant metastases
CS Mets at Dx–Bone	0	No bone metastases
CS Mets at Dx–Brain	0	No brain metastases
CS Mets at Dx–Liver	0	No liver metastases
CS Mets at Dx–Lung	0	No lung metastases
CS Mets Eval	0	Based on clinical assessment
SSF1 CA-125	010	Elevated
SSF2 FIGO Stage	999	FIGO stage not documented
SSF3 Resid Tum Stat/Size after Cytoreduction	000	No gross residual at completion of surgery
SSF4 Tum Location after Cytoreduction	999	Not documented (see comment below)
SSF5 Malig Ascites	999	Ascites not documented

Malignant mixed mesodermal tumor of the ovary is stageable in the TNM system. The only metastases are in the pelvis, in the broad ligament (T2b and CS Extension code 600). The surgeon states that all visible (gross) tumor was removed so SSF3 is 000. However, there is no corresponding code to indicate no residual tumor in SSF4. According to the response to several questions in the CAnswer Forum, use code 999 (not documented) in CS version 0203 when there is no residual tumor after the cytoreduction sugery. In CSv0203, there is not a good code to indicate that there were no ascites, but the response to a question in CAnswer Forum says to use 999 (not documented) as the best available code.

This case will map to pT2b pN0 cM0 Stage Group IIB.

BENIGN, BORDERLINE, AND MALIGNANT BRAIN AND CENTRAL NERVOUS SYSTEM TUMORS

More than 243,000 central nervous system tumors are estimated to be diagnosed in the United States each year. Of these, about two-thirds (180,000) are metastatic and accessioned into registries according to the site of origin. Of the remaining 63,000 primary brain tumors, almost two thirds (over 39,300 or 62%) are benign and borderline, and the balance (estimated at 29,700 for 2010 or 38%) are malignant. Overall, intracranial tumors comprise about 85% of all CNS tumors and spinal cord tumors about 15%. Meningeal tumors are usually reported with the part of the CNS that is involved (cerebral or spinal). Cranial nerve tumors are fairly rare.

Malignant brain tumors have been reportable to cancer registries for decades. It has only been since 2004 that benign and borderline tumors of the brain and central nervous system (CNS) have been reportable to the major population-based cancer registries and the Commission on Cancer, although these tumors have been reportable to various state central registries for a number of years.

CNS tumors as a group constitute about 2% of adult cancers and about 20% of childhood cancers. For both new and experienced registrars, the brain is usually a mystery for several reasons: cases are relatively rare in most facilities and central registries, and the anatomy and terminology are unfamiliar. The diagnosis is frequently made via radiologic studies and the patient may then have to be transferred to a facility with neurosurgical capabilities. Let's start with some basic definitions.

Terms referring to the brain and spinal cord tend to be used interchangeably, but every attempt has been made to use them consistently in this chapter.

- CNS—refers to the central nervous system as a whole (brain and spinal cord)
- Brain—technically refers to the structures within the skull or cranium.
- The word roots for the brain are a combination of Latin and Greek terms.
    - Celphalo-, encephalo-, and cerebro- — the upper part of the brain
    - Cranio- — usually the bony structures that surround the brain
    - Cerebello- — the lower part of the brain
    - Glio- — the cells that make up the brain
- Meningo- — the covering tissues of the brain and spinal cord
- Spino-, myelo- and medullo- — the cord itself
- The spinal cord—the giant nerve—is different from the bony spine or spinal column that surrounds it

This chapter will not cover metastases to the brain from other primary sites, nor tumors of the autonomic nervous system (which manages involuntary actions), the peripheral nervous system in general, or the spinal nerves, all of which are coded to C47._ and are outside the brain and spinal cord.

ETIOLOGY AND NATURAL HISTORY

Little is known about the etiology of CNS tumors. Ionizing radiation, chemicals, and certain genetic syndromes have been associated with an increased risk of tumors. Unfortunately, the five year relative survival rate for malignant CNS tumors is only about 34%.

ICD-O-3 CODES

ICD-O-3	TERM
Cerebral Meninges	
C70.0	Cerebral meninges
C70.1	Spinal meninges
C70.9	Meninges, NOS
Brain	
C71.0	Cerebrum
C71.1	Frontal lobe
C71.2	Temporal lobe
C71.3	Parietal lobe
C71.4	Occipital lobe
C71.5	Ventricle, NOS
C71.6	Cerebellum, NOS
C71.7	Brain stem
C71.8	Overlapping lesion of brain
C71.9	Brain, NOS
Spinal cord and other central nervous system	
C72.0	Spinal cord
C72.1	Cauda equina
C72.2	Olfactory nerve
C72.3	Optic nerve
C72.4	Acoustic nerve
C72.5	Cranial nerve, NOS
C72.8	Overlapping lesion of brain and central nervous system
C72.9	Nervous system, NOS

ANATOMY OF THE CENTRAL NERVOUS SYSTEM

Figure 1 shows the structure of a typical neuron. This basic introduction to the structure of individual neurons will help you understand the anatomy of the central nervous system.

Figure 1. Structure of a Neuron

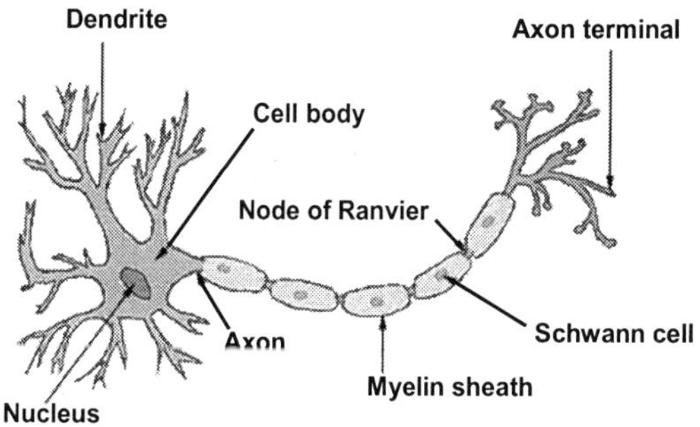

A neuron is comprised of a cell body containing the cell nucleus and long projections called either dendrites or axons.

- The cell body contains a number of structures necessary to maintain cell life. In the brain, the cell bodies form the "grey matter" on the outer surface of the brain. The cell body's nucleus does not divide and multiply as occurs in most other cells. Consequently, damage to one or more neurons is very slow to heal and, in fact, may never heal. There are several different types of neurons, each of which has a specific function within various locations in the body.
- The long nerve fibers extending from the cell body are of two types.
  - The branch-like dendrites receive impulses from other neurons.

Anatomy, ***continued***

  - The longer axon carries nerve impulses away from the cell. Axons can be as long as three feet in humans. In the brain, the axons and their supporting cells form the "white matter" of the brain itself.
- The axon terminals or synaptic knobs contain sacs of chemicals called neurotransmitters that transmit impulses from one cell to another across tiny spaces called synapses.

Neurons do not commonly develop tumors. Instead, tumors generally originate in the the support (glial) cells. For example, the myelin sheath formed by support cells consists of concentric layers of white fatty substance that help insulate and protect the axons. The myelin sheath is interrupted at regular intervals by the nodes of Ranvier, which also help conduct nerve impulses.

Figure 2. Central Nervous System: Brain and Spinal Cord

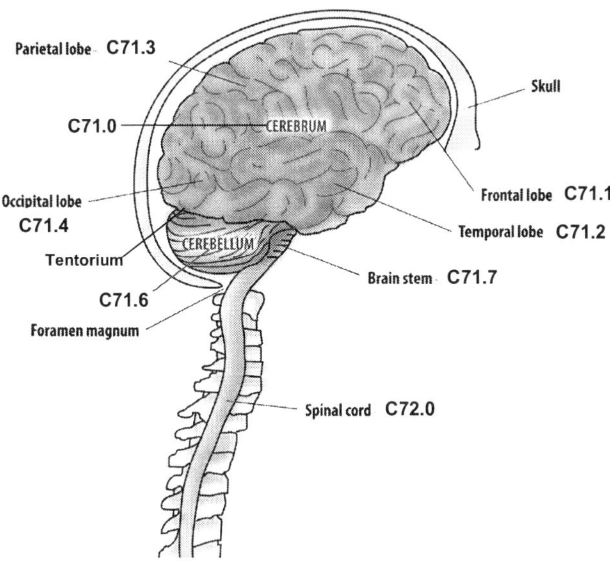

The central nervous system includes the brain, cranial nerves, and spinal cord (Figure 2), plus the intracranial endocrine glands (pineal and pituitary) and the meninges covering the brain and spinal cord. The sites within the brain are coded to C71._, and the spinal cord and cranial nerves are coded to C72._. Meninges are coded to C70._, and the intracranial endocrine glands are coded to C75._.

The major parts of the brain are the ***cerebrum*** and ***cerebellum***, ***diencephalon*** (thalamus and hypothalamus) and ***brainstem***. All of the parts of the brain are encased by bone.

Figure 3. Posterior View of Central Nervous System

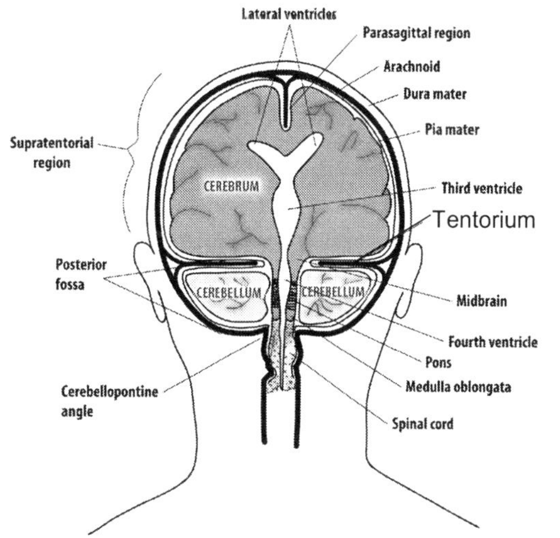

Figure 3 is a view from the back of the head looking forward and shows an important landmark in the brain: the ***tentorium cerebelli.*** This is a flap or sleeve of meninges between the cerebrum and cerebellum.

- Structures above the tentorium cerebelli are called *supratentorial*.
- Structures in the cerebellum and brain stem are called *infratentorial* or posterior fossa.
- Problems arise when tumors start to expand inside the bony skull that protects the brain. Intracranial space is much more limited below the tentorium than it is above the tentorium, and smaller tumors in

Note: Unless otherwise identified, the source of the illustrations in this chapter is: Centers for Disease Control and Prevention. *Data Collection of Primary Central Nervous System Tumors. National Program of Cancer Registries Training Materials.* Atlanta, Georgia: Department of Health and Human Services, Centers for Disease Control and Prevention, 2004. Used with permission.

Anatomy, ***continued***

the cerebellum and brain stem have a much greater effect on surrounding tissues than tumors above the tentorium.

- Understanding whether a tumor is infra- or supratentorial is important in Summary Staging as well as the Collaborative Stage Data Collection System (CS).
- 70% of childhood brain tumors are infratentorial, while 70% of adult brain tumors are supratentorial.
- Also visible in Figure 3 is another landmark, the ***cerebellopontine angle***. This is the point where the cerebellum and brain stem connect with the spinal cord.

Figure 4. Intracranial CNS: Cerebrum and Supratentorial Structures

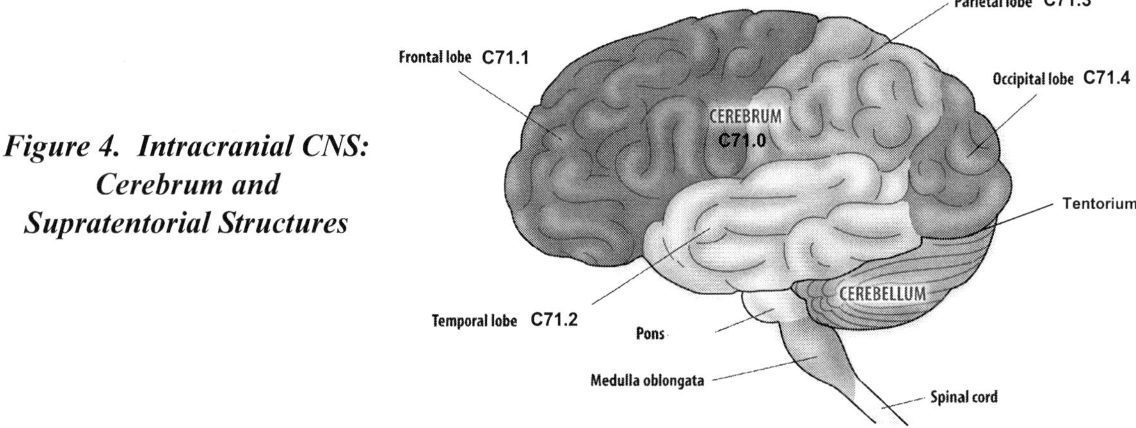

Figure 4 shows the larger, upper part of the brain. This is the ***cerebrum***, which is what most people think of when they hear the term brain. The cerebrum is the largest area of the brain and consists of four pairs of lobes. The lobe names correspond to the bones of the skull that protect them: frontal, parietal, temporal and occipital. Each lobe of the cerebrum has its own ICD-O-3 code.

- The ***frontal lobe*** (C71.1) is associated with motor activity, speech, thought, emotion and skilled movement.
- The ***parietal lobe*** (C71.3) handles body sensitivities (pain, touch, temperature).
- The ***temporal lobe*** (C71.2) is the primary region of the acoustic (hearing) system, handling memory storage and the recognition of sounds.
- The ***occipital lobe*** (C71.4) is the primary region detecting and processing visual images.

The lobes are separated by valleys or grooves called sulci (if shallow) or fissures (if deep). There is a central longitudinal fissure that divides the cerebrum into right and left hemispheres. The raised areas of the brain are called gyri, convolutions or ridges. The more pronounced of these gyri and sulci have specific names that you may read in the operative report.

Figure 5. Functional Areas of Cerebrum

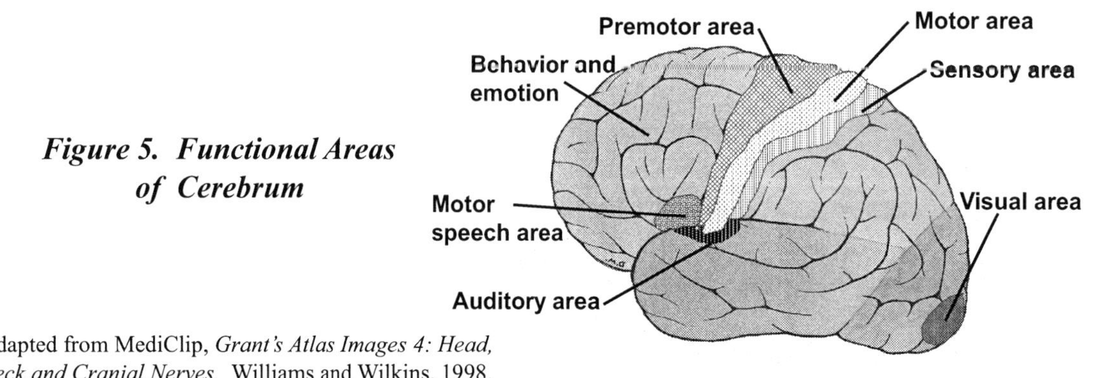

Adapted from MediClip, *Grant's Atlas Images 4: Head, Neck and Cranial Nerves.* Williams and Wilkins, 1998.

Anatomy, ***continued***

The functional areas of the cerebrum have been mapped (Figure 5), and the functions do not always fall neatly into a single lobe. The sensory area processes physical sensations like touch and pain. The visual area in the occipital lobe processes color, shape, movement, and visual association. The auditory area in the temporal lobe recognizes pitch and rhythm as speech, music or noise and helps translate words into thoughts. This is also the memory bank area of the brain. The motor area spans the posterior frontal and anterior parietal lobes and controls voluntary contractions of muscles (basically crude movements). The premotor area in the frontal lobe controls fine movements and learned movements like typing or writing. At the bottom of Figure 6 is the cerebellum, which is infratentorial and not part of the cerebrum. The cerebellum controls motor function and movement, such as posture, walking, and balance.

Because the functions of various areas of the brain have been mapped, the patient's symptoms can contribute information for localizing the site of the tumor. In general, seizures, weakness, headaches, and nausea and vomiting are an indication of increased intracranial pressure (indicating the presence of a space-occupying lesion), but that doesn't help localize the tumor. Sensory changes can give more clues—whether there are auditory or visual disturbances, pain, memory loss, or confusion. All of these symptoms indicate a supratentorial lesion.

Problems with basic walking, spastic movement, and gait disturbances indicate an infratentorial lesion. Increased intracranial pressure from hydrocephalus, an accumulation of excess cerebrospinal fluid caused by a blockage in the normal CNS circulation, also indicates an infratentorial lesion.

Figure 6. Intracranial CNS: Cerebellum and Infratentorial Structures

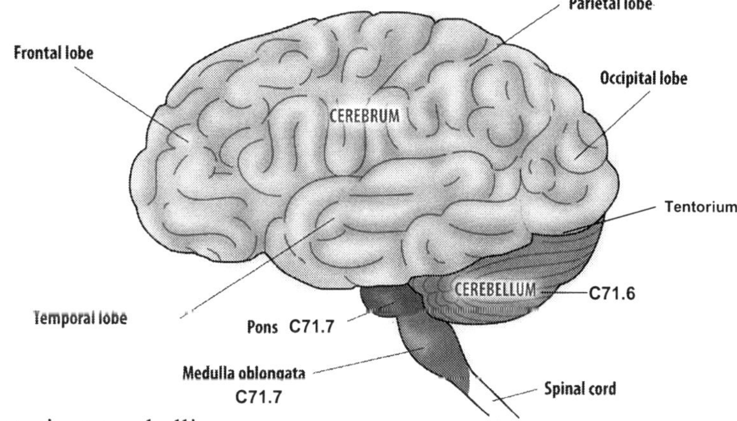

The primary structures below the tentorium cerebelli are the ***cerebellum***, ***pons***, and ***medulla oblongata*** (Figure 6). The cerebellum controls the body's muscle tone and intentional motor functions like walking or repetitive hand movements (like typing). The pons handles expression and eye movement and the medulla handles autonomic functions.

Figure 7 focuses on the ***brain stem***. The brain stem consists of the midbrain, pons, and medulla oblongata.

- The brain stem keeps the brain awake, regulates breathing, heart rate, hunger, thirst, sleep, posture and many other reflex activities including swallowing and vomiting. Damage to even a small area of the brainstem can be fatal.

Figure 7. Brain Stem

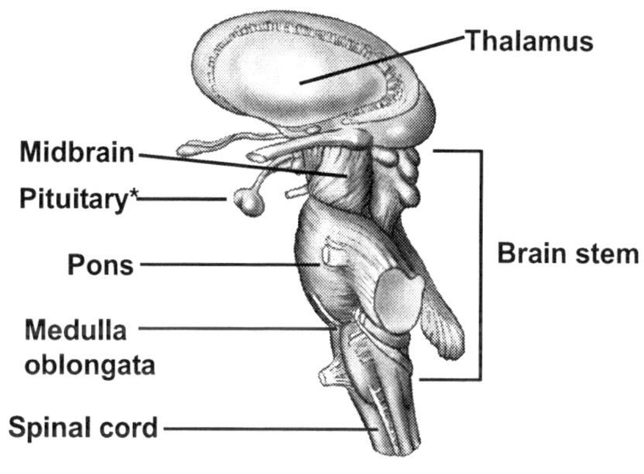

Adapted from MediClip, *Color Anatomy 2*. Williams and Wilkins, 1998.

Nervous Sys

Anatomy, *continued*

- ◦ The midbrain controls visual and auditory reflexes.
- ◦ The medulla oblongata takes care of regulating the heart rate and breathing rate.
- The spinal cord carries nerve impulses to all other parts of the body.
- The thalamus at the top of the brainstem is the relay center between the cerebrum, brain stem and spinal cord. Below the thalamus is the droplet shaped hypo-thalamus. These are discussed in more detail with the next figure.

Figure 8. Central Brain

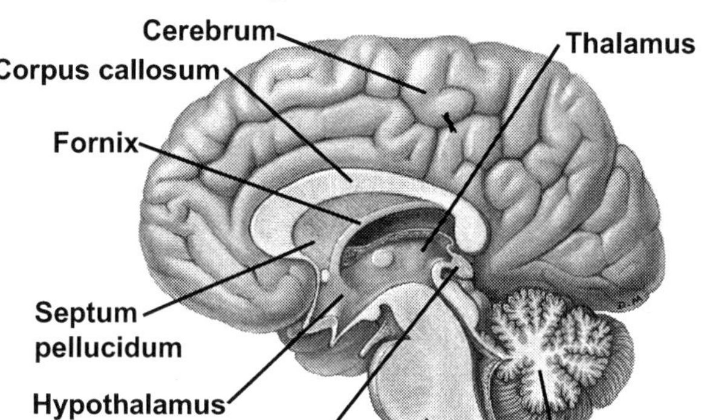

Adapted from MediClip, *Grant's Atlas Images 4: Head, Neck and Cranial Nerves.* Williams and Wilkins, 1998.

Deep within the innermost part of the brain (Figure 8) is the limbic system or central brain, home of the "fight or flight" reflex, survival behavior and other functions, such as memory, rage, and fright.

- The hypothalamus and thalamus, deep in the center of the brain, are parts of the diencephalon. These structures control mood, homeostasis and endocrine functions. The pituitary and pineal glands are part of this area as well.
  - ◦ The centrally located thalamus is the information relay center among all parts of the brain and the brain stem.
  - ◦ The hypothalamus, which is about the size of a lump of sugar, controls automatic body processes. Together with the pituitary gland, the hypothalamus regulates body temperature, food intake, water-salt balance, blood flow and the sleep-wake cycle.
- The hippocampus is for memory storage and learning.
- The fornix is the nerve pathway between the hippocampus, limbic system, and mammillary body and the thalamus.
- The corpus callosum is a bundle of nerve fibers in the center of the brain where impulses transfer from one hemisphere of the cerebrum to the other.
- Below that is the pituitary gland or "master gland" that controls the body's other endocrine glands. More on that later.
- At the lower left of Figure 8 is a cross section of the cerebellum, which looks much different from the gyri and sulci of the cerebrum.

The ventricular system (Figure 9) consists of four cavities and two narrow drains that allow the circulation of CSF.

- In the cerebrum, the right and left lateral ventricles contain thin-walled capillaries lined with epithelial cells. These tissues are the choroid plexuses that produce the cerebrospinal fluid (CSF). CSF drains from each of the lateral ventricles into the single third ventricle via the intraventricular foramen or foramen of Monro.
- Between the supratentorial third ventricle and the smaller

Figure 9. Ventricular System

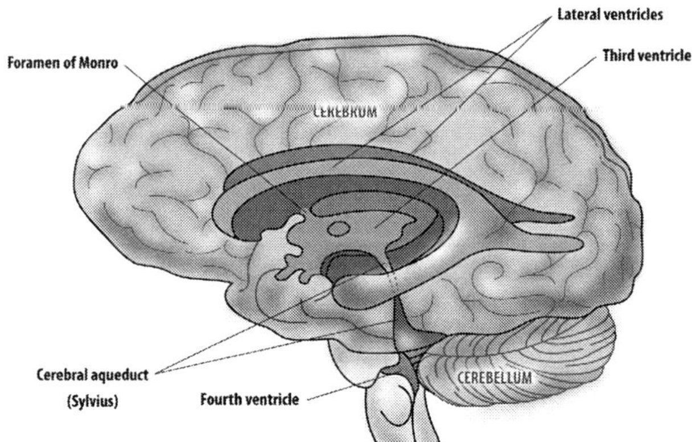

Figure 10. Circulation of Cerebrospinal Fluid

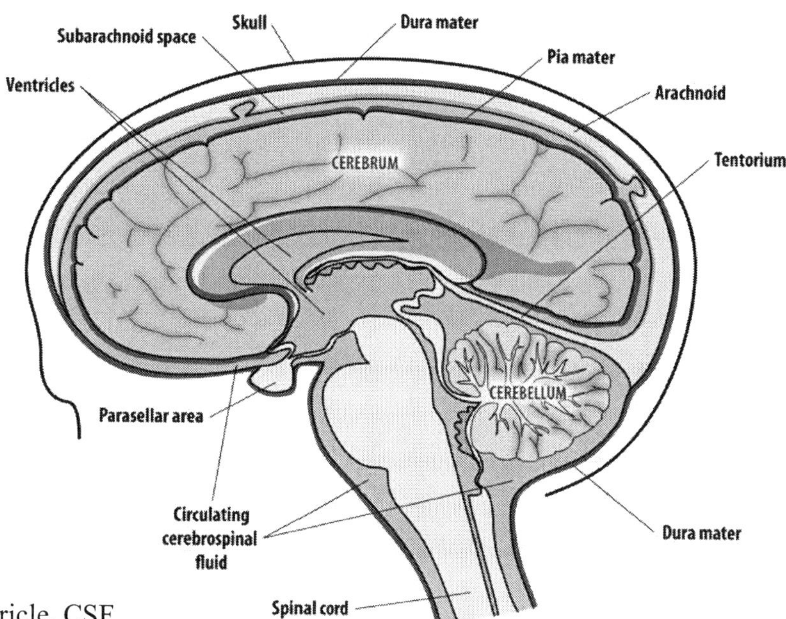

Anatomy, ***continued***

infratentorial fourth ventricle, CSF drains via the cerebral aqueduct or cerebral canal, also called the Aqueduct of Sylvius.

- A different view of the ventricles is shown in Figure 3. There you can see the relationships of the two lateral ventricles and the single third and fourth ventricles.

Figure 10 shows the many areas that are bathed in cerebrospinal fluid, which contains the glucose to nourish brain cells. The fluid also provides a cushion for the brain, supporting the weight of the brain and protecting it from injury during head trauma. As mentioned, CSF is made in the ventricles in the central part of the brain and specific areas called choroid plexus. CSF circulates all the way down to the end of the spinal cord. This is the path for "drop" metastases, which are malignant cells shed from intracranial tumors that filter out like sediment in the spinal cord and grow there as secondary sites.

A landmark that you may read about is the sellar or parasellar area. The pituitary gland (see Figure 15) sits in a deep pocket in the sphenoid bone called the sella turcica because it resembles a Turkish saddle. The name for the general area of the pituitary gland, parasellar area, comes from this structure.

Twelve pairs of ***cranial nerves*** attach to the base of the brain on the underside (Figure 11). Each pair innervates specific areas of the head, neck, and thorax. Some of these nerves relay sensory information, some motor information, some both. Remembering the 12 cranial nerves in order as shown in the figure has been a medical student's challenge for decades. One of the most common memory aids is 'On Old Olympus' Towering Tops A Finn And German Viewed Some Hops,' but there are a variety of others.

Figure 11. Cranial Nerves

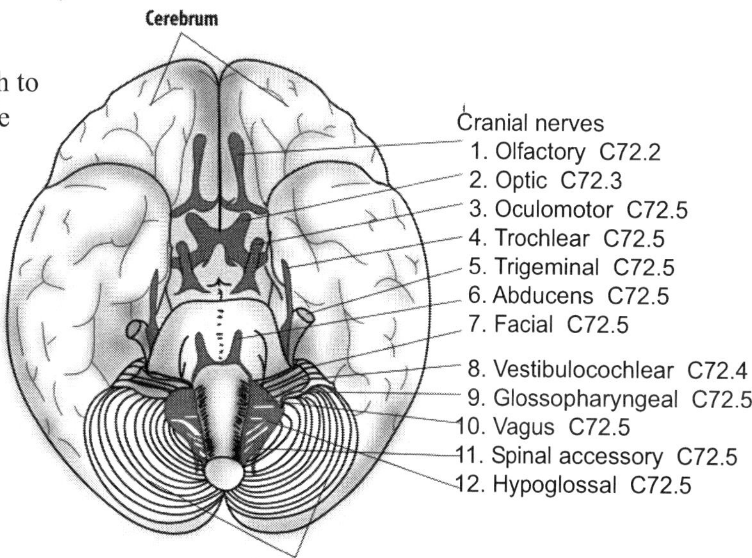

Anatomy, *continued*

In general, cranial nerve tumors are rare, but the type of sensory symptoms can provide clues as to which nerve is affected. Because most of these are long, cord-like nerves, the most likely type of tumor is the Schwannoma, originating from the Schwann cells that wrap around, insulate, and support the nerve axon. MPNST, malignant peripheral nerve sheath tumors, can develop in the peripheral nerves as well as the cranial and spinal nerves.

Meninges cover all parts of the central nervous system—cerebrum, cerebellum, brain stem and spinal cord. There are actually three layers—or *mater*—of meninges. Figure 12 is a cross section of the meningeal layers overlying the brain; the layers surrounding the spinal cord are discussed below.

- The ***dura*** (hard or tough) mater is the fibrous, tough, relatively thick outer layer that lines the skull. The dura mater contains the blood supply for the cranial bones.
- The middle layer of meninges, the ***arachnoid*** mater, is a spider-like web of tissue containing the blood vessels that service brain tissue.
- Between the arachnoid and the pia mater is the subarachnoid space that is filled with cerebrospinal fluid.
- The innermost layer, the ***pia*** (tender) mater is the delicate and highly vascular inner layer in direct contact with the brain and spinal cord.

The meninges are the tissue that develops meningiomas. Meningiomas are most common in adults and rare in children. Females tend to have more meningiomas than males.

Figure 12 also shows the relationship of the meninges, grey matter and white matter in a portion of brain.

- The thick dura mater is visible next to the skull bone.
- The pia mater is a very thin line right next to the grey matter.
- In between are the reticulated or web-like arachnoid and the subarachnoid space that contains the cerebrospinal fluid and blood vessels. The arachnoid projections in the upper left of the figure reabsorb CSF for recirculation. The large venous sinus is a widened area of a vein within the dura mater.
- In the brain itself, the grey matter is 2 - 6 millimeters thick and made up of groups of nerve cell bodies. There are over 300 million nerve cell bodies and their axons in the brain.

Figure 12. Layers of Meninges (Cross Section) with Grey Matter and White Matter

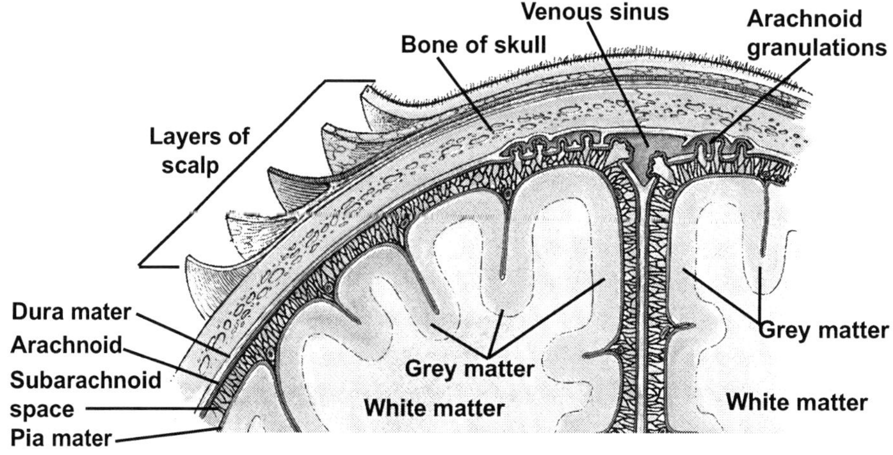

Adapted from MediClip, *Grant's Atlas Images 4: Head, Neck and Cranial Nerves.* Williams and Wilkins, 1998.

Figure 13. Cross Section of Spinal Cord and Vertebra

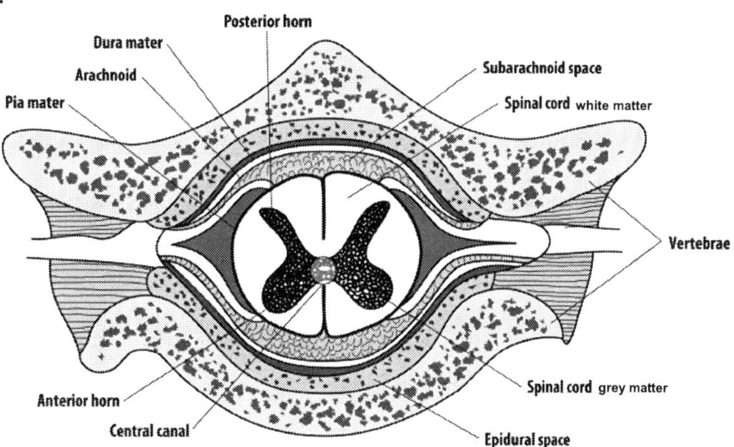

Anatomy, ***continued***

- The white matter consists of myelin covered axons (nerve fibers) extending from the nerve cell bodies in the grey matter. These axons or nerve fibers are insulated by myelin sheaths to speed transmission of nerve impulses from the brain.

Figure 13 shows a horizontal slice through the spinal cord and vertebra. The bone, the contents of the spinal cord itself, and the three layers of meninges that surround the spinal cord can be seen, along with the sub-arachnoid space that contains the circulating cerebrospinal fluid.

- Unlike the brain, the grey matter (the nerve cell bodies) is on the inside of the spinal cord while the white matter is on the outside. The white matter contains the tracts of myelinated axons that relay impulses between the spinal cord and brain. The grey matter includes both axons and glial cells.

Figure 14 shows the spinal nerves and cauda equina.

- The spinal cord is about 17 inches long, about as thick as a finger, and occupies the upper two-thirds of the vertebral column.
- At the end of the spinal cord is the cauda equina, a collection of spinal roots that descend from the lower part of the spinal cord and occupy the vertebral canal below the cord. Their appearance resembles the tail of a horse. The cauda equina has a different ICD-O-3 topography number than the spinal cord. Benign, borderline and malignant tumors of the spinal cord and cauda equina are reportable to all cancer registries.
- Along the spinal cord there are 31 pairs (right and left) of spinal nerves that carry nerve impulses to all parts of the body. Each side of each pair consists of a sensory nerve root to carry sensation (position, pain) to the spinal cord and a motor nerve root to conduct impulses from the central nervous system to control both voluntary and involuntary movement. Tumors of the spinal nerves are not reportable as central nervous system tumors; only malignant tumors of the spinal nerves are reportable, and are coded to C47._.

Figure 14. Spinal Nerves and Cauda Equina

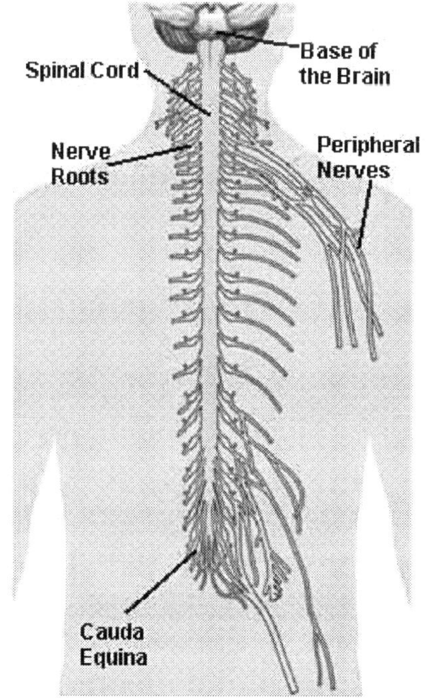

Source: training.seer.cancer.gov

Nervous Sys

Figure 15. Pineal and Pituitary Glands

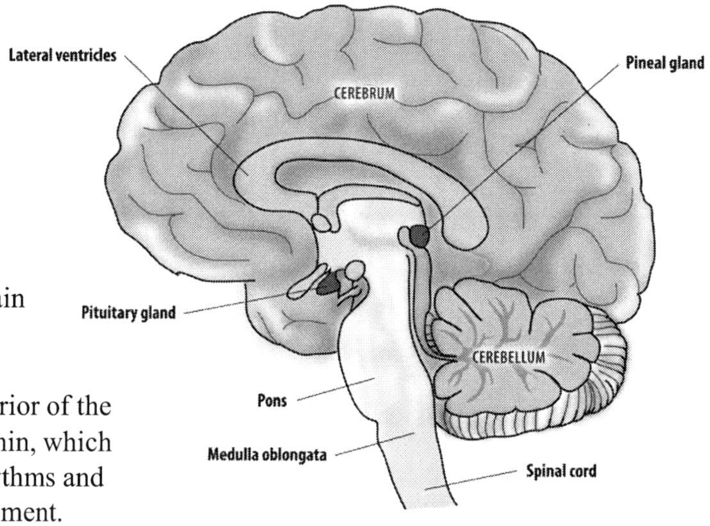

Anatomy, *continued*

Two endocrine glands deep in the brain (Figure 15) can develop papillomas, adenomas, and carcinomas.

- The pineal gland in the posterior of the central brain secretes melatonin, which regulates biological body rhythms and contributes to sexual development.
- The pituitary gland is pea sized but is commonly called the "master gland" because it secretes hormones that control other endocrine glands in the body when instructed by the hypothalamus. Despite its size, there are two major functional areas, the anterior and posterior pituitary. The pituitary gland is enormously complex because each of the hormones is created by unique type of cell. For example, the anterior pituitary contains at least six distinctive endocrinocytes. The cells that secrete thyroid-stimulating hormone do not also secrete growth hormone, and they have receptors for thyroid-releasing hormone, not growth hormone-releasing hormone. Therefore, a variety of endocrine tumors can develop in the pituitary gland.

MULTIPLE PRIMARY RULES

There are separate multiple primary and histology coding rules for benign/borderline and malignant central nervous system tumors. The benign/borderline rules were established when benign and borderline CNS tumors became reportable in 2004. The 2007 rules bring malignant CNS tumors into parallel with the benign/borderline rules.

Unique Features Of Malignant CNS Tumor Rules

- 10 multiple primaries rules
- Time between diagnoses is not a factor for malignant CNS tumors.
- Malignant/invasive CNS tumors are counted separately from benign/borderline CNS tumors.
- Progression of a malignant glial tumor to glioblastoma multiforme is not abstracted again as a new primary.
- Histology coding rules in TWO sections (11 rules total)
  - 6 rules (H1 – H6) in Single Tumor
  - 5 rules (H7 – H11) in Multiple Tumors Abstracted as a Single Primary
- Histology coding rules refer to two tables in the site-specific Terms and Definitions
  - Table 1. Neuroepithelial Malignant Brain and Central Nervous System Tumors
  - Table 2. Non-neuroepithelial Malignant Brain and Central Nervous System Tumors

Summary of Malignant Multiple Primary Rules

This is only a summary of the multiple primary rules for malignant brain and central nervous system. Details of the rules are provided in the official published documents available from www.seer.cancer.gov/tools/mphrules. Refer to the General Instructions for information about coding more specific terms, missing pathology or cytology reports, and other aspects of the rules for this and

Multiple Primary Rules, *continued*

other sets of site-specific rules. ***Always*** refer to the site-specific rules themselves in your preferred format when determining how many abstracts to prepare or the correct histology code for an individual abstract. The published rules include more discussion, examples, and notes. In the rules, the term "brain" includes all parts of the central nervous system.

The standard three modules of the multiple primaries rules are present: unknown if single or multiple tumors, single tumor, and multiple tumors.

- Count only macroscopic, non-metastatic tumors when deciding which module applies.

The first module, unknown if single or multiple tumors, includes an additional rule because of the reportable benign and borderline tumors that also develop in the central nervous system:

M1. Invasive (/3) brain tumor(s) and either benign (/0) or borderline (/1) = always multiple
M2. Number of tumors (single or multiple) can't be determined = single

The CNS rules for single tumors are the same as most other sets of rules:

M3. Single tumor = single

The multiple tumors module therefore starts at rule M4. Many of the determinants for the multiple tumors rules are based on the histology of the individual tumors. The priority of the multiple tumors rules is as follows:

M4. Invasive (/3) brain tumor(s) and either benign (/0) or borderline (/1) = always multiple
M5. Topography different at second or third character = multiple
M6. Glioblastoma multiforme following any glial tumor = single
M7. Histology codes in same branch of Chart 1 or Chart 2 = single
M8. Histology codes in different branches of Chart 1 or Chart 2 = multiple
M9. Histology codes other than in Chart 1 or chart 2 that are different at 1st, 2nd, or 3rd digit = multiple
M10. All other scenarios = single

Summary of Benign/Borderline Multiple Primary Rules

The benign/borderline multiple primary rules were republished in late 2007 in the same format as the malignant multiple primary rules for CNS and other solid tumors.

The first module, unknown if single or multiple tumors, is similar to the rule in most other site-specific modules.

M1. Number of tumors (single or multiple) can't be determined = single

The CNS rules for single tumors are the same as most other sets of rules:

M2. Single tumor = single

The benign/borderline multiple tumors rules are very similar to the malignant multiple tumors rules. They are based on the histology of the individual tumors, but also take into consideration the laterality and the exact locations of the multiple tumors. The priority of the multiple tumors rules is:

M3. Invasive (/3) brain tumor(s) and either benign (/0) or borderline (/1) = always multiple
M4. Topography different at 2nd, 3rd, or 4th character = multiple
Note: The original rule was corrected in an errata published in February 2008 adding the 4th character difference to the multiple primaries rule for benign/borderline tumors.
M5. Different laterality (Table 1) = multiple
M6. Choroid plexus tumors: atypical 9390/1 after 9390/0 = single
M7. Neurofibromatosis 9540/1 after neurofibroma 9540/0 = single
M8. Histology codes in same branch of Chart 1 = single

Multiple Primary Rules, ***continued***

M9. Histology codes in different branches of Chart 1 = multiple
M10. Histology codes where one is not in Chart 1 = multiple
M11. Histology codes are different at 1st, 2nd, or 3rd digit = multiple
M12. All other scenarios = single

HISTOLOGIC CELL TYPES OF CNS TUMORS

Tumors of the central nervous system are grouped by their tissue of origin. The majority of tumors arise in neuroepithelial tissue, the large category that includes astrocytomas and ependymomas.

Malignant neuroepithelial tumors include:

- Gliomas (938_–948_)—represent more than 50% of all primary tumors. Astrocytomas are the most prevalent within this category, comprising 20% of all brain tumors. Astrocytomas are most common in adults. Astrocytes are so-named because their numerous dendrites make the cells look like stars. Astrocytes are the most common of the support cells in the CNS. Some of the dendrites in an astrocyte connect with capillaries and help regulate the flow of substances between neurons and the blood. Others connect to other astrocytes and neurons to protect and support the neurons.
  - Juvenile or pilocytic astrocytoma (9421/1)—a slow-growing tumor that occurs most frequently in children. Until the implementation of ICD-O-3, juvenile or pilocytic astrocytoma was considered malignant. And now, even though it is coded as borderline in ICD-O-3, in North America it is still to be reported as a malignancy for historical consistency (9421/3).
  - Low-grade astrocytomas—more aggressive than pilocytic astrocytomas but less aggressive than anaplastic astrocytomas.
  - Anaplastic astrocytomas (9401)—highly aggressive.
  - Glioblastoma multiforme (9440)—the most aggressive, rapidly growing tumor of this group. Glioblastomas account for 30% of all intracranial tumors.
  - Ependymomas (9391 for NOS)—arise from the cells that line the ventricles and can occur in all ages.
  - There are several subtypes of ependymomas: myxopapillary (9394), papillary (9393), and subependymoma (9383).
- Oligodendrogliomas (9450, 9451, 9460)—vary in grade of malignancy, and prognosis is related to grade. Oligodendrocytes have branchlike extensions that wrap around axons in the central nervous system. They form the myelin sheaths that cover more than one axon at a time. Oligo- means "few"; there are fewer dendrites on this type of glial cell than on an astrocyte.
- Mixed gliomas (9382)—can be combinations of two or even three cell types—astrocytoma, ependymoma, and/or oligodendroglioma. The proportion of the various cells determines prognosis.
- Medulloblastoma (9470, 9471)—a type of primitive neuroectodermal tumor that arises in the posterior fossa, usually in children and young adults, and grows rapidly, sometimes spreading to the spinal axis.

Ependymomas, oligodendrogliomas, and medulloblastomas comprise 9% of all primary brain tumors. Ependymal cells are generally cuboidal ciliated cells that line the cavities of the brain and spinal canal in a single layer. The cilia or "hairs" help circulate the cerebrospinal fluid. Specialized ependymal cells in the ventricles are part of the choroid plexus that generates cerebrospinal fluid, but the choroid plexus itself is considered non-glial.

Histologic Cell Types, *continued*

Primitive neuroectodermal tumor (PNET) (9473) is an embryonal subtype of neuroepithelial tumor, also known as central or supratentorial PNET because of its most common location. Do not confuse central PNET with the pathologically and clinically distinct peripheral primitive neuroectodermal tumor, (pPNET, but also sometimes abbreviated as PNET; 9364), which arises in the soft tissues of the chest, pelvis and other sites. Be aware of the site of origin—do not code all PNETs to 9473.

Other types of neuroepithelial tumors include malignant DNET (dysembryoplastic neuroepithelial tumor), astroblastoma, desmoplastic infantile ganglioglioma, and neurocytoma.

Benign and borderline neuroepithelial (glial) tumors consist of the ependymomas (subependymoma 9383/1; myxopapillary ependymoma 9394/1 and choroid glioma 9444/1) and the neuronal and neuronal-glial neoplasms (subependymal giant cell astrocytoma 9384/1, desmoplastic infantile astrocytoma 9412/1, dysembryoplastic neuroepithelial tumor {DNET} 9413/0, gliofibroma 9442/1, ganglioglioma 9505/1, and central neurocytoma 9506/1).

Malignant non-neuroepithelial tumors include:

- Meningiomas (953_)—arise from the coverings of the brain and spinal cord and account for 18% of all CNS tumors. They are slow growing and vary in behavior from well-differentiated to very aggressive. There are many descriptive terms and several ICD-O-3 codes for various types of meningiomas: meningoepithelial, fibrous, psammomatous, angiomatous, hemangioblastic. Most meningiomas are benign, but some are borderline (atypical meningiomas) and a few are malignant.
- Hemangiopericytoma (9150)—related to meningioma.
- Schwann cells—also called neurolemmocytes and form the myelin sheaths around axons in the peripheral nervous system and cranial nerves. In contrast to an oligodendrocyte, a Schwann cell covers only a single axon. The tumors may be called either Schwannomas or neurilemomas (9560) and may be associated with neurofibromatosis.
- Craniopharyngioma (9350, 9351, 9352)—arises from the remains of a structure found in the developing embryo near the pituitary gland.
- Germ cells—include germinoma, embryonal carcinoma, choriocarcinoma and teratoma that can develop in embryologic remnants in the central nervous system.
- Lymphomas—can develop in the brain even though there are no intracranial lymph nodes. Primary lymphoma of the brain is staged according to the lymphoma staging systems. CNS lymphomas are associated with AIDS.

Benign and borderline non-neuroepithelial tumors include primarily nerve sheath tumors: neurofibromas (several histologic types), neurothekeomas (9562), neuromas (9570), neurinomatosis (9560) and perineuriomas (9571).

Glandular Tumors

- Pineal tumors—slow-growing pineocytomas (9361) and more aggressive pineoblastomas (9362)
- Pituitary tumors—usually benign glandular tumors (adenomas). They are common in adults but rare in children. Because of the many functional cell types in the pituitary gland, there are many descriptors for pituitary adenomas, including chromophobe, acido-, basophil, and prolactinoma.

HISTOLOGY CODING RULES

For the malignant CNS tumors, there are two modules based on number of tumors to be coded. The first one or two rules may seem repetitive, but this was done on purpose to avoid having the reader jump from one place to another in the rules. The 2007 Histology Coding Rules include two important new concepts.

1. Progression of tumor – After a glial tumor is diagnosed and treated, it may recur in a more malignant form with a different name, such as glioblastoma multiforme. The fact that the new name has a different code number does not make it a new primary; rather, the tumor retains its original histology code. However, the progression should be noted in a remarks field on the abstract or in follow-up/recurrence information notes.
2. There are two charts in the site-specific general rules that show the relationships among the various cell types. Chart 1 is for neuroepithelial tumors, Chart 2 is for non-neuroepithelial tumors. Rule H5 for single tumors and rule H10 for multiple tumors refer to these tables; remember to consult them when applying the rules.

Malignant Histology Coding Rules
Single Tumor

- H1. If no pathology/cytology report available, code histology stated by clinician.
- H2. Code histology from a metastatic site if there is no tissue or cytology from the primary site.
- H3. Code as mixed glioma (9382/3) when at least two of the following cell types are described in a single tumor: astrocytic, oligodendroglial, or ependymal.
- H4. If only one histology is stated, code that.
- H5. Code the more specific type when there is a non-specific and a more specific term in the same branch of Chart 1 or Chart 2.
- H6. If no other rule applies, use the ICD-O-3 code for the numerically higher histology as a last priority.

Multiple Tumors Abstracted as a Single Primary

- H7. If no pathology/cytology report available, code histology stated by clinician. This is the same rule as H1 but applies to multiple tumors abstracted as a single primary.
- H8. Code histology from a metastatic site if there is no tissue or cytology from the primary site.
- H9. If only one histology is stated, code that.
- H10. Code the more specific type when there is a non-specific and a more specific term in the same branch of Chart 1 or Chart 2.
- H11. If no other rule applies, use the ICD-O-3 code for the numerically higher histology as a last priority.

Benign/borderline Histology Coding Rules
Single Tumor

- H1. If no pathology/cytology report available, code histology stated by clinician.
- H2. If only one histology is stated, code that.
- H3. Code the more specific type when there is a non-specific and a more specific term in the same branch of Chart 1 or Chart 2.
- H4. If no other rule applies, use the ICD-O-3 code for the numerically higher histology as a last priority.

Multiple Tumors Abstracted as a Single Primary

- H5. If no pathology/cytology report available, code histology stated by clinician. This is the same rule as H1 but applies to multiple tumors abstracted as a single primary.
- H6. Code multiple meningiomas of uncertain behavior to 9530/1. (This is a rare condition.)
- H7. If only one histology is stated, code that.

Histology Coding Rules, ***continued***

H8. Code histology from the original diagnosis.
H9. Code the more specific type when there is a non-specific and a more specific term in the same branch of Chart 1.
H10. If no other rule applies, use the ICD-O-3 code for the numerically higher histology as a last priority.

NPCR CENTRAL NERVOUS SYSTEM SITE AND HISTOLOGY CODING GUIDELINES

In October 2007, the National Program of Cancer Registries (NPCR) of the Centers for Disease Control and Prevention (CDC) published the results of a central nervous system audit and guidelines for correct coding of primary site and histology based on the audit. These guidelines have not been widely distributed, but in general, they are common-sense statements that will enhance the accuracy of coding central nervous system and related tumors.

- Always use the behavior code listed in the ICD-O-3 unless otherwise directed by a pathologist.
- **Site-specific Histology Codes.** Code as follows unless otherwise directed by a pathologist.
  - ***Meningiomas*** (many subtypes with unique codes)—code to meninges (C70._). Meningioma of the choroid plexus is rare, and intraparenchymal meningioma is very rare.
  - ***Choroid plexus tumors***—code to ventricle (C71.5)
  - ***Pituitary adenoma*** (8272/0) and ***pituitary carcinoma*** (8272/3)—code to pituitary (C75.1)
  - ***Craniopharyngiomas*** (9350/1)—very few actually arise in the craniopharyngeal duct; all are non-malignant. Code to suprasellar (C71.9 Brain, NOS), or third ventricle (C71.5) as appropriate.
  - ***Pineal parenchymal tumors***—code to pineal gland (C75.3). Applies to pineocytoma (9361/1), pineoblastoma (9362/3), mixed pineocytoma-pineoblastoma (9362/3) and pineal astrocytoma (9400/3).
  - ***Carotid body tumor*** or ***chemodectoma***—code to carotid body (C75.4)
  - ***Paragangliomas*** and ***glomus tumors***—arise from paraganglionic tissue; reportable only if intracranial; code to aortic body and other paraganglia (C75.5). Includes
    - 8680/_ Paraganglioma
    - 8681/1 Sympathetic paraganglioma*
    - 8682/1 Parasympathetic paraganglioma*
    - 8693/_ Extra-adrenal paraganglioma
    - 8690/1 Glomus jugulare tumor*
    - 8691/1 Aortic body tumor*
    - 8710/3 Glomangiosarcoma**
    - 8711/_ Glomus tumor
    - 8712/0 Glomangioma*
    - 8713/0 Glomangiomyoma*
  - ***Solitary fibrous tumor*** (8815/_)—a rare, usually dural-based lesion that occurs in the cranium or spinal canal, and sometimes in the lateral ventricle or spinal cord. Code to meninges (C70._).
  - ***Vascular tumors***—if in brain or spinal cord, code to CNS site of occurrence, not to blood vessel (C49._). Includes
    - 9120/0 Hemangioma, NOS*
    - 9121/0 Cavernous hemangioma*
    - 9150/0 Hemangiopericytoma, benign*
    - 9150/1 Hemangiopericytoma, NOS*
    - 9161/1 Hemangioblastoma*
    - 9120/3 Angiosarcoma**
    - 9130/3 Hemangioendothelioma**
    - 9150/3 Hemangiopericytoma**

* reportable only for CNS sites
** reportable anywhere in body

Nervous Sys

NPCR CNS Coding Guidelines, *continued*

- ◦ ***Nerve sheath tumors***
    - Malignant (reportable anywhere in body)—code to nerve of origin (C47._ or C72._)
    - Non-malignant (reportable only for intracranial segment of cranial nerves only)—code to nerve of origin (C72.2, .3, .4, and .5)
- ***Germ cell tumors***—code to site of origin, which is usually pineal gland (C75.3), suprasellar region (C71.9 brain, NOS or specific lobe), or posterior third ventricle (C71.5).
    - ◦ ***Teratoma***—report malignant teratomas anywhere in body; report non-malignant teratomas only for CNS sites
- ***Dermoid*** or ***dermoid cyst*** (9084/_)—report malignant dermoids anywhere in the body; report non-malignant dermoids only for CNS sites
- ***Pacinian tumor*** (9507/0)—a non-malignant peripheral nerve tumor; report only if arising intracranially
- ***Neurofibroma, neurilemoma, neuroma***—arise in peripheral nerves; report only if primary is a cranial nerve or nerve root

- **Non-CNS Tumors of the Head**
    - ◦ ***Chordomas*** (9370–9372)—malignant *bone* tumors that arise in base of skull and clivus (C41.0), lower end of vertebral column (C41.2), and occasionally parasellar and sellar area. The parasellar and sellar areas are other names for base of skull (C41.0). Chordomas are always reportable; code to bone of origin.
    - ◦ ***Chondrosarcoma***—malignant cartilage tumor that can develop in the skull base, clivus, parasellar area, cerebellopontine angle, or paranasal sinuses. Chondrosarcomas are always reportable; code to bone of origin, usually bone of skull (C42.0), C3 to L5 spine (C41.2) or sacrum (C41.4).
        - Chordomas and chondrosarcomas of the clivus may extend into the sella turcica, nasopharynx, posterior fossa, foramen magnum and may affect the cranio-cervical junction at C1–C2.
    - ◦ ***Chondroma*** (9220/0, 9221/0)—rare, nonmalignant tumors of bone (usually skull base or paranasal sinuses) reportable only if the primary site is intracranial; code to bone of skull (C41.0).
    - ◦ ***Desmoid tumor***—nonmalignant fibrous tumor commonly found in neck; not reportable—does not occur intracranially
    - ◦ ***Nerve sheath myxoma*** (9562/0)—never occurs intracranially; may be confused with a scarred-over meningioma

GRADING

The most important thing for a registrar to understand about the World Health Organization (WHO) grade for central nervous system tumors is that it does not parallel the ICD-O-3 grade code in the 6th digit of the morphology code. As Figure 16 shows, Grade I in the WHO system is roughly equivalent to a behavior code of benign in ICD-O-3. ICD-O-3's grade codes compare to WHO grades III and IV.

- It is very important that the WHO grade NOT be used as the ICD-O-3 code.
- Remember to assign the ICD-O 6th digit according to the coding rules by coding the words in the diagnosis.
- These are examples of the differences in the way WHO grade and ICD-O 6th digit grade should be coded.

Figure 16. Comparison of WHO Grade and ICD-O-3 Behavior and Grading (6th Digit)

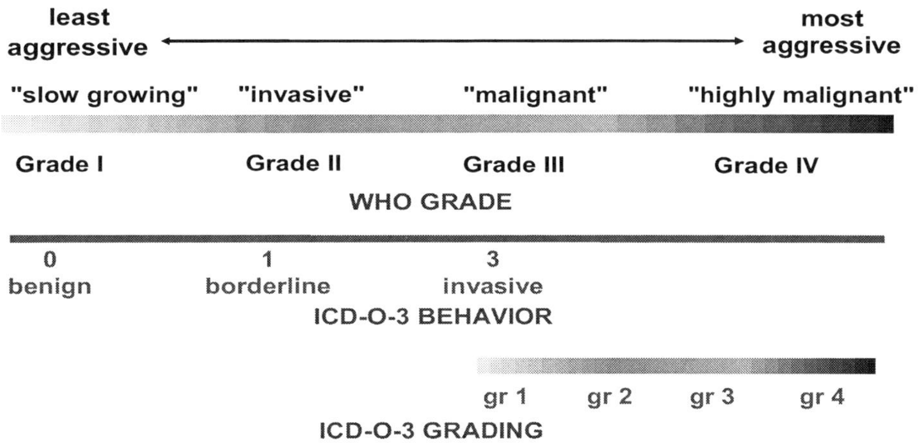

Grade, ***continued***

Histology	WHO Grade	ICD-O 6th digit
Pilocytic astrocytoma	1	9
Well-differentiated low grade astrocytoma	2	1
Anaplastic astrocytoma	3	4
Glioblastoma multiforme	4	9

Note: When there is no tissue diagnosis, it may still be possible to establish the grade of a tumor through magnetic resonance imaging (MRI) or positron emission tomography (PET). In particular, it is now possible to grade brain tumors by this method. Thus if there is no tissue, and grade or differentiation is listed on the MRI or PET report, code the grade based on the report. If there is a tissue diagnosis, grade should be coded from the pathology report only.

BRAIN AND CENTRAL NERVOUS SYSTEM TUMORS ABSTRACTING GUIDELINES

Diagnosing a brain or spinal cord tumor involves taking a careful medical history and evaluating the patient's symptoms to rule out other diagnoses that could cause similar symptoms. The diagnostic pathway includes a complete neurological examination, imaging, and a biopsy of the lesion.

HISTORY

The signs and symptoms that bring the patient to a doctor are a valuable part of the diagnostic work-up for brain and CNS tumors. As noted previously in the anatomy section of this chapter, the symptoms may help to localize the cancer to a specific area of the nervous system. A careful history is important to establish both the type and duration of symptoms. Symptoms may be due to causes other than tumors, and it is the clinician's responsibility to rule out other causes. In addition, symptoms on one side of the body may be related to a tumor on the opposite side of the brain. Common symptoms of brain and CNS tumors (and other conditions) include:

- Headaches (46% of surveyed CNS tumor patients reported this symptom)—non-specific to brain tumors
- Nausea and vomiting (22%)—non-specific to brain tumors
- Vision problems (25%)—any change in vision should be evaluated

History, *continued*

- Seizures (10%)—involuntary change in muscle control, consciousness, behavior or sensation on one or more occasions. Seizures can include twitching, shaking of a limb, violent convulsions of the entire body, difficulty speaking, and altered vision.
- Changes in sensation (16–25%)—sometimes called paresthesias; weakness of limbs, numbness or strange feelings in head or hands
- Behavior or cognitive changes—memory problems, especially short-term memory; inability to concentrate; loss of inhibition; inappropriate actions, emotions, or speech
- Increased intracranial pressure (IICP)—a general term for symptoms caused by something growing or expanding within the confines of the skull, which can include tumor, abscess, hydrocephalus, infection, inflammation and other conditions

Where to look in the patient's record

- History and physical exam report
- Consultation report(s)
- Physician's progress notes

What information to select and record

Pertinent findings relating

- Type and duration of specific symptoms. Table 1 lists focal (limited) symptoms by location of the tumor.

PHYSICAL EXAM

A complete physical examination is necessary to check for any evidence of another tumor that may be causing the CNS symptoms; in other words, to rule out metastases to the brain from another primary site. The physical exam also checks for the patient's general health and ability to withstand potential surgery to remove the CNS tumor. Along with the general physical examination, a complete ***neurological examination*** should be conducted, preferably by a neurologic specialist. The neurological exam supplements the information provided by imaging and lab tests and helps to isolate the part of the nervous system that is malfunctioning. The neurological examination consists of a series of questions answered by the patient and simple activities, such as movements, repeating sentences or performing math problems, regarding

- Mental status—state of consciousness; mood; thought content; appearance and general behavior; intellect (memory; judgment; comprehension; attentiveness; abstract reasoning)
- Cranial nerves—visual function; peripheral vision; eyelid strength; hearing; strength of facial muscles; gag reflex; ability to smell and taste; sensation in head, neck and face
- Motor system—strength of major muscle groups; Babinski response; exam to evaluate muscle atrophy, twitching or abnormal movements
- Sensory system—assessment of responses to pain, temperature, pressure, position using pinpricks or warm and cold objects
- Deep tendon reflexes DTRs or muscle stretch reflexes, usually using a rubber hammer gently struck on a muscle tendon to test involuntary movements
- Coordination and cerebellar function—assessment of voluntary movements such as repeated finger-to-nose movements and tapping fingers rhythmically
- Gait—observing the ability to walk by having the patient walk heel-to-toe in a straight line, walk on toes, walk on heels, and other activities

Other Exams

- **Visual field examination—**a test to determine any defects in the patient's vision, which in turn may reveal the location of a brain tumor. Tumor in different brain sites causes specific visual field alterations.

Table 1. Symptoms by Tumor Location (adapted from American Brain Tumor Association)

Abbreviations: IICP–increased intracranial pressure N&V–nausea and vomiting

C70._ **Meninges**—Seizures, IICP, other symptoms specific to location of tumor
C71.0 Cerebrum
Hypothalamus—Disruption of body functions such as thirst, sleep, body temperature, appetite, and blood pressure, as well as emotional control
Thalamus—Sensory loss on side of body opposite the tumor, including muscle weakness; decreased sense of touch; decreased intellect; vision problems; speech difficulties; loss of urinary control; headache, N&V, and difficulties in walking due to obstructive hydrocephalus.
Basal ganglia—Unilateral paralysis
C71.1 **Frontal lobe**— One-sided paralysis, seizures, short-term memory loss, impaired judgment and personality or mental changes; urinary frequency and urgency; gait disturbances and communication problems; loss of smell, impaired vision, or swollen optic nerve
C71.2 **Temporal lobe**—Seizures; loss of depth perception and sense of time; loss of sound recognition; impaired vision
C71.3 **Parietal lobe**—Seizures; language and reasoning disturbances; loss of ability to read or do arithmetic; difficulty with body orientation in space or recognition of body parts; difficulty with spatial perception
C71.4 **Occipital lobe**—Seizures, blindness in one direction, and other visual disorders
C71.5 **Ventricles**
Third ventricle—Hydrocephalus; IICP; leg weakness; fainting; impaired memory
C71.6 **Cerebellum**—Headaches due to tumor and/or hydrocephalus; N&V; IICP; swollen optic nerve; gait disturbances such as a clumsy, uncoordinated walk, swaying, and staggering; dizziness; tremors; difficulty with speech; double vision; tilting of the head
Cerebellopontine angle—Ringing/buzzing in ear; deafness; facial weakness; dizziness
C71.7 **Brain stem** (midbrain, pons, medulla oblongata)—Vomiting; uncoordinated walk, unilateral muscle weakness of face; difficulty swallowing; slurred speech; double vision; headache; head tilt; hearing loss; personality changes; drowsiness
C71.8 **Overlapping lesion of brain**
Corpus callosum—Impaired judgment; defective memory; behavioral changes
Midline—Headaches; nausea; IICP; abnormal eye movements; visual defects; personality changes
C72.3 **Optic nerve**—Visual defects including eye movement disorders, impaired vision, and abnormal pupil reactions
C72.9 **Other parts of nervous system**
Skull base tumors (deep in head where brain tissue meets the base of the skull)—Slurred speech, difficulty swallowing, double vision; facial weakness; balance problems
C75.1 **Pituitary gland**—Headaches; vision changes; hormone disturbances from inappropriate hormone secretions, such as breast enlargement and lactation, abnormal growth, and other body functions affected by hormones; diabetes insipidus
C75.3 **Pineal gland**—IICP due to hydrocephalus; eye movement disorders; precocious puberty and other hormonal disturbances in children

Physical Exam, *continued*

Where to look in the patient's record

- History and physical exam report
- Consultation report(s)
- Physician's progress notes

Physical Exam, ***continued***

What information to select and record (record all dates)
Pertinent findings of what the physician observes during physical exam and neurological testing
- Clinician's conclusions or impression of patient's neurological status
- Use "evidence of" and "no evidence of" statements
- Document both positive and negative findings

IMAGING

Radiology, ultrasound, and computer imaging studies are the most effective way to determine the location, size, and extent of a lesion. Neuroradiologists can often tell the cell type from the imaging results, and registrars can code the cell type from this information.

Key Word
- **Midline shift**—a description by the radiologist that the normal midline of the brain is out of place. This is usually due to an enlarging tumor lesion or peritumoral swelling on one side pushing the midline toward the uninvolved side. A midline shift is *not* an indication that the tumor has crossed the midline.

- **Magnetic Resonance Imaging (MRI)**—better soft tissue resolution than CT scan; can detect edema, hemorrhage, isodense lesions, tumor enhancement, infarction. More accurate for determining tumor size than CT scan. Can be performed with and without dye contrast; superior for assessing spinal cord lesions. There are several types of MRIs.
    - **Magnetic Resonance Angiography (MRA)**—without using a contrast agent, MRA images blood flow and position of blood vessels leading to a tumor; helps surgeon anticipate highly vascular tumors; less invasive than arteriogram. Can also be performed with a contrast agent (contrast-enhanced, CE-MRA).
    - **Flow-sensitive MRI (FS-MRI)**—images flow of cerebrospinal fluid (CSF) through ventricles and spinal cord; useful for assessing tumors that cause hydrocephalus, such as in the spinal cord or base of skull.
    - **Magnetic Resonance Spectroscopy (MRI Spect or MRS)**—images the metabolic activity (choline, lactate, N-Acetyl Aspartate) in the brain tumor. Metabolites in tumors act differently from normal tissue. MRS helps determine type and grade of tumor and post-treatment can distinguish recurrent tumor from radiation necrosis. In some centers, MRS has largely replaced PET scanning due to superior resolution and accuracy.
    - **Perfusion MRI**—uses contrast agents to examine blood flow; can determine grade of some tumors
    - **Diffusion and diffusion-tensor MRI**—images the random motion of water in tissues (diffusion), in particular along nerves; helps surgeon avoid damaging nerve bundles that have been displaced by tumor
    - **Functional MRI**—tracks use of oxygen in brain instantly as it occurs; useful for treatment planning because it identifies critical motor, sensory, and language centers of brain
- **Computed axial tomography (CAT or CT)**—takes less time to perform, better detection of calcifications, skull lesions and recent hemorrhage than MRI; shows combination of blood vessels, bone, and soft tissues. Uses x-rays rather than the magnetic fields of MRI; can be performed with or without a contrast agent.

Other Imaging Tests for CNS Tumors (see also the Diagnostic Tests chapter in this book)
- **Brain scan**—nuclear imaging of the brain using intravenous injection of radioactive material
- **Single-photon emission computed tomography (SPECT)** imaging—three-dimensional nuclear medicine imaging using gamma rays; used for functional analysis of brain

Imaging, ***continued***

- **Positron emission tomography (PET)** scan—measures biologic activity using radioisotope-labeled glucose; used with other scans to determine grade of tumor; can differentiate among scar tissue, recurrent tumor, and radiation necrosis. Detects metastatic and recurrent brain tumor earlier than MRI or CT; can be used to measure response to therapy.
- **Arteriogram or Angiogram**—an older, invasive technique to assess vascularity and blood flow to a brain tumor using a contrast agent injected into an artery in the groin. Angiograms have been largely replaced by less invasive MRI and CT imaging techniques.
- **Myelogram**—an invasive technique in which a contrast agent is injected into the cerebrospinal fluid to look for a tumor in the spinal cord; can be either a standard x-ray or CT scan; largely replaced by less invasive MRI and CT imaging.
- **Electroencephalogram (EEG)**—an older, invasive technique that measures electrical activity in the brain by using electrodes attached to the patients head; indicates how brain function is affected by the lesion.
- **Magnetoencephalography (MEG)**—assessment of the electrical activity in the brain (similar to EEG), by measuring the magnetic field around the electrical impulses; used in conjunction with other imaging techniques to map functional areas of brain. MEG equipment is available only in a limited number of facilities.

What information to select and record (record all dates)

Pertinent findings as stated by the radiologist from each study including:

- Name of study and area of the body being examined (such as CT of brain, spinal cord MRI)
- Tumor location, including subsite(s)
- Laterality
- Tumor size and extent of tumor

LABORATORY TESTS AND TUMOR MARKERS *(see also Diagnostic Tests and Tumor Markers chapter)*

Laboratory tests (blood tests) will help rule out other causes for the tumor symptoms. Tumor markers help differentiate cell types, but most brain tumors do not express tumor markers. Tumor markers taken at the time of diagnosis (baseline) and during follow-up help to assess tumor burden and monitor for recurrence.

- **Chromogranin-A**—monitors tumor bulk in neuroblastoma, APUDoma, VIPoma, pheochromocytoma; non-diagnostic of CNS tumor
- **Ferritin**—monitors cause of disease in neuroblastoma; non-specific in neurogenic tumors
- **HVA-homovanillic Acid**—elevated levels suggest catecholamine-secreting tumor such as neuroblastoma or ganglioneuroma; high levels rule out pheochromocytoma
- **Neuron Specific Enolase (NSE)**—monitors neuroblastoma; non-specific to CNS tumors
- **VMA (Vanillylmandelic Acid)**—elevated levels suggest catecholamine-secreting tumor such as neuroblastoma or ganglioneuroma; non-specific to VMA.
- **Markers for germ cell tumors**—human chorionic gonadotropin (hCG), alpha fetoprotein (AFP), placental alkaline phosphatase (PLAP)
- **Carcinoembryonic antigen (CEA)**—a marker for leptomeningeal (in the arachnoid or pia mater) tumors (usually metastatic); non-specific for brain tumors
- **Markers for pituitary tumors**—prolactin, thyrotropin, thyroxine, adrenocorticotropin, cortisol, LH, FSH, estradiol, testosterone, growth hormone, insulinlike growth factor-1 (IGF-1), and alpha subunit glycoprotein

Laboratory Tests and Tumor Markers, ***continued***

What information to select and record (record all dates)

- Test type
- Test result
- Normal test value/range

OPERATIVE FINDINGS

In addition to the pathology report of the tissues removed during a procedure, the operative report from diagnostic exploratory procedures and/or cancer directed definitive treatment can provide valuable information about the precise location of the primary tumor and any tumor left behind, as well as clinical information that might affect the staging or histologic diagnosis.

What information to select and record (record all dates)

Pertinent findings as described by the surgeon

- Tumor location including site(s)
- Size of tumor/involved area before removal
- Tissues removed—removal of just the tumor or removal of entire lobe
- Areas not included in pathology specimen; estimate of tumor volume left behind

DIAGNOSTIC PROCEDURES

Key Words

- *Stereotactic radiosurgery*—also called Cyberknife, Gamma knife and X-knife; this is very targeted radiation therapy, *not surgery.* Code as radiation therapy, not surgical treatment.

CYTOLOGY REPORTS

The following procedures yield tumor cells that can confirm the diagnosis of a CNS tumor.

- **Fine-needle aspiration (FNA),** fine needle aspiration cytology (FNAC), fine needle aspiration biopsy (FNAB)—Also called closed needle biopsy or stereotactic needle biopsy. After drilling a small hole (burr hole) in the skull over the lesion, the surgeon inserts a thin needle into the lesion or suspicious area to remove fluid and/or cells. A persistent residual mass may require an excisional biopsy. FNA may be guided by computerized tomography or MRI because direct visualization of the lesion is not possible.
- **Lumbar puncture** (spinal tap)—used to identify malignant cells in cerebrospinal fluid
- **CSF studies—**cytologic analysis of cerebrospinal fluid to detect protein and glucose values, as well as bacteria, fungi, or malignant cells

What information to select and record (record all dates)

- Test type and tissue biopsied
- Positive or negative findings
- Cell type, if given

HISTOLOGY

The following procedures yield pieces of tumor that confirm the diagnosis of cancer and can be used to determine the extent of tumor and further treatment.

- **Open biopsy**—Removal of a piece of the skull (craniotomy) to access brain tissue; if only part of the tumor is removed, this becomes an incisional biopsy. The wound is then closed and the piece of skull is put back in place.

Diagnostic Procedures, *continued*

- **Incisional biopsy**—A diagnostic procedure in which the surgeon cuts a sample of tissue from the lesion or suspicious area. Incisional biopsy cuts through tumor; it is performed when complete removal is unnecessary or not possible. Incisional biopsy may also be performed to establish a diagnosis when cancer is suspected or possible and neoadjuvant (preoperative) treatment is being planned.

PATHOLOGY REPORTS

Pathologic evaluation of any resected tissue not only establishes a diagnosis, but also provides important prognostic information. All parts of the pathology report—the gross and microscopic examination of the specimen, the final diagnosis and comments—should be reviewed for staging, grade, and histology information, but only the final diagnosis should be used to code the histology.

If a CAP checklist (outline format provided by the College of American Pathologists) is provided, the information may be easier to find in that section of the pathology report than in the gross and microscopic narrative sections. The CAP checklist is also called a synoptic report or CAP protocol. An example of a CAP protocol is shown in Table 2.

Table 2. Example of College of American Pathologists (CAP) Brain Tumor Protocol

Clinical Information (Verified)
Right temporal lobe frontal brain mass

Specimen Submitted (Verified)
1 Right frontal mass
2 Right frontal mass
3 Right frontal mass

Intraoperative Consult (Verified)
Frozen Section: 1FS) Brain tissue with sparse inflammation. No evidence of tumor or abscess.
2FS) High grade glial neoplasm

Gross Description (Verified)
Specimen #1 consists of two fragments of tissue each measuring 0.4 cm in greatest dimension. The specimen is submitted for frozen sectioning and is then placed in Cassette 1FS for permanent sections. Specimen #2 consists of a 0.7 cm aggregate of soft tissue. Two H&E touch prep slides are obtained. The specimen is submitted for frozen sectioning and is then placed in Cassette 2FS for permanent sections. Specimen #3 consists of a 1.5 cm aggregate of tissue. The specimen is submitted in Cassette 3A for microscopic examination.

Microscopic Description (Verified)
A microscopic examination was performed and the findings justify the diagnosis.

Diagnosis (Verified)
1) RIGHT FRONTAL MASS: Brain tissue with mild gliosis and mild chronic inflammation.
2) RIGHT FRONTAL MASS: Glioblastoma multiforme.
3) RIGHT FRONTAL MASS: Glioblastoma multiforme.

SPECIMEN TYPE: Resection
SPECIMEN SIZE: 1.5 cm
TUMOR SITE: Cerebrum, right frontal lobe
TUMOR SIZE: Cannot be determined
HISTOLOGIC TYPE: Glioblastoma multiforme
HISTOLOGIC GRADE: Grade 4
MARGINS: Cannot be assessed

Pathology Reports, *continued*

What information to select and record (record all dates)

Final Diagnosis

- Histology (cell type)—Follow the histology coding rules for using this information. Remember, for central nervous system tumors (benign, borderline, and malignant), the ICD-O morphology code is based only from the final diagnosis.
- Behavior
  - /0 Benign, /1 Borderline, /3 Malignant, invasive
- Grade
  - WHO grade I – IV

Gross

- Location of tumor (area of CNS) and location of tumor within resected specimen
- Aggregate size of tumor, if provided by pathologist
- Size of largest focus of tumor, if multifocal
- Presence of multiple tumors

Microscopic (primary tumor)

- Histology of tumor and subtype
- Information about mixed histologies
- Depth of invasion and extent of disease (meninges, bone, supporting tissues, another lobe)
- Status of surgical margins

CENTRAL NERVOUS SYSTEM TUMORS DISEASE MANAGEMENT

Benign, borderline and malignant CNS tumors can be treated in a variety of ways, primarily depending on the cell type and tumor grade. Many benign tumors receive no treatment unless they become symptomatic. With a few exceptions, most malignant tumors undergo surgical debulking, if possible, followed by other modalities. A variety of treatments are under clinical evaluation, including radiosensitizers, hyperthermia, interstitial brachytherapy, and intraoperative radiation therapy, as well as new drugs and biological response modifiers.

SURGERY

Complete resection of the tumor is the treatment of choice, if technically possible, to reduce tumor bulk, preserve neurologic function, and improve the patient's outcome. Tumors that produce fluid (hydrocephalus) may be treated palliatively with a shunt.

Key Words

Craniotomy—Craniotomy is an *approach* to brain surgery, not a cancer directed treatment by itself. The craniotomy provides access to the brain by cutting the skull and creating a bone flap. After the surgical resection of the brain tissue, the bone flap is replaced and secured using fine wire. Any direct exposure of brain tissue during surgery may lead to complications of bleeding (hemorrhage), swelling (edema), increased intracranial pressure (IICP), infection, or brain tissue damage. Craniotomy should not be coded as a separate procedure in Surgery of Other Site.

Laminectomy—Laminectomy is an *approach* to spinal cord surgery, not a cancer directed treatment by itself. A laminectomy creates an opening in a vertebra to provide access to the spinal cord. Laminectomy should not be coded as a separate procedure in Surgery of Other Site.

Surgery, *continued*

Brain-mapping—not a cancer-directed treatment; do not code as Surgery of Primary Site. The purpose of this procedure is to identify vital areas of the brain, such as motor function and speech, so that the surgeon can avoid them during resective surgery. During the procedure, the patient is sedated and given local anesthesia so the surgeon can communicate with the patient. Electrodes stimulate nerves in the brain and measure responses, producing a "map" of brain functions.
Stereotactic radiosurgery—*not* a surgical procedure; do not record as tumor destruction. See Radiation Therapy below. Record as code 41 in the radiation treatment fields Regional Treatment Modality or Boost Treatment Modality as appropriate.
Fluorescence-guided surgery—a newer technique in which the patient is given a fluorescent dye preoperatively. The dye is taken up by the tumor and, using special lights during surgery, the surgeon can differentiate tumor from surrounding normal tissue and do a better job of debulking the tumor.

FORDS Surgery of Primary Site Codes for C70–C72 Primaries
The following surgery codes apply to benign, borderline, and malignant tumors of the meninges, brain, spinal cord, and cranial nerves (C70–C72). They correspond to the three-digit codes used to describe surgical resection in CS Site-Specific Factor 7. Code Surgery of Primary Site from the operative report description supplemented by information from the pathology report.

00 None; no surgery of primary site; autopsy only
- Use this code for clinically diagnosed patients and those who had no surgical resection of the primary
- Use this code for a brain tumor primary initially diagnosed at autopsy

10 Tumor destruction, NOS
- SEER Note: also known as local tumor destruction, NOS
- Includes laser microsurgery, in which MRI is used to pinpoint the tumor location and a laser destroys the tumor
- No specimen sent to pathology

20 Local excision (biopsy) of tumor, lesion, or mass; excisional biopsy
- Use this code for diagnostic procedures such as a biopsy, where the intent is not to remove the entire tumor
- Specimen sent to pathology for examination

21 Subtotal resection of tumor, lesion or mass of brain
- Use this code for procedures where a greater portion of tumor is excised but there is gross tumor left behind (including a statement by surgeon that there was residual tumor in brain)
- Removes tumor tissue but not normal brain tissue
- Tumor involves less than half of lobe
- Specimen sent to pathology for examination

22 Resection of tumor of spinal cord or nerve
- Specimen from resection spinal cord or nerve sent to pathology for examination

30 Radical, total, or gross resection of tumor, lesion, or mass in brain
- Use this code for procedures where the surgeon attempts to remove the entire tumor
- Microscopic tumor may be left behind
- Removes tumor tissue but not normal brain tissue
- Tumor involves less than half of lobe
- Specimen sent to pathology for examination

40 Partial resection of lobe of brain
- Use this code for a procedure that removes the tumor and part of the normal tissue in the lobe
- Tumor involves more than half of lobe
- Does not include resection of spinal cord or spinal nerve primary

FORDS Surgery of Primary Site Codes for C70–C72 Primaries, *continued*

55 Gross total resection of lobe of brain (lobectomy)
- Tumor involves more than half of lobe
- Gross total resection of a lobe is rarely performed for a brain tumor; more likely this procedure is performed for intractable seizures.

90 Surgery, NOS
- Use this code in the infrequent situation where the details of surgery are unknown.

FORDS Surgery of Primary Site Codes for C75 Primaries

Key Words
Hypophysectomy—surgical removal of the pituitary gland (hypophysis). The approach may be through the nose or the sinuses (trans-sphenoidal), or by craniotomy and lifting the frontal lobe out of the skull. Stereotactic radiosurgery (radiation therapy) is an alternative to hypophysectomy.

The surgery codes for the intracranial glands (pineal, craniopharyngeal duct, and pituitary; C75.1–C75.3) are part of the codes for "All Other Sites," but the definitions of resections are similar to those for the CNS organs. Many of the "All Other Sites" surgery codes do not apply to the intracranial glands. The most likely codes to be used for these CNS sites are:

10 Local tumor destruction, NOS
14 Laser (no surgical specimen)
20 Local tumor excision, NOS
27 Excisional biopsy
24 Laser ablation (includes local tumor excision or excisional biopsy and surgical specimen)
25 Laser excision (includes local tumor excision or excisional biopsy and surgical specimen)
30 Simple/partial surgical removal of primary site
40 Total surgical removal of primary site
50 Surgery stated to be "debulking"
60 Radical surgery
- Partial/total removal of the primary site WITH resection in continuity of other organs

RADIATION THERAPY

Radiation therapy is an important part of the treatment of most cell types for adult CNS tumors. It may increase the cure rate for initial treatment or be useful in treating recurrences after failure of surgery. However, because of its long-lasting side effects, radiation is usually avoided in children.

Radiotherapy aids in cell destruction for many types of brain tumors, although radioresponsiveness varies according to cell type. Radiation therapy techniques used to treat central nervous system tumors include

- **External beam radiation (EBRT)** is focused on the brain from a radiation source outside the body. While effective at destroying cancer cells, surrounding normal tissue may also be destroyed. Standard external beam radiation is given less commonly where more techniques with more precision (see below) are available. (External beam, NOS is Modality code 20)
- **Three-dimensional Conformal Radiation Therapy (3D-CRT)** uses sophisticated computers to map the brain and the tumor within it. Radiation beams are then calculated and aimed at the brain from several directions. Patients are fitted with a plastic mold similar to a body cast that keeps them still so that the radiation can be aimed more accurately. Conformal or 3-D therapy is Modality code 32.)

Radiation Therapy, *continued*

- **Intensity Modulated Radiation Therapy (IMRT)** is an advanced form of 3D therapy that allows adjustment of the strength (intensity) of the radiation beams in addition to aiming beams from several directions. The purpose is to deliver a higher dose to the brain tumor while minimizing radiation to surrounding sensitive normal tissues. (IMRT is Modality code 31)
- **Stereotactic radiosurgery** is a radiotherapy technique that aims highly focused external radiation at a specific area of the brain from many directions. This technique provides a maximum radiation dose to the tumor while sparing normal brain tissue through which the radiation must pass. Code stereotactic radiosurgery (NOS) as 41 in Regional Treatment Modality or Boost Treatment Modality as appropriate; do not code as Surgery of Primary Site. Also called gamma knife (code 43), cyberknife (code 42), and X-knife (code 41).
- **Conformal proton beam radiation therapy** focuses proton beams on the tumor. Protons are the positive parts of atoms. They cause little damage to tissues they pass through but are effective in killing cells at the end of their path. Proton beam radiation may be able to deliver more radiation to the brain while reducing side effects on nearby normal tissues, but the technique is not widely available in the United States. (Proton therapy is Modality code 40.)
- **Image Guided Radiation Therapy (IGRT)** is similar in concept to IMRT but uses more frequent imaging with CT, MRT, PET, or ultrasound to adjust the field size and dosage for tumors in locations prone to movement, such as the brain. (IGRT is Modality code 31)
- **Craniospinal radiation** (radiation to whole brain and spinal cord) can be given when there is evidence of tumor spread along the meningeal covering of the spinal cord or into the cerebrospinal fluid that circulates throughout the brain and spinal cord. Ependymomas may need craniospinal radiation because of the way in which they spread.

Radiation therapy techniques under clinical investigation include

- Hyperfractionation (several small doses per day)
- Accelerated fraction (increasing doses during course of treatment)
- Radiation assisted by radiosensitizers
- Interstitial brachytherapy (radioactive needles inserted into tumor), usually in conjunction with external beam radiation
- Intraoperative radiation therapy

SYSTEMIC THERAPY

Chemotherapy helps prolong survival for glioma, medulloblastoma, or germ cell tumor patients. Chemotherapy is usually used after surgery or after radiation therapy for high grade tumors, but may be used alone for recurrent brain tumors.

Key Words

Blood-Brain Barrier—A barrier formed between the blood vessels and glia of the brain that prevents large molecules in the blood, such as bacteria and some types of chemotherapy drugs, from entering brain tissue. The blood-brain barrier reduces or blocks the effectiveness of systemic chemotherapy for CNS tumors. The blood-brain barrier can be counteracted by various treatment modalities including intracranial implantation of chemotherapeutic agents. One newer technique is convection enhanced delivery, where tiny tubes are surgically placed directly into the tumor. The chemotherapy is then injected directly into the tumor, overcoming issues with the blood-brain barrier.

Gliadel wafers—Gliadel® wafers are biodegradable discs impregnated with carmustine (BCNU), the most effective of the chemotherapy agents for brain tumors. During a craniotomy, the surgeon places the wafer directly in the tumor bed and closes the skull. This allows the chemotherapy to work over time by direct contact with the tumor.

CHEMOTHERAPY

- Effective for glioblastoma, brainstem glioma, and medulloblastoma
- Drugs used singly or in combination with other drugs or radiotherapy
  - Nitrosoureas
    - Carmustine (BCNU)
    - Lomustine (CCNU)
  - Temozolomide (Temodar)
  - Cisplatin
  - Carboplatin
  - Etoposide
  - Irinotecan
  - Methotrexate
  - Procarbazine
  - Vincristine
- Targeted therapy drugs (anti-angiogenesis agents)
  - Bevacizumab (Avastin)
  - Sunitinib (Sutent)
  - Sorafenib (Nexavar)
- Growth factor inhibitors and hypoxic cell sensitizers are under clinical investigation.
- Chemotherapy regimens
  - PCV (CCNU, procarbazine, vincristine)
  - Other combinations of effective agents listed above

HORMONE THERAPY

Hormones are not useful for anti-cancer treatment of malignant brain tumors; however, some corticosteroids like dexamethasone are used to decrease brain edema as a palliative or supportive measure. Do not code hormones used palliatively or supportively for reducing edema as hormone therapy. The patient may also receive anti-seizure drugs but these should not be coded as anti-cancer treatment.

BIOLOGICAL RESPONSE MODIFIERS/IMMUNOTHERAPY

Immunotherapy and biological response modifiers such as tumor vaccines are under clinical evaluation but at the present time there are no effective immunotherapy agents for brain tumors.

'USUAL' TREATMENT BY HISTOLOGY AND GRADE (from NCI PDQ)

The patient's cell type and the WHO grade of the tumor determine the choice of treatment modalities. Table 3 shows various cell types and how they are usually treated. All patients should be considered for clinical trials.

Table 3. Treatment Options for Adult Brain Tumors by Cell Type

ICD-O Code / Cell Type	Surg only	Surg and RT	Surg, RT, chemo	Surg, chemo	RT only	Other comb
9150 Hemangiopericytoma		X				X*
9350 Craniopharyngioma (WHO gr. I)	X	X				
9361 Pineocytoma (WHO gr. II)		X				X*
9362 Pineoblastoma (WHO gr. IV)			X			X*
9380 Brain stem glioma					X	
9382 Oligoastrocytoma (WHO gr. II)		X	X			X*
9382 Oligoastrocytoma, anaplastic (WHO gr. III)		X	X			X*
9383 Subependymoma (WHO gr. I)	X	X				
9391 Ependymoma (WHO gr. II)	X	X				
9392 Ependymoma, anaplastic (WHO gr. III)		X				X*
9394 Ependymoma, myxopapillary (WHO gr. I)	X	X				
9400 Pineal astrocytoma		X	X			
9400 Astrocytoma, diffuse (WHO gr. II)	X	X	X*			
9401 Astrocytoma, anaplastic (WHO gr. III)		X	X			X*
9421 Astrocytoma, pilocytic (WHO gr. I)	X	X				
9440 Glioblastoma multiforme (WHO gr. IV)		X	X	X		X*
9450 Oligodendroglioma (WHO gr. II)		X				X*
9451 Oligodendroglioma, anaplastic (WHO gr. III)		X	X			X*
9470 Medulloblastoma		X	X*			
9530 Meningioma (WHO gr. I)	X	X			X	
9530 Meningioma (WHO gr. II, III)		X				X*

* Various options under clinical investigation. Clinical trials may include addition of chemotherapy or various trials of hyperfractionated radiation therapy, brachytherapy, intraoperative radiation therapy, hyperthermia, or radiosensitizers in conjunction with external beam radiation therapy.

COLLABORATIVE STAGE DATA COLLECTION SYSTEM (CS)

Three staging schemas cover all the central nervous system tumors.

- Brain and cerebral meninges
- Other parts of central nervous system
- Intracranial gland (pineal gland, pituitary gland, and craniopharyngeal duct)

Default codes or standard tables are used for many fields, as shown below. (NA means not applicable.)

CS Tumor Size		Uses the common or standard tumor size table
CS Extension	100–999	Extension field is discussed below
CS TS/Ext Eval	9	NA for CNS sites* and intracranial glands**
CS Lymph Nodes	988	NA for CNS sites* and intracranial glands**
CS Reg Nodes Eval	9	NA for CNS sites* and intracranial glands**
Reg LN Pos	99	NA for CNS sites* and intracranial glands**
Reg LN Exam	99	NA for CNS sites* and intracranial glands**
CS Mets at Dx		Site-specific table for CNS sites* and intracranial glands**
CS Mets Eval	9	NA for CNS sites* and intracranial glands**

* CNS sites include brain and cerebral meninges, other parts of central nervous system

** Intracranial glands of the central nervous system are the pineal gland, pituitary gland, and craniopharyngeal duct

CS FOR BRAIN AND CEREBRAL MENINGES

CS Extension

With one important exception, CS Extension codes parallel the summary staging system codes and terminology because there are no equivalent T, N, or M categories. The Collaborative Staging code structure is based on what area of the brain is involved (infra- or supratentorial) and how far the tumor has spread.

The Extension field includes a code for non-malignant brain tumors for cases reportable as of 2004.

- The note defines which structures are supratentorial and which structures are infratentorial.
- Code 050 applies to benign or borderline brain tumors, regardless of any additional structures they may have extended to.
- Codes 100 through 120 are for tumors confined to a single location.
- Codes 150 through 300 are still localized but involve specific sites, such as the ventricles or meninges.
- Codes 400 through 510 are regional by direct extension—the tumor either crosses the midline of the brain or extends across the tentorium.
- Code 600 is still regional.
- Code 750 is the equivalent of distant direct extension.
    - Direct extension from the brain or cerebral meninges through bony structures into the nasal cavity, nasal or posterior pharynx may be described as further contiguous extension.
- Circulating cells in the cerebrospinal fluid which allow tumor cells to circulate to both the spinal cord and brain are coded in CS Mets at Dx code 20.

Collaborative Staging, *continued*

CS Lymph Nodes
Lymph nodes are coded as "not applicable" for brain, cerebral meninges, and intracranial glands.

CS Mets at Dx
In this field, other than "none" and "unknown," the choices are limited to "drop" metastasis (circulating cells in the CSF that have settled and begun to grow in the spinal column), extraneural metastases (outside the central nervous system), distant metastases, not further specified, and a combination code.

Site-Specific Factors
Note: Part I Section 2 of the CS Coding Manual Version 02.03 includes extensive discussion of the site-specific factors for every schema. Rather than rewrite those coding instructions for inclusion in this CASEbook chapter, refer to Part I Section 2 documentation if questions arise. The discussion that follows provides more rationale for why those site-specific factors were included in the various central nervous system schemas.

- The schemas for brain and other parts of the central nervous system use eight site-specific factors. The intracranial gland schema uses only the first two. The default code for all other SSFs is 988.

SSF1—World Health Organization (WHO) Grade Classification (for all CNS schemas)
Because of its prognostic significance, the WHO grade is collected as part of the Collaborative Staging System. Site-specific Factor 1 is used to code cases that are reported in the pathology report or radiology as "WHO grade *x*". If the WHO grade is not provided in the medical record, do not code it based on lists of CNS histologies from outside sources. Some histologies are not WHO-graded. Remember too that this is different from the grade/differentiation code for ICD-O-3. Refer to the SSF1 table for other code choices.

010	Grade I
020	Grade II
030	Grade III
040	Grade IV
999	Clinically diagnosed/grade unknown; Not documented in medical record; grade unknown, NOS

SSF2—Ki-67/MIB-1 Labeling Index: Brain
Ki-67 and MIB-1 are monoclonal antibodies that pathologists use for staining brain and other tumor cells to assess the aggressiveness of the tumor. The monoclonal antibody stains proliferating (actively dividing) cells, so this test, also referred to as the Labeling Index (LI), can differentiate slower growing from more rapidly growing tumors. Other terms are growth fraction, proliferation fraction, and proliferation marker. The LI is expressed as the percentage of cells in the tumor specimen that are in various phases of mitosis (proliferating).

Code the percentage as priority in the range 000 to 100. If the percentage is not specified, code the pathologist's statement of whether the labeling index is normal, slightly elevated, or elevated in the range 200–400.

SSF3—Functional Neurologic Status–Karnofsky Performance Scale (KPS)
The patient's usual functional status is an important underlying prognostic factor for central nervous system tumors. If the patient is already debilitated from other causes, recovery from a brain tumor will not be as complete or successful. The Karnofsky Performance Scale (KPS) provides physicians

Site-Specific Factors, *continued*

and nurses to a uniform tool to assess the patient's ability to do normal activities. In other words, the KPS measures whether the patient is able to perform personal care, do active work, and so forth.

KPS is measured in whole numbers (multiples of 10) from 000 (dead) to 100 (normal activities; able to perform activities of daily living without complaint). Note 3 of this site-specific factor lists the definition of each category. This is not a data field that the registrar can infer from the medical record, because observation of the patient is necessary to determine the patient's functional level. Look for a statement of the Karnofsky Performance Score in a physician's note, the admission history, or the discharge summary. If there is no clinician statement, use code 999.

SSF4—Methylation of 0^6-Methylquanine Methyltransferase (MGMT)
MGMT is an enzyme that repairs damaged DNA. If the DNA has been damaged by chemotherapy, the repair counteracts the effect of the chemotherapy, allowing continued tumor cell replication despite treatment. About two-thirds of glioblastoma multiforme brain tumors over-express MGMT.

Methylation is a natural process that "dilutes" or diminishes the repair capabilities of MGMT. The presence of higher levels of methylated MGMT (code 010) is a favorable prognostic factor indicating that the patient may respond to alkylating chemotherapy such as temozolomide (Temodar) or one of the nitrosoureas (BCNU or CCNU) and consequently have a better survival than a patient with low level of methylation (code 020). The test for methylated MGMT may also be used in cases of anaplastic oligodendroglioma and anaplastic astrocytoma.

Code results from a pathology report or laboratory report (in-house or from a reference lab). If no test for methylated MGMT is reported, code as 999.

SSF5—Chromosome 1p: Loss of Heterozygosity (LOH)
SSF6—Chromosome 19q: Loss of Heterozygosity (LOH)
These site-specific factors code information about two genetic tests, both of which are indicators that the patient may respond to certain chemotherapy agents (procarbazine, lomustine, and vincristine—the three drugs in the PCV regimen). 1p LOH and 19q LOH tests are commonly performed together on cases of oligodendroglioma, anaplastic oligodendroglioma, oligoastrocytoma, and anaplastic oligoastrocytoma, but not usually on other cell types such as glioblastoma.

Heterozygosity is the normal status of having two complete copies of each chromosome. In the case of SSF5, part of the short arm (p) of chromosome 1 is missing. In the case of SSF6, part of the long arm (q) of chromosome 19 is missing. This missing chromosomal data is termed "loss of heterozygosity." Other names include allelic loss and gene deletion.

For patients with brain tumors, loss of either of these pieces of a chromosome (code 010) is actually a favorable prognostic factor because it indicates that the patient may respond to chemotherapy. Use code 020 if the report states that the chromosomes are normal (no loss of heterozygosity). Use code 999 for benign and borderline brain tumors as well as for cases where loss of heterozygosity status is not documented.

SSF7—Surgical Resection
This field was added in CS version 0202 for 2010 cases and forward. At the time, the Commission on Cancer's FORDS manual did not have the same codes. FORDS 2011 uses the same codes as CS version 0203, so in many respects this field is redundant with Surgery of Primary Site. The differences between SSF7 and Surgery of Primary Site in FORDS 2011 are:

Site-Specific Factors, *continued*

- Surgery of Primary Site is a two digit field; SSF7 is a three-digit field having the same codes with a leading zero (21 in FORDS, 021 in SSF7).
- SSF7 code descriptions include a statement whether the tumor involves less than or greater than half of the lobe. This information is not usually available.
- SSF7 is not required by any of the standards setters; Surgery of Primary Site is required for completion of the cancer abstract.
- Code 22 (resection of spinal cord or nerve) is not used in the brain schema, but is included in the Other CNS schema

The purpose of this field is to document the completeness of surgical resection for primary brain tumors as a predictor of outcome: the more tumor that can be removed, the more effective adjuvant radiation or chemotherapy will be. Refer to the Surgery section earlier in this chapter for a more detailed discussion of the codes and definitions. In brief, however, the codes in SSF7 have the following intent:

- Code 020 is really intended for biopsies and procedures where no attempt is made to remove the entire tumor.
- Code 021 is for attempted but incomplete resection (the surgeon indicates that gross tumor was left behind). Most cases will be coded here or in code 030.
- Code 030 is for complete or total resection as noted by the surgeon, although the pathologist may indicate that there was microscopic tumor left at the margins.
- Codes 040 and 055 are rarely performed because they remove normal brain tissue as well as the tumor.

SSF8—Unifocal vs. Multifocal Tumor

This field codes the number of primary tumors in the brain as single/solitary/unifocal (code 001) or multiple/multifocal/multicentric (code 002). Patients with multifocal tumors have a worse prognosis than patients who have a solitary brain tumor. The number of primary tumors also has prognostic value in determining treatment.

Code any statement of single versus multiple tumors—*excluding metastases*—in the medical record. If the number of tumors is determined intraoperatively or on resection, the pathology report takes priority. The number of tumors may also be determined clinically (on imaging or MRI).

CS FOR OTHER PARTS OF CENTRAL NERVOUS SYSTEM

CS Extension

The Extension field for other central nervous system sites (mostly the cranial nerves and spinal meninges) is less detailed. The basic code groups are 050 (benign and borderline), 100 and 300 (localized), 400 to 600 (regional direct extension), and 700–800 (distant).

- Adjacent connective tissue (code 500) is defined in Part I Section 1 of the CS coding instructions.

CS Mets at DX

This field is similar in structure to CS Mets at DX for most solid tumor schemas.

Site-Specific Factors 1–8

The CNSOther schema uses the same eight site-specific factors as brain.

CS FOR INTRACRANIAL GLANDS

CS Extension
The code structure is similar to that for Other Parts of Central Nervous System, with code 050 specified as applying only to pituitary gland, craniopharyngeal duct, and pineal gland.

CS Mets at DX
The code structure is similar to that for Other Parts of Central Nervous System.

Site-Specific Factors 1–2
The Intracranial Gland schema uses only SSF1 (WHO Grade Classification) and SSF2 (Ki-67/MIB-1 Labeling Index).

OTHER STAGING SYSTEMS

SUMMARY STAGE

The Summary Staging classification for the brain, cerebral meninges, and other parts of the central nervous system is found in the Summary Staging Manual 2000 on pages 266 - 268. Because there is no TNM staging system for central nervous system tumors, you should be familiar with summary staging definitions, as they form the basis of the code definitions in Collaborative Staging.

Summary Stage 2000

Code	Brief Description (see Summary Staging Manual 2000 for details)
1—Local	Confined to: ° one hemisphere in one part of brain (infra- or supratentorial) ° more than one lobe in same hemisphere (supratentorial) ° meninges (malignant), NOS ° confined to ventricles or invading/encroaching on ventricular system ° hypothalamus; thalamus
5—Regional, NOS	Crossing midline or tentorium ° invades bone, blood vessels, nerves, spinal cord
7—Distant	Circulating cells in CSF Extension to nasal cavity, nasopharynx, posterior pharynx; outside CNS
8—Not applicable	**Note:** code 8 was added to Summary Stage 2000 effective January 1, 2004 specifically to allow coding of benign and borderline central nervous system tumors, including non-malignant meningiomas.

AJCC (TNM)

There is no AJCC stage for the central nervous system tumors. The *AJCC Cancer Staging Manual* seventh edition discusses various risk and prognostic factors for brain tumors and provides lists of the WHO Classification of brain tumors with their ICD-O-3 morphology codes as well as WHO grades by histology.

Prognostic Indicators for Central Nervous System Tumors (adapted from *AJCC Cancer Staging Manual*, seventh edition)

- Histologic cell type and grade, including presence or absence of necrosis
- Location of tumor within brain

Prognostic Indicators, *continued*

- Proliferative fraction; presence or absence of cells in mitosis
- Presence of gemistocytes or an oligodendroglial component
- CNS or extraneural metastases
- Age of patient (most important prognostic factor after histology)
- Functional neurologic status
- Type and duration of symptoms before diagnosis
- Patterns of enhancement on imaging
- Extent of resection (biopsy, subtotal, radical excision)
- Molecular factors in resected tissue (1p, 19q deletions; methylated MGMT)

EPIDEMIOLOGY AND ETIOLOGY

- Neuroepithelial CNS tumors are more common in whites than other races.
- Neuroepithelial CNS tumors are more common in men than women.
- Meningiomas are more common in blacks than other races.
- Meningiomas are more common in women than men.
- Most common tumors by age group (non-malignant and malignant combined)

0 – 5	Embryonal/PNET/Medulloblastoma
5 – 19	Pilocytic astrocytoma
20 – 34	Pituitary tumors
35 – 54	Meningiomas
55 – 74	Glioblastomas
75 and older	Meningiomas

- Other risk factors
  - Ionizing radiation (high-dose radiation therapy to head as a child, atomic energy)
  - Chemicals (pesticides, solvents, lead, polyvinyl chloride, petroleum-based chemicals, formaldehyde used by pathologists and embalmers)
  - Genetic disorders (neurofibromatosis type 1 {von Recklinghausen's}, Li-Fraumeni syndrome, tuberous sclerosis, von Hippel-Lindau syndrome)
  - Family history of brain tumor
  - Cell phone use (non-ionizing radiation) has *not* been positively linked to CNS tumors.

Page left blank.

Abstracting, Staging, and Coding Exercises

This section includes twelve single-page brain and central nervous system tumor cases to be coded in ICD-O-3, Summary Stage 2000, and CS version 0203.
(AJCC TNM 7th Edition does not apply to CNS tumors.)
NOTE: For the purposes of these brief cases, assume that all other tests not mentioned in the case are negative for malignancy.

- Identify the primary site and schema.
- Assign the codes for primary site, histology, behavior, and grade.
- Assign codes to all applicable CS fields.
- Assume that your facility does offer a test and that the standards setters for your facility require the data field. In other words, avoid using code 988 (not applicable).
- 20XX is the diagnosis year, and where applicable, 20YY is the following year.

Default values for central nervous sytem tumors (not included in case exercises)

Grade Path Value	Blank	No 2, 3, or 4-grade system available
Grade Path System	Blank	No 2, 3, or 4-grade system available
Clinical/Pathologic T, N, M	88	Not applicable
Clinical/Pathologic Stage Group	88	Not applicable
CS TS/Ext Eval	9	Not applicable
CS Lymph Nodes	988	Not applicable
CS Reg Nodes Eval	9	Not applicable
Reg LN Pos	99	Not applicable
Reg LN Exam	99	Not applicable
CS Mets Eval	9	Not applicable for this schema

CASE 1

HISTORY AND PHYSICAL EXAM
Patient collapsed at home and went into seizures. In the emergency room, physical findings were within normal limits.

X-RAYS AND SCANS
1-4-20XX Brain scan: Abnormal uptake in R temporal lobe.
1-6-20XX CT scan: Large lesion in R temporal lobe extending from inner table of temporal bone deep to thalamus.
1-7-20XX Angiogram: Confirms 3 cm vascular mass in R temporal lobe.

LABORATORY REPORTS
All studies within normal limits.

OPERATIVE REPORTS
1-10-20XX Craniotomy and partial resection of temporal lobe tumor: Deep-seated primary tumor medial to lip of temporal horn of ventricle. Gross tumor left in tumor cavity.

PATHOLOGY REPORT
1-10-20XX Astrocytoma, WHO Grade III, right temporal lobe of brain with hypermethylation.

TREATMENT
1-10-20XX Craniotomy and partial debulking of temporal lobe tumor; implantation of Gliadel wafer in tumor bed

Site Code ___ ___ ___.___	**Date Mult Tumors**	**SSF1 WHO Grade** ___ ___ ___
Histology/Behavior/Grade ___ ___ ___ ___ / ___ ___	___ ___ ___ ___ ___ ___ ___ ___	**SSF2 Ki-67/MIB1** ___ ___ ___
Lymph Vascular Invasion ___	**Date Mult Tumors Flag** ___ ___	**SSF3 Karnofsky Performance Scale** ___ ___ ___
Ambiguous Terminol ___	**Mult Tum Reported as One Prim** ___ ___	**SSF4 MGMT Methyl** ___ ___ ___
Date Conclusive Terminol	**Summary Stage 2000** ___	**SSF5 Chr 1p LOH** ___ ___ ___
___ ___ ___ ___ ___ ___ ___ ___	**CS Tumor Size** ___ ___ ___	**SSF6 Chr 19q LOH** ___ ___ ___
Date Conclus Dx Flag ___ ___	**CS Extension** ___ ___ ___	**SSF7 Surg Resect** ___ ___ ___
Multiplicity Counter ___ ___	**CS Mets at Dx** ___ ___	**SSF8 Multifocality** ___ ___ ___

CASE 2

HISTORY AND PHYSICAL EXAM

4 year old girl with a 3 month history of headache, nausea, vomiting and staring spells. She presented with new onset ataxia and slurred speech. No abnormal physical findings.

X-RAYS AND SCANS

4-21-20XX MRI with contrast: Large enhancing mass in the third ventricle involving the left foramen of Monro. Mass is associated with dilated lateral ventricles, and white matter edema. The fourth ventricle was normal in size. No other cortical or ventricular abnormalities were seen.

LABORATORY REPORTS

No significant findings.

OPERATIVE REPORTS

4-28-20XX Left frontal craniotomy: Lesion arising from the left hypothalamus and extending into the third ventricle. Greater than 99% of the tumor was resected.

PATHOLOGY REPORT

4-28-20XX Subependymal giant cell astrocytoma.

TREATMENT

4-28-20XX Left frontal craniotomy and near-total resection of hypothalamic tumor

Her post-operative course was uneventful and she was discharged home.

Site Code ___ ___ ___.___	Date Mult Tumors ___ ___ ___ ___ ___ ___ ___ ___	SSF1 WHO Grade ___ ___ ___
Histology/Behavior/Grade ___ ___ ___ ___/___ ___	Date Mult Tumors Flag ___ ___	SSF2 Ki-67/MIB1 ___ ___ ___
Lymph Vascular Invasion ___	Mult Tum Reported as One Prim ___ ___	SSF3 Karnofsky Performance Scale ___ ___ ___
Ambiguous Terminol ___	Summary Stage 2000 ___	SSF4 MGMT Methyl ___ ___ ___
Date Conclusive Terminol ___ ___ ___ ___ ___ ___ ___ ___	CS Tumor Size ___ ___ ___	SSF5 Chr 1p LOH ___ ___ ___
Date Conclus Dx Flag ___ ___	CS Extension ___ ___ ___	SSF6 Chr 19q LOH ___ ___ ___
Multiplicity Counter ___ ___	CS Mets at Dx ___ ___	SSF7 Surg Resect ___ ___ ___
		SSF8 Multifocality ___ ___ ___

CASE 3

HISTORY AND PHYSICAL EXAM

8 month history of decreased vision and severe headaches. He also has a history of arteriosclerotic heart disease and cerebrovascular accident (CVA) with right hemiparesis. Physical exam limited by patient's weakness on right side and inability to stand. Karnofsky score 50 on admission.

X-RAYS AND SCANS

2-22-20XX CT scan: Large (5.5 cm) low density lesion of the brain compatible with infarct or tumor.

2-22-20XX Chest x-ray: Negative for metastases.

2-23-20XX Carotid angiogram, right: Abnormal neoplastic mass involving right posterior tempoparietal and occipital regions, most likely a high grade glioma with neovascularity.

LABORATORY REPORTS

All routine laboratory studies within normal limits.

OPERATIVE REPORTS

2-28-20XX Right occipital craniotomy with removal of tumor: Neoplasm appeared to invade the dura at the occipital pole in the occipital lobe. Incompletely excised due to extent of lesion. Size not stated.

PATHOLOGY REPORT

2-28-20XX Ependymoma, WHO Grade II-III, right occipital lobe.

TREATMENT

2-28-20XX Right occipital craniotomy and partial removal of occipital tumor

3-21-20XX Patient referred for consultation regarding external beam radiation therapy to brain

Site Code ___ ___ ___.___	Date Mult Tumors ___ ___ ___ ___ ___ ___ ___ ___	SSF1 WHO Grade ___ ___ ___
Histology/Behavior/Grade ___ ___ ___ ___/___ ___	Date Mult Tumors Flag ___ ___	SSF2 Ki-67/MIB1 ___ ___ ___
Lymph Vascular Invasion ___	Mult Tum Reported as One Prim ___ ___	SSF3 Karnofsky Performance Scale ___ ___ ___
Ambiguous Terminol ___	Summary Stage 2000 ___	SSF4 MGMT Methyl ___ ___ ___
Date Conclusive Terminol ___ ___ ___ ___ ___ ___ ___ ___	CS Tumor Size ___ ___ ___	SSF5 Chr 1p LOH ___ ___ ___
Date Conclus Dx Flag ___ ___	CS Extension ___ ___ ___	SSF6 Chr 19q LOH ___ ___ ___
Multiplicity Counter ___ ___	CS Mets at Dx ___ ___	SSF7 Surg Resect ___ ___ ___
		SSF8 Multifocality ___ ___ ___

CASE 4

HISTORY AND PHYSICAL EXAM

17 year old female with a 3 week history of headaches, nipple discharge, hirsutism, abnormal menstruation.
Physical exam: No adenopathy, organomegaly or abnormal skin lesions. Gynecologic exam within normal limits for adolescent female.

X-RAYS AND SCANS

6-15-20XX MRI scan: 1.5 cm enhancing lesion in the sella turcica with compression of normal pituitary gland.

LABORATORY REPORTS

Prior to admission: Serum prolactin: 146 ng/ml (normal range 0–15 ng/ml). Thyroid function tests within normal limits. Serum leutinizing hormone (LH) was 2.2 IU/l (normal), follicle-stimulating hormone (FSH) was 3.5 IU/l (normal), and morning cortisol was 14.5 μg/100 ml (normal).

OPERATIVE REPORTS

6-20-20XX Stereotactic guided excision of pituitary tumor: No report.

PATHOLOGY REPORT

6-20-20XX Pituitary tumor: Monotonous cells with round nuclei, prominent nuclei and moderate blue-gray cytoplasm, displacing normal pituitary architecture. Immunoperoxidase stain for oncocytes is positive in the neoplastic cells.
Final diagnosis: Well-differentiated pituitary oncocytic carcinoma.

TREATMENT

6-20-20XX Stereotactic-guided excision of pituitary tumor
6-25-20XX Started replacement hormonal therapy

Site Code ___ ___ ___ . ___	**Date Mult Tumors Flag** ___ ___
Histology/Behavior/Grade ___ ___ ___ ___ / ___ ___	**Mult Tum Reported as One Prim** ___ ___
Lymph Vascular Invasion ___	**Summary Stage 2000** ___
Ambiguous Terminol ___	**CS Tumor Size** ___ ___ ___
Date Conclusive Terminol ___ ___ ___ ___ ___ ___ ___ ___	**CS Extension** ___ ___ ___
	CS Mets at Dx ___ ___
Date Conclus Dx Flag ___ ___	**SSF1 WHO Grade** ___ ___ ___
Multiplicity Counter ___ ___	**SSF2 Ki-67/MIB1** ___ ___ ___
Date Mult Tumors ___ ___ ___ ___ ___ ___ ___ ___	

CASE 5

HISTORY AND PHYSICAL EXAM

Eleven year old female found by her mother to have a firm bump on her head over the left frontal region.
Neurologic exam: No history of headache, nausea, vomiting, dizziness or tenderness of the lump. Papilledema noted on eye exam. Remainder of physical findings were within normal limits.

X-RAYS AND SCANS

9-18-20XX CT scan: Left frontoparietal bony erosion and thickening by large extra-axial tumor mass that extended into the brain.
9-19-20XX MRI: 7 cm left frontoparietal mass appeared to arise from the region of the dura and bone and extended both intra- and extra-cranially. Overlying bone markedly thickened. Gadolinium enhancement of intracranial portion of tumor with lesser enhancement of extracranial portion. Differential diagnoses: Primary chondrosarcoma, PNET, metastatic neuroblastoma, meningioma.

LABORATORY REPORTS

No abnormal findings

OPERATIVE REPORTS

9-21-20XX Resection of tumor: Expansive mass attached to dura. Peeled away from pia mater and periosteum with some difficulty.

PATHOLOGY REPORT

9-21-20XX Frontoparietal tumor mass: Loosely defined nests of cohesive meningothelial cells with whorl formation and psammoma body formation. Numerous areas of micronecrosis. Occasional mitotic figures. No significant pleomorphism or areas of increased cellularity. Numerous sections of the cerebral surface of the tumor showed no brain invasion. The bone showed diffuse expansion by the tumor, which extended entirely through the outer table of the skull in the area corresponding grossly to bony softening. Final diagnosis: Atypical meningioma.

TREATMENT

9-21-20XX Left frontoparietal craniotomy and excision of subdural tumor

Site Code ___ ___ ___.___	Date Mult Tumors ___ ___ ___ ___ ___ ___ ___ ___	SSF1 WHO Grade ___ ___ ___
Histology/Behavior/Grade ___ ___ ___ ___ / ___ ___	Date Mult Tumors Flag ___ ___	SSF2 Ki-67/MIB1 ___ ___ ___
Lymph Vascular Invasion ___	Mult Tum Reported as One Prim ___ ___	SSF3 Karnofsky Performance Scale ___ ___ ___
Ambiguous Terminol ___	Summary Stage 2000 ___	SSF4 MGMT Methyl ___ ___ ___
Date Conclusive Terminol ___ ___ ___ ___ ___ ___ ___ ___	CS Tumor Size ___ ___ ___	SSF5 Chr 1p LOH ___ ___ ___
Date Conclus Dx Flag ___ ___	CS Extension ___ ___ ___	SSF6 Chr 19q LOH ___ ___ ___
Multiplicity Counter ___ ___	CS Mets at Dx ___ ___	SSF7 Surg Resect ___ ___ ___
		SSF8 Multifocality ___ ___ ___

CASE 6

HISTORY AND PHYSICAL EXAM
Headaches with nausea. Neuro deficits, left hemiplegia, balance problems. No abnormal physical findings.

X-RAYS AND SCANS
3-13-20XX CT head: Consistent with tumor, probably primary.
3-13-20XX Chest x-ray: No evidence of disease.
3-15-20XX MRI brain: Right temporal mass consistent with high grade glioma, size 6 cm.

LABORATORY REPORTS
Routine laboratory tests normal.

OPERATIVE REPORTS
3-16-20XX Resection of brain tumor: Right temporal lobe grossly abnormal with evidence of tumor; grossly debulked.

PATHOLOGY REPORT
3-16-20XX Biopsy of brain: Anaplastic glioma.
Resection of brain tumor: Glioblastoma multiforme in right temporal lobe. Labeling index 12%. MGMT methylation not identified.

TREATMENT
3-16-20XX Gross resection of brain tumor
4-18-20XX to 5-31-200X 4000 cGY to brain

Site Code ___ ___ ___.___	**Date Mult Tumors** ___ ___ ___ ___ ___ ___ ___ ___	**SSF1 WHO Grade** ___ ___ ___
Histology/Behavior/Grade ___ ___ ___ ___/___ ___	**Date Mult Tumors Flag** ___ ___	**SSF2 Ki-67/MIB1** ___ ___ ___
Lymph Vascular Invasion ___	**Mult Tum Reported as One Prim** ___ ___	**SSF3 Karnofsky Performance Scale** ___ ___ ___
Ambiguous Terminol ___	**Summary Stage 2000** ___	**SSF4 MGMT Methyl** ___ ___ ___
Date Conclusive Terminol ___ ___ ___ ___ ___ ___ ___ ___	**CS Tumor Size** ___ ___ ___	**SSF5 Chr 1p LOH** ___ ___ ___
Date Conclus Dx Flag ___ ___	**CS Extension** ___ ___ ___	**SSF6 Chr 19q LOH** ___ ___ ___
Multiplicity Counter ___ ___	**CS Mets at Dx** ___ ___	**SSF7 Surg Resect** ___ ___ ___
		SSF8 Multifocality ___ ___ ___

CASE 7

HISTORY AND PHYSICAL EXAM

53 year old male presenting with bilateral claudication pain and radiating pain to right quadriceps. General physical exam: No adenopathy, organomegaly or physical signs.

X-RAYS AND SCANS

Prior to admission MRI spine: 6 x 5 x 4 mm intradural neural tumor at L2 with L2-3 stenosis and lateral recess stenosis worse on left than right.

7-5-20XX MRI lumbar spine with and without gadolinium enhancement: Small mass 9 x 8 x 8 mm centered to right of midline at L2 level. Differential diagnostic considerations would include meningioma vs. nerve root or nerve sheath tumor vs. drop metastasis.

LABORATORY REPORTS

None significant.

OPERATIVE REPORTS

7-7-20XX Laminectomy and removal of intradural neural tumor: No significant findings reported.

PATHOLOGY REPORT

7-7-20XX 1) Soft tissue, L2: Schwannoma.
2) Bone and ligament, L2-L3: Dense fibrous tissue and corticomedullary bone with no histopathologic abnormalities.

TREATMENT

7-7-20XX L2 laminectomy with removal of intradural neural tumor with microdissection and intraoperative somatosensory and motor evoked potential monitoring. L3 laminectomy. Bilateral L2-3 lateral recess and central decompression performed at second level for distinct pathology and separate diagnosis.

Site Code __ __ __.__	Date Mult Tumors __ __ __ __ __ __ __ __	SSF1 WHO Grade __ __ __
Histology/Behavior/Grade __ __ __ __ / __ __	Date Mult Tumors Flag __ __	SSF2 Ki-67/MIB1 __ __ __
Lymph Vascular Invasion __	Mult Tum Reported as One Prim __ __	SSF3 Karnofsky Performance Scale __ __ __
Ambiguous Terminol __	Summary Stage 2000 __	SSF4 MGMT Methyl __ __ __
Date Conclusive Terminol __ __ __ __ __ __ __ __	CS Tumor Size __ __ __	SSF5 Chr 1p LOH __ __ __
Date Conclus Dx Flag __ __	CS Extension __ __ __	SSF6 Chr 19q LOH __ __ __
Multiplicity Counter __ __	CS Mets at Dx __ __	SSF7 Surg Resect __ __ __
		SSF8 Multifocality __ __ __

CASE 8

HISTORY AND PHYSICAL EXAM
49 year woman with progressive bitemporal visual field loss particularly affecting the right eye. No abnormal physical findings.

X-RAYS AND SCANS
11-2-20XX MRI: Large suprasellar pituitary extension measuring 24 x 21 x 16 mm with displacement of the optic chiasm, deformation of the third ventricle, and some lateral spread on the right side.

LABORATORY REPORTS
Essentially normal.

OPERATIVE REPORTS
11-5-20XX Trans-sphenoidal hypophysectomy.

PATHOLOGY REPORT
11-5-20XX Final diagnosis: Chromophobe adenoma.

FURTHER TREATMENT
Postoperative radiotherapy of pituitary region, total treatment dose of 4680 cGy in 25 daily fractions over five weeks.

Site Code	___ ___ ___.___	**Date Mult Tumors Flag**	___ ___
Histology/Behavior/Grade	___ ___ ___ ___ / ___ ___	**Mult Tum Reported as One Prim**	___ ___
Lymph Vascular Invasion	___	**Summary Stage 2000**	___
Ambiguous Terminol	___	**CS Tumor Size**	___ ___ ___
Date Conclusive Terminol	___ ___ ___ ___ ___ ___ ___ ___	**CS Extension**	___ ___ ___
		CS Mets at Dx	___ ___
Date Conclus Dx Flag	___ ___	**SSF1 WHO Grade**	___ ___ ___
Multiplicity Counter	___ ___	**SSF2 Ki-67/MIB1**	___ ___ ___
Date Mult Tumors	___ ___ ___ ___ ___ ___ ___ ___		

CASE 9

HISTORY AND PHYSICAL EXAM
Patient presented with right jaw pain, facial pain, headache, and hypertension.

X-RAYS AND SCANS
10-2-20XX MRI Brain and IACS [internal auditory canals]: Normal MRI of the seventh and eighth cranial nerve complex and origin/proximal trigeminal nerves. The ventricles, sulci, and cisterns are increased in size compatible with atrophy. No mass effect nor midline shift is identified. Findings are compatible with small vessel disease. Two dural based masses are present. The larger is on the right measuring 1.4 x 1.3 cm in transverse and cephalocaudad dimensions. The slightly smaller one is on the left measuring 0.9 x 0.6 cm in the frontoparietal region in cephalocaudad and transverse dimensions respectively. These are isointense on T1 weighted images and enhance homogeneously. They are slightly hypointense on the FLAIR and T2 weighted images. Findings are compatible with small meningiomas.

LABORATORY REPORTS
Routine laboratory tests within normal limits.

OPERATIVE REPORTS
None.

PATHOLOGY REPORT
None.

TREATMENT
Patient referred for bilateral IMRT

Site Code ___ ___ ___.___	**Date Mult Tumors**	**SSF1 WHO Grade** ___ ___ ___
Histology/Behavior/Grade ___ ___ ___ ___ / ___ ___	___ ___ ___ ___ ___ ___ ___ ___	**SSF2 Ki-67/MIB1** ___ ___ ___
Lymph Vascular Invasion ___	**Date Mult Tumors Flag** ___ ___	**SSF3 Karnofsky Performance Scale** ___ ___ ___
Ambiguous Terminol ___	**Mult Tum Reported as One Prim** ___ ___	**SSF4 MGMT Methyl** ___ ___ ___
Date Conclusive Terminol	**Summary Stage 2000** ___	**SSF5 Chr 1p LOH** ___ ___ ___
___ ___ ___ ___ ___ ___ ___ ___	**CS Tumor Size** ___ ___ ___	**SSF6 Chr 19q LOH** ___ ___ ___
Date Conclus Dx Flag ___ ___	**CS Extension** ___ ___ ___	**SSF7 Surg Resect** ___ ___ ___
Multiplicity Counter ___ ___	**CS Mets at Dx** ___ ___	**SSF8 Multifocality** ___ ___ ___

CASE 10

HISTORY AND PHYSICAL EXAM

Difficulty with memory and speech.
Physical exam: Unremarkable.

X-RAYS AND SCANS

9-8-20XX CXR: LUL mass, no hilar or mediastinal adenopathy.
Repeat CXR showed resolution of mass—likely pneumonitis.
9-8-20XX CT brain: Large 3.8 cm lesion L posterior frontal and temporal region extending across midline.

LABORATORY REPORTS

Routine laboratory tests normal.

OPERATIVE REPORTS

9-11-20XX Excision of brain tumor: Brain very edematous. Frozen section biopsies positive for glioma. Incomplete excision.

PATHOLOGY REPORT

9-11-20XX Left frontotemporal region: Poorly differentiated gliosarcoma. Ki-67 elevated.
Chromosomes 1p and 19q normal (not mutated)

TREATMENT

9-11-20XX Excision of brain tumor
10-2-20XX to 11-17-20XX 7200 rads to frontotemporal area

Site Code ___ ___ ___.___	Date Mult Tumors ___ ___ ___ ___ ___ ___ ___ ___	SSF1 WHO Grade ___ ___ ___
Histology/Behavior/Grade ___ ___ ___ ___/___ ___	Date Mult Tumors Flag ___ ___	SSF2 Ki-67/MIB1 ___ ___ ___
Lymph Vascular Invasion ___	Mult Tum Reported as One Prim ___ ___	SSF3 Karnofsky Performance Scale ___ ___ ___
Ambiguous Terminol ___	Summary Stage 2000 ___	SSF4 MGMT Methyl ___ ___ ___
Date Conclusive Terminol ___ ___ ___ ___ ___ ___ ___ ___	CS Tumor Size ___ ___ ___	SSF5 Chr 1p LOH ___ ___ ___
Date Conclus Dx Flag ___ ___	CS Extension ___ ___ ___	SSF6 Chr 19q LOH ___ ___ ___
Multiplicity Counter ___ ___	CS Mets at Dx ___ ___	SSF7 Surg Resect ___ ___ ___
		SSF8 Multifocality ___ ___ ___

CASE 11

HISTORY AND PHYSICAL EXAM
Elderly patient saw personal MD with complaints of dizziness and headache. No physical examination performed.

X-RAYS AND SCANS
8-16-20XX Emergent CT Brain without contrast: Small partially calcified 1 cm mass in the right frontal lobe abutting the cortex, most likely reflecting a meningioma. Follow-up MRI is suggested.

8-20-20XX MRI Brain with and without contrast: Enhancing extra-axial right frontal lobe mass with apparent dural tail measuring 1 cm AP x 1.1 cm transverse x 1.2 cm craniocaudally. No significant surrounding edema. Findings most compatible with meningioma. There is no increased diffusion weighted signal to suggest an area of acute infarction. There is no definite acute intracranial hemorrhage. Ill-defined linear area of enhancement left frontal region without adjacent inflammation, likely reflecting venous angioma. Six month follow-up advised to ensure stability and exclude other etiology. The visualized paranasal sinuses are grossly clear. There is suggestion of a small area of nodularity in the right parotid gland superiorly coronal image #11 of uncertain significance.

LABORATORY REPORTS
None.

OPERATIVE REPORTS
None.

PATHOLOGY REPORT
None.

TREATMENT
None reported

Site Code ___ ___ ___.___	**Date Mult Tumors**	**SSF1 WHO Grade** ___ ___ ___
Histology/Behavior/Grade ___ ___ ___ ___ / ___ ___	___ ___ ___ ___ ___ ___ ___ ___	**SSF2 Ki-67/MIB1** ___ ___ ___
Lymph Vascular Invasion ___	**Date Mult Tumors Flag** ___ ___	**SSF3 Karnofsky Performance Scale** ___ ___ ___
Ambiguous Terminol ___	**Mult Tum Reported as One Prim** ___ ___	**SSF4 MGMT Methyl** ___ ___ ___
Date Conclusive Terminol	**Summary Stage 2000** ___	**SSF5 Chr 1p LOH** ___ ___ ___
___ ___ ___ ___ ___ ___ ___ ___	**CS Tumor Size** ___ ___ ___	**SSF6 Chr 19q LOH** ___ ___ ___
Date Conclus Dx Flag ___ ___	**CS Extension** ___ ___ ___	**SSF7 Surg Resect** ___ ___ ___
Multiplicity Counter ___ ___	**CS Mets at Dx** ___ ___	**SSF8 Multifocality** ___ ___ ___

CASE 12

HISTORY AND PHYSICAL EXAM

41 year old woman evaluated for post-operative nausea and vomiting. MRI of brain performed as part of search for source of vomiting; mass identified in floor of fourth ventricle.

5-25-20XX Neurologic exam: Patient alert and oriented. No focal cranial nerve abnormalities; no trouble swallowing; normal speech patterns; shoulder shrug intact. No facial asymmetry or numbness. Full occular motions noted; visual acuity intact. No dysmetria, tremor or nystagmus.

X-RAYS AND SCANS

Prior to admission MRI brain: Mass in floor of fourth ventricle extending from posterior brainstem into fourth ventricle. No associated hydrocephalus or associated obstruction or mass effect. Impression: Possible fourth ventricular ependymoma versus choroid plexus papilloma or other exophytic glial tumors of the posterior brainstem.

LABORATORY REPORTS

No significant abnormalities.

OPERATIVE REPORTS

5-31-20XX Removal of infratentorial tumor: partial resection of deep seated brainstem tumor.

PATHOLOGY REPORT

5-31-20XX Open biopsy, infratentorial brain: Unremarkable cerebellum.
Brain stem tumor: Anaplastic astrocytoma, WHO grade 3. MGMT methylation present. MIB-1 labeling index 28.7%

TREATMENT

5-31-20XX Image-guided navigational suboccipital craniotomy for removal of infratentorial tumor with microdissection. Intraoperative monitoring performed with facial nerve emphasis.

7-2-20XX 3D conformal treatment with MRI fusion. 45 Gy to brainstem in 25 doses with 9 Gy boost. Total cumulative dose: 54 Gy.

8-16-20XX Concurrent Temodar

Site Code ___ ___ ___.___	**Date Mult Tumors** ___ ___ ___ ___ ___ ___ ___ ___	**SSF1 WHO Grade** ___ ___ ___
Histology/Behavior/Grade ___ ___ ___ ___ / ___ ___	**Date Mult Tumors Flag** ___ ___	**SSF2 Ki-67/MIB1** ___ ___ ___
Lymph Vascular Invasion ___	**Mult Tum Reported as One Prim** ___ ___	**SSF3 Karnofsky Performance Scale** ___ ___ ___
Ambiguous Terminol ___	**Summary Stage 2000** ___	**SSF4 MGMT Methyl** ___ ___ ___
Date Conclusive Terminol ___ ___ ___ ___ ___ ___ ___ ___	**CS Tumor Size** ___ ___ ___	**SSF5 Chr 1p LOH** ___ ___ ___
Date Conclus Dx Flag ___ ___	**CS Extension** ___ ___ ___	**SSF6 Chr 19q LOH** ___ ___ ___
Multiplicity Counter ___ ___	**CS Mets at Dx** ___ ___	**SSF7 Surg Resect** ___ ___ ___
		SSF8 Multifocality ___ ___ ___

ANSWERS TO BRAIN AND CENTRAL NERVOUS SYSTEM STAGING EXERCISES

Note: All cases will map to T NA N NA M NA Stage Group NA (not applicable)

—— CASE 1 ——

Primary Site	C71.2	Temporal lobe
Histology	9400/39	Astrocytoma, NOS; histologic grade not stated. Do not code WHO grade here.
Lymph Vascular Invasion	9	Lymph-vascular invasion not mentioned in path report
Ambiguous Terminology	0	Conclusive terminology
Date Conclusive Terminol	Blank	Diagnosis made by conclusive terminology
Date Conclus Dx Flag	11	Not applicable
Multiplicity Counter	01	One tumor only
Date Multiple Tumors	Blank	Not applicable
Date Mult Tumors Flag	15	Single tumor only (multiplicity counter is coded 01)
Type Mult Tum as 1 Prim	00	Single tumor
Summary Stage	1	Localized
CS Schema	Brain	
CS Tumor Size	030	3 cm vascular mass
CS Extension	100	Confined to right temporal lobe
CS Mets at Dx	00	Physical exam normal
CS Mets at Dx–Bone	0	No bone metastases
CS Mets at Dx–Brain	0	No brain metastases
CS Mets at Dx–Liver	0	No liver metastases
CS Mets at Dx–Lung	0	No lung metastases
SSF1 WHO Grade	030	WHO grade III
SSF2 Ki-67/MIB1 LI	999	Unknown, not documented
SSF3 Karnofsky Scale	999	Unknown, not documented
SSF4 MGMT Methyl	010	Hypermethylation is another name for elevated levels of methylation
SSF5 Chr 1p LOH	999	Unknown, not documented
SSF6 Chr 19q LOH	999	Unknown, not documented
SSF7 Surg Resection	021	Partial debulking (subtotal resection)
SSF8 Multifocality	001	Unifocal

—— CASE 2 ——

Primary Site	C71.0	Hypothalamus
Histology	9384/19	Subependymal giant cell astrocytoma, no grade
Lymph Vascular Invasion	9	Lymph-vascular invasion not mentioned in path report
Ambiguous Terminology	0	Conclusive terminology
Date Conclusive Terminol	Blank	Diagnosis made by conclusive terminology
Date Conclus Dx Flag	11	Not applicable
Multiplicity Counter	01	One tumor only
Date Multiple Tumors	Blank	Not applicable
Date Mult Tumors Flag	15	Single tumor only (multiplicity counter is coded 01)
Type Mult Tum as 1 Prim	00	Single tumor

Case 2, continued

Summary Stage	8	Not applicable (borderline tumor)
CS Schema	Brain	
CS Tumor Size	999	Size not stated
CS Extension	050	Borderline tumor (even though it extended into third ventricle)
CS Mets at Dx	00	No abnormal physical findings
CS Tumor Size	030	3 cm vascular mass
CS Extension	10	Confined to right temporal lobe
CS Mets at Dx	00	Physical exam normal
CS Mets at Dx–Bone	0	No bone metastases
CS Mets at Dx–Brain	0	No brain metastases
CS Mets at Dx–Liver	0	No liver metastases
CS Mets at Dx–Lung	0	No lung metastases
SSF1 WHO Grade	999	WHO grade not documented
SSF2 Ki-67/MIB1 LI	999	Unknown, not documented
SSF3 Karnofsky Scale	999	Unknown, not documented
SSF4 MGMT Methyl	999	Unknown, not documented
SSF5 Chr 1p LOH	999	Unknown, not documented
SSF6 Chr 19q LOH	999	Unknown, not documented
SSF7 Surg Resection	030	Stated as greater than 99% of tumor resected
SSF8 Multifocality	001	Unifocal

—— CASE 3 ——

Primary Site	C71.8	Overlapping lesion of brain per angiogram; occipital lobe was biopsied and partially debulked, but was not the complete primary site
Histology	9391/39	Ependymoma, histologic grade not stated. Do not code WHO grade here.
Lymph Vascular Invasion	9	Lymph-vascular invasion not mentioned in path report
Ambiguous Terminology	0	Conclusive terminology
Date Conclusive Terminol	Blank	Diagnosis made by conclusive terminology
Date Conclus Dx Flag	11	Not applicable
Multiplicity Counter	01	One tumor only
Date Multiple Tumors	Blank	Not applicable
Date Mult Tumors Flag	15	Single tumor only (multiplicity counter is coded 01)
Type Mult Tum as 1 Prim	00	Single tumor
Summary Stage	1	Localized (invasion of dura not confirmed)
CS Schema	Brain	
CS Tumor Size	055	5.5 cm on CT
CS Extension	600	Appears to invade dura; see comment
CS Mets at Dx	00	Physical exam and lab work essentially negative
CS Mets at Dx–Bone	0	No bone metastases
CS Mets at Dx–Brain	0	No brain metastases
CS Mets at Dx–Liver	0	No liver metastases
CS Mets at Dx–Lung	0	No lung metastases
SSF1 WHO Grade	030	WHO grade III—use higher number
SSF2 Ki-67/MIB1 LI	999	Unknown, not documented
SSF3 Karnofsky Scale	050	KPS reported on admission

Case 3, continued

SSF4 MGMT Methyl	999	Unknown, not documented
SSF5 Chr 1p LOH	999	Unknown, not documented
SSF6 Chr 19q LOH	999	Unknown, not documented
SSF7 Surg Resection	021	Stated as partial removal of tumor
SSF8 Multifocality	001	Unifocal

"Appears to" is an ambiguous term that is considered involvement. The ambiguous terms are listed on page 22 of Part I Section 1 in the CS User Documentation. In this case "appears to" is part of the stage description. Conclusive terminology (ependymoma) was used to code the diagnosis.

—— CASE 4 ——

Primary Site	C75.1	Pituitary gland
Histology	8290/31	Oncocytic carcinoma, well differentiated
Lymph Vascular Invasion	9	Lymph-vascular invasion not mentioned in path report
Ambiguous Terminology	0	Conclusive terminology
Date Conclusive Terminol	Blank	Diagnosis made by conclusive terminology
Date Conclus Dx Flag	11	Not applicable
Multiplicity Counter	01	One tumor only
Date Multiple Tumors	Blank	Not applicable
Date Mult Tumors Flag	15	Single tumor only (multiplicity counter is coded 01)
Type Mult Tum as 1 Prim	00	Single tumor
Summary Stage	1	Localized
CS Schema	Intracranial Gland	
CS Tumor Size	015	1.5 cm lesion on MRI
CS Extension	100	Confined to pituitary gland
CS Mets at Dx	00	Physical exam normal
CS Mets at Dx–Bone	0	No bone metastases
CS Mets at Dx–Brain	0	No brain metastases
CS Mets at Dx–Liver	0	No liver metastases
CS Mets at Dx–Lung	0	No lung metastases
SSF1 WHO Grade	999	WHO grade not stated
SSF2 Ki-67/MIB1 LI	999	Unknown, not documented

—— CASE 5 ——

Primary Site	C70.0	Cerebral meninges. Tumor is in the meninges, not the frontoparietal lobe itself.
Histology	9539/19	Atypical meningioma, borderline, no grade
Lymph Vascular Invasion	9	Lymph-vascular invasion not mentioned in path report
Ambiguous Terminology	0	Conclusive terminology
Date Conclusive Terminol	Blank	Diagnosis made by conclusive terminology
Date Conclus Dx Flag	11	Not applicable
Multiplicity Counter	01	One tumor only
Date Multiple Tumors	Blank	Not applicable
Date Mult Tumors Flag	15	Single tumor only (multiplicity counter is coded 01)
Type Mult Tum as 1 Prim	00	Single tumor
Summary Stage	8	Not applicable (borderline tumor)
CS Schema	Brain	
CS Tumor Size	070	7 cm mass on MRI

Case 5, continued

CS Extension	050	Borderline tumor. Also, path report shows no brain invasion.
CS Mets at Dx	00	Physical findings within normal limits
CS Mets at Dx–Bone	0	No bone metastases
CS Mets at Dx–Brain	0	No brain metastases
CS Mets at Dx–Liver	0	No liver metastases
CS Mets at Dx–Lung	0	No lung metastases
SSF1 WHO Grade	999	WHO grade not stated
SSF2 Ki-67/MIB1 LI	999	Unknown, not documented
SSF3 Karnofsky Scale	999	Unknown, not documented
SSF4 MGMT Methyl	999	Unknown, not documented
SSF5 Chr 1p LOH	999	Unknown, not documented
SSF6 Chr 19q LOH	999	Unknown, not documented
SSF7 Surg Resection	021	Excision not stated as radical or total; coded as subtotal
SSF8 Multifocality	001	Unifocal

—— CASE 6 ——

Primary Site	C71.2	Temporal lobe
Histology	9440/39	Glioblastoma multiforme (use the diagnosis from the larger resection)
Lymph Vascular Invasion	9	Lymph-vascular invasion not mentioned in path report
Ambiguous Terminology	0	Conclusive terminology
Date Conclusive Terminol	Blank	Diagnosis made by conclusive terminology
Date Conclus Dx Flag	11	Not applicable
Multiplicity Counter	01	One tumor only
Date Multiple Tumors	Blank	Not applicable
Date Mult Tumors Flag	15	Single tumor only (multiplicity counter is coded 01)
Type Mult Tum as 1 Prim	00	Single tumor
Summary Stage	1	Localized
CS Schema	Brain	
CS Tumor Size	060	6 cm on MRI
CS Extension	100	Confined to temporal lobe
CS Mets at Dx	00	No abnormal physical findings
CS Mets at Dx–Bone	0	No bone metastases
CS Mets at Dx–Brain	0	No brain metastases
CS Mets at Dx–Liver	0	No liver metastases
CS Mets at Dx–Lung	0	No lung metastases
SSF1 WHO Grade	999	WHO grade not stated in medical record
SSF2 Ki-67/MIB1 LI	012	Labeling index stated as 12%
SSF3 Karnofsky Scale	999	Unknown, not documented
SSF4 MGMT Methyl	020	Methylation not identified (gene status unmethylated)
SSF5 Chr 1p LOH	999	Unknown, not documented
SSF6 Chr 19q LOH	999	Unknown, not documented
SSF7 Surg Resection	030	Gross resection of brain tumor; grossly debulked
SSF8 Multifocality	001	Unifocal

—— CASE 7 ——

Primary Site	C72.0	Spinal cord
Histology	9560/09	Schwannoma; benign, no grade
Lymph Vascular Invasion	9	Lymph-vascular invasion not mentioned in path report
Ambiguous Terminology	0	Conclusive terminology
Date Conclusive Terminol	Blank	Diagnosis made by conclusive terminology
Date Conclus Dx Flag	11	Not applicable
Multiplicity Counter	01	One tumor only
Date Multiple Tumors	Blank	Not applicable
Date Mult Tumors Flag	15	Single tumor only (multiplicity counter is coded 01)
Type Mult Tum as 1 Prim	00	Single tumor
Summary Stage	8	Not applicable (benign tumor)
CS Schema	Other CNS	
CS Tumor Size	009	9 mm on second MRI
CS Extension	050	Benign tumor
CS Mets at Dx	00	No physical findings of metastases
CS Mets at Dx–Bone	0	No bone metastases
CS Mets at Dx–Brain	0	No brain metastases
CS Mets at Dx–Liver	0	No liver metastases
CS Mets at Dx–Lung	0	No lung metastases
SSF1 WHO Grade	999	WHO grade not stated
SSF2 Ki-67/MIB1 LI	999	Unknown, not documented
SSF3 Karnofsky Scale	999	Unknown, not documented
SSF4 MGMT Methyl	999	Unknown, not documented
SSF5 Chr 1p LOH	999	Unknown, not documented
SSF6 Chr 19q LOH	999	Unknown, not documented
SSF7 Surg Resection	022	Resection of tumor of spinal cord
SSF8 Multifocality	001	Unifocal

—— CASE 8 ——

Primary Site	C75.1	Pituitary gland (the only suprasellar content is the pituitary gland)
Histology	8270/09	Chromophobe adenoma; benign, no grade
Lymph Vascular Invasion	9	Lymph-vascular invasion not mentioned in path report
Ambiguous Terminology	0	Conclusive terminology
Date Conclusive Terminol	Blank	Diagnosis made by conclusive terminology
Date Conclus Dx Flag	11	Not applicable
Multiplicity Counter	01	One tumor only
Date Multiple Tumors	Blank	Not applicable
Date Mult Tumors Flag	15	Single tumor only (multiplicity counter is coded 01)
Type Mult Tum as 1 Prim	00	Single tumor
Summary Stage	8	Not applicable (benign tumor)
CS Schema	Intracranial Gland	
CS Tumor Size	024	Largest measurement on MRI 24 mm = 2.4 cm
CS Extension	050	Benign tumor
CS Mets at Dx	00	No abnormal physical findings
CS Mets at Dx–Bone	0	No bone metastases
CS Mets at Dx–Brain	0	No brain metastases

Case 8, continued

CS Mets at Dx–Liver	0	No liver metastases
CS Mets at Dx–Lung	0	No lung metastases
SSF1 WHO Grade	999	WHO grade not stated
SSF2 Ki-67/MIB1 LI	999	Unknown, not documented

—— CASE 9 ——

Note: This patient has two primaries based on benign multiple primary counting rules.

	Right		Left	
Primary Site	C70.0	Cerebral meninges	C70.0	Cerebral meninges
Histology	9530/09	Meningioma, NOS	9530/09	Meningioma, NOS
Lymph Vascular Invasion	9	LVI not mentioned	9	LVI not mentioned
Ambiguous Terminology	1	Ambiguous terminol	1	Ambiguous terminol
Date Conclusive Terminol	Blank	No conclusive term	Blank	No conclusive term
Date Conclus Dx Flag	15	Ambig term coded 1	15	Ambig term coded 1
Multiplicity Counter	01	One tumor only	01	One tumor only
Date Multiple Tumors	Blank	Not applicable	Blank	Not applicable
Date Mult Tumors Flag	15	Single tumor only (multi counter is 01)	15	Single tumor only (multi counter is 01)
Type Mult Tum as 1 Prim	00	Single tumor	00	Single tumor
Summary Stage	8	Not applicable (benign)	8	Not applicable (benign)
CS Schema	Brain		Brain	
CS Tumor Size	014	1.4 cm on MRI	009	0.9 cm on MRI
CS Extension	050	Benign tumor	050	Benign tumor
CS Mets at Dx	00	PE negative	00	PE negative
CS Mets at Dx–Bone	0	No bone metastases	0	No bone metastases
CS Mets at Dx–Brain	0	No brain metastases	0	No brain metastases
CS Mets at Dx–Liver	0	No liver metastases	0	No liver metastases
CS Mets at Dx–Lung	0	No lung metastases	0	No lung metastases
SSF1 WHO Grade	998	No histologic exam	998	No histologic exam
SSF2 Ki-67/MIB1 LI	998	No histologic exam	998	No histologic exam
SSF3 Karnofsky Scale	999	Not documented	999	Not documented
SSF4 MGMT Methyl	998	No histologic exam	998	No histologic exam
SSF5 Chr 1p LOH	998	No histologic exam	998	No histologic exam
SSF6 Chr 19q LOH	998	No histologic exam	998	No histologic exam
SSF7 Surg Resection	000	No surgery of prim site	000	No surgery of prim site
SSF8 Multifocality	001	Unifocal	001	Unifocal

Both primaries were diagnosed based on ambiguous terminology ("compatible with"). Since there is no indication that the meningiomas were ever histologically confirmed, the ambiguous terminology, date conclusive terminology and date conclusive diagnosis flag fields are all coded to indicate the cases were accessioned based on ambiguous terminology.

—— CASE 10 ——

Primary Site	C71.8	Overlapping lesion of frontal and temporal lobes
Histology	9442/33	Gliosarcoma, poorly differentiated
Lymph Vascular Invasion	9	Lymph-vascular invasion not mentioned in path report
Ambiguous Terminology	0	Conclusive terminology
Date Conclusive Terminol	Blank	Diagnosis made by conclusive terminology

Case 10, continued

Date Conclus Dx Flag	11	Not applicable
Multiplicity Counter	01	One tumor only
Date Multiple Tumors	Blank	Not applicable
Date Mult Tumors Flag	15	Single tumor only (multiplicity counter is coded 01)
Type Mult Tum as 1 Prim	00	Single tumor
Summary Stage	5	Regional, NOS (extending across midline)
CS Schema	Brain	
CS Tumor Size	038	3.8 cm on CT scan
CS Extension	400	Extending across midline on CT
CS Mets at Dx	00	Physical exam and chest x-ray negative for metastases
CS Mets at Dx–Bone	0	No bone metastases
CS Mets at Dx–Brain	0	No brain metastases
CS Mets at Dx–Liver	0	No liver metastases
CS Mets at Dx–Lung	0	No lung metastases
SSF1 WHO Grade	999	WHO grade not stated
SSF2 Ki-67/MIB1 LI	400	Ki-67 stated as elevated
SSF3 Karnofsky Scale	999	Unknown, not documented
SSF4 MGMT Methyl	999	Unknown, not documented
SSF5 Chr 1p LOH	020	Negative for loss of heterozygosity
SSF6 Chr 19q LOH	020	Negative for loss of heterozygosity
SSF7 Surg Resection	021	Operative report states incomplete excision
SSF8 Multifocality	001	Unifocal

—— CASE 11 ——

Primary Site	C70.0	Cerebral meninges (do not code to frontal lobe)
Histology	9530/09	Meningioma, NOS; benign, no grade
Lymph Vascular Invasion	9	Lymph-vascular invasion not mentioned in path report
Ambiguous Terminology	1	Ambiguous terminology
Date Conclusive Terminol	Blank	No conclusive terminology
Date Conclus Dx Flag	15	Ambiguous terminology coded as 1
Multiplicity Counter	01	One tumor only
Date Multiple Tumors	Blank	Not applicable
Date Mult Tumors Flag	15	Single tumor only (multiplicity counter is coded 01)
Type Mult Tum as 1 Prim	00	Single tumor
Summary Stage	8	Not applicable (benign)
CS Schema	Brain	
CS Tumor Size	012	1.2 cm in greatest dimension on MRI
CS Extension	050	Benign tumor
CS Mets at Dx	00	No statement of physical findings (code as negative)
CS Mets at Dx–Bone	0	No bone metastases
CS Mets at Dx–Brain	0	No brain metastases
CS Mets at Dx–Liver	0	No liver metastases
CS Mets at Dx–Lung	0	No lung metastases
SSF1 WHO Grade	998	No histologic examination of primary site
SSF2 Ki-67/MIB1 LI	998	No histologic examination of primary site
SSF3 Karnofsky Scale	999	Not documented

Case 11, continued

SSF4 MGMT Methyl	998	No histologic examination of primary site
SSF5 Chr 1p LOH	998	No histologic examination of primary site
SSF6 Chr 19q LOH	998	No histologic examination of primary site
SSF7 Surg Resection	000	No surgery of prim site
SSF8 Multifocality	001	Unifocal

This case was diagnosed based on ambiguous terminology ("compatible with"). Since there is no indication that the meningioma was ever histologically confirmed, the ambiguous terminology, date conclusive terminology and date conclusive diagnosis flag fields are all coded to indicate the case was accessioned based on ambiguous terminology.

—— CASE 12 ——

Primary Site	C71.7	Brain stem
Histology	9401/34	Anaplastic astrocytoma (code 'anaplastic' in histology as well as grade)
Lymph Vascular Invasion	9	Lymph-vascular invasion not mentioned in path report
Ambiguous Terminology	0	Conclusive terminology
Date Conclusive Terminol	Blank	Diagnosis made by conclusive terminology
Date Conclus Dx Flag	11	Not applicable
Multiplicity Counter	01	One tumor only
Date Multiple Tumors	Blank	Not applicable
Date Mult Tumors Flag	15	Single tumor only (multiplicity counter is coded 01)
Type Mult Tum as 1 Prim	00	Single tumor
Summary Stage	1	Localized
CS Schema	Brain	
CS Tumor Size	999	Tumor size not stated
CS Extension	300	Tumor involves fourth ventricle from brainstem
CS Mets at Dx	00	No statement of physical findings, but patient underwent surgery to primary site
CS Mets at Dx–Bone	0	No bone metastases
CS Mets at Dx–Brain	0	No brain metastases
CS Mets at Dx–Liver	0	No liver metastases
CS Mets at Dx–Lung	0	No lung metastases
SSF1 WHO Grade	030	WHO grade III
SSF2 Ki-67/MIB1 LI	029	MIB-1 labeling index stated as 28.7 (round up)
SSF3 Karnofsky Scale	999	Unknown, not documented
SSF4 MGMT Methyl	010	Stated as MGMT methylation present
SSF5 Chr 1p LOH	999	Unknown, not documented
SSF6 Chr 19q LOH	999	Unknown, not documented
SSF7 Surg Resection	021	Stated as partial resection of brainstem tumor
SSF8 Multifocality	001	Unifocal

Page left blank.

MALIGNANT LYMPHOMA

This chapter focuses on diseases of the lymphatic system. There are literally dozens of different diseases that fall under the broad term 'malignant lymphoma.' Coding and staging of the lymphomas is fairly straightforward because there's no T, N, or M—only a stage group to determine, and only a limited number of Collaborative Staging fields to code. However, the more challenging aspect of these diseases is coding the morphology and, sometimes, identifying and coding the primary site. Even these issues have been improved with the implementation of the Hematopoietic Multiple Primary and Histology coding rules in 2010.

As noted above, malignant lymphoma is a very general term covering both Hodgkin lymphoma and non-Hodgkin lymphoma, each of which is a broad term that covers a number of specific cell types of lymphoma. Non-Hodgkin lymphoma is more than seven times as common as Hodgkin lymphoma. In 2010, there were an estimated 74,030 cases of malignant lymphoma diagnosed in the United States. Of the lymphomas, about 8,500 were Hodgkin lymphoma and over 65,500 were non-Hodgkin lymphoma (NHL). Non-Hodgkin lymphoma ranks as the sixth most frequent cancer in both men and women in the 2010 estimates. The incidence rate for non-Hodgkin lymphoma has been stable in men for the past decade but continues to rise in women. The incidence rate for Hodgkin lymphoma has been fairly stable over the same period.

Stem cells, also called pluripotential cells (meaning that they have the potential to develop into any type of blood or lymphoid cell), are generated in the bone marrow, which is the soft, spongy center of larger bones. When a stem cell divides into two daughter cells, one will remain a stem cell and continue to divide into daughter cells through its natural lifespan. The other daughter cell will embark on the process of maturation. Some stem cells stay in the marrow to mature—these become myeloid cells. Others travel to other parts of the body to mature—these are primarily lymphoid cells.

ETIOLOGY AND NATURAL HISTORY

Most of the known risk factors for non-Hodgkin lymphoma relate to impaired immune function, but the majority of lymphoma diagnoses have no known risk factors. Persons with organ transplants receiving immunosuppressant drugs to prevent transplant rejection are at increased risk, as are people with autoimmune conditions and HIV-infected patients. Human T-cell leukemia/lymphoma virus type I (HTLV-I), Epstein-Barr virus (EBV), and probably hepatitis C (HCV) are all linked to various types of lymphomas. In addition, exposure to chemicals such as herbicides and chlorinated organic compounds are known to increase risk of developing lymphoma. A particular type of lymphoma, mucosa-associated lymphoid tumor (MALT) is associated with *Helicobacter pylori* infection of the stomach.

Unless otherwise indicated, the discussion that follows applies to both Hodgkin lymphoma and non-Hodgkin lymphoma.

ANATOMY OF THE LYMPHATIC SYSTEM AS IT RELATES TO STAGING

LYMPH NODE CHAINS AND LYMPH NODE REGIONS

Malignant lymphoma (ML) is a disease that can arise in almost any organ in the body, but it most commonly occurs in lymph nodes. There are approximately 500 lymph nodes in the human body, organized into 36 major lymph node-bearing stations or lymph node chains. (Refer to the Lymphatic System chapter in this CASEbook for a detailed list.) The lymph nodes act as filters for lymphatic fluid before it is returned to the bloodstream. The lymph nodes also act as immune response centers that defend against infection.

The primary site for malignant lymphoma is determined by which lymph node *chains* or primary organ(s) are involved. ML is staged by the number of lymph node *regions* involved. A lymph node chain is a group of lymph nodes, usually named for their location in a specific area of the body or the blood vessel along which they lie. A lymph node region can be defined in two ways: anatomically as in ICD-O-3, and for staging. The definitions for staging will be discussed in the Collaborative Staging section, below.

Figure 1 and the lists that follow define the lymph node regions above and below the diaphragm as well as the lymph node chains that are part of each region *for purposes of coding the primary site for a nodal lymphoma.*

Figure 1. Lymph Node Regions and Boundaries with ICD-O-3 Codes

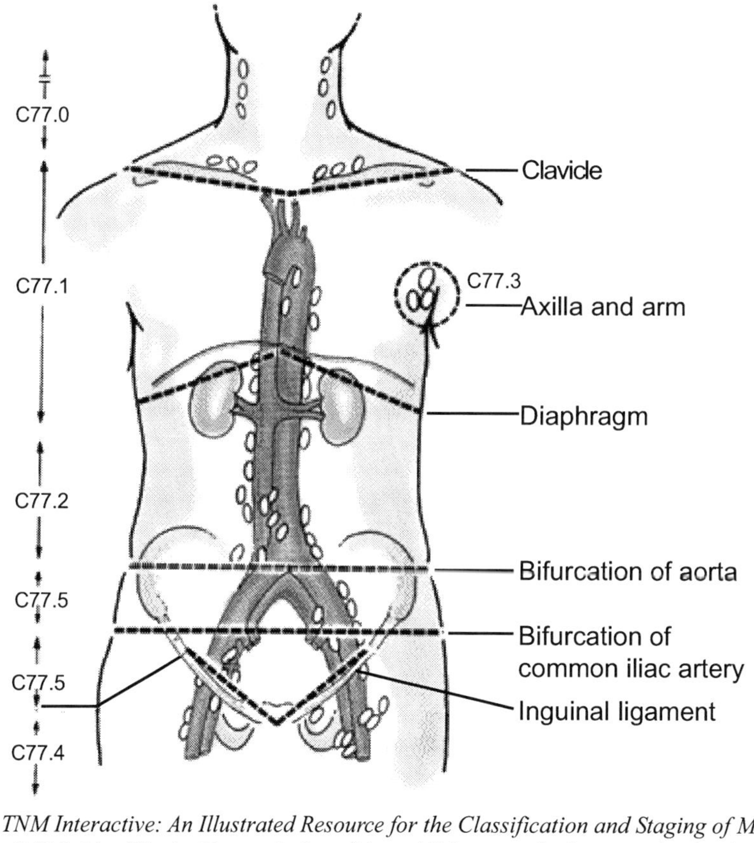

Adapted from *TNM Interactive: An Illustrated Resource for the Classification and Staging of Malignant Tumors*, 1998. Edited by L H Sobin. Used with permission of the publisher; any further reproduction is strictly prohibited.

Lymph Node Chains and Lymph Node Regions, *continued*

ICD-O-3	Definition
C77.0	Lymph nodes of head, face and neck
C77.1	Intrathoracic lymph nodes
C77.2	Intra-abdominal lymph nodes
C77.3	Lymph nodes of axilla or arm
C77.4	Lymph nodes of inguinal region or leg
C77.5	Pelvic lymph nodes
C77.8	Lymph nodes of multiple regions
C77.9	Lymph node, NOS

Lymphomas of these sites are commonly called ***nodal*** lymphomas.

Lymph nodes above the diaphragm
Lymph nodes of head, face and neck (C77.0) auricular, buccal (buccinator), cervical, Delphian (anterior to thyroid isthmus), facial, jugular (superficial and deep), jugulodigastric (subdigastric), laterotracheal (anterior deep cervical), mandibular, occipital, parotid, preauricular, prelaryngeal, pretracheal, postauricular (mastoid), retropharyngeal, scalene, sublingual, submandibular, submaxillary, submental and supraclavicular (transverse cervical)

Intrathoracic lymph nodes (C77.1) bronchial, bronchopulmonary, diaphragmatic, esophageal, hilar (pulmonary root), innominate (bracheocephalic), intercostal, mediastinal, parasternal (internal mammary), peritracheal, pulmonary, pulmonary hilar, thoracic, thymic, tracheal, and tracheobronchial

Lymph nodes of axilla or arm (C77.3) axillary (levels I-III; low/superficial, mid, apical/deep), brachial, cubital, epitrochlear, infraclavicular, interpectoral (Rotter's), pectoral, subclavicular, subscapular, upper limb

Lymph nodes below the diaphragm
Intra-abdominal lymph nodes (C77.2) abdominal, aortic, celiac, colic, common duct, gastric, gastro-omental (gastroepiploic), hepatic, ileocolic, inferior mesenteric, infrapyloric (subpyloric), intestinal, lumbar, mesenteric, midcolic, pancreatic, pancreaticolienal (pancreaticosplenic), para-aortic, periaortic, pericholedochal, peripancreatic, porta hepatis, portal, pyloric, retrocrural, retroperitoneal, splenic (lienal), splenic hilar, superior mesenteric

Lymph nodes of inguinal region or leg (C77.4) femoral (superficial inguinal), inguinal, Cloquet's, groin, lower limb, Rosenmuller's (uppermost deep inguinal), popliteal, subinguinal (deep inguinal), tibial

Pelvic lymph nodes (C77.5) hypogastric (internal iliac), iliac, inferior epigastric, infundibulopelvic (utero-ovarian), intrapelvic, obturator, paracervical, parametrial, pararectal (anorectal), presymphysial, sacral, sacral promontory (Gerota's)

ICD-O-3 RULES FOR CODING PRIMARY SITE FOR NODAL LYMPHOMAS

- Nodal lymphomas are coded to C77.__.
- Code the primary site to the lymph node where the lymphoma originated.
- If more than one lymph node chain is involved, code the primary site to lymph nodes of multiple regions (C77.8). This code is a variation on the ICD-O-3 code Cxx.8 rule for overlapping sites. For other organs like breast and colon, the sites must be adjacent to each other. For lymphoma, the .8 code can be used even when the lymph node regions are not adjacent to each other. A case coded to C77.8 cannot be Stage I.

Coding Primary Site, *continued*

- Note that the primary site is not necessarily the site of the lymph node biopsy. A physician usually elects to biopsy the most accessible lymph node (a lymph node close to the surface) rather than a lymph node biopsy that would require a more extensive surgical procedure such a retroperitoneal lymph node biopsy.

In addition, lymphomas may also develop in other lymphatic tissues, including:

- Spleen (C42.2)
- Thymus (C37.9)
- Lymphoid nodules in the appendix (code to appendix, C18.1)
- Peyer's patches (lymphoid tissue of surface of small bowel) (code to appropriate segment of small intestine, C17._)
- Tonsils (palatine tonsils, C09.9; lingual tonsils, C02.4; pharyngeal tonsils {adenoids}, C11.1)
- Waldeyer's ring (C14.2)—the lymphoid tissues surrounding the throat. If you were to draw an imaginary line connecting lymphoid tissues of the throat—the pharyngeal tonsils located on the back wall of the throat (commonly referred to as adenoids), the palatine tonsils on either side of the throat and the lingual tonsils situated at the base of the tongue—that line would form a circle called Waldeyer's ring. (Heinrich W.G. Waldeyer-Hartz was a 19th century German anatomist.)

Lymphomas of these organs are called ***extranodal*** lymphomas, because they do not start in a lymph node but they are still part of the lymphatic system. Code lymphomas of these sites to the organ of origin.

Additional lymphatic sites above the diaphragm: Waldeyer's ring (tonsils, adenoids, lingual tonsils), thymus

Additional lymphatic sites below the diaphragm: Spleen, Peyer's patches, lymphoid nodules in the appendix

EXTRALYMPHATIC LYMPHOMAS

There are smaller areas of lymphatic tissue in other organs as well. Malignant lymphoma can develop in any organ of the body, but the most common ***extralymphatic*** sites are:

- Stomach (C16._)
- Intestines (C17._, C18._)
- Uterus (usually C54._)
- Brain (C71._)
- Breast (C50._)
- Bone (C40._, C41._)

Note: Sometimes the terms *extranodal* (meaning not in lymph nodes) and *extralymphatic* (meaning not in the major lymphatic tissues) are used interchangeably. Be aware of this as you read medical records. An organ such as the tonsils can be extranodal without being outside of the lymphatic system. The preferred terminology for lymphomas of solid organs like stomach, uterus and brain is *extralymphatic*. Extralymphatic Hodgkin lymphoma is uncommon; extralymphatic non-Hodgkin lymphoma occurs more frequently but is still only about 25% of all NHL.

ICD-O-3 RULES FOR CODING PRIMARY SITE FOR EXTRALYMPHATIC LYMPHOMAS

- Extralymphatic lymphoma is coded to the primary site where it started. For example, a malignant lymphoma of the small intestine, NOS is coded C17.9.
- If only an extralymphatic site is involved and there is no lymph node involvement, code the primary site to the extralymphatic site.
- When both an extralymphatic site and lymph nodes are involved, look for a physician statement or final diagnosis that states this is an extralymphatic/extranodal lymphoma. Usually the lymphoma starts in the extralymphatic site and the lymphoma cells travel to the regional lymph nodes via normal organ drainage patterns. The lymphatic channels that flow into lymph nodes contain tiny one-way valves that do not allow the backflow of lymph into the organ. Therefore, it would be highly unusual for a lymphoma to start in the lymph nodes and migrate backwards against normal lymphatic flow to involve the organ. In fact, the lymphatic system flows only in one direction—from the organ into the node, and then out of the node and on to the next drainage chain, always moving back toward the heart.
- In contrast, a lymphoma can also develop in a lymph node region near an organ and invade the organ directly. This type of lymphoma would be coded to C77._ as the primary site and would have an "E" suffix on the stage group. See the discussion of the "E" suffix in the AJCC (TNM) section of Other Staging and Classification Systems later in this chapter.

When Primary Site Cannot Be Determined

- When the site of origin cannot be determined to be nodal or extralymphatic, code the primary site to Lymph Nodes, NOS C77.9. For example, if no primary site is documented and the only pathology is from a bone marrow biopsy, code the primary site to C77.9. Rule D in ICD-O-3 allows the use of C80.9, unknown primary site for lymphomas where the site of origin cannot be identified and the lymphoma is suspected to be extranodal, but U.S. rules say that the preferred code is C77.9 in most cases. The infrequent situation where, for example, there is lymphoma equally in lungs and stomach without any involvement of lymph nodes would be coded appropriately to C80.9.

  Note: There is a discrepancy between the wording of ICD-O-3 Rule D as printed in the summary of principal rules on page 20 and Rule D as printed in the discussion on page 26. The wording on page 26 is correct.

Note: All lymphomas—nodal, extranodal, or extralymphatic—use the same staging (Ann Arbor system), although the codes differ among summary stage, TNM, and Collaborative Staging.

HEMATOPOIETIC CODING RULES

For diagnosis year 2010 and forward, a new set of coding guidelines was implemented for the malignant lymphomas and other hematopoietic diseases. Formally named the *Hematopoietic and Lymphoid Neoplasm Case Reportability and Coding Manual*, most registrars refer to them as the Heme MP/H rules. The concepts are a continuation of the MP/H rules for solid tumors but are specific to neoplasms in the ICD-O-3 morphology code range 9590 to 9992. The background and details of the heme rules are discussed in the Multiple Primary and Histology Coding Rules chapter of this CASEbook, including the appendices in the coding manual and the use of the hematopoietic data base. This chapter will cover only the rules that apply to the malignant lymphomas.

Hematopoietic Coding Rules, ***continued***

Features of Hematopoietic MP/H Rules

- Four sets of rules
  - Case Reportability—whether the case should be accessioned; unique to the heme diseases (7 of 10 rules apply to lymphomas)
  - Multiple Primary Rules—how many abstracts to prepare (9 of 12 rules apply to lymphomas)
  - Primary Site and Histology Coding Rules (6 of 9 modules apply to lymphomas)
  - Grade Coding Rules—unique to heme rules; coding ICD-O morphology 6th digit (10 of 11 rules apply to lymphomas)
- No time limit between diagnoses
- Histology coding rules refer to a chart in the site-specific Terms and Definitions providing priorities for most specific histology code

Summary of Multiple Primary and Histology Coding Rules

Because lymphoma is a systemic disease, the usual MP/H format of three modules for the multiple primaries rules and two or more modules for histology coding rules does not apply. Instead, there are four sets of guidelines and rules to be applied in order. The heme MP/H rules were designed to collapse into the ICD-O-3 coding rules for international comparisons, so you will see rules similar to the basic ICD-O-3 rules as well as rules that cover specific situations that are not covered in ICD-O-3.

This is only a summary of the multiple primary and histology coding rules that apply to lymphomas. Details of the rules are provided in the official published documents available from www.seer.cancer.gov/tools/heme/index.html. Refer to the Introduction for information about coding more specific terms, missing pathology or cytology reports, and other aspects of the rules. **Always** refer to the site-specific rules themselves in your preferred format when determining how many abstracts to prepare or the correct primary site or histology code for an individual abstract. The published rules include more discussion, examples, and notes.

Case Reportability Instructions

The Case Reportability Instructions are not hierarchical and are presented in text format only. Read through them and if *any* instruction applies, the case is reportable.

1. Report case when only information available is that MD started cancer-directed treatment for reportable neoplasm. Report the case even if diagnostic tests are equivocal, inconclusive, or negative. Cancer-directed treatment options for lymphomas are listed in the National Cancer Institute's Physician Data Query (PDQ) system at www.cancer.gov.
2. Report diagnoses with ambiguous terms (except from cytology or tumor markers): Appears, Apparent(ly), Comparable with, Compatible with, Consistent with, Favor(s), Malignant appearing, Most likely, Presumed, Probable, Suspect(ed), Suspicious (for), Typical (of).
3. Report a clinical diagnosis from anywhere in the medical record.
4. [Multiple myeloma rule]
5. [Leukemia rule]
6. [Newly reportable diagnoses rule]
7. Report case when reportable diagnosis appears in any text or report listed as a definitive diagnostic method in the hematopoietic data base (Heme DB).
8. Report case if described as malignant by clinician but ICD-O-3 code is /1.
   - All lymphomas are /3; this rule will rarely apply to a lymphoma diagnosis.
9. Report all /3 in ICD-O-3 range 9590-9992 plus new terms in WHO Classification
   - There are about 18 new lymphoma or lymphoma/leukemia terms from the latest edition of the WHO Classification.
10. Use Heme DB to check for reportability in situations not listed above.

Hematopoietic Coding Rules, *continued*

Multiple Primary Rules

The multiple primary rules are hierarchical and are presented in the three formats (text, flowchart, and matrix). Start at rule M1 and keep reading until you find the *first* rule that applies to the case.

- For all rules in this module, "same anatomic location" is defined as a single lymph node, single organ, or single area of tissue.

M1. Minimal information = single primary
- Includes death certificate only (DCO) cases; Pathology-Report-Only cases. This rule is primarily for central registry use.

M2. Single histology = single primary
- Based on a definitive diagnostic method

M3. Two or more non-Hodgkin lymphomas in same anatomic location = single primary
- This is a new rule for registrars as of 2010.
- Using the Heme DB for determining multiple primaries in the same location may result in a wrong answer.

M4. Hodgkin and non-Hodgkin lymphoma in same location = single primary

M5. Hodgkin lymphoma in one tissue and non-Hodgkin lymphoma in a different tissue = multiple primaries

M6. NOS diagnosis first, then more specific histology within same histologic grouping = single primary

M7. Acute phase/Chronic phase timing rule part 1—does not apply to lymphomas

M8. Acute phase/Chronic phase timing rule part 2—does not apply to lymphomas

M9. Acute phase/Chronic phase timing rule part 3—does not apply to lymphomas

M10. Transformation rule part 1: Original diagnosis is less aggressive phase/chronic phase AND second diagnosis is blast/acute phase more than 21 days = multiple primaries

M11. Transformation rule part 2: When blast/acute neoplasm reverts to less aggressive/ chronic phase and no indication that patient has been treated = single primary

M12. Transformation rule part 3: Original diagnosis is blast/acute neoplasm AND reverts to less aggressive/chronic phase after treatment = multiple primaries

M13. Use Heme DB to check for multiple primaries in situations not listed above.

Primary Site and Histology Coding Rules

The primary site and histology coding rules consist of nine modules in the three formats. After applying the rules in Module 1, go directly to the appropriate histology-specific module. Start at the first rule in that module and keep reading until you find the *first* rule that applies to the case. Only the modules that apply to lymphomas are discussed here.

- For all rules in this module, "same tissue" is defined as a single lymph node or lymph node region, single organ, or single area of tissue.

Module 1—General Rules

PH1. Code primary site from any report in the medical record or the Heme DB.
- Keep in mind that the biopsy site is not necessarily primary site

PH2. Code the histology diagnosed by definitive diagnostic method in Heme DB as given in any pathology report, laboratory report, or clinical diagnosis.

PH3. If no definitive diagnostic method is available, code primary site and histology from clinician statement on medical record or death certificate

Module 2—Plasma cell neoplasms rules—does not apply to lymphomas

Hematopoietic Coding Rules, *continued*

Module 3—Lymphoma/Leukemia rules

- Some hematopoietic neoplasms can be coded as either a lymphoma or leukemia depending on the tissue from which the diagnosis was made. This module provides detailed rules, but the easiest ways to remember the module's concepts are these:
  - If the diagnostic tissue is "liquid" (in other words, blood or bone marrow), code as a leukemia with bone marrow as the primary site.
  - If the diagnostic tissue is a "lump" (in other words, a lymph node, organ, or other solid tissue), code as a lymphoma with the site of origin (lymph node, organ, tissue) as the primary site.

PH9. If the diagnosis is "B-cell small lymphocytic lymphoma/Chronic lymphocytic leukemia" and the peripheral blood is involved, code as B-cell chronic lymphocytic leukemia (CLL) (9823/3) with bone marrow (C42.1) as the primary site.

PH10. If the diagnosis is "B-cell small lymphocytic lymphoma/Chronic lymphocytic leukemia" and origin in the bone marrow cannot be verified, code as Small lymphocytic lymphoma (SLL) (9670/3) and site of origin (lymph node, organ, tissue) as the primary site.

PH11. Other lymphoma/leukemias: when the only involvement is bone marrow for the specific diagnoses listed, code bone marrow (C42.1) as the primary site and the leukemia histology.

PH12. Other lymphoma/leukemias: when there is involvement of a lymph node region, tissue or organ for the specific diagnoses listed, code the site of origin as the primary site and the lymphoma histology.

Module 4—Preleukemia, smoldering leukemia and myelodysplastic syndrome rules—does not apply to lymphomas

Module 5—Myeloid neoplasms—does not apply to lymphomas

Module 6—Specific lymphomas

PH16. Diffuse large B-cell lymphoma (DLBCL) and follicular lymphoma (FL) in same tissue: code site of origin and 9680/3 (DLBCL).

- These two diagnoses are sometimes found together in the same tissue. DLBCL is the more aggressive cell type and may mask the FL. If FL shows up in the same tissue post-treatment, do not change the histology.

PH17. Follicular lymphoma: code site of origin and appropriate FL histology when diagnosis is diffuse follicular lymphoma.

- FL has four histology codes based on grade (mix of large and small lymphocytes). For FL, grade is not the same as grade/differentiation (sixth digit of ICD-O-3 morphology code).

PH18. Follicle cell lymphoma (9597/3): code 9597/3 and skin as primary site when skin is involved (with or without regional node involvement for that area of skin).

PH19. Large B-cell lymphoma (9680/3): code 9680/3 and skin as primary site when skin is involved (with or without regional node involvement for that area of skin).

PH20. B-cell lymphoma, NOS (9680/3): code 9680/3 and skin as primary site when skin is involved (with or without regional node involvement for that area of skin).

PH21. Composite lymphoma (9596/3): code 9596/3 when both Hodgkin and non-Hodgkin lymphoma are present in the same tissue and code the site of origin as the primary site.

PH22. Two or more non-Hodgkin lymphomas in same tissue: code site of origin as primary site and the numerically highest ICD-O-3 morphology code.

- There is no combination code in ICD-O-3 for mixed non-Hodgkin lymphomas.

PH23. Waldenstrom's macroglobulinemia (WM) (9761/3): code blood (C42.0) as primary site and 9761/3 as histology when diagnosis is lymphoplasmacytic lymphoma (LPL) in bone marrow and IgM monoclonal gammopathy in blood.

Hematopoietic Coding Rules, *continued*

PH24. Lymphoplasmacytic lymphoma (9671/3): code 9761/3 and site of origin when diagnosis is WM or WM and LPL and lymph nodes or lymphoid tissue is involved with or without bone marrow involvement.
- PH 23 and PH 24 are variations of the "liquid/lump" concept. WM and LPL are the same malignant cell with different backgrounds.

Module 7—Primary site for lymphomas

- These rules help assign the primary site for any lymphoma not covered in the previous module. Many are common sense, but this is the first time they have been organized into a list.
  - The "lymph node region" referred to in these rules is the ICD-O-3 subsite, for example C77.0, lymph nodes of head and neck. These rules establish the primary site, not the lymph node regions for staging.

PH25. Code specific lymph node region when only one is involved

PH26. Lymphoma in mediastinal mass = mediastinal nodes (C77.1)

PH27. Lymphoma in retroperitoneal or mesenteric mass = intra-abdominal nodes (C77.2)

PH28. Lymphoma in inguinal mass = inguinal nodes (C77.4)

PH29. Code specific lymph node region when multiple chains involved in same region

PH30. Code C77.8, Lymph nodes of multiple regions, when multiple regions (multiple ICD-O-3 lymph node subsites) involved.

PH31. Code C77.9, Lymph node, NOS, when primary site or lymph node region is not specifically described.

PH32. Code C42.1, Bone marrow, when only bone marrow is involved.

PH33. Code specific organ when lymphoma is only in an organ.

PH34. Code lymph node region when physician says lymphoma started in lymph nodes and extended into organ.
- This pattern of lymphoma spread is uncommon and requires a statement by the physician.

PH35. Code specific organ when lymphoma is in organ and its regional nodes.

PH36. Code C77.9, Lymph node, NOS, when lymphoma present in organ(s) and non-regional nodes and site of origin cannot be determined.

PH37. Code to C80.9, Unknown primary site, when there is no lymphoma in nodes and physician indicates lymphoma may originate in an organ.

Module 8—General histology coding (all histologies including lymphomas)

PH38. Code non-specific histology when one non-specific and multiple specific histologies.
- All diagnoses must be part of same primary in Heme DB.

PH39. Code specific histology when one non-specific and one specific histology.
- Both diagnoses must be part of same primary in Heme DB.

Module 9—Default rules (all hematopoietic and lymphoid neoplasms)

PH40. Use Heme DB to code primary site and histology when PH1–PH39 do not apply.

PH41. When histology cannot be determined from Heme DB, code numerically higher ICD-O-3 morphology code.

Grade Coding Rules

The grade or phenotype (T-cell, B-cell, and so forth) coding rules are unique to the hematopoietic and lymphoid diseases. They allow the sixth digit of the ICD-O-3 morphology (grade/differentiation) to be coded for more lymphomas than the rules prior to 2010.

G1. Code 9 for all myeloid, histiocytic and dendritic cell neoplasms—does not apply to lymphomas (all lymphomas are lymphoid phenotype)

Hematopoietic Coding Rules, *continued*

G2. Code grade or phenotype from any statement in medical record.
G3. Use code range 5–8 and 9 only.
- Do not code well-, moderately-, or poorly-differentiated for lymphomas.
- Do not code grade from diagnosis of follicular lymphoma or nodular sclerosis Hodgkin lymphoma.
- Do not code low-, intermediate-, or high-grade terminology from Working Formulation.

G4. Use code 5 for list of T-cell origin lymphomas and hematopoietic neoplasms.
G5. Use code 5 for variants of T-cell origin terminology.
G6. Use code 6 for list of B-cell origin lymphomas and hematopoietic neoplasms.
- Includes precursor B-cell and mature B-cell neoplasms

G7. Use code 6 for variants of B-cell origin terminology.
G8. Use code 7 for description of null cell, common cell, or non-T non-B.
G9. Use code 8 for list of NK (natural killer) cell lymphoma.
G10. Use code 8 for variants of NK-cell origin terminology.
G11. Use code 9 when cell type is not determined, combined phenotype, or not stated.
- Includes Hodgkin lymphoma cell types, which are not listed in any of the previous rules.

HISTOLOGIC CELL TYPES OF MALIGNANT LYMPHOMAS

Malignant lymphoma is a generic term that includes two distinct types of lymphoma.
- Hodgkin lymphoma – named after Thomas Hodgkin, who first identified patients with enlarged lymph nodes who appeared not to have infections in the 1830s
- Non-Hodgkin lymphoma (NHL) – all the other types of lymphomas

Within each of these two major types of lymphomas are a number of distinct diseases. All of the malignant lymphomas arise from lymphoid cells (lymphocytes), but may develop from either the B-cell maturation line or the T or NK cell lines. These cell lines, or phenotypes form the basis for the current classification of lymphomas, the World Health Organization (WHO) classification.

HODGKIN LYMPHOMA

Hodgkin lymphoma is less common than non-Hodgkin lymphoma (NHL). The characteristic cell that differentiates Hodgkin lymphoma from NHL is the Reed-Sternberg cell, which looks like owl's eyes because of the large double nuclei. Dorothy Reed (1874–1964) was a woman pathologist, one of the first female graduates of Johns Hopkins Medical School. She was the first to distinguish tuberculosis from Hodgkin lymphoma in 1902 by the cell that was named after her. Carl Sternberg (1872–1935) was an Austrian pathologist who described the same cell as one of the identifiers of Hodgkin lymphoma at approximately the same time as Dorothy Reed.

Reed-Sternberg cell
surrounded by normal lymphocytes

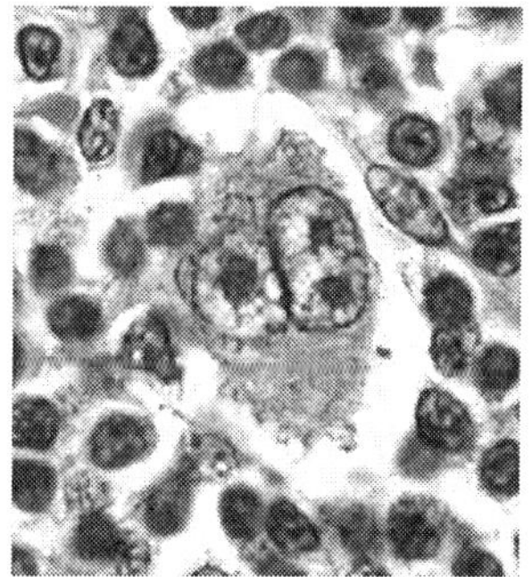

Source: Ed Uthman, MD. Used with permission.

The different cell types of Hodgkin lymphoma include:
- Hodgkin lymphoma, NOS (9650/3) (formerly called Hodgkin's disease)
- Classical Hodgkin lymphoma has four subtypes (introduced by Lukes and Butler; also called the Rye Classification, named after a conference in Rye, New York in 1966). These were the primary Hodgkin cell types known until about 1990.

Histologic Cell Types, *continued*

Hodgkin Lymphoma, *continued*

Classic Hodgkin lymphoma cell types, listed in order from best to worst prognosis:

- Lymphocyte-rich Hodgkin lymphoma (9651/3)—formerly called diffuse lymphocyte predominance Hodgkin's disease; about 5% of Hodgkin lymphomas; most commonly localized to a few lymph nodes (low stage)
- Nodular sclerosing Hodgkin lymphoma (9663/3, 9664/3, 9665/3, 9667/3)—most common subtype in developed countries (60–80% of all Hodgkin lymphomas); incidence higher in younger patients
- Mixed cellularity Hodgkin lymphoma (9652/3)—second most common type (15–30%); incidence higher in older patients
- Lymphocyte depletion Hodgkin lymphoma (9653/3, 9654/3)—about 1% of cases; occurs mainly in older people; diagnosed at higher stage than other lymphomas.

- Hodgkin lymphoma, nodular lymphocyte predominance (9659/3)—recognized as a distinct type of Hodgkin lymphoma about 1990 because of a popcorn-like appearance of Reed-Sternberg cell variants. About 5% of all Hodgkin lymphomas; more common in men that women of any age.

NON-HODGKIN LYMPHOMA

NHL is about three times more common than Hodgkin lymphoma. There is a long evolutionary history behind the current histologic classification of non-Hodgkin lymphomas (see Other Staging and Classification Systems at the end of this chapter).

WHO Classification of Lymphomas

In 1999, the World Health Organization (WHO) Classification adopted the theory of the REAL classification (see end of chapter) that hematopoietic diseases (lymphomas and leukemias) shared the same cell lines. The third edition of the WHO classification served as the basis for reorganizing and modifying hematopoietic and lymphoid histology codes between ICD-O-2 and ICD-O-3. In 2008, a new edition of the WHO classification was published. The fourth edition reorganized the hematopoietic and lymphoid neoplasms. As a result, Table 13 on pages 16–18 of ICD-O-3 is no longer accurate or complete; do not use Table 13 for coding lymphomas. The 2008 WHO classification also added about 30 new entities to the spectrum of hematopoietic and lymphoid neoplasms. The 2010 Hematopoietic MP/H rules include these new entities, but they are not printed in ICD-O-3.

The WHO classification includes both myeloid and lymphoid neoplasms. Due to its length, it will not be repeated here (the complete classification is listed in the Heme MP/H rules). The twelve major categories of the WHO classification are (lymphoma categories are in italics):

Myeloid neoplasms

- Myeloproliferative Neoplasms
- Myeloid and Lymphoid Neoplasms with Eosinophilia and Abnormalities of PDGFRA, PDGFRB or FGFR1
- Myelodysplastic/Myeloproliferative Neoplasms
- Myelodysplastic Syndromes
- Acute Myeloid Leukemia and Related Precursor Neoplasms
- Acute Leukemias of Ambiguous Lineage

Lymphoid neoplasms

- *Precursor Lymphoid Neoplasms*
- *Mature B-Cell Neoplasms*
- *Mature T-Cell and NK-Cell Neoplasms*
- *Hodgkin Lymphoma*
- Histiocytic and Dendritic Cell Neoplasms
- *Post-Transplant Lymphoproliferative Disorders*

Histologic Cell Types, ***continued***

The malignant lymphomas are a subset of the lymphoid neoplasms; there are no myeloid lymphomas. There are 46 lymphoma codes in the WHO classification encompassing over 150 diagnoses. The terms are scattered throughout the range 9590 to 9729 because there were not enough sequential numbers available to reorganize these diseases according to the new WHO classification. About 85% of non-Hodgkin lymphomas are of B-cell origin. Among the more common non-Hodgkin B-cell diagnoses are diffuse large B-cell, follicular, small lymphocytic, mantle cell, marginal zone or mucosa associated (MALT), and Burkitt lymphomas. Among the more common non-Hodgkin T-cell diagnoses are cutaneous T-cell (including mycosis fungoides and Sezary syndrome), anaplastic large cell, peripheral T-cell, and extranodal NK/T-cell lymphoma.

The Hematopoietic MP/H rules discussed previously in this chapter provide rules for selecting the best morphology code and phenotype (grade) for the case. The following general statements apply to coding lymphoma morphology in ICD-O-3.

- The preferred terminology for lymphomas is the WHO Classification.
- All lymphomas have a behavior code of /3.
- When a tumor is sent away for pathologic review, the consulting pathologist may use different descriptive terms because the he or she is using a different classification scheme. If at all possible, code the most specific diagnostic statement given, even though it may not be the higher code number.
- The usual ICD-O-3 rule about coding the highest code number does not apply in the lymphomas and leukemias section of ICD-O-3 because terms had to be inserted where space and unused codes were available.
- Non-specific or less specific terms are usually indicated by NOS, not otherwise specified. The largest category is 9680/3, diffuse large B-cell lymphoma, which has more than 20 synonyms. If you have one of these terms and another, more specific term, code the more specific term even if the code number is lower. The following terms are considered non-specific.

9590/3	Malignant lymphoma, NOS
9591/3	Non-Hodgkin lymphoma, NOS
9650/3	Hodgkin lymphoma, NOS
9680/3	Malignant lymphoma, diffuse large B-cell, NOS
9690/3	Follicular lymphoma, NOS
9702/3	Mature T-cell lymphoma, NOS
9727/3	Precursor cell lymphoblastic lymphoma, NOS

- The Heme DB includes a wealth of details about specific lymphomas, including the new entities from the 2008 WHO classification. Refer to the Heme DB for epidemiologic, diagnostic, and other information useful for abstracting lymphomas.

MALIGNANT LYMPHOMA ABSTRACTING GUIDELINES

A careful diagnostic and staging workup can often differentiate between Hodgkin and non-Hodgkin lymphoma even before tissue is removed for examination. Table 1 compares the general characteristics of both types of lymphoma.

HISTORY

There are no screening tests for malignant lymphoma. The signs and symptoms that bring the patient to a doctor are a valuable part of the diagnostic work-up for malignant lymphomas of all types. A careful history is important to establish both the type and duration of symptoms. Most nodal lymphomas present as a non-painful lump or bump, but extralymphatic lymphoma symptoms may be due to causes other than nodal enlargement, such as abdominal symptoms from a lymphoma of the small intestine. Most symptoms of lymphoma are non-specific, so it is the clinician's responsibility to rule out other causes of lymphadenopathy, such as infections or benign lymph node enlargement. The most common symptom of lymphoma is enlarged lymph nodes, which are discussed under Physical Exam.

B Symptoms

Certain other specific symptoms can affect the patient's prognosis. These are collectively referred to as "B Symptoms", presumably in contrast to being "A" (asymptomatic). B symptoms include any of the following symptoms:

1. Unexplained weight loss—greater than 10% of body weight in 6 months prior to diagnosis
2. Unexplained fever—temperature over 38 degrees Centigrade (100.4 Fahrenheit) that may come and go within the previous month
3. Night sweats (drenching)—recurrent within the previous month; more common with Hodgkin lymphoma

B symptoms are more important prognostically for Hodgkin lymphoma than NHL, but should be recorded whenever they are mentioned. B symptoms are not necessarily diagnostic by themselves. However, if a patient has B symptoms at diagnosis, the physician will have a "sign" to watch for recurrence, because the B symptoms will return.

TABLE 1. CHARACTERISTICS OF HODGKIN AND NON-HODGKIN LYMPHOMAS

	Hodgkin	Non-Hodgkin
Frequency	25% of lymphomas	75% of lymphomas
Age distribution	15–40 and > 55	All ages, but mostly over 50
Sites of origin	Nodal	Extranodal, nodal
Location	90% above diaphragm	30% extralymphatic
Nodal distribution	Axial	Peripheral
Mode of spread	Contiguous	Noncontiguous
Stage at diagnosis	Commonly localized	Infrequently localized
B symptoms	Frequent	Less frequent
Extranodal primaries	Uncommon	More common
Stage distribution	80% stage I or II	85% stage III or IV
Prognosis	75% curable	3 prognostic groups
Pathologic characteristics	Reed-Sternberg cell	B or T cell
Bone marrow involvement	Uncommon	Common for certain histologies

History, ***continued***

Other symptoms that are not part of the "B symptoms" group include

- General fatigue or lack of energy
- Itching (pruritus) or a rash, without an apparent cause, much more severe than that caused by dry skin
- Sensitivity to alcohol causing painful lymph nodes
- Coughing, trouble breathing, or chest pain
- Pain, fullness, or swelling of abdomen

Where to look in the patient's record

- History and physical exam report
- Consultation report(s)
- Physician's progress notes

What information to select and record (record all dates)

- Absence or presence of specific B symptoms
- Duration and intensity of symptoms
- Any other symptoms related to the lymphoma

PHYSICAL EXAM

The physician should visually inspect and palpate all accessible lymph node chains for masses, asymmetry between right and left sides, and abnormal-appearing areas—in other words, any mention of enlarged or abnormal lymph nodes. Also, the physician should look for splenomegaly, hepatomegaly, masses, or other physical symptoms.

- For lymphomas, any mention of lymph nodes is to be interpreted as involvement. Any reference to lymph nodes as *lymphadenopathy*, *adenopathy*, *enlarged*, *rubbery*, *"shotty"*, *matted*, or *"with visible swelling"* should be considered involvement by lymphoma. A reference to a "rock hard" node may mean involvement by carcinoma instead.

Where to look in the patient's record

- History and physical exam report
- Consultation report(s)
- Physician's progress notes

What information to select and record (record all dates)

Pertinent findings as to *what the physician sees and feels* when examining the patient

- Specific involved lymph node chains
- Any organomegaly or other masses
- Use "evidence of" and "no evidence of" statements
- Document both positive and negative findings

IMAGING

Although the most common symptom of malignant lymphoma is enlarged lymph nodes on the surface of the body, it is important that a thorough search for involved deeper lymph nodes and organs be conducted with imaging in order to stage the patient properly. The radiologist should look for and mention any evidence of enlarged or abnormal lymph nodes, as well as abnormalities in other organs such as lung, liver, spleen, or brain, just as on the physical exam. Imaging tests used to determine the extent and stage of lymphomas include:

Imaging, ***continued***

- **Chest x-ray**—assessment of hilar nodes and mediastinal nodes, which are a common site of involvement by lymphoma
- **CT scans** of chest, abdomen, and/or pelvis—more precise evaluation of lymph nodes in body cavities to determine extent of bulky nodal disease
- **PET scan**—a supplemental technique (after CT) useful for determining whether an enlarged node contains lymphoma and for detecting small deposits of lymphoma anywhere in the body. Post-treatment, the PET scan can differentiate between residual lymphoma and scar tissue.
  - **CT/PET fusion imaging**—combining PET's ability to detect lymphoma with CT's detailed images to provide more complete diagnostic and staging information
- **Gallium scans**—using a radioisotope (gallium) to find lymphoma anywhere in the body
- **Liver/spleen scans**—nuclear studies (usually technetium) looking for enlargement or abnormality of either organ
- **Upper GI**—particularly for gastric lymphomas
- **Bone scans**—looking for isolated bone lesions or multiple involved bones
- **Lymphangiography**—also called bipedal lymphography; invasive procedure using contrast media injected into lymphatic vessels in both feet to assess lymph nodes in abdomen and pelvis; infrequently used due to potential morbidity and the accuracy of non-invasive CT and other types of imaging, but best for detecting retroperitoneal lymph node involvement
- **MRI scan**—using electromagnetic radio waves to computer-generate images of internal organs; useful for detecting small but involved lymph nodes and abnormalities in the spleen and other organs
- **Ultrasonography**—assessing the structures in the abdomen and pelvis using images created by sound waves. A probe or transducer is passed back and forth across the surface of the body. The sound waves can delineate lymph nodes, organ enlargement, and masses but can't diagnose lymphoma specifically. .

What information to select and record (record all dates)

Pertinent findings as stated by the radiologist from each study including:

- Name of study and area of the body being examined (for example, CT chest, PET scan, Liver-spleen scan)
- Involved area(s)
- Laterality of involved lymph nodes
- Relationship of lymphoma to other tissues, such as impingement/compression of or extension to other structures (another organ, other lymph node chains)
- Regional or distant spread, including location and number of metastatic lesions

ENDOSCOPY (Scopes)

In general, endoscopy is not useful for diagnosing nodal lymphomas; however it may be helpful in determining the extent of extralymphatic involvement of hollow organs, such as the stomach, small intestine, or large intestine.

What information to select and record (record all dates)

- Name of procedure
- Pertinent findings as described by the physician
- Record both positive and negative findings
- Location of any biopsies

LABORATORY TESTS AND TUMOR MARKERS (See also Diagnostic Tests chapter)

Basic laboratory tests are usually not useful for lymphomas, other than for a general assessment of body system functions. Diagnosis of malignant lymphoma should be made by examination of tissue or cells. Sophisticated tumor markers can help identify the specific lymphoma cell type. Tumor markers taken at the time of diagnosis (baseline) and during follow-up also help to assess lymphoma burden and monitor for recurrence. There are no screening tests to detect lymphoma. Laboratory tests used in the diagnosis and monitoring of lymphoma include:

- **CBC**—a low lymphocyte count and anemia may indicate lymphoma
- **Alkaline phosphatase**—elevated counts may indicate bone or liver involvement
- **LDH** (lactate dehydrogenase or LD)—monitors blood for presence of an enzyme released by heart, liver, kidneys, skeletal muscle, brain, blood cells and/or lungs if tissue is damaged by tumor or other disease; not diagnostic of lymphoma, but can be elevated in higher stages
- **Immunophenotyping**—determines the types of surface molecules (clusters of differentiation or CD) present on cells. The combination of CD marker values determines the specific lymphoma cell type. Examples of different CD marker combinations are shown in Table 2.
- **Immunocytochemistry**—the use of monoclonal antibodies to detect specific antigens on the surface of cells; also called immunohistochemistry
- **Flow cytometry**—measures multiple characteristics on and within individual cells (nucleus and cytoplasm), such as cell size, CD markers, antigens, ploidy, and DNA, to help determine the specific lymphoma cell type
- **Differential Staining Cytotoxicity (DiSC)**—assesses the cytotoxic drug sensitivity of fresh human cells to determine response to various chemotherapy agents before starting full treatment
- **Cytogenetics**—evaluation of the chromosomal structure of the lymphoma. Many of the new entities in the WHO classification are diagnosed on the basis of translocations (*t*), deletions (del or -), inversions (*i*) or other abnormalities of the chromosomes. Cytogenetic testing requires a specialty laboratory and it takes weeks to receive the results.
- **Molecular genetic studies**—evaluation of lymphoma cell DNA using fluorescent in situ hybridization (FISH) or polymerase chain reaction (PCR); even more sensitive than cyto-genetics for detecting abnormal cells

What information to select and record (record all dates)

- Test type
- Test result
  Note: it is not necessary to record each individual CD marker result; a statement of "CD markers reported" will suffice to identify those cases in the registry if a researcher wants to investigate further
- Normal test value/range

Note: A new code was added to the Diagnostic Confirmation field in 2010 to provide more information about highly specialized methods of diagnosis for lymphomas and hematopoietic diseases. Code 3, Positive histology *plus* positive immunophenotyping *and/or* positive genetic studies, is used only for lymphomas and hematopoietic diseases when the positive diagnosis is further defined by a specialized test. When the initial diagnosis is made by one of the procedures in code 1 (positive histology, such as examination of tissue or bone marrow) and additional tests provide a more specific diagnosis based on genetic testing or special stains (immunophenotyping), use code 3. Examples of genetic tests include the Philadelphia chromosome for chronic myeloid leukemia, PDGFRA (platelet-derived growth factor receptor A), FGFR1 (fibroblast growth factor receptor 1), and tests for genetic abnormalities such as

TABLE 2. EXAMPLES OF CELL SURFACE MARKER PATTERNS FOR VARIOUS LYMPHOMAS

	CD5	CD10	CD20	CD23	CD 79a	ALK-FL	Bcl-1	Bcl-2	Bcl-6	C-myc	TdT
Low grade B-cell NHL											
Follicular	-	+	+	-	+	-	-	+/-	+	-/+	-
Sml lym'cytic	+	-	+	+	+	-	-	+	-	-	-
MALT	-	-	+	-	+	-	-	+	-	-	-
Marginal Zone	-	-	+	-	+	-	-	+	-	-	-
High grade B-cell NHL											
Diffuse Lrg Cl	-/+	+/-	+	-	+	-	-	+/-	+	-/+	-
Mantle cell	+	-/+	+	-	+	-	+	+	-	-	-
Burkitt	-	+	+	-	+	-	-	-	+	+	-
Lymphoblastic	-	+/-	-/+	-	-/+	-	-	+/-	-	-	+

Laboratory Tests and Tumor Markers, *continued*

inversions (inv), deletions (del or -) and translocations (t). Examples of immunophenotyping include flow cytometry, immunohistochemical stains, and monoclonal antibodies such as CD4 (there are over 300 CD markers), TdT, Ki-67, Bcl, and C-Myc. The hematopoietic data base lists the definitive diagnostic methods for each type of lymphoma.

Example Initial lymph node biopsy shows B-cell lymphoblastic leukemia/lymphoma [NOS]. Further chromosomal studies show a translocation (t) between chromosomes 9 and 22 for a final diagnosis of B-cell lymphoblastic leukemia/lymphoma with t(9;22)(q34;q11.2) (ICD-O-3 code 9812/3). Because the chromosomal studies provided a more specific diagnosis, use code 3 in the Diagnostic Confirmation field.

OPERATIVE FINDINGS

In addition to the pathology report of the tissues removed during a procedure, the operative report from diagnostic exploratory procedures and/or cancer directed definitive treatment for extralymphatic lymphomas can provide valuable information about the precise location of the primary, any areas of involvement left behind, or clinical information that might affect the staging or histologic diagnosis.

What information to select and record (record all dates)

Pertinent findings as described by the surgeon

- Site(s) of involvement
- Organs and tissues removed—removal of just the tumor or removal of entire primary site
- Involved tissues or areas not included in pathology specimen
- Size of tumor/involved area before removal
- Status of lymph nodes, including anatomic name/chain and laterality
- If no findings are documented, document as "findings not recorded"
- Reason if no cancer-directed surgery was performed

DIAGNOSTIC PROCEDURES

Cytology Reports

The following procedures may yield cells that confirm the diagnosis of lymphoma, although a larger sample from a tissue biopsy is better to provide more precise identification of the specific cell type.

- **Lymph node aspiration**—biopsy procedure using a thin needle to take a sample of tissue or fluid from a lymph node. The procedure is also called fine needle aspiration.

Diagnostic Procedures, *continued*

- **Fine-needle aspiration (FNA)**, fine needle aspiration cytology (FNAC), fine needle aspiration biopsy (FNAB)—insertion of a thin needle into the mass or suspicious area to remove fluid and/or cells for microscopic examination. FNA may be guided by ultrasound or computerized tomography when direct visualization of the lesion is not possible. FNA sample sizes are small and do not provide information about the internal structure of the lymph node, but can differentiate between lymphoma (NOS) and other diseases in the node. An excisional biopsy of a node or other involved tissue is usually required to obtain enough tissue to make the definitive diagnosis of a specific lymphoma cell type.
- **Lumbar puncture**—looking for cerebrospinal fluid involvement by lymphoma; performed infrequently
- **Pleural or peritoneal cytology** (thoracentesis or paracentesis)—removal of fluid from the chest or abdomen; useful for diagnosing primary effusion lymphoma

What information to select and record (record all dates)

- Test type and tissue biopsied
- Positive or negative findings
- Cell type, if given

Histology

The following procedures yield pieces of tumor tissue that confirm the diagnosis of lymphoma and can be used to determine further treatment.

- **Core needle biopsy**—uses a large bore needle to obtain a small amount of tissue for microscopic analysis in a procedure similar to fine needle aspiration (see above). Core needle biopsy may also be image-guided. Use of core needle biopsy is usually limited to patients who cannot tolerate an invasive surgical procedure.
- **Lymph node biopsy**—usually an excisional biopsy (see below) that removes one or more lymph nodes to provide sufficient tissue to diagnose a specific lymphoma cell type
- **Incisional biopsy**—diagnostic procedure in which the surgeon removes a sample of tissue from the mass or suspicious area. Incisional biopsy cuts through tumor; it is performed when complete removal is unnecessary or not possible.
- **Excisional biopsy**—also called surgical, total, or open biopsy. The purpose of an excisional biopsy is to attempt to remove the entire mass or a large portion of the mass for therapeutic as well as diagnostic purposes. Removed tissue is then sent to the pathologist for diagnosis. **Note**: Read the body of the operative report carefully. Frequently surgeons will title the report "biopsy" and the report will describe an excisional biopsy when the intent of the procedure was to excise the entire lesion.
- **Bone marrow aspiration and biopsy**—indicated to rule out Stage IV disease, for diagnosing indolent lymphomas, for further investigation of unusual laboratory test results, and for other reasons. Lymphoma involvement of the bone marrow moves the patient to the highest stage, so bone marrow biopsy is a fairly common diagnostic procedure for lymphoma cases. Low grade or indolent lymphomas are more likely to have bone marrow involvement than higher grade lymphomas. The aspiration retrieves liquid (cells) from the marrow and the biopsy retrieves a sample of the marrow to examine for its structure and the presence of fibrosis or sclerosis.
- **Endoscopic biopsy**—Used for diagnosing extralymphatic lymphomas of hollow organs. Tissue for microscopic examination is removed by means of an endoscope (a fiberoptic cable for viewing inside the body), which is inserted into the body along with sampling instruments. Endoscopy allows the physician to visualize the abnormality and guide the sampling.

Diagnostic Procedures, *continued*

Pathology Reports

Pathologic evaluation of any resected tissue not only establishes a diagnosis, but also provides important staging (and therefore prognostic) information. All parts of the pathology report—the gross examination of the specimen, the microscopic examination, the final diagnosis and comments—should be reviewed for staging, cell type, phenotype (grade), and other histology information, but only the final diagnosis should be used to code the histology. Remember that the site of the biopsy may not be the best site code to use for describing the extent of the lymphoma. Examples of a lymphoma cytology report, a lymphoma pathology report, and a bone marrow biopsy and aspiration report are shown in Table 3.

- **Bone marrow aspiration and biopsy**—may be reported on a special hematology report form rather than a standard pathology report (see description above)
- **Staging laparotomy**—very infrequently performed, because imaging is just as precise and less invasive. See the comments on staging laparotomy under Surgery, below.

If a CAP checklist (outline format provided by the College of American Pathologists) is provided, the information may be easier to find in that section of the pathology report than in the gross and microscopic narrative sections. The CAP checklist is also called a synoptic report or CAP protocol.

What information to select and record (record all dates)

Final Diagnosis

- Specific histology (cell type)—follow the histology coding rules for using this information.
- Phenotype (B-cell, T-cell or NK-cell)
- Behavior
- Mixed histology information, if any

Gross

- Location of lymphoma mass within resected specimen
- Size of largest area of lymphoma

Microscopic (for extranodal and extralymphatic lymphomas)

- Extent of disease—adjacent tissues, adjacent lymph node chains
- Status of surgical margins

Microscopic (for nodal lymphomas)

- Location of involved nodes—name(s) of lymph node chain(s), laterality
- Involvement of node capsule (extracapsular extension—an possible indicator that the "E" suffix should be added to the Stage Group)
- Fixed/matted lymph nodes

Other Information

- Stage as stated by pathologist (Ann Arbor, TNM)
- Results of biopsies of possible metastatic sites

TABLE 3. EXAMPLES OF CYTOLOGY, PATHOLOGY, AND BONE MARROW REPORTS FOR MALIGNANT LYMPHOMA

CYTOLOGY REPORT

SPECIMEN/SITE: FNA Left axillary mass

CLINICAL DATA: 10 cm left axillary mass; ? lymphoma, ? Cancer

GROSS DESCRIPTION:
Prepared 8 slides. Specimen sent for flow cytometry.

DIAGNOSIS:
Smears contain abnormal lymphoid cells with vesicular nuclei and prominent nucleoli. Flow cytometry showed lambda light chain restricted B-cells with the following phenotype, CD19+, CD20+, CD5-, CD10+, CD23-, HLADR+ and CD71+. Immunophenotype is consistent with a monoclonal B-cell lymphoproliferative disorder possibly originating from follicle centre cells and with an increased proliferative potential. Large B-cell lymphoma is included in the differential diagnosis.

PATHOLOGY REPORT

SPECIMEN/SITE: Portion of left axillary node

CLINICAL DATA: Incisional biopsy left axillary node. Probably lymphoma. PLEASE NOTE: Lymphoma protocol was completed on this specimen including LM, EM, flow, and impressions, frozen section.

GROSS DESCRIPTION:
Specimen received fresh labeled "left axillary mass" consists of a portion of pink-tan rubbery lymph node with some fibrofatty tags and measures 2 x 1.2 x 1 cm. (A1, 1 pc used for frozen section; A2 A3, 2 pc each formalin fixed: A4, 2 pc: B5 fixed ax).

MICROSCOPIC DESCRIPTION:
Sections are of tissue showing a diffuse infiltrating including into fat by large abnormal lymphoid cells. No normal lymph node tissue is seen. An area of necrosis is noted.

FLOW CYTOMETRY:
Immunophenotyping confirmed the presence of large-sized monoclonal lambda-restricted B cells (CD19+, CD20+, DR+, CD10+, CD5-, CD23-, and CD71+)

IMMUNOHISTOCHEMISTRY:
Bcl-6, CD10, CD20 – positive, Bcl-2, MUM-1 – negative, CD3 – positive (reactive T cell pattern), Ki67 - >50% cells positive, p53 - >80% cells positive.

DIAGNOSIS:
Non-Hodgkin Lymphoma, large B cell (WHO classification)

COMMENT:
Findings as described above suggest aggressive disease.

Table 3, *continued*

BONE MARROW ASPIRATION AND BIOPSY REPORT

SPECIMEN/SITE: Left PIC bone marrow biopsy

CLINICAL DATA: 33 year old with newly diagnosed NHL.

GROSS DESCRIPTION:
Specimen labeled "left PIC bone biopsy" consists of a core of bone marrow that measures 0.8 cm in length x 0.3 cm in diameter with some hemorrhagic material. (A1, 2 pcs, sent for fix and decal, ax)

MICROSCOPIC DESCRIPTION:
The cancellous bone is normal. The bone marrow cell:fat ratio is at 55:45. All three hematopoietic cell lineages are present and show maturation. Focal areas of fibrosis noted. No morphological evidence of lymphoma seen.

DIAGNOSIS: See microscopic description and comment.

COMMENT: Please see also Bone Marrow aspirate of [date]

BONE MARROW REPORT

SPECIMEN/SITE: Left PIC

	Count %		Count %
Blasts	1.4	Lymphocytes	25.8
Promyelocytes	5.2	Lymphocytes (Immature)	
Myelocytes	5.0	Plasmacytes	8.0
Metamyelocytes	4.6	Plasmacytes (Immature)	
P.M.N. Bands	13.8		
P.M.N. Mature	7.2	Pronormoblast	2.0
Eosinophil (all stages)	2.6	Basophilic Normoblast	5.6
Basophils (all stages)		Polychromatophilic Normoblast	8.2
Promonocytes		Orthochromic Normoblast	8.8
Monocytes	1.8	Unclassified Cells	

Megakaryocytes: Normal Myeloid/Erythroid Ratio: 1.7/1.0

Further Tests: [ ] Immunophenotyping [ ] Cytogenetics [ ] Molecular Pathology
[ ] Electron Microscopy [ ] Culture (Microbiology) [X] Bone Biopsy

Clinical Abstract: 33 year old female with newly diagnosed Non-Hodgkin lymphoma. Bone marrow for evaluation.

Peripheral Blood: HCB 80G/l, hct 0.25 1 l/l, mcv 76.5 fl., MCHC 319 g/L, RDW 15.5% Normochromic normocytic, WBC 3.5 x 109/L, DIFF: Neutrophils 1.225 x 109/L, Bands 0.700 x 109/L, Lymphocytes 1.295 x 109/L, Monocytes 0.245 x 109/L, Metamyelocytes 0.035 x 109/L, Platelet count 176 x 109/L

Bone Marrow Specimen	Satisfactory	Unsatisfactory
Aspirate	[X]	[ ]

Cellularity: Apparently normocellular

Erythropoiesis: Present. M/E ratio 1.7/1.0. Maturation appears normoblastic and haemoglobinisation is unimpaired.

Stored Iron: 4/6, siderocytes rare, sideroblasts normal.

Granulopoiesis: Maturation is seen to the polymorphonuclear stage.

Lymphoplasmacytic complement: There are areas in the slides which show increased lymphocytes which in the main appear to be of mixed morphology. Occasional small irregular ?cleaved cells seen, ?significance.

Megakaryocytes: Present in normal numbers

Diagnosis: Bone marrow aspirate, left PSIS: There is good hematopoietic representation. No diagnostic morphologic findings of lymphoma are seen. Please see description above. Please see also bone marrow biopsy of [date].

MALIGNANT LYMPHOMA DISEASE MANAGEMENT

Treatment for both Hodgkin and non-Hodgkin lymphoma is usually radiation therapy (for early stage disease, Stage I and II) and/or chemotherapy (for stage III and IV cases). Treatment for non-Hodgkin lymphoma depends on the cell type and stage at diagnosis. For example, low grade, low stage NHL may be treated by observation until symptomatic or with radiation only, whereas intermediate grade, low stage NHL should receive radiation and chemotherapy, and high-grade, low stage NHL would probably receive combination chemotherapy only. Current therapy for Hodgkin disease cures over 75% of patients.

For treatment purposes, the National Cancer Institute and other agencies divide non-Hodgkin lymphomas into two categories, indolent and aggressive, and treatment is generally based on these categories. Examples of the major cell types in each category are listed in Table 4.

- Lymphomas, particularly NHL, can convert to a more aggressive form after initial treatment.
- Low grade non-Hodgkin lymphomas respond to chemotherapy and irradiation, but continue to relapse for a long period of time.

TABLE 4. INDOLENT AND AGGRESSIVE LYMPHOMAS

Indolent Lymphomas	Aggressive B-Cell Lymphomas	Aggressive T-Cell Lymphomas
Follicular lymphomas	Diffuse large cell lymphoma	T-cell lymphoblastic lymphoma
Small lymphocytic lymphoma / Chronic lymphocytic leukemia	- Angiocentric lymphoma (pulmonary B-cell)	Anaplastic large cell (Ki-1) lymphoma
Lymphoplasmacytic lymphoma	Large cell immunoblastic lymphoma	Peripheral T-cell lymphomas
- Waldenstrom's macro-globulinemia	Lymphoblastic lymphoma	- T-cell lymphoma / leukemia
Marginal zone lymphoma	Burkitt lymphoma	- Angioimmunoblastic T-cell lymphoma
- MALT lymphoma	Mantle cell lymphoma	- Angiocentric lymphoma (nasal T-cell)
- Nodal marginal zone lymphoma	Primary mediastinal B-cell lymphoma	- Intestinal T-cell lymphoma
- Splenic marginal zone lymphoma	Primary effusion lymphoma	- Peripheral T-cell lymphoma
Cutaneous T-cell / Mycosis fungoides / Sezary syndrome	Primary central nervous system (CNS) lymphoma	NK-cell lymphomas
	- AIDS related lymphoma	Primary central nervous system (CNS) lymphoma
		- AIDS related lymphoma

SURGERY

- **Nodal lymphomas**—The most common surgical procedure for lymphoma is an excisional biopsy of a lymph node (see Diagnostic Procedures–Histology, above). However, the purpose of the excisional biopsy is usually diagnostic rather than therapeutic. In September 2008, a joint statement was released by the Commission on Cancer, National Program of Cancer Registries, and SEER Program providing guidance as to how excisional biopsy of a single lymph node should be coded in the FORDS Surgery of Primary Site codes for lymphoma. The statement reads:

  Use code 25 in Surgery of Primary Site when only one lymph node is involved and the single involved lymph node is removed by an excisional biopsy.

  Rationale: A surgical procedure to a single lymph node when the single lymph node is the primary is usually done for diagnostic purposes, [but may also be treatment in some cases]. COC collects this information as code 02 in the fields Surgical Diagnostic and

Surgery, ***continued***

Staging Procedure and Surgical Diagnostic and Staging Procedure at This Facility when the biopsy is an incisional or needle biopsy or aspiration. Any central registry that wants to continue to collect information on incisional and needle biopsies or aspiration should collect the information in the field RX SUMM—DX/STG PROC, which is not required by either SEER or NPCR.

In other words, for lymphomas, code excisional biopsy of a lymph node in Surgery of Primary Site only when it removes all evidence of the lymphoma (cancer-directed treatment for Stage I). Do not code incisional biopsy, needle biopsy or aspiration of a lymph node in this field. Any excisional biopsy for diagnosis only should be coded in Surgical Diagnostic and Staging Procedure or a similar central registry data field.

- Surgery of Primary Site codes are used infrequently for cancer-directed treatment of lymphomas, because most nodal lymphomas are treated with chemotherapy and/or radiation. The Surgery of Primary Site codes for lymph node primaries include:
  - 25 Local tumor excision, NOS; Less than a full chain; includes an excisional biopsy of a single lymph node
  - 30 Lymph node dissection, NOS
    - 31 One chain
    - 32 Two or more chains
  - 40 Lymph node dissection, NOS PLUS splenectomy
    - 41 One chain
    - 42 Two or more chains
  - 50 Lymph node dissection, NOS and partial/total removal of adjacent organ(s)
    - 51 One chain
    - 52 Two or more chains
  - 60 Lymph node dissection, NOS and partial/total removal of adjacent organ(s) PLUS splenectomy (Includes staging laparotomy for lymphoma)
    - 61 One chain
    - 62 Two or more chains
- **Extranodal and extralymphatic lymphomas**—Surgical procedures for extranodal and extralymphatic lymphomas should be coded using the surgical codes for the involved organ.
- **Staging Laparotomy**—evaluation of the contents of the abdomen for the purpose of determining the extent of disease. Precise staging is important for Hodgkin lymphoma and to a lesser extent non-Hodgkin lymphoma. A staging laparotomy is not routinely done for lymphoma unless the opportunity for obtaining better staging information exceeds the risk of operative morbidity. CT and PET imaging technology can provide nearly as complete staging information with much less risk.

  An adequate staging laparotomy includes abdominal exploration, wedge and needle biopsies of the liver, multiple lymph node biopsies, bone marrow biopsy, and splenectomy. Staging laparotomy is considered a diagnostic procedure rather than surgical treatment. The staging laparotomy is an opportunity to identify landmarks within the abdomen, such as unresectable large nodes or the splenic pedicle, which will affect the design of radiation treatment for the patient.

Note: Surgical resection of an abdominal lymphoma does not meet the definition of a staging laparotomy unless all of the biopsies and splenectomy noted above are part of the procedure.

RADIATION THERAPY

Radiation is commonly used in low stage Hodgkin lymphoma and NHL (Stage I and II). Patients with higher stage disease may be treated with radiation to reduce tumor mass or bulky disease. Usually patients are treated with radiation on only one side of the body (above or below the diaphragm). Radiation may also be given for central nervous system prophylaxis, for intracranial metastases, or for treatment of a primary brain lymphoma.

Specific radiation therapy techniques include:

- Involved field radiation—treating only the involved lymph node areas
- Mantle field radiation—radiation to the neck, chest and mediastinum, and axilla
- Mini-mantle—radiation to the neck, axilla, and upper chest but not to low mediastinum
- Inverted Y—radiation to upper abdomen, spleen, and pelvic nodes
- Total body irradiation (TBI)—low dose radiation to all lymph chains and areas (mantle and inverted Y) for advanced disease

Two therapeutic drugs, Bexxar (tositumomab) and Zevalin (Ibritumomab), are coded as radioisotopes. These two drugs are monoclonal antibodies conjugated to radioactive particles. The monoclonal antibody seeks out and attaches to malignant lymphocytes (lymphoma cells) and the radioactive particles kill the cell. Do not code Bexxar or Zevalin as immunotherapy.

SYSTEMIC THERAPY

CHEMOTHERAPY

Chemotherapy is the principal modality for lymphoma treatment, particularly for higher stage disease. Combination chemotherapy has been investigated in clinical trials since the 1960s. In the past few years, combination chemotherapy has included Rituxan, a monoclonal antibody effective in seeking out and shutting down malignant lymphocytes (non-Hodgkin lymphoma cells). Refer to SEER*Rx for additional regimens and alternative listings of drugs.

Chemotherapy for non-Hodgkin Lymphoma (choice of regimen depends on stage and cell type) More than a dozen drugs are effective for non-Hodgkin lymphoma. Treatment is usually a combination of three or more drugs.

- CHOP—cytoxan, doxorubicin, vincristine, prednisone
- CHOP plus other agents—cytoxan, doxorubicin, vincristine, prednisone plus Rituxan or another drug plus maintenance with methotrexate and 6-mercaptopurine
- C-MOPP—cyclophosphamide, vincristine, procarbazine, prednisone
- C-MOPP—cyclophosphamide, vincristine, procarbazine, prednisone
- CVP—cytoxan, vincristine, prednisone (with or without Retuximab R-CVP)
- CVAD—cyclophosphamide, vincristine, doxourubicin, dexamethasone
- EPOCH—etoposide, prednisone, oncovin, cyclophosphamide, doxorubicin
- FND—Fludarabine, mitoxantrone, with or without dexamethasone
- R-FM—rituximab, fludarabine, mitoxantrone
- R-FCM—rituximab, fludarabine, cyclophosphamide, mitoxantrone

Other combinations used less frequently or in the past

- ACVBP—doxorubicin, cyclophosphamide, vindesine, bleomycin, prednisone
- APO—doxorubicin, vincristine, prednisone, methotrexate, 6-mercaptopurine
- BACOP—bleomycin, doxorubicin, cytoxan, vincristine, prednisone
- CNOP—cyclophosphamide, mitoxantrone, vincristine, prednisone
- COMLA—cytoxan, vincristine, methotrexate with leucovorin rescue, cytarabine
- COPP—cytoxan, vincristine, procarbazine, prednisone

Systemic Therapy—Chemotherapy, *continued*

- MACOP-B—methotrexate with leucovorin rescue, doxorubicin, cytoxan, vincristine, prednisone, bleomycin
- m-BACOD—intermediate-dose methotrexate, bleomycin, doxorubicin, cytoxan, vincristine, dexamethasone
- ProMACE-CytaBOM—cytoxan, etoposide, doxorubicin, prednisone, alternating with cytarabine, bleomycin, vincristine, intermediate-dose methotrexate
- ProMACE-MOPP—cytoxan, etoposide, adriamycin, methotrexate, and folinic acid, alternating with mechlorethamine, vincristine, procarbazine and prednisone
- Cytoxan as a single agent
- Chlorambucil as a single agent

Note: Do not code antibiotic therapy or proton pump inhibitors as treatment for MALT lymphoma. Although the lymphoma will respond to these treatments, they do not meet the definition of cancer-directed treatment. Instead, antibiotics and stomach acid blockers eliminate the stimuli that cause the MALT lymphoma to grow.

Chemotherapy for Hodgkin Lymphoma (choice of regimen depends on stage and cell type)

- ABV—doxorubicin, bleomycin, vinblastine
- ABVD—doxorubicin, bleomycin, vinblastine, dacarbazine
- AV—doxorubicin, vinblastine
- AVD—doxorubicin, vinblastine, dacarbazine
- BEACOPP—bleomycin, etoposide, doxorubicin, cyclophosphamide, vincristine, procarbazine, prednisone
- CEC—cyclophosphamide, lomustine, vindesine, melphalan, prednisone, epidoxorubicin, vincristine, procarbazine, vinblastine, bleomycin
- COPP/ABVD—cyclophosphamide, vincristine, procarbazine, prednisone alternating with doxorubicin, bleomycin, vinblastine, dacarbazine
- MOPP—mechlorethamine, vincristine, procarbazine, prednisone
- MOPP/ABV—mechlorethamine, vincristine, procarbazine, prednisone alternating with doxorubicin, bleomycin, vinblastine
- MOPP/ABVD—mechlorethamine, vincristine, procarbazine, prednisone alternating with doxorubicin, bleomycin, vinblastine, dacarbazine
- MOPPEVBCAD—mechlorethamine, vincristine, procarbazine, prednisone, epidoxorubicin, bleomycin, vinblastine, lomustine, doxorubicin, vindesine
- Stanford V—doxorubicin, mechlorethamine (nitrogen mustard), vincristine, vinblastine, bleomycin, etoposide, prednisone (with radiation therapy)

Other combinations used less frequently or in the past

- LOPP—chlorambucil, vincristine, procarbazine, prednisone
- MVPP—mechlorethamine, vinblastine, procarbazine, prednisone
- MVVPP—mechlorethamine, vincristine, vinblastine, procarbazine, prednisone
- ChlVPP—chlorambucil, vinblastine, procarbazine, prednisone
- CVPP—cytoxan, vinblastine, procarbazine, prednisone
- PAVe—procarbazine, melphalan, vinblastine
- BCVPP—bleomycin, cytoxan, vinblastine, procarbazine, prednisone

Note: Multidrug regimens such as ProMACE-CytaBOM and MOPP/ABV alternate drugs over a number of weeks of therapy to allow the organs affected by the chemotherapy agents to recover between treatments. These regimens should be recorded as a single course of therapy. For example, do not record these regimens as ProMACE for first course, CytaBom as second course, ProMACE (again) as third course, and CytaBOM (again) as fourth course.

Systemic Therapy—Chemotherapy, *continued*

Newer agents for Hodgkin lymphoma include targeted therapies such as lenalidomide (Revlimid) and bortezomib (Velcade), which are useful in plasma cell neoplasms; rituximab (Rituxan), which targets lymphocytes and is known to be effective for non-Hodgkin lymphoma; tositumomab (Bexxar), a monoclonal antibody conjugated to a radioisotope (code as radioisotope under Radiation Therapy); brentuximab vedotin (SGN-35), a monoclonal antibody conjugated to a cell poison (in clinical trials).

Bortezomib (Velcade) and temsirolimus (Torisel) are targeted therapies effective in non-Hodgkin lymphoma. These drugs work by blocking cell reproduction processes and essentially shutting down tumor growth. Alemtuzumab (Campath) is a monoclonal antibody used to treat some types of peripheral T-cell lymphoma. Ofatumumab (Arzerra), a monoclonal antibody used to treat chronic lymphocytic leukemia, is being studied for certain types of lymphomas. Bendamustine (Treanda) was recently approved for non-Hodgkin lymphoma treatment.

HORMONE THERAPY

Lymphoma patients usually receive a corticosteroid such as prednisone, dexamethasone, or decadron, as part of a combination chemotherapy regimen. Although corticosteroids are defined as hormones, they do not work in the body in the same way that hormone treatment for breast or prostate cancer works. Corticosteroids have antitumor effect for lymphomas and other lymphocytic diseases by controlling white cell (lymphocyte) proliferation. Therefore, prednisone and other corticosteroids are coded as hormone therapy rather than ancillary or supportive care for lymphomas, lymphocytic leukemias, and multiple myelomas. Occasionally hormone therapy alone is used in older lymphoma patients with comorbidities that make chemotherapy risky; hormones may be given alone to see if the patient responds to treatment.

BIOLOGICAL RESPONSE MODIFIERS/IMMUNOTHERAPY

Many new drugs are being developed for treatment of lymphoma, including several monoclonal antibodies that target cell markers on lymphocytes. Consult SEER*Rx (available free from www.seer.cancer.gov/tools/seerrx) to determine whether the drug being used should be coded as chemotherapy, immunotherapy, or a radioisotope.

Biovax/DTM is in clinical trials for the treatment of non-Hodgkin lymphoma, more specifically follicular lymphoma. This vaccine is created from the patient's lymphoma cells, which are mixed with immune system stimulants and injected back into the patient to fight the lymphoma. Interferon may be an option for certain types of lymphomas, but other than these two drugs, at present there are no effective immunotherapies for lymphoma.

HEMATOLOGIC TRANSPLANT AND ENDOCRINE PROCEDURES

Stem Cell Transplant

High-dose chemotherapy and stem cell transplant are indicated for Hodgkin lymphoma that responds incompletely to standard treatment. There are two basic types of stem cell transplants.

Autologous—the patient's own stem cells are collected prior to high-dose chemotherapy and given back to patient after treatment
Allogenic—stem cells from a donor (relative or unrelated) are given to the patient after treatment

- Non-myeloablative (also called mini-transplant or reduced intensity transplant)—uses lower doses of chemotherapy that does not wipe out bone marrow followed by an allogenic transplant.

USUAL TREATMENT BY PROGNOSTIC GROUP AND STAGE (from NCI PDQ)

The following options are based on the Ann Arbor/TNM Stage Group and prognostic category for Hodgkin or non-Hodgkin lymphoma. See the Chemotherapy section above for definitions of the various combination chemotherapy regimens.

HODGKIN LYMPHOMA

Early Stage Favorable Adult Classic Hodgkin Lymphoma (Stage I or II without risk factors)
- 2 cycles ABVD plus involved field radiation therapy
- 4 to 6 cycles ABVD
- Radiation therapy only in selected cases

Early Stage Unfavorable Adult Classic Hodgkin Lymphoma (Stage I or II with any risk factor*)
- 4 to 6 cycles ABVD or Stanford V
- 2 cycles ABVD plus involved field radiation therapy

* B symptoms; extranodal involvement; 3 or more lymph node areas involved; elevated ESR; large mediastinal mass.

Advanced Stage Favorable Adult Classic Hodgkin Lymphoma (Stage III or IV with 3 or fewer risk factors**)
- 6 to 8 cycles ABVD
- 6 to 8 cycles ABVD plus involved field radiation therapy for bulky disease

Advanced Stage Unfavorable Adult Classic Hodgkin Lymphoma (Stage III or IV with > 3 risk factors**)
- 6 to 8 cycles ABVD
- BEACOPP (increased dose)

** Male sex; age > 44; Stage IV; Albumin <4.0 g/dL; Hgb <10.5 g/dL; WBC at least 15,000/mm3; absolute lymphocyte count <8% of total WBC

Nodular Lymphocyte Predominant Hodgkin Disease

Early stage (no B symptoms, limited involvement)
- Radiation therapy alone
- Close observation in selected patients

Advanced disease (B symptoms)
- Rituximab with or without additional chemotherapy (under clinical investigation)

NON-HODGKIN LYMPHOMA

Indolent, Stage I and Contiguous Stage II Adult Non-Hodgkin Lymphoma
- Involved field radiation therapy
- Watchful waiting (active surveillance)
- Chemotherapy with radiation therapy
- Extended field radiation therapy to cover adjacent prophylactic lymph nodes
- Rituximab alone or with combination chemotherapy
- Other therapies used for patients with advanced stage lymphoma

Aggressive, Stage I and Contiguous Stage II Adult Non-Hodgkin Lymphoma
- Chemotherapy (R-CHOP) with or without involved field radiation therapy

Usual Treatment, *continued*

Indolent, Non-Contiguous Stage II/III/IV Adult Non-Hodgkin Lymphoma

- Careful observation in selected patients
- Rituximab alone or with combination chemotherapy
- Fludarabine or cladribine
- Cytoxan, chlorambucil, or bendamustine
- Combination chemotherapy
- Zevalin or Bexxar
- Other chemotherapy options and clinical trials with or without radiation therapy

Aggressive, Non-Contiguous Stage II/III/IV Adult Non-Hodgkin Lymphoma

- R-CHOP
- CHOP alone
- Autologous bone marrow or stem cell transplant for high risk patients

STAGING OF LYMPHOMAS

Staging for both Hodgkin and non-Hodgkin lymphoma is based on the number and location of involved lymph node regions, as well as extranodal/extralymphatic, splenic, and bone marrow involvement. Regardless of the location of the lymphoma (nodal, extranodal, or extralymphatic), all lymphomas use the same staging systems.

The traditional staging for both Hodgkin and non-Hodgkin lymphoma was initially presented at the Ann Arbor Symposium on Staging of Hodgkin's Disease, in April, 1971. For the Ann Arbor System, clinical staging includes all of the non-invasive procedures; pathologic staging is based on findings made as a result of invasive procedures such as laparotomy or mediastinotomy.

The definitions of the Ann Arbor staging system were adopted into the TNM system and then into Collaborative Staging. T, N, and M elements are not used for this disease.

CS Extension = AJCC/UICC 7th edition = Ann Arbor Staging

LYMPH NODE REGIONS FOR STAGING PURPOSES

The Ann Arbor staging of lymphomas (as well as the TNM stage group and the Collaborative Stage Data Collection System {CS}) counts involved lymphatic (lymph node regions) and extralymphatic sites to determine stage. Figure 2 is a picture of what we call "Lymphoma Man." This illustration appeared in the original article describing the Ann Arbor staging classification for Hodgkin lymphoma. You can see from the illustration that various lymph chains were grouped into regions for counting during the staging process. These are not anatomically related lymph nodes but the groupings have been agreed upon by oncologists and they apply to this day.

Note that the lymph node regions identified in Lymphoma Man are not the same as the ICD-O-3 lymph node regions pictured in Figure 1. For example, both the mediastinal and hilar lymph nodes are part of C77.1, intrathoracic lymph nodes, but they are counted separately for Ann Arbor staging. Similarly, the mesenteric and para-aortic lymph nodes are separate regions for the purposes of staging within C77.2 of ICD-O. This is an important concept to understand when determining the stage.

When staging lymphomas, follow these guidelines.

- Any mention of lymph nodes is considered involvement (see comments in Physical Exam, above)

Staging, ***continued***

- The spleen is considered clinically involved if there is palpable splenomegaly that is confirmed by x-ray/scan.
- According to the Ann Arbor staging system, lymph node chains in the central (axial) part of the body are only counted once when it comes to determining a stage, even though both right side and left side lymph nodes may be involved. Axial (central) lymph nodes are mediastinal, hilar, paraaortic, internal mammary, and mesenteric. The same guideline applies to the TNM stage group and Collaborative Stage.
- On the other hand, peripheral lymph nodes (to the sides of the body rather than along the center line) are counted separately for each involved side. Peripheral lymph nodes include axillary and intramammary, inguinal, femoral, infraclavicular, pelvic, and cervical (supraclavicular, occipital, preauricular). For example, if the left axillary lymph nodes are involved, the case is Stage I. If both the right and the left axillary lymph nodes are involved, the case is Stage II. The same guideline applies to the TNM stage group and Collaborative Stage.
- Involvement of soft tissue adjacent to a lymphoma site doesn't alter the staging.
- Extranodal sites within the lymphatic system (tonsils, spleen, thymus) are counted as single lymph node regions for the purposes of staging.
- If an extralymphatic site is involved, the suffix E is added to the stage. A primary brain lymphoma would be stage IE.
- The suffix "S" is used to indicate spleen involvement either pathologically or clinically. If the spleen is palpable and visible on x-ray, the spleen is defined as being clinically involved.
- The "E" and "S" suffixes are coded in the Clinical Stage Descriptor field in FORDS if used for TNM and are part of the derived stage in CS.

Figure 2. Anatomical Regions for Staging of Lymphoma

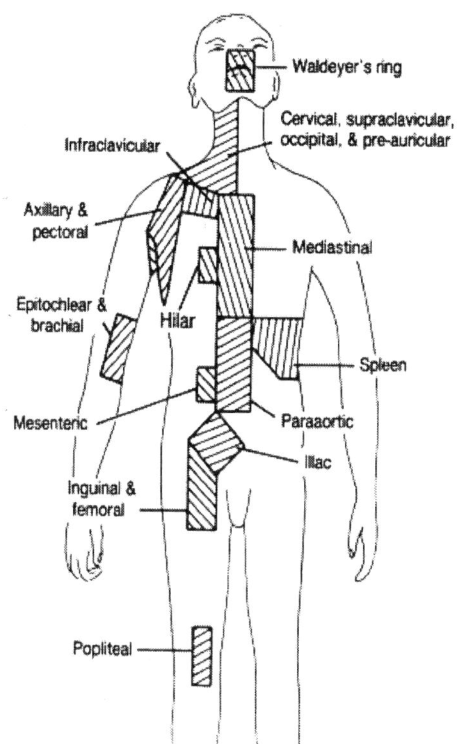

Image source: Wikipedia article "Lymph Node" and other internet sites.

Distinguishing Stage IE from Stage IV Disease

Sometimes it is difficult to determine the stage of a lymphoma because of its unusual presentation. To decide between Stage IE and Stage IV disease, look at the location of the primary tumor and the number of lesions.

- If the site of origin is *stomach, colon, brain or uterus*, the lymphoma is most likely extralymphatic (IE, or IIE if regional nodes are also involved).
- If *bone or lung,* look carefully for multiple lesions. If multiple areas of involvement are present, the lymphoma is most likely Stage IV.
- If the site of origin is *liver, bone marrow, pleura, or cerebrospinal fluid,* by definition the lymphoma is Stage IV. Malignant pleural or pericardial effusion is also Stage IV.
- A single lesion in *stomach, colon or another extranodal site* would be Stage IE (extranodal). However if there is more than one extranodal site involved, the lymphoma is Stage IV.

Staging, *continued*

The following are examples of various lymphoma stages. Illustrations of the stages are shown in the Collaborative Stage Data Collection System section.

- MALT lymphoma of stomach: Stage IE
- Malignant lymphoma of bilateral testes: Stage IE (bilateral involvement of a single extralymphatic organ is stage IE)
- Small lymphocytic lymphoma of tonsil and cervical lymph nodes: Stage II (tonsil is an extranodal lymphatic structure—no suffix E is used)
- Enteropathy-type T-cell lymphoma of the appendix and pericolic lymph nodes: Stage IIE
- Nodular sclerosing Hodgkin lymphoma of the iliac and periaortic lymph nodes: Stage II (separate lymph node regions on one side of the diaphragm)
- Follicular lymphoma grade 2 of the parotid gland: Stage IE
- Diffuse large B-cell lymphoma of bilateral axillary lymph nodes and spleen: Stage IIIS (each axilla is counted as one lymph node region; the spleen is on the opposite side of the diaphragm and also gets a suffix S)
- Hodgkin lymphoma, mixed cellularity, of the mediastinal and periaortic lymph nodes: Stage III (lymph nodes are on both sides of the diaphragm)
- Hepatosplenic gamma-delta T-cell lymphoma of spleen with involvement of liver: Stage IV
- Lymphoma diagnosed in bone marrow only (no evidence of lymphoma elsewhere): Stage IV (code primary site to C77.9)

COLLABORATIVE STAGE DATA COLLECTION SYSTEM (CS)

Malignant lymphomas of all sites use the same coding schema. This schema is used for both Hodgkin lymphoma and non-Hodgkin lymphoma regardless of where in the body they develop. The schema includes code 9823, chronic lymphocytic leukemia/small lymphocytic lymphoma, when the primary site associated with this code is anything except blood (C42.0), bone marrow (C42.1), or hematopoietic system, NOS (C42.4).

Make sure that your CS manual is complete by downloading any replacement pages from www.cancerstaging.org/cstage/manuals/index.html. Review carefully the notes preceding each table of the malignant lymphoma schema in the Collaborative Stage Data Collection System Coding Instructions version 02.03.02. Use the notes and comments in this section to supplement the information in the CS documentation. Remember that all of the general rules in Part I of the CS documentation apply to the site schema.

Most of the CS fields are defaulted (not used).

CS Tumor Size	988	Not applicable. Tumor size is not a factor in lymphoma staging.
CS Extension	100–999	Extension field is discussed below
CS TS/Ext Eval		Used only for staging laparotomy or autopsy staging; see below
CS Lymph Nodes	988	Not applicable. This field is not used for lymphoma.
CS Reg Nodes Eval	9	Not applicable for this schema
Reg LN Pos	99	Not applicable
Reg LN Exam	99	Not applicable
CS Mets at Dx	98	Not applicable. All disease is coded in CS Extension.
CS Mets Eval	9	Not applicable for this schema
SSF1		Associated with HIV/AIDS; see below
SSF2		B-symptoms; discussed below
SSF3		International Prognostic Index; see below
SSF4		Follicular Lymphoma International Prognostic Index; see below
SSF5		International Prognostic Score; see below

Collaborative Staging, *continued*

CS Extension Code Examples

These are examples only. Consult the Collaborative Stage Coding Instructions for complete definitions for each code.

Stage I
Cervical nodes only

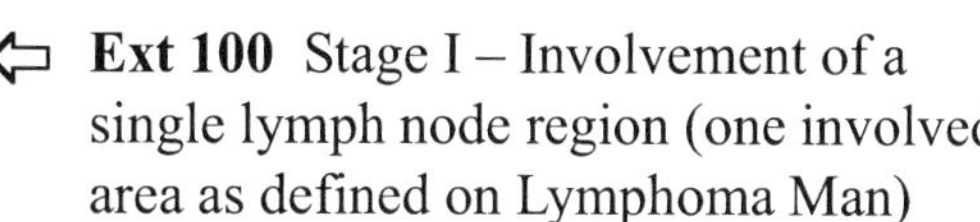

Ext 100 Stage I – Involvement of a single lymph node region (one involved area as defined on Lymphoma Man)

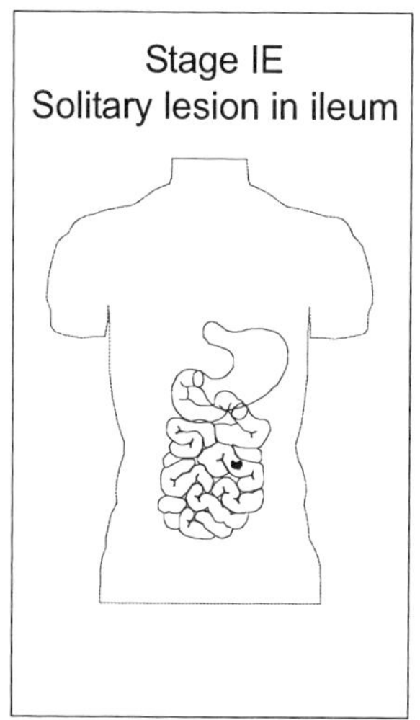

Ext 110 Stage IE – Involvement of a single extralymphatic organ or site (for example, stomach or brain or lung)

Ext 120 Stage IS – Involvement of spleen only

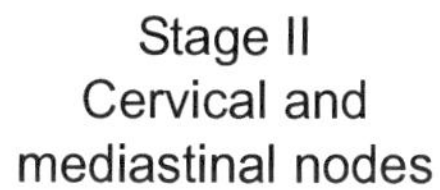

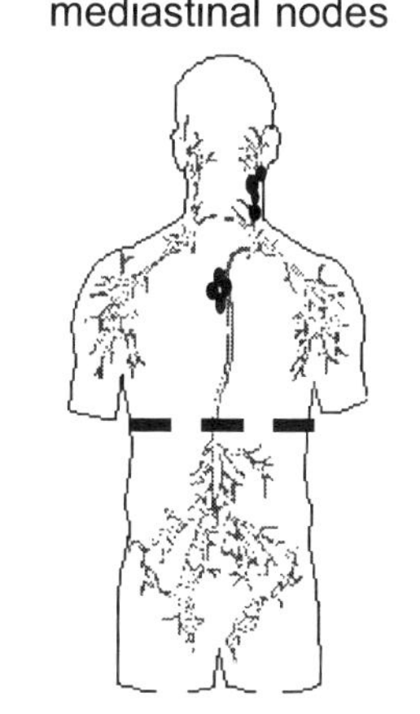

Ext 200 Stage II – Involvement of two or more lymph node regions on the same side of the diaphragm (such as involved cervical and mediastinal nodes)

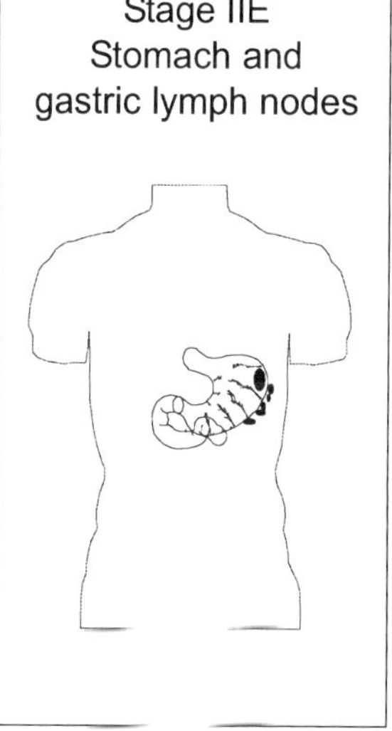

Ext 210 Stage IIE – Localized involvement of a single extralymphatic organ or site and its regional lymph node(s) with or without other lymph node regions on the same side of the diaphragm (such as a lymphoma of the stomach and perigastric lymph nodes)

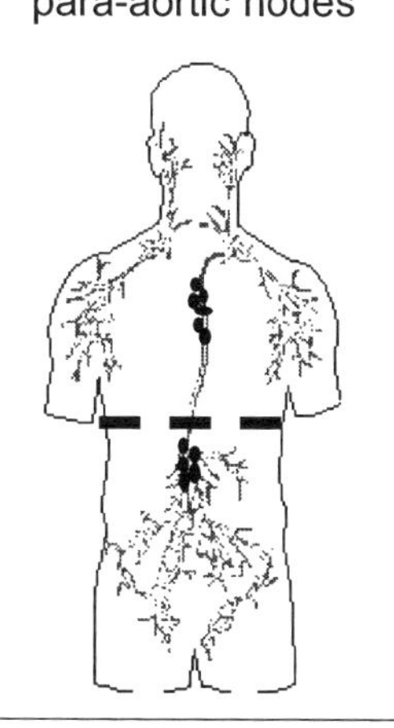

Ext 300 Stage III – Involvement of lymph nodes regions on both sides of the diaphragm (such as involved axillary, mediastinal and periaortic lymph nodes)

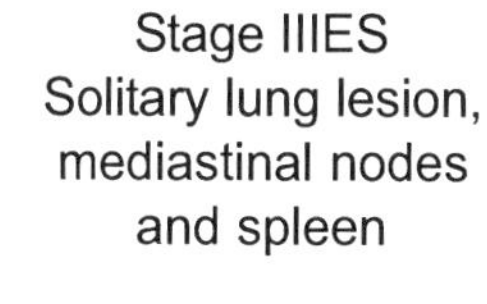

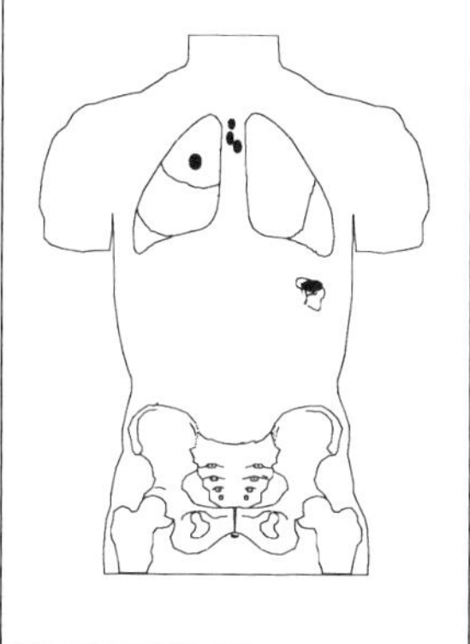

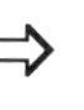

Ext 330 Stage IIIES – Involvement of an extralymphatic organ or site and lymph node regions on both sides of the diaphragm OR involvement of an extralymphatic organ or site and lymph nodes above the diaphragm plus spleen (shown)

Lymphoma

CS Extension Code Examples, *continued*

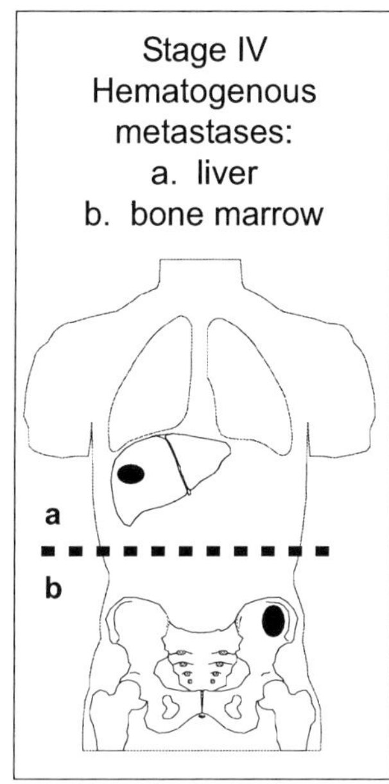

Ext 800 Stage IV – Isolated extra-lymphatic organ involvement (hematogenous spread) (such as lymphoma diagnosed in liver or bone marrow only)

Ext 800 Stage IV – Disseminated (multi-focal) involvement of one or more extra-lymphatic organ, with or without associated lymph node involvement (for example, nodular involvement of lungs)

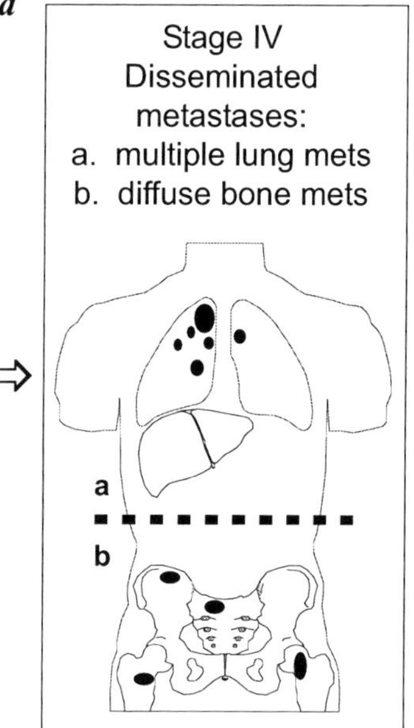

CS Extension

- The extension codes are based upon the Ann Arbor stage/AJCC Stage Grouping. Each possible combination of stage group, extralymphatic (E) and spleen (S) suffixes (for example, Stage I, Stage IE, Stage IS) has its own extension code. Review Notes 1-4.
- Note 1 defines the structures that are lymphatic and extralymphatic. Any lymphatic structure is to be coded and counted the same as a lymph node region.
- Note 2 explains that "S" is used to indicate spleen involvement.
- Note 3 says to assume there is no lymph node involvement if there is no mention of extranodal involvement but several diagnostic procedures were done, including laparotomy.
- Note 4 adds another guideline that involvement of adjacent soft tissue does not alter the classification.

CS TS/Ext Eval

This field has a very limited use in Collaborative Staging—to identify those few patients who undergo complete staging laparotomy. Only codes 0 (not done), 2 (autopsy for suspected or diagnosed tumor), 3 (staging laparotomy done), 8 (autopsy diagnosis) and 9 (unknown; not documented) can be used in this field. A staging laparotomy consists of multiple lymph node and organ biopsies and thorough abdominal exploration (see Surgery, above). Simple abdominal lymph node biopsies do not meet the definition of staging laparotomy.

SITE-SPECIFIC FACTORS 1–5

Note: Part I Section 2 of the CS Coding Manual Version 02.03 includes extensive discussion of the site-specific factors for every schema. Rather than rewrite those coding instructions for inclusion in this CASEbook chapter, refer to Part I Section 2 if questions arise. The discussion that follows provides more rationale for why those site-specific factors were included in the lymphoma schema.

- Both Hodgkin and non-Hodgkin lymphoma use the same five site-specific factors.

SSF1—Associated with HIV/AIDS

Because several types of lymphoma are associated with HIV infection, this field is used to indicate HIV/AIDS status.

000 No – Not associated with HIV/AIDS; HIV negative

Site-Specific Factors, *continued*

010 Yes – Associated with HIV/AIDS; HIV/AIDS present; HIV positive
999 Unknown if HIV/AIDS present; insufficient information; not documented in patient record

- In order to code 000, there must be a statement in the record that the patient has been tested for HIV/AIDS and is negative. Do not assume the patient is HIV negative based on age, gender, or lack of a statement in the medical record.
- If there is no mention of HIV or AIDS in the medical record, use code 999.
- Some central registries have given instructions to their reporting registrars that this field should always be coded as 999 to protect the confidentiality of the patient.

SSF2—Systemic Symptoms at Diagnosis

This field is used to code the presence or absence of specific "B" symptoms.

- When the computer algorithm is run, the letter A (code 000) is added to the stage group to indicate that there are no B symptoms present, for example, Stage IIA.
- When the computer algorithm is run, the letter B (coded 010) is added to the stage group to indicate any of the following symptoms:
    1. Unexplained weight loss more than 10% of body weight in 6 months prior to diagnosis
    2. Unexplained fever above 38 degrees Centigrade recurring over at least a month
    3. Night sweats (drenching)

  Example: Stage IB indicates that a patient has localized lymphoma with B symptoms present.
- Pruritus is generalized itching and is not considered a B symptom by itself. Pruritus has its own code 020 and maps to "asymptomatic." Any combination of pruritus and other B symptoms is coded to 030 and maps to B symptoms.

Site-Specific Factors 3–5 Prognostic Indices and Scores

Three different estimates of prognosis have been developed for the malignant lymphomas based on histology, patient age, stage, and other risk factors. This point system approach to assessing risk factors has not been completely accepted by clinicians, but supplements traditional anatomic stage information with laboratory values and assessments of the patient's general condition.

Review the medical record for a statement of a prognostic index or score; do not calculate the score from documentation in the chart. If the score is named, code the value in the appropriate site-specific factor and code the other two as 999. If the score is not named and is less than 5, code SSFs 3–5 as 999. If the score is 6 or higher, assume that it is the International Prognostic Score for Hodgkin lymphoma. Code the value in SSF5 and code SSFs 3 and 4 as 999.

SSF3—International Prognostic Index (IPI) Score

The International Prognostic Index (IPI) score was introduced in the sixth edition of the *AJCC Cancer Staging Manual* and included in CS version 1. The IPI score is discussed in some detail in the AJCC Cancer Staging Manual, seventh edition. Originally intended to assist clinical decision making and estimate prognosis for aggressive lymphomas, its use has expanded to other non-Hodgkin subtypes as well. To determine the IPI score, the clinician looks at the patient's history, medical status and stage of disease and scores one point for each adverse risk factor. Risk factors include:

- Age 60 or older
- Stage III or IV disease
- More than one area of extranodal involvement
- Poor performance status (needs a lot of help with daily activities)
- Elevated serum lactate dehydrogenase (LDH)

Site-Specific Factors, *continued*

The sum of the adverse prognostic factors is converted into a risk group: 0 or 1 is low risk, 2 is low intermediate, 3 is high intermediate, and 4 or 5 is high risk.

Code the sum of the risk factors as stated by the clinician. If no point value is given, code a statement of risk (low, intermediate, or high). If there is no mention of an IPI score, code this field as 999, unknown or not documented.

SSF4—Follicular Lymphoma International Prognostic Index (FLIPI) Score
The Follicular Lymphoma International Prognostic Index (FLIPI) score published in 2004 is a modification of the IPI score (see site-specific factor 3) developed for estimating the prognosis of less aggressive follicular lymphomas. This site-specific factor was introduced with CS version 2. To determine the FLIPI score, the clinician looks at the patient's history, medical status and stage of disease and scores one point for each adverse risk factor. Risk factors are similar to the IPI and include:

- Age 60 or older
- Stage III or IV disease
- More than four nodal areas involved
- Elevated serum lactate dehydrogenase (LDH)
- Serum hemoglobin concentration less than 12 g/dL

The sum of the adverse prognostic factors is converted into a risk group: 0 or 1 is low risk, 2 is intermediate risk, and 3–5 is high risk.

Code the sum of the risk factors as stated by the clinician. If no point value is given, code a statement of risk (low, intermediate, or high). If there is no mention of a FLIPI score, code this field as 999, unknown or not documented.

SSF5—International Prognostic Score (IPS)
The International Prognostic Score (IPS) is similar to the International Prognostic Index for non-Hodgkin lymphomas, but is specific to Hodgkin lymphoma. Of the seven risk factors in this system, four are laboratory values of blood serum. The IPS risk factors are:

- Age 45 and above
- Stage IV
- Male gender
- Serum hemoglobin < 10.5 g/dL
- Serum albumin < 4 g/dL
- White blood count $\geq 15{,}000/mm^3$
- Lymphocytopenia $\leq 600/mm^3$ or $< 8\%$ of white cell count

Unlike the IPI and FLIPI, the risk factor points of the IPS are not translated into a statement of low, intermediate, or high risk. Code the point total as stated by the clinician. If there is no mention of an IPS score, code this field as 999, unknown or not documented.

OTHER STAGING AND CLASSIFICATION SYSTEMS

SUMMARY STAGE

- Page 277 in the *Summary Staging Manual 2000* lists the lymph nodes and lymphatic structures above and below the diaphragm. This is important as the diaphragm serves as a landmark when staging lymphomas.
- Disregard the list of morphology codes at the top of page 278, because it is no longer complete.
- Review the staging definitions for Localized (code 1), Regional, NOS (code 5), Distant (code 7), and Unstaged, Not Stated (code 9). Notice that for lymphomas there is only Regional, NOS (code 5). For lymphomas, code 2, Regional Direct Extension and code 3, Regional Lymph Nodes are not used.
- The definitions listed within each SEER Summary Stage include references to the Ann Arbor stage, i.e. Stage I, Stage II, Stage III and Stage IV. Also review Notes 1–6 on page 279.

AJCC (TNM)

AJCC TNM staging for Hodgkin and non-Hodgkin lymphoma is different from other primary sites.

- For malignant lymphomas, individual T, N, and M categories are not assigned. Only a Stage Group is documented. It is important to identify how many groups of lymph nodes and/or how many organs are involved with lymphoma, and this information is represented by the Stage Grouping, which is virtually the same as Ann Arbor Staging.
    - On the cancer registry abstract, the T, N, and M fields for both clinical and pathologic staging are coded "88" (not applicable).
- AJCC staging for malignant lymphomas is primarily clinical. A pathologic stage group is assigned only when a staging laparotomy is performed.
- The letter E is used with the Stage Grouping to indicate "Extralymphatic." This identifies the site of origin as something other than lymph nodes or lymphatic structures. The "E" suffix may be written in the medical record or on the staging form.
    - On the cancer registry abstract, the "E" information is coded in the fields Clinical and Pathologic Stage (Prefix/Suffix) Descriptor.
- The AJCC Cancer Staging Manual, sixth and seventh editions, use "E" to designate lymph node involvement with extranodal extension directly invading other organs. This includes lymphoma that directly extends from a lymph node mass to an organ and lymphoma that directly extends from an organ to its adjacent lymph nodes. This concept is also used in CS. Examples:
    - Stage IE: primary parotid lymphoma involving entire gland (a single extralymphatic site)
    - Stage IIE: primary lung lymphoma with hilar and mediastinal involvement presenting as separate masses (lung and lymph nodes)
    - Stage IIE: lymphoma of mediastinal lymph nodes that have involved adjacent lung tissue by direct extension (new use of "E")
- Notice that the diaphragm is used as a landmark in staging malignant lymphomas. It is important to know the lymph node regions and chains located above and below the diaphragm.
- The suffix "S" is used to indicate spleen involvement either pathologically or clinically. If the spleen is palpable and visible on x-ray, the spleen is defined as clinically involved.
- The AJCC Cancer Staging Manual discusses several additional issues relating to lymphoma staging, such as definitions of spleen and liver involvement, and the A and B symptoms.

AJCC (TNM), *continued*

- The Lymphoid Neoplasms chapter of the AJCC Cancer Staging Manual also includes information about staging of mycosis fungoides, multiple myeloma, and pediatric lymphoid malignancies. Mycosis fungoides and multiple myeloma have separate schemas in CS.

HISTORIC MORPHOLOGIC CLASSIFICATION SYSTEMS

Gall and Mallory

This was one of the earliest lymphoma classifications, from the 1940s. The terminology of this classification still appears in ICD-9 and ICD-10, and the terminology is still used by veterinarians.

- Lymphosarcoma
- Reticulum cell sarcoma

Rappaport Classification

The Rappaport Classification was published in 1966 and was widely used until the mid 1980's. The Rappaport classification is based upon the histologic appearance of the malignancy (size and shape). The terminology used in the Rappaport Classification includes:

- Lymphocytic lymphoma (small like a lymphocyte cell)
- Histiocytic lymphoma (larger like a histiocyte cell, but not a true lymphoma of histiocytes)
- Mixed lymphocytic and histiocytic lymphoma (mixed small and large cell)

Lukes-Collins Classification

Around 1974 another NHL classification was published. The Lukes-Collins classification was based on the microscopic physical appearance of the lymphoma cells. Terms used in the Lukes-Collins Classification include:

- Small lymphocytic lymphoma
- Small cleaved or small non-cleaved lymphoma (the cell has or does not have a cleft or crack; in other words, the cell has "cleavage")
- Large cleaved or large non-cleaved lymphoma
- Histiocytic lymphoma

Working Formulation

The Working Formulation was developed in 1982 as a means for translation of terms from Rappaport to the Lukes-Collins and other classifications. However, it became a classification of its own and has been used by many pathologists. For example, the following diagnoses describe the same disease:

Rappaport: Nodular mixed lymphocytic-histiocytic
Lukes-Collins: Mixed small cleaved and large cleaved follicular center cell, follicular type
Dorfman: Follicular, mixed small and large lymphoid
Kiel: Centroblastic/centrocytic
Working Formulation: Follicular, mixed small cleaved and large cell

REAL Classification

The REAL classification (Revised European American Lymphoma) was developed in 1994 and represented a major shift in the medical understanding of lymphoid and hematopoietic diseases. The REAL classification is based on cell lineage (T- or B-cell lymphocytic, myeloid, plasma cell, etc.) rather than on the disease (lymphoma, leukemia, myeloma). It includes some lymphoma subtypes not listed in the Working Formulation and new ones identified by cytogenetics, phenotyping and other molecular genetic markers. It evolved into the current WHO Classification of Lymphoid Tumors.

EPIDEMIOLOGY AND ETIOLOGY

- Lymphoma incidence is highest in North America, followed by Australia and New Zealand and northern Europe.
- Lymphoma incidence is lowest in south-central and eastern Asia and Eastern Europe.
- Non-Hodgkin lymphoma is increasing faster than any other malignant disease except melanoma. Incidence rates for Hodgkin lymphoma have been steady for many years.
- Lymphoma is slightly more common in men than women.
- All types of lymphoma are more common in whites than blacks or Asians.
- The median age at diagnosis is 67 for NHL and 37 for Hodgkin lymphoma.
    - Hodgkin lymphoma actually has a bimodal age distribution: 15-34 and over age 55.
- Lymphoma is the third most common childhood cancer.

Risk Factors

- No known *preventable* risk factors, other than avoiding viral infections listed below
- Viral infections—HTLV-1 (T-cell lymphoma); EBV virus (Burkitt lymphoma); HIV (diffuse large B-cell lymphoma and others); human herpes virus 8 (HHV8) (primary effusion lymphoma); hepatitis C virus
- Bacterial infection H. pylori (MALT lymphoma)
- Medical conditions—immunosuppression resulting from HIV/AIDS; organ transplants; inherited immune deficiency syndromes; autoimmune diseases (lupus, sprue, rheumatoid arthritis)
- Chemicals—Benzene, weed or insect killers, Dilantin®
- Radiation exposure (nuclear accidents or radiation therapy for other cancers)
- Genetics—parents, children, and siblings of CLL patients at higher risk
- Cancer Therapy—patients with a history of chemo- and/or radiotherapy at slightly greater risk

Page left blank.

Abstracting, Staging, and Coding Exercises

This section includes twelve brief malignant lymphoma cases to be coded in ICD-O-3, Summary Stage 2000, TNM seventh edition (clinical and pathologic), and CS version 0203.

NOTE: For the purposes of these brief cases, assume that all other tests not mentioned in the case are negative for malignancy.

- Identify the primary site and schema.
- Assign the codes for primary site, histology, behavior, and grade.
- Assign codes to all applicable CS fields.
- Assume that your facility does offer a test and that the standards setters for your facility require the data field. In other words, avoid using code 988 (not applicable).
- 20XX is the diagnosis year, and where applicable, 20YY is the following year.

Default values for malignant lymphomas (not included in case exercises)

Lymph Vascular Invasion	8	Not applicable
Multiplicity Counter	88	Lymphoma diagnosis
Date Multiple Tumors	Blank	Not applicable
Date Mult Tumors Flag	11	Not applicable (multiplicity counter is coded 88)
CS Tumor Size	988	Not applicable
CS Lymph Nodes	988	Not applicable
CS Reg Nodes Eval	9	Not applicable
Reg LN Pos	99	Not applicable
Reg LN Exam	99	Not applicable
CS Mets at Dx	98	Not applicable
CS Mets Eval	9	Not applicable for this schema

CASE 1

PHYSICAL EXAM
49 year old female with right cervical lymph nodes palpably enlarged. No axillary or inguinal lymphadenopathy. Abdomen: No organomegaly or masses.

X-RAYS AND SCANS
6-2-20XX CT chest/abdomen/pelvis: No lymphadenopathy identified. Spleen normal.

PROCEDURES
6-6-20XX Biopsy of enlarged cervical lymph node.

PATHOLOGY REPORTS
6-6-20XX Biopsy of cervical lymph node: Small lymphocytic lymphoma.

6-10-20XX Bone marrow biopsy: Negative.

TREATMENT
6-14 to 7-10-20XX Radiation therapy to right cervical region

Site Code ___ ___ ___.___	**Collaborative Staging Schema**	**SSF3 Internat Prognos Index (IPI)** ___ ___ ___
Histology/Behavior/Grade ___ ___ ___ ___/___ ___	**CS Extension** ___ ___	**SSF4 Follic Lymph IPI (FLIPI)** ___ ___ ___
Summary Stage 2000 ___	**CS TS/Ext Eval** ___	**SSF5 Internat Prognos Score (IPS)** ___ ___ ___
TNM Stage Group (clinical) ______	**SSF1 Assoc with HIV/AIDS** ___ ___ ___	
	SSF2 B Symptoms ___ ___ ___	

CASE 2

PHYSICAL EXAM
62 year old male complaining of night sweats, abdominal pain and 35 pound weight loss over last two months. Upper abdominal mass felt to supraumbilical area. No organomegaly or other masses felt.

X-RAYS AND SCANS
11-21-20XX CT chest/abdomen/pelvis: No hepatosplenomegaly. No lymphadenopathy.

PROCEDURES
11-24-20XX Partial gastrectomy: Mass in greater curvature of stomach. Entire mass removed. Liver normal. No grossly enlarged lymph nodes identified.

PATHOLOGY REPORTS
11-24-20XX Stomach: Grade 3 follicular lymphoma with transformation to diffuse large B cell lymphoma, see comment.
Comment: This is a grade 3 follicular lymphoma with areas of transformation to diffuse large B cell lymphoma; approximately 25% of tissue examined shows features of follicular lymphoma which are highlighted by the BCL-2 positive germinal centers.

Case 2, continued

TREATMENT
11-24-20XX Partial gastrectomy
Referred to medical oncologist for consideration of combination chemotherapy. Due to age and overall medical condition, considered low intermediate risk on International Prognostic Index.

Site Code __ __ __.__	Collaborative Staging Schema	SSF3 Internat Prognos Index (IPI) __ __ __
Histology/Behavior/Grade __ __ __ __/__ __	CS Extension __ __	SSF4 Follic Lymph IPI (FLIPI) __ __ __
Summary Stage 2000 __	CS TS/Ext Eval __	SSF5 Internat Prognos Score (IPS) __ __ __
TNM Stage Group (clinical) ______	SSF1 Assoc with HIV/AIDS __ __ __	
	SSF2 B Symptoms __ __ __	

CASE 3

PHYSICAL EXAM
16 year old male complaining of flu-like symptoms, fever, night sweats, weight loss. Physical exam essentially unremarkable.

X-RAYS AND SCANS
2-2-20XX Chest x-ray: Mediastinal mass
2-10-20XX CT chest: Lungs clear. Mediastinal lymph nodes enlarged.
2-10-20XX CT abdomen/pelvis: Enlarged celiac lymph nodes.

ENDOSCOPY
2-15-20XX Mediastinoscopy: Biopsy of enlarged mediastinal node taken.

PROCEDURES
2-16-20XX Bone marrow aspiration and biopsy.

PATHOLOGY REPORTS
2-15-20XX Mediastinal lymph node biopsy: Hodgkin lymphoma, nodular sclerosing type.
2-16-20XX Bone marrow biopsy: Negative.

TREATMENT
2-20-20XX Started 2 cycles ABVD
2-26 to 3-22-20XX Mini-mantle radiation therapy to mediastinum

Site Code __ __ __.__	Collaborative Staging Schema	SSF3 Internat Prognos Index (IPI) __ __ __
Histology/Behavior/Grade __ __ __ __/__ __	CS Extension __ __	SSF4 Follic Lymph IPI (FLIPI) __ __ __
Summary Stage 2000 __	CS TS/Ext Eval __	SSF5 Internat Prognos Score (IPS) __ __ __
TNM Stage Group (clinical) ______	SSF1 Assoc with HIV/AIDS __ __ __	
	SSF2 B Symptoms __ __ __	

CASE 4

PHYSICAL EXAM

Patient noted slowly increasing rubbery mass in right testicle. Not painful, no prior trauma. Mass is not translucent.

X-RAYS AND SCANS

7-12-20XX CT chest and abdomen: Negative for lymphadenopathy.

PROCEDURES

7-14-20XX Excision of right testis with cord.
7-17-20XX Bone marrow aspiration and biopsy.

PATHOLOGY REPORTS

7-14-20XX Right orchiectomy: Malignant lymphoma, high grade lymphoplasmacytic, right testis and extratesticular soft tissue.
7-17-20XX Bone marrow biopsy: Negative.

TREATMENT

7-24-20XX Started m-BACOD combination chemotherapy

Site Code ___ ___ ___.___	**Collaborative Staging Schema**	**SSF3 Internat Prognos Index (IPI)** ___ ___ ___
Histology/Behavior/Grade ___ ___ ___ ___/___ ___	**CS Extension** ___ ___	**SSF4 Follic Lymph IPI (FLIPI)** ___ ___ ___
Summary Stage 2000 ___	**CS TS/Ext Eval** ___	**SSF5 Internat Prognos Score (IPS)** ___ ___ ___
TNM Stage Group (clinical) ________	**SSF1 Assoc with HIV/AIDS** ___ ___ ___	
	SSF2 B Symptoms ___ ___ ___	

CASE 5

HISTORY

64 year old female with 1 week of swelling, right leg. Swelling resolves after lying down at night. No other symptoms.

PHYSICAL EXAMINATION

1-20-20XX Abdominal mass on pelvic exam.

X-RAYS AND SCANS

1-22-20XX Barium enema prior to admission: Negative for colon mass.
1-24-20XX IVP: Right pelvic mass.
1-24-20XX CXR: Negative

PROCEDURE

1-27-20XX Abdominal exploration, omentectomy, TAH and BSO, dissection of L iliac nodes: Omentum stuck to tumor, which extends far lateral to iliac vessels and from inguinal ligament to bifurcation of aorta. Liver/spleen: No disease.

Case 5, continued

PATHOLOGY REPORTS

1-27-20XX Iliac lymph nodes: Follicular, small cleaved cell lymphoma. Inguinal lymph nodes: No tumor. Uterus: Atrophic. Tubes/ovaries: Serosal adhesions; no tumor

1-30-20XX Bone marrow aspiration biopsy: Follicular, small cleaved cell lymphoma infiltrating bone marrow.

TREATMENT

2-8-20XX Started CVP combination regimen

Site Code ___ ___ ___.___	Collaborative Staging Schema	SSF3 Internat Prognos Index (IPI) ___ ___ ___
Histology/Behavior/Grade ___ ___ ___ ___/___ ___	CS Extension ___ ___	SSF4 Follic Lymph IPI (FLIPI) ___ ___ ___
Summary Stage 2000 ___	CS TS/Ext Eval ___	SSF5 Internat Prognos Score (IPS) ___ ___ ___
TNM Stage Group (clinical) ________	SSF1 Assoc with HIV/AIDS ___ ___ ___	
	SSF2 B Symptoms ___ ___ ___	

CASE 6

HISTORY

78 year old male with COPD x 9 months. Noted swelling in low cervical region for 3 months.

PHYSICAL EXAMINATION

7-28-20XX Matted nodes, right neck

X-RAYS AND SCANS

7-28-20XX CXR: Scattered ill-defined nodular densities in both lung fields; unknown etiology; however, metastatic lesions cannot be entirely excluded. Scattered granulomatous residuals may present similarly. Pleural reactive changes right base.

7-29-20XX Liver scan: WNL.

7-29-20XX Bone survey: WNL.

7-30-20XX Abdominal CT scan: Negative.

PROCEDURE

8-1-20XX Excision of cervical node mass.

PATHOLOGY REPORTS

8-1-20XX Cervical lymph nodes: Lymphocyte depletion Hodgkin's disease.

8-15-20XX Bone marrow aspiration biopsy: Hyperplasia; no tumor.

TREATMENT

8-18-20XX IPS: 3. In view of age, started prednisone only

9-1 to 9-10-20XX Radiation therapy to cervical region. 1000 rads total

Case 6, continued

Site Code ___ ___ ___.___	Collaborative Staging Schema	SSF3 Internat Prognos Index (IPI) ___ ___ ___
Histology/Behavior/Grade ___ ___ ___ ___ / ___ ___	CS Extension ___ ___	SSF4 Follic Lymph IPI (FLIPI) ___ ___ ___
Summary Stage 2000 ___	CS TS/Ext Eval ___	SSF5 Internat Prognos Score (IPS) ___ ___ ___
TNM Stage Group (clinical) ________	SSF1 Assoc with HIV/AIDS ___ ___ ___	
	SSF2 B Symptoms ___ ___ ___	

CASE 7

HISTORY
30 year old female complaining of irregular bouts of abdominal pain. Patient had lost 20 pounds without trying (usual weight 150).

PHYSICAL EXAMINATION
10-12-200X No lymphadenopathy. HEENT: WNL. On admission, noted persistent fever.

X-RAYS AND SCANS
10-14-20XX Liver scan: Negative.
10-14-20XX CXR: Negative for masses.
10-15-20XX GI series: Mass in jejunum.
10-15-20XX Barium enema: Negative for abnormalities.

SCOPES
None.

PROCEDURES
10-17-20XX Abdominal exploration, proximal jejunal resection: No regional lymph node involvement. 7 cm mass involving small bowel wall and mesentery. Liver and spleen appeared free of disease.

PATHOLOGY REPORTS
10-17-20XX Jejunal tissue: Mucosa-associated lymphoid tissue (MALT) lymphoma. Mesenteric lymph nodes: No evidence of tumor

TREATMENT
10-17-20XX Proximal jejunal resection

Site Code ___ ___ ___.___	Collaborative Staging Schema	SSF3 Internat Prognos Index (IPI) ___ ___ ___
Histology/Behavior/Grade ___ ___ ___ ___ / ___ ___	CS Extension ___ ___	SSF4 Follic Lymph IPI (FLIPI) ___ ___ ___
Summary Stage 2000 ___	CS TS/Ext Eval ___	SSF5 Internat Prognos Score (IPS) ___ ___ ___
TNM Stage Group (clinical) ________	SSF1 Assoc with HIV/AIDS ___ ___ ___	
	SSF2 B Symptoms ___ ___ ___	

CASE 8

HISTORY
Asymptomatic 65 year old male with bilateral axillary lymph node masses noted on physical.

PHYSICAL EXAM
7-31-20XX Bilateral axillary nodes palpable. 1.5 x 6.0 cm right inguinal mass fixed to fascia. Smaller nodes also palpable in R inguinal region grouped into 7 x 4 x 3 cm mass. Left groin nodes palpable. No abdominal masses.

X-RAYS AND SCANS
8-2-20XX Chest CT scan: No mediastinal or bronchial adenopathy.
8-2-20XX Liver scan: Hepatomegaly.
8-6-20XX Lymphangiogram: Lymphoma in inguinal, pelvic and periaortic nodes.

PROCEDURES
8-19-20XX Excision, right groin nodes.
8-27-20XX Right axillary node dissection.

PATHOLOGY REPORTS
8-19-20XX Inguinal lymph nodes: Nodular histiocytic lymphoma.
8-27-20XX Right axillary nodes: R/O lymphoma. Slide consultation: Follicular large cell lymphoma.

TREATMENT
9-5-20XX Started CVP
Radiation therapy planned after patient returns from vacation.

Site Code ___ ___ ___.___	Collaborative Staging Schema	SSF3 Internat Prognos Index (IPI) ___ ___ ___
Histology/Behavior/Grade ___ ___ ___ ___ / ___ ___	CS Extension ___ ___	SSF4 Follic Lymph IPI (FLIPI) ___ ___ ___
Summary Stage 2000 ___	CS TS/Ext Eval ___	SSF5 Internat Prognos Score (IPS) ___ ___ ___
TNM Stage Group (clinical) ________	SSF1 Assoc with HIV/AIDS ___ ___ ___	
	SSF2 B Symptoms ___ ___ ___	

CASE 9

HISTORY
70 year old male with gradual swelling in left neck. Saw MD when his wife complained about how bad it looked.

PHYSICAL EXAM
5-2-20XX Few matted cervical nodes. No other nodes or masses.

X-RAYS AND SCANS
5-7-20XX CXR: Unsatisfactory due to patient movement.
5-8-20XX CT Chest: Lobular right superior mediastinal masses consistent with clinical diagnosis of Hodgkin disease in paratracheal nodes; lungs clear.
5-10-20XX Bone scan: Negative.
5-11-20XX Liver scan: WNL.

Case 9, continued

PROCEDURES

5-17-20XX Staging laparotomy and splenectomy: No visible tumor in liver, spleen or abdominal nodes.

PATHOLOGY REPORTS

5-12-20XX L cervical node biopsy: Hodgkin lymphoma, mixed cellularity.

5-17-20XX Liver biopsy: Negative. All node biopsies negative. Bone biopsy: Negative. Spleen: Mixed cellularity Hodgkin lymphoma.

TREATMENT

6-8-20XX Started 4MeV to mantle field and periaortic nodes

Site Code ___ ___ ___.___	**Collaborative Staging Schema**	**SSF3 Internat Prognos Index (IPI)** ___ ___ ___
Histology/Behavior/Grade ___ ___ ___ ___ / ___ ___	**CS Extension** ___ ___	**SSF4 Follic Lymph IPI (FLIPI)** ___ ___ ___
Summary Stage 2000 ___	**CS TS/Ext Eval** ___	**SSF5 Internat Prognos Score (IPS)** ___ ___ ___
TNM Stage Group (clinical) ________	**SSF1 Assoc with HIV/AIDS** ___ ___ ___	
	SSF2 B Symptoms ___ ___ ___	

CASE 10

HISTORY

23 year old HIV-positive male with complaints of difficulty breathing while lying flat in bed. Admitted after fainting while stooping over. One month prior to admission, developed cold and non-productive cough. In past six weeks, night sweats and fever occurred regularly.

PHYSICAL EXAM

11-12-20XX Knot-like swelling in left neck that hurts when he coughs. Bilateral anterior cervical adenopathy. HEENT normal, except thyroid not palpated. Chest had slight dullness to percussion. Abdomen soft, nontender. Liver about 9 cm to percussion. Spleen tip not palpable. No other masses or tenderness.

X-RAYS AND SCANS

11-14-20XX Chest x-ray: Right upper lobe infiltrate may be due to inflammatory process secondary to partial airway obstruction, but possibility of lymph node involvement cannot be excluded. Bilateral hilar and mediastinal enlargement most likely due to lymph-adenopathy. Findings are compatible with lymphoma compressing trachea.

11-15-20XX Gallium scan: Massive lymph node involvement in mediastinum and possible lymph node involvement in periaortic region.

11-16-20XX L/S scan: No changes suggestive of metastases.

11-16-20XX IVP: Normal

11-18-20XX Abd CT scan: Definite periaortic lymphadenopathy consistent with below-the-diaphragm involvement by lymphoma.

SCOPES

11-22-20XX Mediastinoscopy: Matted nodes in mediastinum compressing trachea.

PROCEDURES

11-19-20XX Biopsy of left neck abscess.

Case 10, continued

PATHOLOGY REPORTS
11-19-20XX Left neck: Grade 2 follicular lymphoma.
11-22-20XX Endoscopic biopsies of mediastinum: Follicular lymphoma, NOS. FLIPI low risk
11-30-20XX Bone marrow aspiration biopsy, right superior iliac crest: Negative for tumor.

TREATMENT
11-23 to 11-26-20XX Palliative radiation therapy to superior mediastinum (1000 rads)
12-1-200X Started MOPP regimen

Site Code ___ ___ ___.___	Collaborative Staging Schema	SSF3 Internat Prognos Index (IPI) ___ ___ ___
Histology/Behavior/Grade ___ ___ ___ ___/___ ___	CS Extension ___ ___	SSF4 Follic Lymph IPI (FLIPI) ___ ___ ___
Summary Stage 2000 ___	CS TS/Ext Eval ___	SSF5 Internat Prognos Score (IPS) ___ ___ ___
TNM Stage Group (clinical) ________	SSF1 Assoc with HIV/AIDS ___ ___ ___	
	SSF2 B Symptoms ___ ___ ___	

CASE 11

HISTORY
Patient presented with "bumps" in armpit and neck.

PHYSICAL EXAM
9-2-20XX Gross adenopathy in both axilla and cervical lymph nodes. No enlargement of spleen or liver.

X-RAYS AND SCANS
9-5-20XX CT Pelvis: Possible mass in terminal ileum.
9-5-20XX CT Chest: Extensive axillary and cervical adenopathy.

PROCEDURES
9-7-20XX Biopsy of cervical lymph node.
9-10-20XX Colonoscopy to terminal ileum with biopsy.
9-15-20XX Bone marrow aspiration and biopsy.

PATHOLOGY REPORTS
9-7-20XX Cervical node: Diffuse large B-cell lymphoma.
9-10-20XX Biopsy of terminal ileum: Diffuse lymphoma, large B-cell type.
9-15-20XX Bone marrow aspiration and biopsy: Negative for lymphoma.

TREATMENT
Patient referred to medical oncologist for combination chemotherapy

Site Code ___ ___ ___.___	Collaborative Staging Schema	SSF3 Internat Prognos Index (IPI) ___ ___ ___
Histology/Behavior/Grade ___ ___ ___ ___/___ ___	CS Extension ___ ___	SSF4 Follic Lymph IPI (FLIPI) ___ ___ ___
Summary Stage 2000 ___	CS TS/Ext Eval ___	SSF5 Internat Prognos Score (IPS) ___ ___ ___
TNM Stage Group (clinical) ________	SSF1 Assoc with HIV/AIDS ___ ___ ___	
	SSF2 B Symptoms ___ ___ ___	

CASE 12

HISTORY

26 year old male presented to primary care MD with 1 year history of gradually enlarging lumps on both sides of neck. Referred immediately to medical oncologist.

PHYSICAL EXAM

4-7-20XX Multiple rather small 1 to 1.5 cm lymph nodes along sternocleidomastoid muscle at all levels of neck bilaterally. Palpable bilateral supraclavicular lymphadenopathy. No axillary, or inguinal lymphadenopathy. Chest clear to auscultation. Abdomen soft and nontender; no masses or organomegaly.

X-RAYS AND SCANS

4-12-20XX CT Neck: 3 x 2 cm opacity in posterior cervical region superior to hyoid bone. 2.9 x 2.6 cm opacity in left supraclavicular region.

4-12-20XX CT Thorax: Significantly enlarged, ill-defined lymph nodes measuring up to 2 cm in short axis dimension in superior mediastinum, especially anteriorly, extending up into the lower neck. No pleural fluid. Respiratory artifact in lung images.

4-12-20XX CT Abdomen and Pelvis: Imaging limited by barium within large bowel. Liver not enlarged; no focal lesions. Spleen is within normal limits for length and AP diameter; no focal lesions. No gross retroperitoneal lymphadenopathy. No lymphadenopathy within pelvis. No destructive bone lesions in regions assessed.

4-14-20XX Whole body gallium scan with SPECT of head, neck and thorax: Increased gallium activity in left side of neck consistent with gallium avid lymph nodes. Remainder of examination is unremarkable.

PROCEDURES

4-7-20XX Ultrasound guided core biopsy, left cervical lymph node.

4-13-20XX Excisional biopsy, left neck node.

4-15-20XX Bone marrow aspiration and biopsy.

PATHOLOGY

4-7-20XX Core biopsy, L cervical node: Atypical cellular infiltrates.

4-13-20XX Excisional biopsy, left neck node: Nodal marginal zone B-cell lymphoma, CD20 and CD10 positive.

4-15-20XX Bone marrow aspiration and biopsy: Negative for lymphoma.

TREATMENT

4-20-20XX 6 cycles of R-CHOP

4-25-20XX to 5-30-20XX Radiation to left neck, supraclavicular nodes, and superior mediastinum. Total 70 Gy.

Site Code ___ ___ ___.___	**Collaborative Staging Schema CS Extension** ___ ___	**SSF3 Internat Prognos Index (IPI)** ___ ___ ___
Histology/Behavior/Grade ___ ___ ___ ___ / ___ ___	**CS TS/Ext Eval** ___	**SSF4 Follic Lymph IPI (FLIPI)** ___ ___ ___
Summary Stage 2000 ___	**SSF1 Assoc with HIV/AIDS** ___ ___ ___	**SSF5 Internat Prognos Score (IPS)** ___ ___ ___
TNM Stage Group (clinical) ________	**SSF2 B Symptoms** ___ ___ ___	

ANSWERS TO LYMPHOMA CASES

—— CASE 1 ——

Primary Site	C77.0	Cervical lymph nodes
Morphology	9670/3	Small lymphocytic lymphoma, NOS
Grade	6	B-cell per Grade rules
Summary Stage	Localized	
TNM Stage Group	IA	
CS Extension	100	Single lymph node region
CS TS/Ext Eval	0	No staging laparotomy
SSF1 AIDS/HIV	999	No information
SSF2 B symptoms	000	Asymptomatic; no B symptoms mentioned
SSF3 IPI	999	No information
SSF4 FLIPI	999	No information
SSF5 IPS	999	No information

This case maps to Stage IA.

—— CASE 2 ——

Primary Site	C16.6	Greater curvature of stomach
Morphology	9680/3	Diffuse large B-cell lymphoma Heme MP/H rule PH16
Grade	6	B-cell
Summary Stage	Localized	
TNM Stage Group	IBE	
CS Extension	110	Lymphoma confined to stomach (single extralymphatic site)
CS TS/Ext Eval	0	No staging laparotomy (abdominal surgery is not the same as a staging laparotomy)
SSF1 AIDS/HIV		
SSF2 B symptoms	010	Night sweats, 35 pound weight loss in two months = B symptoms
SSF3 IPI	991	Stated as low intermediate risk
SSF4 FLIPI	999	No information
SSF5 IPS	999	No information

This case maps to Stage IBE.

—— CASE 3 ——

Primary Site	C77.8	Lymph nodes of multiple regions
Morphology	9663/3	Hodgkin lymphoma, nodular sclerosis, NOS
Grade	9	No phenotype stated
Summary Stage	Distant	Involvement of lymph nodes on both sides of diaphragm
TNM Stage Group	IIIB	
CS Extension	300	Mediastinal nodes above diaphragm; celiac nodes below diaphragm = Stage III
CS TS/Ext Eval	0	No staging laparotomy

Case 3, continued

SSF1 AIDS/HIV	999	No information
SSF2 B symptoms	010	Fever, night sweats, weight loss = B symptoms
SSF3 IPI	999	No information
SSF4 FLIPI	999	No information
SSF5 IPS	999	No information

This case maps to Stage IIIB.

—— CASE 4 ——

Primary Site	C62.9	Testis, NOS
Morphology	9671/3	Malignant lymphoma, lymphoplasmacytic
Grade	6	B-cell per Grade rules; do not code "high grade" for lymphomas
Summary Stage	Localized	
TNM Stage Group	IAE	
CS Extension	110	Involvement of a single extralymphatic site (testis)
CS TS/Ext Eval	0	No staging laparotomy
SSF1 AIDS/HIV	999	No information
SSF2 B symptoms	000	Asymptomatic; no B symptoms mentioned
SSF3 IPI	999	No information
SSF4 FLIPI	999	No information
SSF5 IPS	999	No information

This case maps to Stage IAE. (E suffix includes extratesticular soft tissue extension)

—— CASE 5 ——

Primary Site	C77.5	Iliac lymph node (pelvic lymph node region)
Morphology	9695/3	Follicular lymphoma, small cleaved cell
Grade	6	B-cell per Grade rules
Summary Stage	Distant	Bone marrow involvement
TNM Stage Group	IVA	
CS Extension	800	Bone marrow biopsy positive
CS TS/Ext Eval	0	No staging laparotomy
SSF1 AIDS/HIV	999	No information
SSF2 B symptoms	000	Asymptomatic; no B symptoms mentioned
SSF3 IPI	999	No information
SSF4 FLIPI	999	No information
SSF5 IPS	999	No information

This case maps to Stage IVA.

—— CASE 6 ——

Primary Site	C77.0	Cervical lymph nodes involved
Morphology	9653/3	Hodgkin lymphoma, lymphocyte depletion, NOS
Grade	9	No phenotype stated
Summary Stage	Localized	
TNM Stage Group	IA	
CS Extension	100	Single lymph node region—cervical lymph nodes
CS TS/Ext Eval	0	No staging laparotomy
SSF1 AIDS/HIV	999	No information
SSF2 B symptoms	000	Asymptomatic; no B symptoms mentioned
SSF3 IPI	999	No information
SSF4 FLIPI	999	No information
SSF5 IPS	003	Stated as IPS 3

This case maps to Stage IA.

The ill-defined bilateral nodular densities in the lungs are too non-specific to be considered metastases from the lymphoma, and the patient's treatment was appropriate to Stage I disease.

—— CASE 7 ——

Primary Site	C17.1	Jejunum
Morphology	9699/3	MALT lymphoma
Grade	6	B-cell per Grade rules
Summary Stage	Localized	
TNM Stage Group	IBE	
CS Extension	110	Single extralymphatic site (small intestine)
CS TS/Ext Eval	0	No staging laparotomy (abdominal resection and resection is not the same as a staging laparotomy)
SSF1 AIDS/HIV	999	No information
SSF2 B symptoms	010	B symptoms present (unexplained weight loss > 10% of body mass)
SSF3 IPI	999	No information
SSF4 FLIPI	999	No information
SSF5 IPS	999	No information

This case maps to Stage IBE.

—— CASE 8 ——

Primary Site	C77.8	Lymph nodes of multiple regions (bilateral axillary C77.3 and inguinal C77.4)
Morphology	9698/3	Follicular large cell lymphoma (the consultant's diagnosis is more specific)
Grade	6	B-cell per Grade rules
Summary Stage	Distant	Lymph nodes on both sides of diaphragm
TNM Stage Group	IIIA	

Case 8, continued

CS Extension	300	Lymph node involvement on both sides of diaphragm; bilateral axillary counts as two regions above diaphragm plus inguinal nodes below diaphragm
CS TS/Ext Eval	0	No staging laparotomy
SSF1 AIDS/HIV	999	No information
SSF2 B symptoms	000	Stated as asymptomatic
SSF3 IPI	999	No information
SSF4 FLIPI	999	No information
SSF5 IPS	999	No information

This case maps to Stage IIIA.

—— CASE 9 ——

Primary Site	C77.8	Lymph nodes of multiple regions; cervical nodes and mediastinal (paratracheal) nodes above diaphragm plus spleen (a lymphatic site) below diaphragm
Morphology	9652/3	Hodgkin lymphoma, mixed cellularity
Grade	9	No phenotype stated
Summary Stage	Distant	Lymph nodes above diaphragm and extranodal lymphatic site below diaphragm
TNM Stage Group	IIIS	
CS Extension	320	Lymph node involvement above diaphragm plus spleen
CS TS/Ext Eval	3	Staging laparotomy performed
SSF1 AIDS/HIV	999	No information
SSF2 B symptoms	000	Asymptomatic; no B symptoms mentioned
SSF3 IPI	999	No information
SSF4 FLIPI	999	No information
SSF5 IPS	999	No information

This case maps to Stage IIIS.

—— CASE 10 ——

Primary Site	C77.8	Lymph nodes of multiple regions (cervical, hilar, mediastinal, and periaortic)
Morphology	9691/3	Grade 2 follicular lymphoma
Grade	6	B-cell per Grade rules (do not code grade for follicular lymphoma in 6th digit)
Summary Stage	Distant	Lymph nodes above and below diaphragm
TNM Stage Group	IIIB	
CS Extension	300	Lymph node involvement on both sides of diaphragm
CS TS/Ext Eval	0	No staging laparotomy
SSF1 AIDS/HIV	010	Stated as HIV-positive
SSF2 B symptoms	010	B symptoms (night sweats and fever) reported
SSF3 IPI	999	No information
SSF4 FLIPI	990	Stated as low risk
SSF5 IPS	999	No information

This case maps to Stage IIIB.

— CASE 11 —

Primary Site	C77.9	Lymph node, NOS
Morphology	9680/3	Diffuse large B-cell lymphoma
Grade	6	B-cell phenotype
Summary Stage	Distant	Ileum plus lymph nodes on opposite side of diaphragm
TNM Stage Group	IIIE	
CS Extension	310	Involvement of an extralymphatic organ (ileum) plus lymph nodes on the other side of the diaphragm (cervical and axillary)
CS TS/Ext Eval	0	No staging laparotomy performed
SSF1 AIDS/HIV	999	No information
SSF2 B symptoms	000	Asymptomatic; no B symptoms mentioned
SSF3 IPI	999	No information
SSF4 FLIPI	999	No information
SSF5 IPS	999	No information

This case maps to Stage IIIE.

The ileum is not the site of origin of this lymphoma because the regional nodes are not involved. When the primary site can't be determined, code the primary as C77.9

— CASE 12 —

Primary Site	C77.8	Lymph nodes of multiple regions; bilateral cervical nodes, bilateral supraclavicular nodes, and mediastinal
Morphology	9699/3	Nodal marginal zone lymphoma
Grade	6	B-cell phenotype stated
Summary Stage	Regional, NOS	Two or more lymph node regions on same side of diaphragm
TNM Stage Group	IIA	
CS Extension	200	Involvement of two or more lymph node regions on same side of diaphragm (bilateral cervical, bilateral supraclavicular and mediastinal)
CS TS/Ext Eval	0	No staging laparotomy performed
SSF1 AIDS/HIV	999	No information
SSF2 B symptoms	000	Asymptomatic; no B symptoms mentioned
SSF3 IPI	999	No information
SSF4 FLIPI	999	No information
SSF5 IPS	999	No information

This case maps to Stage IIA.

Even if the bilateral cervical lymph nodes were the only areas of involvement, the case would still be Stage II because of the bilaterality.

Page left blank.